the Injured
Athlete

Daniel N. Kulund, M.D.

Assistant Professor of Orthopedic Surgery
Adjunct Professor of Physical Education
Director of the Runners' Clinic
University of Virginia Medical Center, Charlottesville, Virginia
Fellow of the American Academy of Orthopedic Surgeons
Member of the American College of Sports Medicine
Advisory Member, National Athletic Trainer's Association
Member, National Strength and Conditioning Association
Associate Editor, The Physical Education Index

Illustrated by
Ronald J. Ervin, B.F.A., A.M.I.

University of Virginia Medical Center
Charlottesville, Virginia

With 8 Additional Contributors

the Injured Athlete

J. B. LIPPINCOTT COMPANY Philadelphia
Toronto

Sponsoring Editor: Sanford J. Robinson
Manuscript Editor: Leslie E. Hoeltzel
Indexer: Deborah A. Ziwot
Art Director: Maria S. Karkucinski
Designer: Patrick Turner
Production Assistant: George V. Gordon
Compositor: Ruttle, Shaw & Wetherill, Inc.
Printer/Binder: Halliday Lithograph Corp.

The authors and publisher have exerted every effort to ensure that drug selection and dosage set forth in this text are in accord with current recommendations and practice at the time of publication. However, in view of ongoing research, changes in government regulations, and the constant flow of information relating to drug therapy and drug reactions, the reader is urged to check the package insert for each drug for any change in indications and dosage and for added warnings and precautions. This is particularly important when the recommended agent is a new or infrequently employed drug.

3 5 6 4

Library of Congress Cataloging in Publication Data

Main entry under title:

The Injured Athlete.

  Bibliography.
  Includes index.
  1. Sports—Accidents and injuries. 2. Sports medicine. I. Kulund, Daniel N. [DNLM: 1. Physical education and training—Methods. 2. Sports medicine. QT 260 I515]
RD97.I55   617′.1027   81-20931
ISBN 0-397-50449-7   AACR2

Printed in the United States of America

Dedicated to
my dad, Nicholas Kulund;
my mentors,
A.A. Savastano and
Frank C. McCue III;
and my family,
Sandy, Patrick, and David

Contents

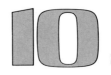

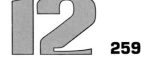

13

The Elbow, Wrist, and Hand   295

FRANK C. McCUE III

14

The Torso, Hip, and Thigh   331

15

The Knee   361

16

The Leg, Ankle, and Foot   425

Appendix A—
The Spectrum of Sport   473

Appendix B—
The Sports Medicine Team   475

Contributors

Associate Professor of Physical Education and
Assistant Professor of Orthopedics
Director of the Biomechanics Laboratory
University of Virginia
Charlottesville, Virginia

Clifford E. Brubaker, Ph.D.

Assistant Professor
School of Education
Head Athletic Trainer
University of Virginia
Charlottesville, Virginia
College Trainer of the Year, 1979

Joe H. Gieck, R.P.T., A.T.C., Ed.D.

Professor of Orthopedic Surgery,
Plastic Surgery, and Surgery of the Hand
University of Virginia Medical Center
Team Physician
University of Virginia
Charlottesville, Virginia

Frank C. McCue III, M.D.

Associate Professor of Medicine
Director, Non-Invasive Cardiology Laboratory
Division of Cardiology
University of Virginia Medical Center
Charlottesville, Virginia

Randolph P. Martin, M.D.

Associate Professor
Director, Human Performance Laboratory
Department of Physical Education
Blatt Physical Education Center
College of Health
University of South Carolina
Columbia, South Carolina

Russell R. Pate, Ph.D.

Associate Professor of Education
Director of Sports Psychology
Department of Health and Physical Education
University of Virginia
Charlottesville, Virginia

Robert J. Rotella, Ph.D.

Athletic Training Consultant
The Aerobic Performance Center
Charlotte, North Carolina

Thomas H. Soos, M.Ed., A.T.C.

Exercise and Biomechanics Consultant
Former Olympian and United States Olympic Team Coach
Research Associate
University of New Mexico
Albuquerque, New Mexico

Miklós Töttössy, M.A., M.S.

Preface

In our increasingly athletic society, youths, women, prime-age athletes, older athletes, and handicapped persons are running, swimming, training with weights, and competing in a wide variety of individual, dual, and team sports. Sports medicine, the scientific study and care of people in the context of exercise and sport, has grown with this boom in athletics. Simultaneously, a need has developed for a clinically useful sports medicine book to aid the physician who sees some, many, mostly, or only athletes in his practice, and for other members of the sports medicine team. *The Injured Athlete* has been written to fill this need.

The reader is first shown how to perform a complete preparticipation examination and how to treat the medical problems of athletes. Russell Pate then discusses the principles of training and differences in the training of youths, women, and prime-age and older athletes. Next, Cliff Brubaker describes how to evaluate fitness, and Randy Martin reviews the effects of exercise on the cardiovascular system. After an up-to-date chapter on strength and power training, Professor Töttössy discusses the importance of warming up and provides pictures from which one may design a warm-up program for athletes.

The athletic trainer plays a key role in the rehabilitation of the injured athlete. Joe Gieck describes the trainer's duties, including how to fit protective equipment and the steps in rehabilitating injured athletes. Tom Soos then shows how the trainer uses adhesive tape. There is also a psychological side to athletic injuries, and sports psychologist Bob Rotella details the coping strategies that athletes may use to help in psychological rehabilitation.

The Injured Athlete is foremost a clinically useful guide to the prevention, diagnosis, and treatment of athletic injuries. To this end, Ron Ervin has combined dynamic illustrations and action photographs to depict injury mechanisms, disrupted anatomy, diagnostic methods, and treatment. The injury chapters range from the head to the foot and include a comprehensive chapter on athletic injuries to the elbow, wrist, and hand by Frank McCue and discussions of throwing, running, and cycling. Finally, along with useful tables, the appendices contain the position statements of our American College of Sports Medicine.

Daniel N. Kulund, M.D.

Acknowledgments

My thanks to Dr. Arthur J. Helfet, orthopedic surgeon, sportsman, and advisor;

Ron Ervin, the "Wizard of Air," who worked so closely with me to produce dynamic illustrations;

Allan J. Ryan, the clearest voice and driving force in sports medicine;

The many orthopaedic and other pioneers in sports medicine;

Physicians who read and critiqued sections: Peyton Eggleston, Fritz Dreifuss, Munsey Wheby, Ken Greer, John Shrum, Alan Rogol, Richard Winn, J.A. Fogle, Michael Johns, George Minor, Jim Chandler, and Art Wyker;

David Brody, "the runner's doctor," and Katherine Braun;

Sports orthodontist Richard Kaufman;

The Orthopaedic Chairman at the University of Virginia, Warren Stamp, his son Marcus, and the members of our Orthopaedic staff: Charles Frankel, Robert McLaughlin, Mary Williams Clark, and Michael Sussman;

Bob Cronin, my friend and colleague, Bill Ober, and Bob Fritz;

Coaches Mark Bernardino, Ron Good, Dennis Craddock, Bill Dunn, Billy Williams, and Reg Roberts;

All-around champion Jim "Gym" Gibson, Dan McCoy, tennis professional Phil Rogers, and the masterful C. Alphonso Smith;

Athletic trainers Bill Nelson, Bernie DePalma, and Ellen Malloy;

Photographers Dan Grogan and John Atkins; Pat Pugh and Ursula Ziolkowski, who developed and printed the pictures;

Aniko Töttössy, Jan Jensen, and Marianne Schwartz, who worked diligently on the warm-up section;

George Paul and Nell Fuller of the Claude Moore Health Sciences Library;

Jennifer Carter, my hard-working and trusted secretary, who cheerfully handled so many tough jobs and typed the manuscript;

Don Young for his typing help, and Irene Lawhorne and Kathy Bailey for their assistance; and

The J. B. Lippincott team of J. Stuart Freeman, Jr., Sanford Robinson, Richard Heffron, and Leslie E. Hoeltzel who worked so well with us to produce this book.

As athletes of all ages have entered sports in recent years, athletic diversity has become the norm. Sport beckons the young, the prime-age athletes, women, older people, the handicapped, and even those who may be suffering from disease. A sports physician will be asked to make evaluations and to treat patients according to the type of athlete, the particular sport, and the athlete's goals; to design fitness programs; and to give advice on cardiovascular fitness, strength training, warming up, and protective gear. The prevention, treatment, and rehabilitation of athletic injuries, including musculoskeletal problems, will be fundamental to one's practice.

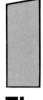

The Athlete's Physician

The athlete is generally a healthy and well-motivated person. However, an injury that might be insignificant to another patient may be a serious handicap to him, and for this reason the sports physician must appreciate the value the athlete places on sport. If, for example, an athlete is told to stop exercising and to rest, he will often resist this advice and seek help elsewhere, for "REST" in athletic medicine means to *Resume Exercise* below the *Soreness Threshold*. Depending upon his sport, the athlete may avoid pain-producing activities by decreasing his mileage, by switching to another swim stroke, or by using a temporary orthosis. With an injury to a lower extremity, he may stay fit by exercising in a pool or on a bicycle with his sound leg clipped to a pedal. In general, slings and casts are to be avoided because immobilization reduces proprioception and increases rehabilitation time.

It should be remembered that the rehabilitation of an injured athlete is both physical and psychological and that, unlike a nonathlete, he soon is exposed to the same forces that caused his injury. His flexibility and strength, therefore, must be greater when he returns to practice and competition than they were before treatment. His rehabilitation will be aided by his understanding of exercise and by his willingness to work hard. The athlete expects, and should be given, an explanation of his injury and the options for treatment and should be told how he may help his recovery. Psychological rehabilitation is also important, although psychological scars may not be as apparent as physical scars. This effort will be reinforced by systematic desensitization techniques that allow the athlete to relax and to concentrate when he returns to his sport.

The athlete's physician must keep fully informed of the newest research in his field by reading and attending seminars (*see* Appendix). Also recommended is that he set a good example and gain trust by training and being fit.

The Team Physician

The team physician may be a doctor who takes a turn sitting on the bench at Friday-night football games. Occasionally, he may be a parent of one of the players and may attend games and practices, but only as long as his child is on the team. This is not a desirable situation, for the team physician should be under contract to the school. He should be responsible for the athletes' health care and committed to setting up comprehensive programs for preseason evaluation, conditioning, health education, and injury prevention, treatment, and rehabilitation. He is usually a generalist because most problems in sports medicine are common ones, such as upper respiratory infections.[19, 39] The team doctor will, however, need specialist consultants to assist him in the treatment of injuries.

Legal Aspects of Sports Medicine

Current trends in litigation have made the team physician very vulnerable to legal liability. In fact, awards of up to $2 million have been rendered in sports injury cases. Because the team physician may have to make fast decisions under pressure, he needs to exercise good judgment, to be conscientious, and to follow established guidelines to avoid liability problems.[24, 32, 37, 45]

Negligence

When the physician treats athletes, a doctor–patient relationship is established between him and the members of the team under his care. He must treat the athletes as he would his own private patients. It is immaterial under the law whether diagnoses and treatments are provided for a fee or *gratis*. Moreover, the statute of limitations is no safeguard against action by a minor because a suit for negligence can be withheld until the young athlete reaches maturity, at which time he may file suit.

Obviously, sports injuries are common and may be devastating. In one instance, a high school quarterback was tackled on a "quarterback sneak." He lay on the field, and his coach, suspecting a neck injury, checked the young man's grip and found it functioning. The coach then asked eight young men to carry the athlete to the sidelines, which they did without the aid of a stretcher. There the athlete was found to be quadriplegic. Consequently, both the coach and the doctor were found negligent: the coach for failing to wait for the doctor to come onto the field, and the doctor for failing to act promptly after the injury.[45]

The team physician may become involved in legal action through tort liability or direct malpractice suits. Because most courts do not hold coaches and trainees responsible for the diagnosis and treatment of sports injuries, this responsibility must be assumed by a physician. Hence, the team physician will be the major defendant in most cases of litigation. These cases are mostly "tort liability" ones, where liability for personal injury is allegedly a result of the defendant's negligence. Currently, there is a trend to expand the areas in which tort liability is applicable and to increase the size of tort awards. For this reason, the team physician should take every precaution to avoid becoming a defendant in a tort liability case, and he should have liability insurance that covers athletic contests.

The principal charge against which the team physician will have to defend is that of negligence on his part. Negligence is defined as failure to act as a prudent physician would under similar circumstances. An example of negligence would be failure to follow standard procedures and established methods for treating an injury. One should keep in mind that negligence may consist of inaction as well as action. Actionable negligence comprises four elements, and a cause of action in tort requires proof that all four elements be present. The elements are

[1] that the defendant had a duty to act to avoid unreasonable risk to others; [2] that the defendant breached said duty with failure to observe that duty; [3] that failure to observe the duty was the proximate cause of the damage; and [4] that actual damage or injury occurred.

A doctor is not an ensurer of the success of all treatments and procedures. He is not held liable for honest mistakes of judgment, as when the proper treatment is open to reasonable doubt and his action conforms to the standards of good medical practive in his community. However, the standard of care is measured in terms of the doctor's specialty, and the conduct of a physician specializing in sports injuries who treats such an injury could be judged negligent even though the same conduct by a general practitioner might not be.

Legal defenses against the charge of negligence include *assumption of risk* and *contributory negligence.* An athlete, for example, assumes some risk when undertaking to wrestle or to play tackle football, and athletes may act in a negligent manner, thereby contributing to an injury.

To help avoid tort liability, the physician should do the following.

Follow established guidelines.
Have a contract drawn up with the school.
Secure an athletic trainer.
Design and conduct a thorough preparticipation physical examination with attention to disqualifying defects.
Use sound judgment for allowing athletes to return to competition after injury or illness.
Institute proper care early if an injury occurs.
Seek informed consent for treatment.
Be careful about releasing information.

The Contract

When a physician becomes a team doctor, it is often a labor of love. He should, however, insist on an agreement with school officials that spells out his responsibilities. The school must, in turn, vest the physician with the authority to make medical judgments relating to students' participation in school sports. Since the health of the athletes will be the physician's prime concern, his must be the final word on all medical decisions.

Good communication is important, and for this reason the team physician should meet with athletes and their parents before the start of the season. A suit-conscious public may have the notion that protective equipment always prevents injury and may therefore charge negligence if an athlete is injured. This notion can be dispelled at the preseason meeting if the limitations of protective equipment are explained. Athletes and parents should also be told how the doctor, trainer, coaches, and athletes propose to reduce the chance of injury.

At this time the team physician should also meet with the coaches to establish guidelines for injury control and to assist in the development of conditioning programs. Dangerous coaching practices, such as the teaching of head tackling and butt blocking, should be forbidden. Descriptive terms such as "punishment drill," "crucifixion," "suicide," "hamburger," "meatgrinder," and "gauntlet" are best avoided.[4] Athletes must be made aware of the risks of participation, and the mechanics of catastrophic injury should be clearly demonstrated and explained.

The Athletic Trainer

The athletic trainer is a key person in the high school athletic program, and if the school does not have a trainer one should be recruited. The trainer's sole concern is safety of the athletes. He carries out injury-control programs and attends practices and games, activities that the team physician often is unable to perform. The trainer fits protective equipment, makes sure it is worn in practices and games, and checks it at least once a week, since the equipment occasionally loosens or parts break. The same good-quality equipment worn in games should be worn in practices. It is also the trainer's duty to be sure that the playing facilities and gym equipment are properly cared for, and he shares with the physician the responsibility to point out dangers in practice areas, on the playing field and in the gym, that may be overlooked by others. The trainer administers first aid with the aim of keeping minor injuries from causing major disability. He should also recognize more serious injuries and take proper first aid steps to avoid compounding such injuries.

The trainer works under, and follows the directives of, the team physician. For this reason, he is almost always regarded as an agent of the team physician; thus negligence on his part is often imputed to the doctor. Good rapport between the physician and the trainer is essential, and guidelines should be clearly established and respected.

The Preparticipation Examination

The preparticipation examination is an important duty of the team physician, and tort liability may be applied to this procedure. The examination includes a complete history that covers previous illnesses and allergies and that will serve as a base for medical records and may affect later treatment. The examination should be a thorough one, in accord with guidelines for the examination of athletes, and the findings should be disclosed to the athlete, the athlete's parents, and the athlete's family physician.

Courts have noted that athletes erroneously have been found physically qualified to participate in sports.[21, 25] The physician should avoid guaranteeing or giving assurance that it will be safe for a team member to participate in a sport. Instead he may record, "I can find no medical reason why the athlete should not participate," or, "The examination failed to disclose anything that would prevent the youngster from participating in athletics."

If the physician decides that a disqualifying defect, such as one kidney, one eye, or one testicle, warrants that an athlete not participate in a sport, he should not allow anyone to persuade him to change his decision. A defect occasionally may be found in a youngster who has participated in athletics since grade school, and the athlete and his parents may be unable to understand why the defect is now considered disqualifying. Although they may offer to sign a release, the law gives *the parents no authority to release future claims on behalf of the child.* The parents, family doctor, athlete, and school or college should be informed of the findings and the physician's decision. If, contrary to the physician's recommendation, the athlete is allowed to participate in the sport, the physician should repeat his objection to continued participation.

Emergency Care of Athletic Injuries and Return to the Game

The team physician should be available during practice sessions and be present at games, alert for injuries. He should be well versed in the proper care of major injuries, such as those to the head, eyes, neck, and significant musculoskeletal injuries.[12, 43] Proper aids, such as backboards and splints, must be available. There should be no hesitation if an athlete needs to be carried from the field on a stretcher. Every athlete should understand that leaving the field on a stretcher is not a sign of weakness.

The team physician often will have to make on-the-spot decisions as to whether an athlete who has been injured during a game should be allowed to continue playing.[18] An overcautious appraisal may mean a loss for the home team. If, however, the risk of allowing an injured athlete to re-enter a game is taken, the injury may worsen and result in permanent harm to the athlete. *"When in doubt, keep the athlete out."* The team physician must never let anyone pressure him into allowing an athlete who has not fully recovered from an illness or an injury to play. His prime concern must be the health of those under his care. To prevent athletic injuries from going undetected, a firm and inflexible rule should be established that all injuries, no matter how trivial, be reported to the trainer or team physician. An early, accurate diagnosis will ensure prompt treatment and faster recovery.

Transportation for injured athletes, including routes to and from the playing and practice fields, should be arranged ahead of need. If an athlete suffers a major injury during a game and must be taken to the hospital, the team physician should accompany him. If the injury is not life-threatening, however, the trainer may accompany the injured athlete; the physician should remain at the field in case a major injury does occur. In most cases, emergency medical technicians will be especially helpful in providing for the care and transportation of injured athletes or ill spectators.

Explaining Treatment to the Athlete

To care properly for an athlete's injuries and to avoid claims of negligence, the nature of the injury and the treatment alternatives must be explained to the athlete and his parents. This information should be sufficient for them to make an intelligent choice as to whether treatment is necessary. The dangers, if any, and the advantages of alternative treatments should be carefully laid out. If drugs are needed, their effects should be described and any alternative measures explained. A new treatment must not be implemented without a full explanation to the athlete and his parents, for a court may regard such treatment as experimentation.

X-rays of the injured area must be taken because their absence may be regarded as negligence. Good medical records are important, and athletes must be followed closely with full control over their treatment. Treatment should not be prematurely ended, but if an athlete terminates treatment before being medically discharged, he must be persuaded to resume treatment, if possible. Failure to follow up an athlete who is under treatment may be construed by the courts as abandonment of treatment. Moreover, athletes should not be allowed to return to competition in any sport after an injury or illness unless recovery is complete. If a case is a difficult one, advice should be sought from a consultant. No firm promise or guarantee of result should be given, nor any assurance that there will be no residual limitations or disabilities.

Releasing Information

The doctor-patient relationship is a confidential one, and medical information about the athlete's condition should not be disclosed without his specific written consent. Even with consent, the physician may be subject to liability if his statements turn out to be inaccurate. If a statement of opinion is made with the knowledge that another will act upon it, the giver of the opinion may be held responsible for damage incurred because of the inaccuracy of his opinion, even though it was rendered in good faith and gratuitously.[42] If consent is given for release of information, any disclosure should be limited to the objective facts of the injury, leaving the team with the burden of determining the current fitness of the athlete.

Obviously, the position of team physician is a demanding one, with liability potential. To render tort liability less likely, the physician must use good judgment, follow established guidelines, and be aware of the latest research and developments in the field of sports medicine. The responsible team physician should also educate athletes and their parents, coaches, and medical personnel about good health practices and the prevention and care of athletic injuries.

Preseason Examination

On first entry into a sports program, each athlete needs a comprehensive history and physical examination.[7, 9, 26, 33] The examination establishes baselines for later comparisons, uncovers deficiencies, and evaluates limitations relative to the given sport. The team physician can locate and quantify inherent or acquired musculoskeletal weaknesses that may predispose the athlete to injury. Also, the injury-prone athlete can be identified, as can those who have histories of concussion or heat stroke, rendering them more susceptible to these conditions.

The examination should be performed before the season starts to allow time to arrange further evaluations and to design and implement exercise programs to remedy deficiencies.[40] When undue risks are anticipated for athletes with potentially disqualifying conditions, the athletes should be counseled and guided into alternative activities. Balanced competition requires that youths be matched according to their levels of maturity.

The preseason examination is a course in health education, especially when youngsters with asthma, diabetes mellitus, or a convulsive disorder are being advised. These children need highly individualized examinations with explanations of how exercise can benefit their asthma or diabetes and how they can help to control the medical condition.

How often should preseason examinations be conducted? As noted above, a comprehensive medical examination should precede the entry of a young athlete, such as a high school freshman, into a sports program. After this examination, problem-oriented medical attention is appropriate, with a check on intervening problems before each new sports season. In this continuing medical care, the emphasis should be on quality, not frequency.

When should the preseason examination be conducted? A good time is 4 to 6 weeks before conditioning programs or preseason practice begins, because early examinations allow time to obtain consultations and accomplish treatment. There are three types of such examinations: the *individual* examination, the *mass* examination, and the *group* examination. A thorough, private, individual examination by the athlete's family doctor can provide an excellent assessment of fitness for sport because the doctor knows the youngster's medical history. He may, however, be unfamiliar with the medical aspects of sport, and hence be inclined to be conservative. In other instances, the doctor may pass over health conditions that should limit participation in certain sports. As doctors learn more about sports medicine, better individual preseason examinations will result, reducing the potential for injury as greater understanding of the physical requirements for particular sports events is acquired.

Each year, millions of young athletes undergo hasty and superficial mass examinations by volunteer doctors in noisy, crowded locker rooms. These examinations endanger the athlete, generating a low opinion of doctors and the importance of health care and physical fitness. The place for the examination is usually determined by local conditions, but ideally the examination will be conducted in an appropriate setting by doctors who are trained to administer a thorough examination and who take care to check for those factors that may predispose a young athlete to injury or illness.

Because of the large number of athletes who must be examined and the limited number of physicians qualified to conduct such examinations, a carefully organized group examination with a team approach is recommended. The team should consist of doctors, trainers, nurses, and others who may assist with various routines, such as maintaining discipline and directing traffic. The doctors may include specialists, generalists, residents, and medical students.

The group examination usually is conducted in a large area, such as a physical therapy department.[5] Audiology booths may be used when absolute quiet is needed, as during the heart examination. Boys should wear shorts and girls halter tops or swimsuit tops. An overall health inventory is the first item to be completed. After weights are recorded, the athletes will proceed through a series of stations labeled with large signs. These will include medical, dental, eye and ear, musculoskeletal, orthopedic, and review stations. When the examinations have been completed, the team physician will confer with the school nurse and coaches to review and analyze the findings.

The History for the Preparticipation Examination

Because it will be an important part of the athlete's medical record throughout his career, the history taken at the preparticipation examination must be thorough. A number of typical questions are listed below. Answers should be supplied by the athlete and his parents, and information may also be obtained from the family physician. An instructor will explain the questions, and parents should assist in filling out the form to be certain that all questions are answered properly and no important omissions occur. Any circled answers or "yes" responses should be explained or described. Because there is no standard history form, questions will differ depending on the group examined and the purpose of the examination.

History for Preparticipation Examination

Name _____ Age _____ Birthdate _____

Home address _____

Phone number _____

Phone numbers where parents can be reached at work:

_____

List the sports that you plan to participate in this year:

   Fall: _____

   Winter: _____

   Spring: _____

   Summer: _____

What are your long range goals?

   Academic: _____

   Vocational: _____

   Athletic: _____

What are your personal goals in athletics? _____

_____

_____

What other sports do you participate in? _____

_____

Have you ever been told by a physician to restrict your sports activity

   or not to participate in a sport? _____

Are your currently under a doctor's care? _____

Dates of Immunizations

   Measles _____ Smallpox _____

   Diphtheria _____ Poliomyelitis _____

   Typhoid _____ Tetanus toxoid booster _____

History for Preparticipation Examination (Continued)

Medicines and Allergies

Do you take any medications? _____ If so, list them: _____

_____

Have you ever had a reaction (allergy) to medication? _____

Have you ever had a severe reaction to an insect bite or sting?

_____

Have you ever had asthma, hay fever, or hives? _____

Family History

Has anyone in your family had diabetes, cancer, bleeding tendencies, a stroke, heart trouble, high blood pressure, lung disease or

tuberculosis? _____

_____

Review of Your Illnesses

Have you ever had a skin problem, such as acne, herpes, eczema, scarlet fever, ''jock itch'', ''athlete's foot'', or other skin condition(s)? _____

_____

Have you ever had epilepsy (convulsions), asthma, hay fever, diabetes, hepatitis, jaundice or mononucleosis? _____

_____

Have you ever had anemia or blood disease, sickle cell trait, or a

bleeding tendency (bruise easily)? _____

Have you ever been given a blood transfusion? _____

Have you ever had heart disease, rheumatic fever, high or low blood pressure, emphysema, tuberculosis, pneumonia, stomach or intestinal trouble, kidney disease, kidney or bladder infection, venereal disease, or arthritis? _____

_____

Have you ever been pregnant? _____ Number of times _____

Any miscarriages? _____

Do you have any loss or impaired function of any paired organ?

    Eyes: ⎯⎯⎯

    Ears: ⎯⎯⎯

    Lungs: ⎯⎯⎯

    Kidneys: ⎯⎯⎯

    Testes: ⎯⎯⎯

Have you had any illness that lasted longer than a week? ⎯⎯⎯

Have you had any illness that would interfere with your best perfor-

    mance? ⎯⎯⎯⎯⎯⎯⎯⎯⎯⎯

Have you ever been treated for mental illness or "nerves"? De-

    scribe: ⎯⎯⎯⎯⎯⎯⎯⎯⎯⎯

Review of Injuries

Have you ever had an injury that caused limitation of activity or

    required medical attention? ⎯⎯⎯⎯⎯⎯⎯⎯

Any injury to bone, muscle, ligament, tendon or joint? ⎯⎯⎯⎯

    Was medical attention required? ⎯⎯⎯⎯⎯⎯⎯

    How long were you disabled? ⎯⎯⎯⎯⎯⎯⎯

Are you currently suffering from an injury? ⎯⎯⎯⎯⎯⎯

Do you have an injury that may interfere with your best perfor-

    mance? ⎯⎯⎯⎯⎯⎯⎯⎯⎯

Have you had any problems in the past in being rehabilitated after

    an injury and returning to competition? ⎯⎯⎯⎯⎯⎯

Have you ever gone to an emergency room or a doctor for x-rays?

⎯⎯⎯⎯⎯⎯⎯⎯⎯⎯⎯⎯⎯⎯⎯

Have you ever had any operations, even minor ones? ⎯⎯⎯⎯

    Give details: ⎯⎯⎯⎯⎯⎯⎯⎯⎯⎯

⎯⎯⎯⎯⎯⎯⎯⎯⎯⎯⎯⎯⎯⎯⎯

⎯⎯⎯⎯⎯⎯⎯⎯⎯⎯⎯⎯⎯⎯⎯

History for Preparticipation Examination (Continued)

Review of Systems

Have you ever fainted or "blacked out"? _____

    Was this during exercise? _____

Have you ever had a skin rash? _____

The Head

Have you ever had convulsions (epilepsy)? _____

    How many times? _____

Have you had dizzy spells, recurrent headaches, lightheadedness,

    or memory loss from a blow to your head? _____

Have you ever been unconscious (knocked out)? _____

The Neck

Have you had neck pain or pain in your shoulder or down an arm?

_____

Gums and Teeth

When did you last visit a dentist? _____

Do you have bridge work or wear dental braces or dentures? _____

Eyes

Have you ever been examined by a vision specialist? _____

    If yes, how long has it been since the examination? _____

Do you have any difficulties with your eyes, such as blurred distance

    vision, blurred near vision, double vision, or headaches? _____

    If you have headaches, describe them: _____

_____

Do you have frequent styes, watering, redness, eye pain, light sen-

    sitivity, trouble judging distances, burning, squinting to see,

    twitching of your eyelids, or trouble seeing as it gets dark or at

    night games? _____

_____

Do you normally wear eyeglasses? _____

    For practice? _____

    For contests? _____

    Do you have a spare pair? _____

Do you normally wear contact lenses? _____

   For practice? _____

   For contests? _____

   Are these hard or soft lenses? _____

   Do you have a spare pair? _____

If you do wear glasses or contact lenses, how long have you been

   using the present pair? _____

Ears

Do you have trouble hearing? _____

Do you have ringing in your ears? _____

Do your ears itch? _____

Nose

Does your nose run? _____

Has it ever been broken? _____

Any trouble breathing through your nose? _____

Shoulder

Any shoulder pain, especially when you throw, serve, or swim? ___

_____

Do you ever feel as if your shoulder is giving out? _____

_____

Have you ever had a shoulder separation or dislocation? _____

_____

Chest

Have you ever had rib cage pain? _____

Have you ever had chest pain? _____

Any skipped beats or racing heartbeat? _____

Do you have a chronic cough, recurrent colds, or shortness of

   breath? _____

Does exercise cause you to cough or become short of breath more

   so than other athletes? _____

History for Preparticipation Examination (Continued)

**History for
Preparticipation
Examination
(Continued)**

Back

Have you had upper back pain? _____

Have you had lower back pain? _____

Do you feel low back pain when your spine is jolted on landings or
when you overextend your spine? _____

Pelvis

Do you have a hernia (rupture)? _____

Do you have pelvic or groin pain? _____

Do you have burning when you urinate? _____

Do you urinate frequently? _____

Have you had albumin or sugar in your urine? _____

Menstrual History

Date of your first menstrual period _____, 19 ____

Are your periods regular or irregular? _____

How many periods have you had in the last 90 days? _____

When was your last period? ____ / ____ /19 to ____ / ____ /19

Does your athletic performance suffer during any phase of the menstrual cycle? _____

Do you take pills for birth control or for regulation of your menstrual
cycle? _____

If so, what type are they, how long have you been taking them,
and in what dosage? _____

_____

Do you have a vaginal discharge? _____

Bowels

Do you have frequent constipation or diarrhea? _____

Have you ever noticed blood in your stools or black stools? _____

_____

Do you have hemorrhoids? _____

Hips and Thighs

Did you have hip pain? _____

Have you ever had a "Charlie horse" (bruised thigh) or pulled

hamstring? _____

Knee

Have you ever had a swollen knee? _____

Ever had pain in or around your knee? _____

Ever had an unstable knee with giving way, clicking, popping,

catching, or locking? _____

Do your kneecaps catch or slide out of place? _____

Do your knees hurt when you run or jump? _____

Legs and Ankles

Do you have leg pains? _____

Do you have large, swollen leg veins? _____

Have you ever sprained an ankle? _____

If so, how many times? _____

Does your ankle give way or swell? _____

Feet

Do you have painful feet? _____

Do you have flat feet? _____

Do you wear orthotics? _____

If so, where did you obtain them? _____

Obtained for what reason? _____

What is your shoe size? _____What kind of shoes do you prefer

for training, competition, and for everyday walking? _____

History for Preparticipation Examination (Continued)

Muscles

Do you suffer from muscle cramps? _____

Do you have recurrent swelling or instability in your

Neck, shoulder, elbow, wrist, or hand? _____

Spine, pelvis, knee, leg, ankle, or foot? _____

Do you have any pain, catching, grinding, slipping, sliding, giving

way, rubbing, bumps, lumps, or bones anywhere that you think

may be abnormal? _____

_____

Sleep History

How many hours of sleep do you need? _____

Do you sleep well or do you have difficulty sleeping? _____

_____

Do you wake up tired? _____

How do you manage to fall asleep when you are having difficulty

falling asleep? _____

Are you familiar with relaxation techniques? _____

Do you develop motion sickness while traveling? _____

Meals

What is your ''best weight''? _____

How much do you weigh now? _____

Has your body weight recently increased or decreased? _____

By how many killigrams (pounds)? _____

How is your appetite? _____

Describe your meals yesterday and today (including snacks):

_____

_____

_____

_____

_____

Do you have what some people may call "dietary fads"? _____

_____

Do you have any favorite food supplements? _____

Describe the kind of meal you prefer before a contest: _____

_____

Are there any foods that make you sick, especially before a game or

contest? _____

Do coffee, tea, or caffeine-containing soft drinks make you jittery or

upset your stomach? _____

Your Training Program

Do you know how to perform a complete warm-up for competition

in your sport? _____

Describe your warm-up: _____

_____

_____

_____

Describe your strength training program: _____

_____

_____

_____

Describe your aerobic conditioning program: _____

_____

_____

_____

Do you have any specific recurrent pains when you warm up, lift

weights, or run? _____

Are there any exercises that hurt you or that you are unable to

perform, although many of your teammates can? _____

_____

Are there any areas of your body that you believe are not very

flexible? _____

History for Preparticipation Examination (Continued)

**History for
Preparticipation
Examination
(Continued)**

Are there any areas of your body that you believe are weak? _____

_____

Are there any additional comments that you wish to make about

your medical history? _____

_____

_____

_____

Do you have any worries about your health or any other questions

that you would like to discuss with the doctor? _____

_____

_____

_____

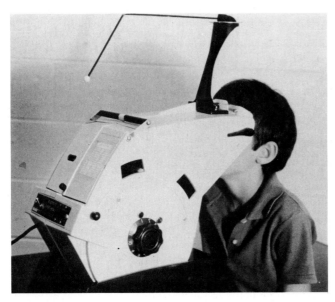

FIG. 1-1
The Titmus machine is
used for vision testing.

Preseason Examination of the Eyes

While poor vision may account for dropped passes, similar errors, and poor performance, the athlete may not know that his vision is abnormal. The Titmus machine (Fig. 1-1), which may be found in a Department of Motor Vehicles, should be used for vision tests because youths with poor vision have been known to memorize the Snellen chart to bluff their way through an informal examination.

An athlete who has only one useful eye is best excluded from contact sports. Athletes with significant amblyopia should also be barred because trauma to the better eye could be devastating. Athletes with high degrees of myopia are notoriously susceptible to retinal detachment, and this tendency may be brought out by contact sports. Some myopic persons have considerable chorioretinal degeneration, but others with an equivalent myopia have ostensibly normal retinas. Thus, the visually deficient athlete's eyes must be closely examined, and the procedure should include a dilated fundus examination for any spectacle-dependent myopic person. It should be noted that angioid streaks of retinal degeneration are warnings of an increased danger of detachment and that contact sports are not permitted after repair of retinal detachment.

Preseason Examination of the Teeth

Preventive dentistry includes a mouth mirror examination to reduce the chances that a player will be lost during the season because of a toothache. The preparticipation examination is also a good occasion to check for temporomandibular joint imbalances and to start a mouthguard program.

Preseason Musculoskeletal Examination

The musculoskeletal system examination should draw attention to those areas most prone to injury. Blyth and Mueller found that 46% of all injuries to high school football players were injuries to the lower extremity; 24% to the upper extremity; 13% to the trunk; 13% to the head and neck; and less than 1% internal.[6] More specifically, 19% of the injuries were at the knee; 15% at the ankle; 8% at the shoulder; and 8% involved the hand. Obviously, these areas should be carefully examined because they are at high risk for injury. Signs of old injury should not be overlooked since weak links in the limbs may increase the potential for new injury.

Neck

Neck length should be measured with a tape measure from the occiput to the vertebra prominens, which is the spinous process of C-7. The neck circumference is then measured just below the larynx and the neck motion checked. The athlete first must lower his chin to his chest with his mouth closed, because an open mouth will add about 15° to the flexion. If there is a gap of one fingerwidth between the athlete's chin and chest, there will be 10° of restricted motion.

To check neck extension, the athlete should lean his head backwards until his forehead is parallel to the ceiling, a position that yields 35° to 50° of next extension. For lateral flexion testing, the athlete should bend his head toward his shoulder without shrugging. This measurement depends on the athlete's musculature, which can block the movement, but 40° to 45° of lateral flexion is desirable. For measurement of neck rotation, the athlete should turn his neck as far as he can to each side.

Shoulder

In the shoulder examination, strength is estimated, range of motion is checked, and any contractures are detected. The player moves his arms against manual resistance to determine whether any strength measurement is less than normal. If there is insufficient strength, a program for improvement should be established. To check for winging of the scapula, the athlete should do a wall push-up (Fig. 1-2A).

For shoulder range of motion, especially important for swimmers and baseball players, the athlete lies supine (Fig. 1-2B), and the scapula is controlled by its proximity to the table. An inward shoulder rotation of about 90° is normal. The scapula is tilting if the athlete must lift his shoulder off the table as he presses down toward the table with his hands.

An athlete may develop internal rotation contractures of the shoulder from off-season bench presses. To check for this condition, the

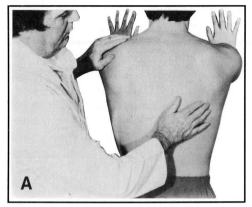
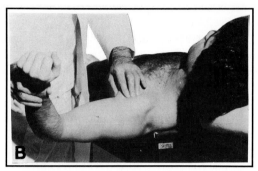

FIG. 1-2
The examiner feels for winging of the scapula as the athlete does a wall push-up (*A*). With the athlete supine, he checks for limited external rotation of the shoulder (*B*).

athlete should flex his hips and knees and then place his arms back over his head. If the lower back arches, the latissimus and pectoralis are tight.

Elbow

The carrying angle of the elbow is usually about 20° of valgus. Some flexion deformity will usually be found in the elbows of pitchers, tennis players, and boxers, and even a Little League baseball pitcher's forearm may lack full supination.

Back

For a back examination, the athlete should bend forward, a position that normally produces a good curve to the spine (Fig. 1-3A). If the athlete has tight hamstrings, his lower back will flatten.

The distance between C-7 and S-1 is measured while the athlete is standing straight. The athlete fully flexes forward, and the change in distance between the two points is measured—usually a difference of about 10 cm (4 in). A measurement of less than 10 cm is a sign of decreased flexibility of the lower back, and if the bending measurement remains about the

same as the upright one, ankylosing spondylitis should be suspected.

A sit-and-reach test may be used to determine general spinal flexibility. Lordosis (swayback) increases an athlete's susceptibility to lower back strain, and when this condition appears, postural exercises are prescribed to help remedy the lordotic posture. The physician checks for leg-length inequality by resting his hands on the athlete's iliac crests and noting whether his hands are at the same level (Fig. 1-3B).

Scoliosis

The preparticipation examination is a good occasion to screen for scoliosis or spinal curvature. This condition is seen mostly in 9- to 14-year-old girls, who may even have a substantial curve that their parents may not have noticed. Since secondary curves may balance the head in line with the pelvis, the spine may not, at first glance, appear crooked. The early discovery of scoliosis is essential so that proper bracing and, where necessary, surgery can be done to prevent large curves that may affect cardiopulmonary function and decrease life expectancy.

When checking for scoliosis, ascertain that the shoulders are level before checking elbow height. Waist and flank symmetry are observed, and the subject then bends forward to have the alignment of the spinous processes and the symmetry of the thorax checked. Curves of less than 15° should not limit a youngster's activities. But where a curve exceeds 20°, especially in the lumbar region, contact sports such as football or tumbling may lead to further back trouble. Although scoliosis may produce some disability later in life, the activity of the young competitor need not be restricted except for contact sports because future problems may bear no relation to earlier sports activities. Youngsters with large curves may wear a scoliosis brace to prevent progression of the curvature. The brace may be removed for bathing and exercise and also for swimming. Full athletics may be permitted with the athlete wearing the brace except for contact sports, where a brace may be a hazard to opponents. Brace-free athletic participation promotes well-adjusted and physically fit youngsters and need not necessarily lead to an increase in the scoliotic curve. The development of better muscle tone through athletics may well hinder curve progression, especially if sport is combined with free gymnastic exercises designed to counteract the curve.

Youngsters with vertebral epiphysitis (Scheuermann's disease) have standing lateral spine films that show vertebral wedging and undulation of their vertebral end-plates. The wedging produces a round back deformity that may be progressive. These youngsters should avoid activities like the butterfly stroke and bench presses, which develop the pectoral muscles and act to increase the humpback. Progression of the deformity is combated by postural and back extensor strengthening exercises and by bracing, where needed.

Hips

Hip flexor strength may be tested with the athlete in a sitting position with crossed arms so that he cannot press down on the examining table. He then lifts his knee against the examiner's resistance while the examiner tries to break the athlete's hip flexion manually. In addition to rating the strength of hip flexion, this test reflects muscular strength around the knee. The examiner next checks for hip adductor tightness (Fig. 1-4A) by abducting the athlete's hips without hiking them. With the knee and toes pointing toward the ceiling, each leg should abduct about 45°.

Daily sitting and riding in cars tightens hip flexors, and this can be corrected by stretching. With one knee bent onto the chest, the athlete's other knee is allowed to flex over the table

FIG. 1-3
The length of the athlete's spine as he stands is compared with that as he bends over (*A*). A leg-length discrepancy may be found during a check for pelvic tilt (*B*).

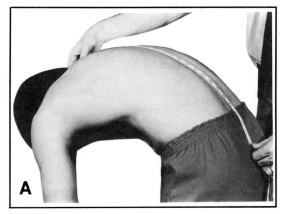

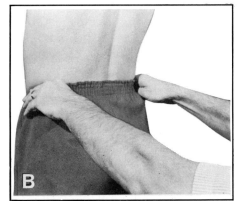

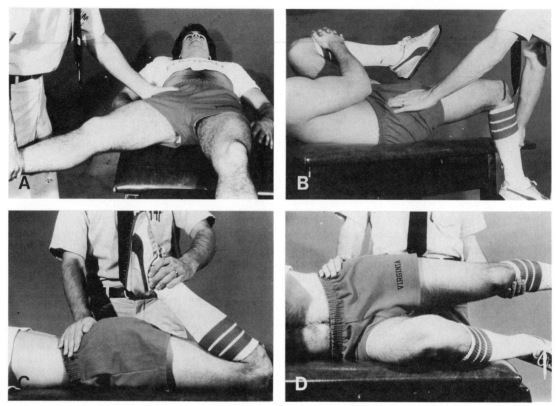

FIG. 1-4
The examiner checks for adductor tightness (*A*), a tight rectus femoris
(*B, C*), and a tight iliotibial band (*D*).

edge. Refusal of the lowered knee to flex to 90°, with some extension of the knee instead, connotes hip flexor tightness. Such tightness resides in the rectus femoris (Figs. 1-4B, 1-4C), which crosses both the hip and knee joints. Hip flexor tightness may also be tested with the athlete prone. The athlete first maximally flexes his knee, then the examiner passively flexes the knee further to see if the anterior-superior iliac spine on the same side rises. This normally occurs at about 130° of knee flexion, but if the pelvis rises earlier this indicates that the rectus femoris is tight.

Knee

The athlete's hamstrings demand evaluation because tightness or weakness promotes muscle pulls. Tight hamstrings stimulate patella problems, such as tendinitis and chondromalacia. They also hinder easy knee extension, causing the knee to follow the path of least resistance into injurious rotary movements.

A neutral pelvis position is needed for hamstring testing, but tight hip flexors will arch the low back and tilt the pelvis anteriorly. To establish a neutral position, a pillow is placed under the athlete's thigh to flatten his lower back. The opposite thigh is placed flat on the table to fix the pelvis and to keep it from rotating. The tested hip is flexed to 90° (Fig. 1-5A), and the athlete then actively extends the knee (Fig. 1-5B), aiming for 180° of knee extension.

The athlete's knee ligaments should be examined for laxity and the knee checked for bowlegs, knock-knees, and recurvatum. The

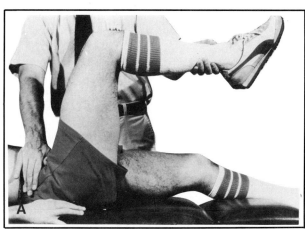

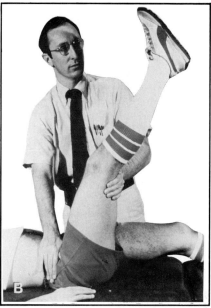

FIG. 1-5
Hamstring tightness is assessed by having the athlete flex his hip (A) and then asking him to extend his knee (B).

FIG. 1-6
The circumference of the athlete's thigh is measured about 18 cm (7 inches) above his knee joint (A). A gross test for knee strength is achieved by having the athlete flex his hip against the examiner's resistance (B).

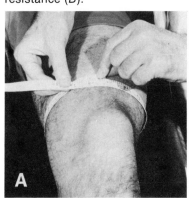

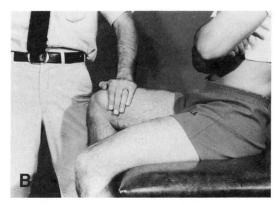

patella position should be noted and its tracking inspected. The thigh circumference should then be measured about 18 cm above the knee joint and also around the kneecap (Fig. 1-6A). If there is a difference of more than 2.5 cm (1 in) in the circumference of the thighs, a knee strengthening program is advisable.

Iliotibial Tract

The iliotibial tract courses from the pelvis to the tibia. In a runner, tightness of this band may lead to lateral hip and knee pain. To test for tightness, the athlete must lie on his side with the tested limb raised (Fig. 1-4D). The back is flattened by flexing the lower hip, and the tested knee is then flexed to 90°, the hip extended, and the knee pressed down toward the table. If the band is not tight, the knee should reach the table without extending. Alternatively, the lower knee may be flexed, with the tested limb allowed to drop. The foot will normally fall below the level of the table if the band is not tight.

Ankle

A lack of ankle dorsiflexion freedom predisposes the athlete to inversion sprains. Ankle motion should range from 10° to 20° dorsiflexion to about 50° plantar flexion. Dorsiflexion is first tested with the knee flexed to 90° to measure the soleus component of the heel cord. The knee is then fully extended and ankle dorsiflexion is retested to measure the gastrocnemius portion. To test ankle dorsiflexion more dynamically, the athlete should crouch and lean forward with his heel on the ground. The angle between the leg and the vertical thus becomes a measure of ankle dorsiflexion.

All athletes, especially those with tight heel cords, should stretch on a stair step or on an incline board, and should use a wobble board program to develop and maintain proprioception.

The Feet

The team physician or a team podiatrist can help to prevent foot problems, to evaluate footwear, and to provide inserts and orthoses. The athlete's feet should be thoroughly evaluated with checks for imbalances, calluses, corns, warts, blisters, athlete's foot, and ingrowing toenails. A check of everday walking, training, and competition shoes is also recommended.

Loose-Joints or Tight-Joints

Studies have shown that loose or tight joints in an athlete have a bearing on injuries.[30] An increased occurrence of knee sprains has been found in loose-jointed athletes, whereas more muscle tears have occurred in tight-jointed professional football players.[30] After screening these players, specific exercises have been designed to increase the strength of the loose-jointed players and the flexibility of the tight-jointed ones. The flexibility screening has served as a means of reducing knee injuries in contact sports and high-velocity athletics. Tests for flexibility include supination of the hand with shoulder rotation, flexion of the spine, assumption of the lotus position, hip rotation, and knee recurvatum.

When systematic flexibility testing was tried with high school players, however, no correlation was found between the frequency of knee and ankle injuries and the looseness of the players' joints. This difference between high school players and professional athletes may be related to developmental phenomena. For example, as the high school athlete matures, his loose joints become tighter, so the loose-jointed sophomore may become a tight-jointed senior.

When joint flexibility was studied in 2817 West Point cadets, no statistical relation was found between joint flexibility and joint injuries sustained in general athletic competition. Also, no relation was found between subjective joint laxity tests and objective biomechanical knee ligament examinations. Since no correlation appears to exist between ligamentous laxity and the type of injury, it may be a disservice to restrict a high school athlete from participating on the basis of ligament laxity testing.

What about psychological factors and injury? Personality factors have been found to correlate well with injury rates and severity,[20] and Cattell's 16-personality factor questionnaire (16-PF) has been useful in assessing this variable. Factor A contrasts reserved, detached, critical, and cool persons to outgoing, warmhearted, easygoing, and participating persons. The former types sustained the most severe injuries. Factor one contrasts dependent, overprotective, sensitive athletes to tough-minded, self-reliant ones. The tender-minded were more likely to be injured. Whether this test has the potential to predict tackle football injuries is not known, but the possibility exists.

Each athlete should possess the essential fit-

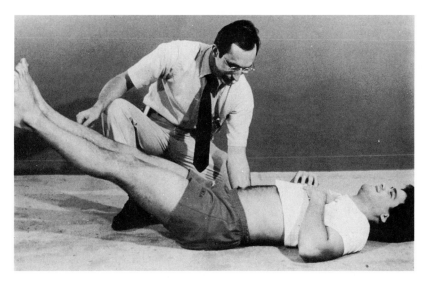

FIG. 1-7
Abdominal strength is assessed by seeing how far the athlete can lower his legs without arching his back.

ness base of strength, flexibility, endurance, and proper warm-up technique because a strong and flexible athlete has the best chance of avoiding injury.

Strength

During the preseason physical examination, the athlete's muscular strength may be measured manually or with weights or machinery. Manual muscle testing requires experience, and gross weaknesses may be noted by comparing sides. A single maximal effort on a particular lift with standard weights or a strain gauge measurement of isometric contractions are the best strength indicators.

The grip dynamometer will provide a rough gauge of overall body strength. In this procedure, the athlete stands with his arm hanging comfortably at his side. After one practice squeeze he is asked to squeeze again and release, and the measurement is recorded.

The Cybex isokinetic machine may be used to measure strength at different speeds, and also peak torque, total work, and muscular endurance, but this machine is expensive.

Upper abdominal muscular endurance is measured with timed sit-ups, and lower abdominal endurance with leg raises and abdominal hangs. During a sit-up, the abdominal muscles stabilize the trunk to enable the athlete to sit up. The hip flexors work for the remainder of the sit-up, making it unnecessary for the youngster to do a full sit-up to condition the upper abdominal muscles, since total trunk flexion is achieved by 30°.

Lower abdominal muscle strength is ascertained with the athlete lying on his back. As he flexes his hips to 90°, his lower back flattens against the floor, and he is instructed to lower his legs while keeping his lower back flat (Fig. 1-7). Weak abdominal muscles will cause the pelvis quickly to tilt anteriorly, putting stress on and arching the lower back. The athlete with strong abdominal muscles will be able to lower his legs closer to the ground without arching his back.

Preseason Cardiac Examination

A relatively simple cardiovascular screening examination will usually rule out any significant pathologic states.[38, 41] The examiner aims to detect any unusual body build, such as that associated with Marfan's syndrome, or the facial features characteristic of the person with congenital aortic valvular disease. The chest is inspected for abnormal cardiac pulsations or an abnormal chest wall configuration. Substantial moment-to-moment variations in the resting heart rate of the young person are not uncommon.

The sitting blood pressure is a screen for hypertension. Long arms or large biceps, however, may produce abnormal readings if the cuff of the sphygmomanometer is too narrow. The blood pressure bladder should cover at least two thirds of the upper arm and be long enough to circle not less than one half of the circumference of the arm. The total length of the cuff should be long enough to be wrapped around the arm several times.

A child younger than 10 years old should generally not have a blood pressure higher than 130/75 mm Hg.[41] For youths 10 to 15 years of age, the maximum blood pressure should not exceed 140/80 mm Hg. Persons with mild elevation of their blood pressure should be rechecked often to ensure that the elevated blood pressure is not a transient one resulting from anxiety. However, persistent primary hypertension is a sign that further cardiologic evaluation is needed. Youngsters with moderate hypertension must be advised not to engage in primary isometric exercises since these cause marked increases in both systolic and diastolic blood pressures.

Examination for coarctation of the aorta is made by simultaneously palpating the femoral and brachial arteries. A weak or absent lower extremity pulse or a notable delay in the femoral pulse compared to the brachial pulse will alert the physician to this possibility. Also, if the child has high blood pressure in the upper extremities, the femoral pulse and lower extremity blood pressure should be measured to check for possible coarctation of the aorta.

Many youngsters and endurance-trained athletes will normally have a systolic ejection-type murmur. The examiner should listen for the normal first and second heart sounds, ejection and nonejection clicks, and third and fourth heart sounds. If the first heart sound is easily heard and there is no holosystolic murmur, it is unlikely that the youngster has a significant ventricular septal defect. The second heart sound normally splits with inspiration. If both components of this sound are of normal intensity and split normally with inspiration, this will usually rule out a significant abnormality. Aortic insufficiency causes a high-pitched diastolic blowing murmur, whereas a patent ductus arteriosus will produce a continuous heart murmur.

Any situation that increases cardiac output will increase the intensity of heart sounds and murmurs. Thus, harmless small flow murmurs may sound quite prominent in an anxious youngster or in one with an elevated temperature. Also, it is not uncommon for an anxious child to have ectopic atrial beats. There is some ambiguity on the significance of resting premature ventricular contractions (PVCs), and resting PVCs have a variable response to exercise in children and young adults. However, a significant coupling of PVCs, or frequent PVCs, may be associated with a myocarditis. For this reason, any question about the type or significance of premature beats should be referred to a pediatric-cardiologist or cardiologist for evaluation.

The examiner must take care not to create a cardiac neurosis in a youngster. Consultation with a cardiologist familiar with the heart problems of children is suggested by American Academy of Pediatrics experts before excluding any youngster from competition.

Scrotum and Testes

Hydrocele

A hydrocele is an accumulation of straw-colored fluid between the two layers of the tunica vaginalis. A bright light will show through the hydrocele sac, and in larger hydroceles, the tunica vaginalis may have to be excised. A hydrocele occurring in a person older than 5 years of age may signal a malignancy.

Varicocele

Scrotal varicoceles contain an abnormally dilated pampiniform plexus of veins. The varicocele is caused by defective valves in the internal spermatic vein and is almost always found on the left side.

The athlete with a varicocele feels dull scrotal pain that disappears when he lies down. Exercise may distend the varicocele to cause pain. When a varicocele is painful, the pain may be relieved by wearing an athletic supporter with the scrotum up front instead of stuck between the legs. If the pain is severe, however, the internal spermatic vein may be ligated near the internal inguinal ring.

The Athlete with One Testis

An athlete is considered to have one testis if the other is maldescended, is atrophied from mumps orchitis, or if there has been torsion of one testis. Some doctors will exclude a youngster with a maldescended testis from contact sports, reasoning that a testis may be easily injured. Contact sports may be allowed after the maldescended testis has been replaced in the scrotum. Other physicians will allow the youngster to enter contact sports on the assumption that injury to a testis is rare if an athlete supporter and protective cup are worn. If an athlete with one testis is allowed to participate, however, the athlete, his parents, and the school authorities should be informed of the risk to the remaining healthy testis.

Cryptorchidism (Maldescended Testes)

The testes normally descend from the gonadal ridge to the inguinal ring, enter the inguinal canal, and, by birth, move into the scrotum. In 3% of all male infants, however, a testis fails to descend. There are three types of maldescended testes: the retractile, the ectopic, and the true undescended. Most are *retractile,* caused by an active cremasteric reflex that draws the testis out of the scrotum during examinations. These testes are histologically normal and usually descend into the scrotum by puberty.

The *ectopic* testis resides outside the normal pathway between the abdominal cavity and the scrotum, near the superficial inguinal ring, pubopenile or perineal. These testes also are histologically normal, requiring surgical placement into the scrotum where they must reside to mature and to produce healthy spermatazoa. Because body temperature is 2° higher than in-

trascrotal temperature, developing spermatazoa will not mature at body temperature.

The true undescended testis lies outside the scrotum but at some point along the pathway of descent. These testes, unlike other types, are histologically abnormal and have an increased incidence of cancer, regardless of whether they are brought down into the scrotum. Most surgeons prefer to place the undescended testis into the scrotum, where it can be palpated, or to remove it. Surgery should be done before the age of 10 and usually is done in the fifth year, before the child starts school.

Hernia

Hernias should be diagnosed in the preparticipation examination and repaired early to avoid later problems. If repair is ignored, vigorous athletic activity may force omentum and bowel down into the hernia sac, and both may incarcerate and strangle.

There are several types of hernias, and each type should be searched for. Indirect hernias result from a congenital weakness of the athlete's internal abdominal ring. The neck is narrow, and the bowel may be trapped and can strangle. These hernias should be repaired before allowing competition, especially if the sac comes down into the inguinal canal. Repair is needed even when the sac does not come down to the scrotum. Umbilical and epigastric hernias should also be repaired because omentum may become incarcerated in them. Femoral hernias are relatively more frequent in women than in men and may be responsible for mysterious groin pains. They are difficult to identify, but when one is found it should be repaired. A graduated exercise program will allow the athlete to return to practice about 4 weeks after hernia repair.

Hemorrhoids

Athletes should be checked for hemorrhoids during the preparticipation physical examination. Hemorrhoidal veins are the only valveless veins below the heart, and if a contracted sphincter traps some of these veins outside, they may swell and occasionally thrombose. When a thrombosis occurs, the clot must be evacuated and a stool softener prescribed.

Anal fissures and sentinel piles are treated twice a day with a soothing balm and hydrocortisone suppositories. Cold witch hazel packs used externally will help to relieve discomfort.

Laboratory Tests

The young athlete's capillary blood hemoglobin must be checked, especially in postpubertal girls and youngsters from low-income families. Athletes who use aspirin occasionally have microscopic blood loss from subacute gastritis that may leave them anemic. Prepubertal youngsters normally have about 11.5 g of hemoglobin/dl of their blood, but a postpubertal boy will have 14 g/dl or more and a postpubertal girl, 12 g or more. If a boy has less than 13 g or a girl less than 12 g, he or she should have a complete blood count.[29]

A dip stick analysis of each athlete's urine is also done at the comprehensive preseason examination.

Proteinuria

Protein in the urine may be related to posture or represent a normal response to exercise.[35] Nonrenal causes of proteinuria include fever, emotional stress, or exposure to excessive heat or cold.

Postural proteinuria associated with a prolonged exaggerated lordotic posture may be a presenting sign of renal disease. The lordosis may cause renal vasoconstriction and venous congestion leading to renal ischemia, although the condition usually has a good prognosis and most patients do not present with active renal disease. However, renal biopsy will show some changes in about one half of these patients. It is important to follow up on this disorder because treatment may slow the progress of renal disease.

Exercise-Induced Proteinuria

A functional proteinuria normally follows rigorous exercise.[8] This occurs because blood is shunted to the exercising muscles and renal ischemia results from renal vasoconstriction and venous congestion. The renal blood flow drops together with a smaller drop in glomerular filtration rate and an increased filtration fraction.

During the Commonwealth Games of 1976, proteinuria was often found in athletes after endurance events. Inulin and creatinine clearance of athletes with proteinuria and those without the condition were identical, and hemodynamic changes in renal function were also identical regardless of whether the athletes had proteinuria. The condition was probably a physiologic response of the tubules or glomerulus to the relative drop in blood flow during exercise rather than a pathologic condition. Perhaps the proteinuria reflects a combination of changes in blood flow, pH, and relative hydration states, which in turn effect changes in the basement membrane that allow more protein to pass across the membrane than can be reabsorbed by the tubules.

Urinary Protein

A normal adult passes an upper limit of 150 mg of protein in his urine each day, when reclining, the quantity is much less. Children pass from 35 mg to 70 mg of protein daily. Two thirds of the protein usually is globulin and one third albumin. Heavy outputs of 750 mg or more in 24 hours probably reflect underlying renal disease.

Dipstick Screening

The dipstick is an effective screening test. It contains a pH sensitive dye, tetrabromophenol, which turns from blue to green when albumin in normally acid urine prevents hydrogen ions from acting on the dye. A dipstick "trace" means less than 30 mg/dl or protein. If the urine is strongly akaline, it may give a false-positive reading. For this reason, when urine is protein positive and akaline, the result should be checked against a precipitation method such as sulphosalicylic acid. If a dipstick test shows a trace it is usually discounted, but if it is more strongly positive another specimen should be obtained.

What To Do If There Is Protein in the Urine

If an adolescent or a young adult has 1+ to 4+ proteinuria on a routine dipstick analysis, the examiner should determine whether the proteinuria is intermittent or continuous. Serial samples are collected. The athlete voids at bedtime and discards the sample. He then voids on rising and labels this sample #1. His next sample is taken when his daily routine is underway and is labeled #2. The tubes should be left in the refrigerator, not in a freezer, since freezing may confuse the precipitation readings. This schedule is repeated for 2 additional days before the samples are brought to the laboratory.

If there is no protein in the morning sample and later samples are positive, benign orthostatic proteinuria is probable. The urine should be rechecked in about 6 months. The finding of proteinuria in all samples suggests renal disease. Urine sedimentation, blood urea nitrogen concentration, and creatinine clearance should then be ascertained and an intravenous pyelogram performed.

Exercise in Renal Disorders

Renal blood flow decreases by about 50% during exercise and may leave the tubules in a weakened state. Because of this decrease, exercise should be limited for patients with impaired kidney function and those with a history of acute or chronic renal parenchymal disease. A premature return to vigorous exercise after acute nephritis may lead to further kidney damage.

Proteinuria preceded by a severe sore throat leads to a suspicion of postinfectious glomerulonephritis. However, an athlete in training who has a positive throat culture for streptococcus and protein and sediment in his urine may have only a throat infection and a normal renal response to exercise.

Paperwork and Permission Slips

At the time of the preparticipation examination, permission slips and information cards must be completed in triplicate, with the original for the school records, a copy for the parents, and another one for the athlete's personal physician. Formal consent must be obtained for the preparticipation physical examination, for emergency care on the field, and to allow treatment of the child at a medical center in the event of injury. Resumes of medical records are kept on 5 in × 8 in cards, including listings of previous injuries and treatment, allergies, where to contact parents at work and home, family doctor's phone number, and signed consent for emergency medical care. These cards are carried to all games away from home.

Balanced Competition (Maturity Matching)

Although balanced competition reduces injuries, it is difficult to arrange in early adolescence, as most school competition is arranged by grade level and most community-sponsored activiities are organized by age group. Unfortunately, age is not a completely satisfactory index of the young athlete's physical capability or of his susceptibility to injury.

At age 13, boys may vary physically from 40 kg (90 lbs) of baby fat and peach fuzz to 100 kg (220 lbs) of muscle and moustache.[17] The early adolescent's strength, stamina, coordination, body composition, and, to some extent, skills are more closely related to sexual maturation than to age. For this reason, maturity matching assumes importance in grades 7 through 12, where youngsters range in age from 12 to 19 years.

Maturity matching of girls is best attained by the menarchal method. Regardless of their chronological age, all girls in the United States are considered to have a developmental age of 12½ years at the time of their first menstrual period. Thus, a girl who had her first menstrual period 3 years ago is considered to have a developmental age of 12½ years plus 3 years, or 15½ years.

For boys, a series of drawings is used to grade the growth of facial, axillary, and pubic hair on a scale of one to five. The results may be recorded in a master log, and these athletes may then be channeled into competition with others at the same stage of maturity.

Other methods for assessing developmental age are wrist x-rays and grip strength. Wrist x-rays may be compared to skeletal growth x-rays in a radiologic atlas, and grip strength measurement is a fairly reliable index of a person's physical maturity.[13, 40]

Maturity matching should become more popular as more educators and physicians become aware of its benefits in reducing injuries and promoting fair competition.

On-the-Field Responsibilities

The team physician should be readily available before, during, and after games and practices. If he cannot attend, he must delegate authority to another doctor. The team physician should check the training room after each practice and enforce the rule that all injuries be reported. Because athletic injuries demand prompt attention for optimum results, treatment of the injured athlete should not be delayed.

Contents of The Team Physician's Bag

Stethoscope
Blood pressure cuff
Disposable syringes
Needles
Alcohol swabs
Tourniquet
Intravenous tubing
A large-bore (#15) needle
Two-way radio pager or walkie-talkie
Dimes for pay phone
Pencils
Notebook or pad of paper
Oral screw
Ophthalmoscope and otoscope
Fluorescein strips
Pen light
Tongue blades
Padded tongue blade
Percussion hammer
Thermometer
Examination gloves
Cotton swabs
Kocher clamps
Tape measure
Aluminum finger splints
Multigadget Swiss army knife
Safety pin

Bandage scissors
Sterile suture set
Sterile gloves
Tincture of benzoin
Band aids, butterflies, and Steri-strips
Adhesive tape
Gauze pads, roller bandage, and elastic wraps

Medicines

Ringer's lactate
Dextrose solution
Xylocaine
Epinephrine
Lanoxin
Propanalol
Atropine
Dopamine
Sodium bicarbonate
Lasix
Valium
Dextrose (50% solution)
Decadron
Compazine
Antivert
An antihistamine
Benadryl
Ammonia capsules

THE YOUNG ATHLETE **29**

Robaxin
Aspirin
Ascription
Acetaminophen
Codeine
Antacid tablets
Maalox
Lomotil
Hydrogen peroxide
Betadine
Neosporin ointment
Xylocaine injectable

On the Doctor's Person
Oral screw
Tongue forceps
Airway
Tongue depressors
Bandage scissors
Penlight
Paper bag (for rebreathing)
Sterile gauze pads
Tape 2.5 to 3.75 cm (1 to 1½ in)
Band Aids
Multipurpose Swiss Army knife

Return to Competition

It is the team physician's responsibility to decide whether an athelete may return to practice or games after an injury or illness. Overcautious appraisals may mean lost games, but failure to be cautious enough may mean serious harm for the athlete. His injury may worsen with play, converting a minor hurt into a major disability, or the first injury may lead to a second one, as when a dazed athlete is unable to protect himself.

After each injury, a firm diagnosis should be made before the athlete is allowed to return to competition.[16] For example, a single ligament ankle sprain is more informative than a "swollen ankle." Normally, an athlete should not return to the game if he has been knocked out, is dazed, or has inappropriate responses for more than 10 seconds after having been struck on the head. Additional symptoms that bar return to play are numbness, tingling, obvious swelling or bleeding, limited range of motion, or need for assistance to leave the field. Before re-entering a game, the athlete must be functioning normally and satisfy performance criteria such as starts, cuts, jumps, and blocks.

The athlete may return to practice after an injury if he is not favoring the injured part and has met performance criteria. After a knee injury, for example, he must regain full strength and flexibility and run figure-eights, cariocas (cross-over-step-runs) and 40-yard sprints without a limp.

The injured athlete's pain should never be masked by shots, pills, or nerve stimulators to allow him to participate. If a player claims injury and asks to be excused from play, he should not return to the game, no matter what the medical staff and coaching staff think of the injury. It is the team physician's responsibility to analyze the circumstances and suggest preventive programs after every injury.

The Young Athlete

The growth plates of young athletes, especially at the elbow, hip, and knee, are susceptible to acute injury and overuse, and either type of injury can lead to long-term problems. Further, a youth's ability to develop strength depends on his physical maturity. An immature youth with open epiphyses and a thin and weak neck should therefore refrain from collision sports such as tackle football. A teenager also has less flexibility when going through a growth spurt, and in such periods the youngster should avoid collision sports and speed work but continue to stretch daily. Such immature youths can train on a Hydra-Gym circuit; they may also work on technique for Olympic-style weightlifting with a lightly loaded bar. Power lifting should be disallowed because it emphasizes heavy weights. Other problems for children arise in wrestling, when a grappler tries to make weight, and in gymnastics, where hard training and a low food intake may stunt growth. Each young athlete should wear appropriate top-grade protective gear, such as mouth guards, when practicing or competing in sports.

Based on their own experience and because of budget cuts, many citizens and school boards are questioning the value of physical education in schools, classes that usually include a monotonously repetitive playing of touch football, basketball, and softball. Children often participate wearing their school clothes, do not shower, and return to class sweaty and dirty. Time spent on these traditional team sports should be de-emphasized and replaced by health education, wherein the youngsters acquire the skills, knowledge, and attitudes for a lifetime of activity. Physicians may join with health and physical educators in designing and implementing these programs: This marriage was made years ago in Greek mythology when Asclepius, the god of medicine, married Hygieia, the goddess of health.

The fitness concepts of a modern physical education program are best taught through activity, and cognitive material is built into the activity setting. Lecturing is kept to a minimum, and only after a period of vigorous physical activity. The physical educator can systematically incorporate ample cognitive material into the curriculum during just 3 minutes of class. Three minutes twice a week for 40 weeks a year over 10 years adds up to 40 hours of cognitive material.

In addition to the cognitive aspects of the physical education curriculum, some parts may be coordinated with the curricula of other courses. Physical education may also serve as the "lab" for certain topics in biology and health education. Just as in other courses, homework, out-of-class projects, and term papers should be required. Fitness testing can be a cognitive experience if the youth is told why he is being tested, what the results mean, how the results will be used, and how he can improve his performance.

A modern physical education program for young people will produce favorable attitudes toward physical fitness and serve as a base for intramural sports. Quality and quantity are important because a variety of activities will allow each participant to gain from sport at his level. Interscholastic competition allows physically talented athletes to compete against other talented ones, with the better athletes providing examples for others to emulate. While physicians have given most of their attention to this talented group, intramural athletes need similar supervision because they are generally less proficient, use inferior equipment, and play on poorer fields.

The fitness value of competitive sports is obvious, but there are other lasting benefits. Sports satisfy the young athlete's need for adventure and help him to learn self-discipline and the relation between hard work and success. He also learns how to accept and meet challenges, how to win and lose, and how to work with others toward goals.[9]

The Female Athlete

Because of their social conditioning, most women have been relatively inactive and have shown little interest in athletics. Those who did participate usually did not perform well because they were poorly conditioned and had inexperienced coaches. The larger number of women competing today are stronger, are more skillful and aggressive, and are bringing their physiologic capabilities to a new peak.

Unconditioned women entering athletics have a high injury rate, whereas the injury rate for conditioned female athletes is equal to that of their male counterparts, although the spectrum of injuries differs. The difference in injuries is related to women's anatomic peculiarities and relaxed joints. Shoulder injuries are common because the arms are relatively weak. Lordosis puts more strain on the back, and a wide pelvis requires that the hips move more during walking and running, a movement that puts more strain on the back and promotes pelvic pain and greater trochanteric bursitis.

The female athlete is predisposed to knee problems by knock knees, increased "Q angles" (the angle that the patellar tendon makes with the long axis of the limb), flat kneecaps, and shallow intercondylar grooves. Compared to men, a woman's foot is generally flatter and prone to arch pain. Her metatarsals are smaller, and she suffers stress fractures. A woman also develops bunions more readily and has more frequent pains at the metatarsophalangeal joint of the great toes.

Women normally prefer to wear minimal protective equipment, and the rules are designed to limit contact and injuries. A player in field hockey, for example, may not swat a high ball with her stick, although she may block it. Strict officiating is the key to keeping today's stronger and more aggressive players in these games free of encumbering, unattractive protective gear.

Athletic Infertility

Young women who train strenuously in activities like ballet, modern dancing, running, and gymnastics often menstruate later than do their less active peers and also have a higher prevalence of menstrual irregularities and secondary amenorrhea. One of five elite female distance runners who train 104 km (65 miles) or more per week will fail to menstruate at all or do so no more frequently than one or two times a year. These problems may be associated with physical stress or the emotional stress of competition, diversion of blood flow away from the ovaries during exercise, or an altered body core temperature owing to a low percentage of body fat.

A minimum level of about 17% body fat seems to be needed for the onset and maintenance of menses in the human female, and when body fat is low the reproductive system shuts down preventing conception. A weight loss of 10% to 15% below normal represents a loss of about one third of body fat and can cause amenorrhea. When weight is regained, the menstrual cycles resume. Many questions, however, remain unanswered: What are the long-term consequences of the athletic amenorrhea? How many women athletes fail to resume menses after hard training? Does the amenorrhea preclude a normal development of the endocrine system or harm the development of the reproductive organs?

Although women show considerable variability in menstrual flow, most need not alter their training, competing, and even swimming during a menstrual period. Although personal records have been set at all phases of the cycle, some women must reduce their activity before and during the menstrual period because they do not feel well.

Pregnancy

Exercise is advisable during pregnancy, and a fit woman usually has a better labor. She may, however, be too nauseated to train during the first trimester, and during the third trimester the uterus is large, the fetus bounces, and the breasts swell, making exercise uncomfortable and often causing backache.

As the pregnancy advances, there is a progressive decline in a woman's circulatory reserve owing to peripheral pooling of blood and obstruction of venous return by the large, gravid uterus. If there is already some compromise of the umbilical circulation, moderately severe maternal exercise may harm the fetus by temporarily reducing uterine blood flow and fetal PO_2.

Thus, a pregnant woman should train at a comfortable pace. If she trains too hard, expends too many calories, and fails to gain the recommended 11 kg (25 lbs), her baby's nutrition may be compromised. She must therefore be advised to titrate her exercise, cutting back on hard training and avoiding exhaustion and excessive heat.

Although the fetus is well protected by the mother's pelvis and later by a cushion of amniotic fluid, contact sports and downhill skiing are best avoided in the later stages of the pregnancy. Most sports may be resumed about 2 weeks after delivery and swimming may be resumed at about 3 weeks post-partum when the cervix has closed.

The Older Athlete

Older people are now eagerly entering sports, but many of them are unprepared. Even former athletes will find that training techniques have changed. Most injuries in older athletes are due to improper warm-up, training errors, and poor technique.

The older athlete should develop a fitness foundation before competing rather than competing to become fit. Fatigue can result in poor concentration and injury and the older person may also suffer from arthritis and degenerated tendons. He usually has poor flexibility and diminished proprioception. Injuries commonly occur during plyometric activities owing to the switch from an eccentric to a concentric contraction, when stress is the greatest.

The physician often is asked to construct fitness programs for older athletes and to counsel them about competitive sports, such as cycling, tennis, track and field, and swimming. Local coaches and physical educators may instruct the older athlete in warm-up and training techniques and see that they have adequate gymnasium and pool time.

I have had the opportunity to study many veteran Bikecentennial cyclists, "Super Senior" tennis players, masters track and field athletes, and masters swimmers. I was pleased to find athletic competition healthful and wholesome for men and women of all ages, even those older than 80 years of age. The Bikecentennial veterans each averaged 2 million pedal strokes in cycling 7200 km (4500 miles) from Reedsport, Oregon, to Yorktown, Virginia.* During and after the tour, the knees of this group felt better than ever.[22] The Super Senior tennis players averaging 50 years of playing experience, participate each year in the United States Tennis Association's National Clay Court 70, 75, and 80 Championships in Charlottesville, Virginia.† Their good stroke mechanics and fitness help to keep injuries to a minimum, although they all have "tennis shoulder," a drooped, hypertrophied racquet arm, and other normal responses to heavy use.[23]

Masters track and field athletes also compete in age groups. These athletes often lack coaching and proper warm-up and occasionally are injured while trying events, such as hurdles or the pole vault, for which they lack the necessary strength or skills.

Each year, the only Masters swim camp in America is held in Virginia.‡ Swimmers come from all parts of the country to learn contemporary approaches to training for competition. They are taught flexibility and strengthening programs and stroke drills, their strokes are videotaped, and they receive individualized instruction from collegiate coaches.

REFERENCES

1. ALYEA EP, PARISH HH, JR: Renal response to exercise—renal findings. JAMA 167:807–813, 1958
2. APPENZELLER H: Athletics and the Law. Charlottesville, Virginia, The Michie Company, 1975
3. BAILEY RR et al: What the urine contains following athletic competition. NZ Med J 83:809–813, 1976
4. BALL RT: Capable coach is best defense against threat of litigation. First Aider, Cramer 48:1, February 1979
5. BLACKBURN TA (ed): Guidelines for Pre-Season Athletic Participation Evaluation. Ad Hoc Committee on Pre-Season Athletic Participation Evaluation. Alexandria, Virginia, Sports Medicine Section, American Physical Therapy Association, 1979
6. BLYTH CS, MUELLER FO: When and where players get hurt. Football injury survey: Part I. Phys Sportsmed 2(9):45–52, 1974
7. CLAYTON ML et al: Football: the pre-season examination. J Sports Med 1:19–24, 1973
8. COLLIER W: Functional albuminuria in athletes. Br Med J 1:4–6, 1907
9. CRAIG TT (ed): Comments in Sports Medicine. Chicago, American Medical Association, 1973
10. FAIRBANKS LL: Return to sports participation. Phys Sportsmed 7(8):71–74, 1979
11. DECOF L, GODOSKY R: Sports Injury Litigation. Litigation and Administrative Practice Series, No. 139. New York, The Practicing Law Institute, 1979
12. DUDA vs. BAINES, 12, New Jersey Superior Court, 326, 79A, 2d 695
13. FLEISHMAN EA: The Structure and Measurement of Physical Fitness. Englewood Cliffs, New Jersey, Prentice-Hall, 1968
14. FLYNN TG et al: Injuries to young athletes. Committee on Pediatric Aspects of Physical Fitness, Recreation and Sports. Pediatrics 65:649–650, 1980

* Bikecentennial, P.O. Box 8308, Missoula, MT 59807.
† Super Seniors Tennis Players, C. Alphonso Smith, President, 2512 Woodhurst Road, Charlottesville, VA 22903.
‡ Masters Swim Camp; contact Mark Bernardino, U.S. Camps, P.O. Box 6546, Charlottesville, VA 22906.

15. GARDNER KD JR: "Athletic psuedonephritis"—alteration of urine sediment by athletic competition. JAMA 161:1613–1617, 1956

16. GARRICK JG: Sports medicine. Ped Clin North Am 74:737–747, 1977

17. GOMLAK C: Problems in matching young athletes: baby fat, peach fuzz, muscle and mustache. Phys Sportsmed 3(5):96–98, 1975

18. HALE VS. DAVIES, 86 Georgia Appellate, 126, 70 S.E. 2d 923

19. HIRSCH FJ: The generalist as team physician. Phys Sportsmed 7(8):89–95, 1979

20. JACKSON DW et al: Injury prediction in the young athlete: a preliminary report. Am J Sportsmed 6(1):6–14, 1978

21. KERBY VS. ELK GROVE UNION DISTRICT, 1 California Appellate 2d 246, 36, P. 2d 431

22. KULUND DN, BRUBAKER CE: Injuries in the Bikecentennial Tour. Phys Sportsmed 6:467–478, 1978

23. KULUND DN et al: The long-term effects of playing tennis. Phys Sportsmed 7(4):87–94, 1979

24. LOWELL CH: Legal responsibilities and sportsmedicine. Phys Sportsmed 5(7):60–68, 1977

25. LUCE VS. BOARD OF EDUCATION OF JOHNSON CITY, 2 Appellate Division 2d 502, 157, New York State 2d 123

26. MARSHALL JL, TISCHLER HM: Screening for sports: guidelines NY State J Med 78:243–251, 1978

27. MARSHALL JL et al: Joint looseness: a function of the person and the joint. Med Sci Sports Exerc 12:189–194, 1980

28. MAYNE BR: If sports medicine is your bag—equip it well. Phys Sportsmed 3(9):67–69, 1975

29. NATHAN DC, OSKI FA: Hematology of Infancy and Childhood, p 98. Philadelphia, WB Saunders, 1974

30. NICHOLAS JA: Injuries to knee ligaments: relationship to looseness and tightness in football players. JAMA 212:2236–2239, 1970

31. NICHOLAS JA: A study of thigh muscle weakness in different pathological states of the lower extremity. Am J Sports Med 4:241–248, 1976

32. OBREMSKEY M: Courts set legal guidelines for physical education instructors. First Aider, Cramer 46:4, December 1976

33. PERCY EC: The physician and the athlete. Can Med Assoc J 102:137–138, 1970

34. RYAN AJ (moderator): Guidelines to help you in giving on-field care. Phys Sportsmed 3(9):50–63, 1975

35. RYAN AJ (moderator): Proteinuria in the athlete. Phys Sportsmed 6(7):45–61, 1978

36. RYAN AJ (moderator): Qualifying exams: a continuing dilemma. Phys Sportsmed 8(8):10, 1980

37. SAVASTANO AA: The team physician and the law. RI. Med Soc J 51:558–565, 1968

38. SCHELL NB: Cardiac evaluation of school sports participants. NY State J Med 78:942–943, 1978

39. SHAFFER TE: So you've been asked to be the team physician? Phys Sportsmed 4(12):57–63, 1976

40. SHAFFER TE: The health examination for participation in sports. Phys Sportsmed 7(10):27–40, 1978

41. THORNTON ML et al: Cardiac Evaluation for Participation in Sports. Policy Statement. Evanston, Illinois, American Academy of Pediatrics, 1977

42. WEISTART JC, LOWELL CH: The Law of Sports. Charlottesville, Virginia, Merrill, 1979

43. WELCH VS. DUNSMUIR. Joint Union High School District, 326, P. 2d 633, California 1958

44. WILKINS E: The uniqueness of the young athlete: musculoskeletal injuries. Am J Sport Med 8:377–381, 1980

45. WILLIS GC: The legal responsibilities of the team physician. J Sportsmed 1:28–29, 1972

46. ZARICZNYJ B et al: Sports-related injuries in school-aged children. Am J Sports Med 8:318–324, 1980

The Handicapped Athlete

Handicapped athletes include those who are blind, deaf, or paralyzed; amputees; the mentally retarded; and those with other neuromuscular or skeletal disease. The handicapped person who participates in athletics acquires skills and confidence, drops body weight, subdues depression, increases his mobility and endurance, and rehabilitates atrophied muscles. Handicapped sports are not just rehabilitation, but sporting events in their own right. The 1976 Olympiad for the Physically Disabled attracted 1500 athletes from 38 countries.[29] This was the first Olympiad with full competition for blind, paralyzed, and amputee athletes.

When the handicapped athlete competes in his own class, the competition is rewarding for the athlete and exciting for spectators.[13] There is a tendency, however, for outsiders to compare the performance of the handicapped to that of able-bodied athletes. Even against such standards, the performance of a handicapped athlete may be spectacular.[29] A one-legged high jumper, for example, has hopped up to the bar and cleared 1.85 m (6 ft, 1 3/4 in), a wheelchair athlete has done a metric mile in 5 hours and 15 seconds, a blind athlete has run 100 m in 11.6 seconds guided by the voice of his coach at the end of the track, and a paraplegic weightlifter has bench-pressed 263 kg (585 pounds).

The handicapped person's physician is best suited to channel his patient into sports programs because the physician is best informed about his patient's disabilities.

There is a great need for a national organization to oversee all sport for the disabled and to unify it with able-bodied sport. Pools, gymnasiums, and coaches should be readily accessible to disabled athletes, who are entitled to opportunities for physical education, recreation, and interscholastic and intercollegiate sports comparable to those of able-bodied athletes.

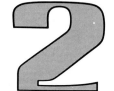

2

Special Athletes, Medical Problems, Nutrition, and Drugs

The Blind Athlete

All blind athletes are legally blind, but some are completely blind and others have partial sight. The athlete with partial sight has the advantage of being able to perceive light and dark and appreciate shadows.

Wrestling, track, and swimming have long been the favorite sports of the blind athlete, but other sports for the blind include bowling, skiing, and track-and-field events such as the pentathlon.[46] He may also participate in beep baseball, golf, tandem bicycling, and even archery.

In track, the athlete runs with a sighted companion who holds a short line or the runner listens to his coach calling instructions. Blind bowlers use a portable, 3.6-m (12-ft) long, waist-high guide rail. In downhill skiing, a sighted skier trails closely behind the blind athlete (Fig. 2-1). The sighted skier calls signals, touches the blind skier with a ski pole, or uses clap sticks to guide the blind skier audibly. In beep baseball, a regulation softball with a battery in it emits a beep. Although many beep baseball players do not wear protective gear, all players should be encouraged to wear face masks and chest protectors.

The Deaf Athlete

Profound deafness is usually due to sensorineural defects rather than conduction defects. Most often, the athlete's mother had rubella during the first trimester of pregnancy, but sometimes the deafness results from Rh incompatibility of the parents, meningitis, viral infection, or a congenital malformation. If the athlete has cochlear damage but little semicircular canal or vestibular apparatus damage, he probably will escape equilibrium problems.

If his vestibular mechanism is damaged, the deaf athlete must work extra hard to achieve balance and coordination.[51] For example, it will be difficult for the athlete to walk on a balance beam, do rapid spins, or do sharp turns. The deaf athlete may also have major problems with communication. He must constantly look around to ascertain the position of teammates and has to develop his peripheral vision. Signals, such as dimming the lights in a hockey rink rather than blowing a whistle, are used.

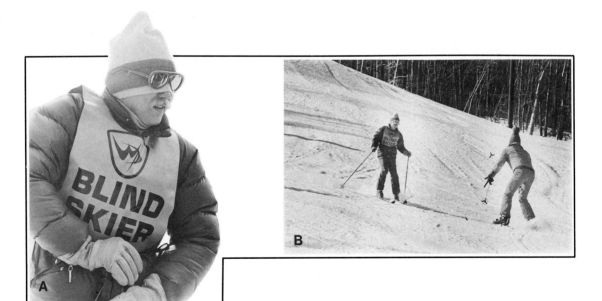

FIG. 2-1
A blind skier (*A*) is guided by instructions from a sighted companion (*B*).

Because deaf athletes appear to be normal, public interest in and support for athletic programs for the deaf is lacking. However, Gallaudet College, a liberal arts college for the deaf in Washington, D.C., sponsors a full athletic program for deaf athletes.

The Paralyzed Athlete

The first international sporting event for paralyzed athletes took place in 1952 at Stoke-Mandeville Hospital in England, the home of the National Spinal Injury Center, directed by Sir Ludwig Guttman. The competition consisted only of archery, but more events and more competitors were added later, and a medical classification system was developed. In 1960, the Wheelchair Olympics moved to the site of the Olympic Games in Rome. In 1964, they were held 1 week after the able-bodied Olympics in Tokyo, and in 1968 the games were held in Israel. In 1972, Heidelberg hosted the games a few weeks before the able-bodied Olympics in Munich. The year 1976 marked the first Olympiad for physically disabled, blind, paralyzed, and amputee athletes held in Toronto 1 week after the Montreal games.[29]

Wheelchair games include track and field, swimming, weightlifting, slalom, archery, pentathlon, and table tennis. There is also competition in fencing, rifle shooting, snooker, precision javelin (throwing a javelin into a large target), darchery (a combination of darts and archery), and basketball. The National Wheelchair Athletic Association is headquartered at the Bulova School of Watchmaking in New York.

Spinal-cord-injured athletes are not the only participants at the wheelchair games; also included are athletes with neurologic or paralyzing disorders, such as polio and meningomyelocele. Some amputees also compete in wheelchairs. Paralyzed persons are introduced to athletics at regional spinal cord injury centers before joining the National Wheelchair Athletic Association or park and recreation department programs.

Doctors and therapists classify paralyzed athletes because proper classification is important to assure fair competition, and the disability of an athlete may improve or worsen with time, requiring reclassification. Quadriplegic atheltes are classified according to whether they lack triceps function, have some triceps, or have some hand function (Table 2-1).[13] The paraplegic's trunk muscles, abdominal muscles, and hip extensors and flexors are also checked although classification may be difficult when patterns of disability vary so widely. Classification for the National Wheelchair Athletic Association differs from that for the National Wheelchair Basketball Association (Table 2-2). Both equitable team competition and participation in basketball by severely disabled players are encouraged by the rule limiting the number of player points each team may have in a game to 12 (points being equal to the class of each player, that is, class I = 1 point, class II = 2 points, and so forth).[13]

Wheelchair athletes have a low injury rate. At the National Wheelchair Games, the athletes have had very few shoulder problems from propelling the wheelchair (Fig. 2-2), but sometimes their skin has broken down in sensitive areas, especially on the hands. Some quadriplegic athletes have suffered heat exhaustion, partly because of their decreased sweating ability.

The Amputee Athlete

Amputee games include track and field, swimming, skiing, slalom, riflery, pentathlon, football-kicking, table tennis, and bowling.

There are 12 categories of amputee athletes, defined by combinations of loss of one or both legs, whether above or below the knee, and by various levels of loss of the upper extremity.[27] Amputee sports not only benefit the competitors, but the search for better prostheses for competition may lead to advances in materials and fittings for all amputees.

Although most amputee athletes compete with a prosthesis, some compete without this device, whereas others use a wheelchair. A skier may ski with or without a prosthesis, and some skiers "three-track" with an outrigger that has a short ski tip and a swivel (Fig. 2-3).

TABLE 2-1.

Classification for National Wheelchair Athletic Association Competitions

Class	Equivalent Spinal Cord Level	Function Present	Function Absent
IA	C-6 or higher	Wrist extensor	No better than fair triceps; nothing distally; no balance or lower extremity function
IB	C-7	Good or normal triceps	No finger flexors of extensors; no balance or lower extremity function
IC	C-8	Finger flexors and extensors	No intrinsics; no balance or lower extremity function
II	T-1→T-5	Normal upper extremity function	No better than poor abdominal muscles; no useful balance or lower extremity function
III	T-6→T-10	Upper abdominal muscles	Some balance but not normal; no lower extremity function
IV	T-11→L-2	Normal abdominal strength	No better than poor quadriceps; nothing distally
V	L-3→S-5	Fair or better quadriceps	Lower extremity weakness "significant and permanent"
VI		(Swimming only; ability to push off a wall with lower extremities L-5→S-5)	

TABLE 2-2.

Classification for National Wheelchair Basketball Association*

Player Points	Class	Equivalent Spinal Cord Level	Function Present	Function Absent
1	I	T-7 or higher		Impaired balance; no lower abdominal muscles or lower extremity function
2	II	T-8→L-2	May have hip flexors graded good, adductors graded fair, and quadriceps graded poor	No useful lower extremity function (this class includes those with bilateral hip disarticulation but otherwise normal muscles)
3	III	L-3 or lower	Quadriceps fair or better; all other lower extremity disabilities (including amputation)	

* A team (five players) may not total more than 12 points at any time in a game.

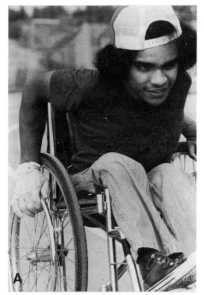
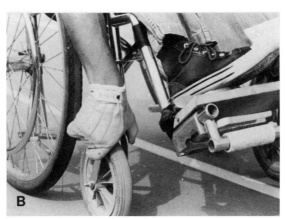

FIG. 2-2
A wheelchair athlete (*A*), with just one usable hand, can steer by reaching down to the caster wheel (*B*).

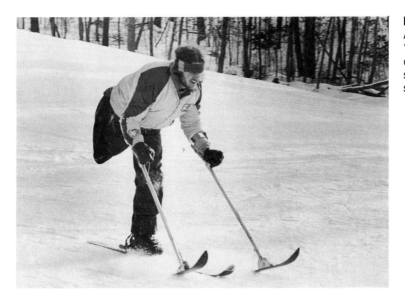

FIG. 2-3
An amputee skier can "three-track" with outriggers that have a short ski tip and a swivel.

The "Special Olympics"

The "Special Olympics" are open to all mentally retarded athletes 7 years of age or older,[7] and this group now totals more than 400,000 special olympians and 150,000 volunteers. An International Special Olympics is held every 4 years, and each year thousands of local and area meets are conducted. Official sports in the Special Olympics include track and field, swimming and diving, gymnastics, floor hockey, basketball, ice skating, bowling, volleyball, and wheelchair events.

Supervisors at these competitions must be

alert for seizures and be sure that the competitors take their preventive medicines. At the 1975 International Games in Michigan, there were 15 recorded grand mal seizures. Also, although some mentally retarded athletes have good control, others may not know when to stop because of a lack of judgment and therefore, need constant supervision in social situations.

Ice Skating Therapy

Because balance is lost and regained on a hard and slippery surface, ice skating helps youngsters with physical or mental disabilities to gain confidence and self-control.[1] Their body awareness is enhanced as their anxiety level drops and their muscle tension decreases.

Ice skating therapy benefits children with minimal brain dysfunction because the skating refines precision movement. Obstacle courses may be set up to improve task completion skills for youngsters who have difficulty controlling their behavior and attention. Skating also elevates the kinesthetic awareness of children with learning disabilities and is especially beneficial for youngsters with spastic cerebral palsy and mild to moderate hemiplegia and for the mentally retarded.

Ice skating therapy demands good balance but requires less power and strength than walking.[1] The structural and motor requirements for participation include a stable spine, extensor and abductor stability of the hips and extensor stability of the knee, good quadriceps, and the absence of marked knee flexion contractures. Children should have some dorsiflexion and plantar flexion stability of the ankle, which an ankle-foot orthosis could help, and motor power across their ankle joints. Their feet should be relatively plantigrade.

The skate shoes should fit snugly. Off-the-ice walking on perfectly fitted skates is a good exercise before attempting the ice. The skater should use single blades without toe picks. An outrigger skate aid—a figure skating blade mounted on a Lofstrand-type crutch—can increase his base of support.

The Hein-A-Ken skate aid (Fig. 2-4) is based on the principle of learning to skate with a chair[1] but is more stable than an ordinary chair. It is especially helpful for children unable to propel themselves with a reciprocal action. The aid allows children to make more effective use of the motor power in the sound leg and to shift their weight away from the affected side in a scooter motion. Eventually they begin stroking and gliding and are gradually weaned from the skate aid.

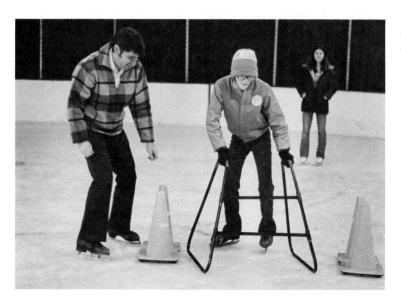

FIG. 2-4
The skate aid permits a young skater to develop his skating technique and gain confidence.

Medical Problems

Diabetes Mellitus

Exercise is beneficial for the athlete with diabetes mellitus because it lowers blood glucose levels. Diabetic persons who exercise are usually in better control, and an exercise program often stimulates diabetics to comply with proper management of the diabetes.[15]

Most experienced diabetics do not change their insulin doses with exercise but increase their food intake instead. However, the insulin-dependent diabetic who starts an exercise program should first decrease his insulin by 20% to 40%. Abdominal sites should be used for insulin deposit, and the diabetic person should avoid injecting into exercised extremities, since increased circulation in the exercised part allows insulin to be absorbed too rapidly. The insulin-dependent diabetic should take glucose supplements every hour during sustained exercise because these athletes are more likely than are other diabetics to become ketoacidotic or hypoglycemic. Insulin is needed to support the life of these athletes, who usually have an onset of the disease at younger than 20 years of age and who do not become very overweight.

A diabetic's precompetition meal should be high in carbohydrate and relatively low in fat and protein. The timing of the meal is important, and it should be eaten several hours before exercising. If the athlete drinks a strong sugar solution 30 minutes before exercising, his liver will shut off its glucose output. The intestine cannot meet the demands placed on it, and the athlete becomes hypoglycemic after the exercise begins.

Diabetic persons should take responsibility for their own care, bringing food to practices and competitions.[8] The food should be put aside so that others will not snack on it. Doctors, trainers, and coaches should be well informed on diabetes, as injuries to diabetics must be treated carefully. Coaches and teammates must be alert for trouble signs and symptoms and be aware of treatment procedures. Trainers must avoid use of excessively hot or cold modalities on the diabetic athlete, and diabetic persons should avoid using counterirritants on their legs. Footwear should be especially checked so that sores may be prevented.

Diabetic coma is caused by too much sugar and acetone in the blood with too little insulin. The athlete may feel sick, have a stomach ache, be confused or lethargic, have a fruity breath odor, and have a fast pulse. He should be asked if he has eaten and if he has taken his insulin. Ketoacidosis takes time to develop, so it is unlikely to occur during a game.

Insulin shock may be caused by an overdose of insulin, too much exercise, or too little food. The athlete will be fatigued and irritable; he may have slurred speech, a headache, dizziness, hunger, and poor coordination; his hands may tremble; and he will feel faint and may even lose consciousness. In contrast to diabetic coma, there is no fruity breath odor, and the pulse is normal. The athlete should be given sugar in the form of sweet drinks or candy and be allowed to rest so that the sugar can be absorbed.

Addison's Disease

Athletes with well-controlled Addison's disease may participate in all sports. These athletes add extra salt to the evening meal if they have sweated a lot or if they anticipate heavy perspiration. Sometimes extra prednisone is taken before competition.

Hemophilia

Concentrates of Factor VIII are available, as cryoprecipitate or as commercially available products, that will allow hemophiliacs to participate in athletics.[52] However, even though Factor VIII concentrates are effective, hemophiliacs are best advised to participate in noncontact sports and to avoid tackle football because of the danger of intracranial bleeding.

In the past, a cast was applied when a hemophiliac's joint was injured. The limb then quickly atrophied, weakened, and became unstable, further bleeding occurred, and the joint finally collapsed. When a hemophiliac is injured today, he is given an early booster shot of Factor VIII concentrate. There is time for the booster because the athlete's bleeding will be at a normal rate. Factor VIII concentrate averts most serious bleeding and is followed by physical therapy.

Concentrates of Factor VIII may be transported in a small freezer and kept in a refrigerator at camps and gymnasiums. The drug may be infused by a trained layman or by the athlete himself. If the hemophiliac must take other drugs, he usually ingests them.

Sickle Cell Trait

Sickle cell disease includes sickle cell anemia (hemoglobin S-S) and the less severe hemoglobin S-C and hemoglobin S-Thal conditions. With two abnormal genes for hemoglobin S, persons with sickle cell anemia will be anemic, with a hemoglobin rarely higher than 7 g. This results in problems before the youth is old enough to consider athletic participation.

The athlete with sickle cell trait inherits one abnormal gene for hemoglobin (S) and one normal gene (A) to form an AS genotype. Ten percent of American blacks have sickle cell trait, which is 50 times more common than sickle cell anemia. The athlete with this disorder is at risk for sickling or sickle cell crisis when at high altitude (greater than 1200 m, or 4000 feet) or under the stress of environmental heat.[56] Decreased oxygen causes red blood cells to deform, elongate, and assume a crescent or sickle shape. These cells then have reduced oxygen-transporting capacity and may lodge in blood vessels and vital organs, such as the spleen, and cause pain.

Black athletes and athletes of dark Mediterranean origin may be screened with a simple screening kit test based on turbidity or with a sickle cell preparation test. If the test findings are positive, the athlete should have a hemoglobin electrophoresis done for a definitive diagnosis, and genetic counseling should be offered. Subjects should be made aware of the early symptoms of sickle crisis, which include sudden pain under the lower left ribs, hematuria, weakness, and nausea.

The athlete with sickle cell trait need not be restricted from sports, as he can prevent dehydration by taking fluids before and during practice and contests while avoiding heavy anaerobic work and performing adequate and gradual warm-ups.

Colds

A cold is an infectious disease spread by coughing, sneezing, talking, or contact. The chance of contracting a cold depends on the frequency and degree of exposure to the virus, coupled with the athlete's relative immunity. Colds are not prevented by being in "good shape," and a trained athlete can catch a cold just as easily as a nonathlete.

The chance of a cold spreading through a team can be reduced if athletes avoid community drinking cups, using dispenser squeeze bottles instead. In cold weather, athletes should stay warm and avoid leaving practice sessions with wet hair after showers or saunas. Chills may be prevented by keeping hair shorter during the winter and by using a hair dryer. Wool stocking hats should be worn in cold weather.

Colds cannot be worked off by vigorous exercise. Instead, exercise puts an extra demand on the athlete's body when he needs all of his resources to fight the infection. He should rest, eat well, and drink plenty of fluids, keeping away from the team to prevent the cold from spreading. A serious communicable disease may start with symptoms that resemble a simple cold, and pills or capsules will reduce the symptoms of a cold but will not effect a cure.

It is better for an athlete to miss a few practices and return strong than to drag through drills for a week. Athletes with a mild cold may compete but should not do so if fever is present. Poor athletic performance may be due to an illness such as a low-grade tonsillitis. Also, a myocarditis may accompany some viral illnesses, and if the athlete with this disorder trains or competes he may suffer an arrhythmia and die suddenly.

Infectious Mononucleosis

The Epstein-Barr virus causes infectious mononucleosis but only in those persons who lack antibodies to this virus. Better sanitation and hygiene have lowered the prevalence of infectious mononucleosis in children, but more mononucleosis is now found in high school and college athletes, where the virus finally infects them at a later age.[48]

The incubation period ranges from 42 to 49 days. Signs and symptoms of the illness include malaise, sore throat, headache, aching, fever (which may be very high), occasionally jaundice, sometimes encephalitis and neuritis, and rarely abdominal pain that mimics acute appendicitis. Early signs include small white spots on the anterior pillars of the tonsils and lymphadenopathy. Toward the 14th day, physical signs are at their zenith. The spleen enlarges and may rupture easily, so it must be examined gently and infrequently.[19, 47]

The blood of an athlete with mononucleosis contains a relative lymphocytosis of at least 50% lymphocytes and a total lymphocytosis. A concurrent acute bacterial infection may abolish the relative lymphocytosis, but the total lymphocyte count will be at least 3500/ml. More than 10% of these lymphocytes are atypical ones. Usually, a positive heterophil test clinches the diagnosis, but the test may not be positive until the third week. Liver function test findings are also sometimes abnormal.

The athlete should stay in his room until his temperature falls, whereupon he may return to class. His lymph gland size and breathing should be checked. Although the side effects of steroids may outweigh their good effects, steroids may be needed if lymph glands block the pharynx. The athlete must be restricted from sport since his spleen may easily rupture owing to lymphocytic infiltration and softness. At the height of the disease, a small increase in intraabdominal pressure can cause rupture. The spleen must be two or three times larger than normal to be palpated. Its size may be checked with ultrasound or on a plain film of the abdomen, and 3 weeks later the study should be repeated to see if the size has changed.[11, 55] A radionuclide scan or computerized axial tomography may also be used to determine spleen size.[20, 27, 53]

How long should the athlete be restricted from sports after mononucleosis? Early return is dangerous because a large spleen is more tense than normal and projects below the ribs. It thus loses the natural protection of the ribs, rendering it more susceptible to injury and rupture. For this reason, the athlete may return to sport only when he feels well, laboratory test findings are normal, and the spleen has returned to a normal size—a recovery that may be delayed for 3 to 6 months.

Infectious Hepatitis

Type A hepatitis virus is transmitted by a fecaloral route to cause infectious hepatitis.[32] Serum hepatitis, on the other hand, is usually more serious and is transmitted by a type B virus.

The incubation period for infectious hepatitis is 2 to 6 weeks. The *preicteric phase* of fever and gastrointestinal discomforts precedes an *icteric phase* of liver tenderness and jaundice. Bilirubin and liver enzyme levels rise. Jaundice disappears during the *convalescent phase,* and the person becomes immune to subsequent infectious hepatitis but not to serum hepatitis.

In a 1969 college-football-team outbreak, the attack rate of infectious hepatitis was 92%.[12, 40, 60] The team could only play two games the entire season because passive immunization had been administered too late. A football team is a relatively closed population, and if hepatitis occurs all of the other players will need human immune serum globulin injected into each gluteal region to achieve passive immunity to the disease.

Because enzyme changes may be a normal concomitant of vigorous exercise, high creatinine phosphokinase and lactic dehydrogenase levels in a distance runner do not necessarily reflect a pathologic condition but may instead be related to muscle damage from running.

Epilepsy

Epilepsy is not a disease but a symptom. The cause of idiopathic, self-generating seizures and the precise location in the brain where the electrical stimulus begins are unknown.[2]

Genetic factors predispose a person to seizures if he inherits a low seizure threshold. Hypoglycemia, adrenalin release, or cerebral metabolic changes associated with hyperventilation may precipitate seizures. There is no evidence that vigorous physical activity or fatigue after sports precipitates epilepsy.

Head injuries may result in structural alterations in the brain, and stresses to an athlete may trigger seizures from this area. Since seizures arise somewhere in the brain, some doctors consider it unwise for an epileptic person to risk repeated head trauma.[38] Although this seems logical, there is no proof that repetitive physical contact, even to the head as in tackle football, causes more seizures in an epileptic than usually occur when the same athlete is asleep in bed. In fact, many seizures occur nocturnally as the person sleeps.

Participation In Sports

The supposed adverse effect of head injury on the course of pre-existing epilepsy probably has been exaggerated and may not exist.[2] Injury rates for epileptics in full athletic programs are identical to those of nonepileptic persons in full athletic programs—programs that include soccer, tackle football, and boxing.[14] Livingston has studied 20,000 epileptics in his seizure clinic over the past 40 years.[34-36] He allows his patients to participate fully in athletics and has reported no adverse effect from sports activity, including tackle football.

Nonetheless, an individualized approach is still best for determining the suitability of an epileptic for contact sports. No restrictions are recommended for athletes with only nocturnal epilepsy, whereas the frequency of other sei-

zures must first be ascertained. If they are daily or weekly, contact sports should be prohibited. If the seizures are uncontrolled, horseback riding or high altitude climbing should be ruled out even if seizures are infrequent. Partial complex seizures may have bizarre motor or psychic manifestations. If an initial seizure has been clearly associated with head trauma, the physician should be reluctant to allow participation in sports that hold a significant risk of head injury. Also, contact sports should be prohibited when seizures are followed by a prolonged postconvulsive state.

Vigorous physical activity does not alter the metabolism of antiepileptic drugs, which will control about 60% of seizures, although in most instances their site and mode of action has not been ascertained. Epileptic youths should be continued on anticonvulsive drug therapy through adolescence, as this is the time when many controlled epileptics have a recurrence of their seizures.

The team physician, trainer, and coach must identify epileptic athletes and be familiar with seizure patterns. When a seizure occurs, the athlete should be kept from hurting himself.

Exercise-Induced Asthma

Exercise-induced asthma is an asthma attack that occurs after exercise. When mild, the athlete may only cough frequently or appear unusually dyspneic, but when severe, the athlete will wheeze and be very short of breath, with fatigue and anxiety interfering with his athletic activity. Most chronic asthmatics have exercise-induced asthma, as do many people with allergies. The condition also intensifies with seasonal allergies, high pollen counts, smoke and other irritants, fatigue, coldness, emotional upset, stress, and upper respiratory infections. The severely asthmatic person will have a stronger reaction to exercise than will the person with a mild asthmatic condition.

Exercise-induced hyperventilation of the trachea is more severe in winter. Normally by the time air reaches the larynx, it has been brought to body temperature and is fully humidified.

During exercise and dyspnea, however, the lower airway must heat and humidify the air. Mucosal cooling may initiate vagal reflexes that release chemical mediators from mucosal mast cells, with an effect resembling that of an immediate hypersensitivity reaction of the bronchial smooth muscle.

Asthmatic athletes adapt normally to exercise for at least 5 to 10 minutes, and as their ventilation rate and tachycardia subside after the exercise bout, they become symptomatic. With longer exertion, symptoms may begin during the exercise period. However, sport helps the person with exercise-induced asthma by upgrading his fitness and lowering his heart rate and ventilatory rate.[31] The athlete is then able to do more without inducing asthma.

Diagnosis

When an athlete wheezes and is very short of breath, the diagnosis presents little problem, but an athlete with mild exercise-induced asthma may have only a hacking cough and mild dyspnea. Pulmonary functions may be diminished by 20% to 30%, yet there may be no frank wheezing. A severe attack, however, may come later. To diagnose exercise-induced asthma, the physician should give the athlete an exercise challenge in the form of the exercise that provoked the attack.

A sound, practical approach to the diagnosis of mild exercise-induced asthma is to assume exercise-induced asthma if an athlete coughs frequently or seems unusually dyspneic. The physician should treat the subject with a bronchodilator and observe him to see if his symptoms resolve. The physician should also bring a stethoscope to practices and listen for wheezes. Special attention must be given to asthmatic athletes who have had a cold, because their airway remains irritable and their lung functions are depressed for as long as a week after a cold.

Selection of a Sport

Many asthmatic athletes select sports that emphasize skill and coordination. They tailor their involvement to short activities rather than endurance sports like soccer or time-consuming activities like tennis, which may precipitate exercise-induced asthma.

Endurance sports differ in their tendency to induce asthma, with running and cycling causing asthma twice as often as does swimming. Encouragingly, several world class swimmers are asthmatic, and asthmatics have won Olympic gold medals. In swimming, regular forced deep breathing promotes maximum emptying of the lungs, and belly-breathing and exhaling against resistance eliminate trapped air; the swimmer also breathes at the water's humid surface.

Coping with the Disorder

Simple breathing methods may prevent asthmatic attacks. The athlete breathes with his diaphragm, forcing expiration against a closed glottis when the first symptoms of asthma appear. During exertion he should breathe through his nose rather than through his mouth, to help warm the air. In cold weather, a ski mask may be worn and a lightweight surgical mask added if needed.

"Running through" an attack allows the asthmatic athlete to participate in basketball, hockey, and soccer, as asthmatic attacks are less severe after 12 to 16 minutes of exercise than after 6 to 8 minutes of exercise.[26] The severity of the attack reaches a plateau at about 6 minutes before gradually diminishing. The mechanism for this is poorly understood. In addition, if the athlete resumes exercising in less than 90 minutes, the second exercise bout causes less severe attacks than the first. Thus, by vigorously warming up an hour or so before an event, the asthmatic athlete may compete in a more refractory state.

Drug Treatment

The most effective way to inhibit exercise-induced asthma is by pharmacologic pretreatment.[21] The drug must be taken *before* exercise. The most effective medicines are epinephrine, isoetherine, isoproterenol, metaproterenol, terbutaline, and theophylline. Cromolyn sodium and atropine are effective for some asthmatic persons but not for others. Corticosteroids are not helpful in preventing exercise-induced asthma, nor are antihistamines. Propranalol worsens the condition.

Most drugs are inhaled just before exertion, and the effects may last for hours. Oral drugs are taken 1 to 2 hours before exercise to attain therapeutic levels, and their timing and dosage may be adjusted to produce optimal effects. Inhaled adrenergic drugs are effective in small doses that only occasionally produce paradoxical bronchospasm, tachycardia, and tachyarrhythmia. Oral adrenergic agonists are given in higher doses than when inhaled, but the inotropic and chronotropic effects of these agents increase the risk of tachyarrhythmia during exercise. Among the commonly used drugs, metaproterenol produces fewer cardiac effects, and its duration of action is longer than that of isoproterenol or epinephrine. Athletes in strenuous competitive sport and those with cardiovascular problems should use cromolyn sodium as the drug of first choice. The mechanism of action of cromolyn sodium is unknown, but it is thought to inhibit the release of mediators from mast cells. If the athlete does not respond to cromolyn, an inhaled, selective beta-2-adrenergic agent such as isoethrane may be a second choice. Ephedrine, isoproterenol, and metaproterenol are banned by the Medical Commission of the International Olympic Committee.[41] However, atropine, cromolyn sodium, glucocorticoids, the beta-2-agonist terbutaline, and theophylline are acceptable.

Nonprescription medications that contain epinephrine, such as Primatene mist and Bronkaid mist, are usually safe, but these medicines may be abused during strenous events. Athletes should be cautioned to use good judgment when taking a drug after an attack has started during competition, as potentially toxic doses of epinephrine can be inhaled from metered dose inhalers. The combination of lactic acidosis, hypoxia, and increased endogenous catecholamines, plus a burst of adrenergic agonist entering the body by inhalation, may be lethal. The athlete and his parents must be alerted to this combination and the dangers of abusing nonprescription drugs.

Sex Before Sports

Some coaches recommend abstinence from sexual intercourse during training or on the night preceding a contest, believing that it diminishes athletic performance by sapping strength and interfering with the athlete's rest pattern. There is, however, no physiologic evidence that sexual activity saps strength. In fact, a 70 kg athlete expends an average of only 4 to 6 calories per minute during intercourse, an amount roughly equivalent to a brisk walk around a city block. Moreover, sex may be an effective outlet for pre-event jitters and provide the athlete with a good night's sleep.

The Athlete's Skin

The athlete's skin may be damaged by heat, cold, viruses, bacteria, fungi, and contact with clothing or other objects. The sun can burn an athlete, and a hot, sweating athlete may develop miliaria or cholinergic urticaria.

Sunburn

Sunburn is generally viewed as a sign of health and vigor, but this condition is actually a dermatitis that damages and ages the athlete's skin. Sunburn is a hazard not only in the summertime, but also during sunny, spring skiing if the skier wears only a T-shirt and shorts. There is less atmosphere at pollution-free, high-altitude ski areas to screen out the ultraviolet rays, and the snow also reflects these rays.

Athletes should stay out of the bright sun during the hottest part of the day to prevent sunburn. Gradual adaptation to the sun may be achieved by applying a sunscreen that contains benzoate to partly absorb ultraviolet rays and permit slow tanning. If the athlete is going in and out of water, he should use a sun screen in an alcoholic vehicle that will penetrate the skin and not be washed off by perspiration or swimming. Sun protectors contain para-amino benzoic acid, which blocks most of the ultraviolet light.

If an athlete's skin is burned, a soothing lotion that contains a mild anesthetic should be applied, and soothing tub baths may be taken in boric acid solution. If sunburn worsens after a surface anesthetic has been applied to a sunburn, even though the athlete is avoiding the sun, the surface anesthetic must be discontinued because it may be causing an allergic reaction.

Sunbathing is not recommended, especially on competition days, because prolonged exposure to the warm sun has an enervating effect. Sun screens and sun blockers should be available when athletes travel from one area of the country to another.

Miliaria

Miliaria, or heat rash, may affect well-tanned persons when they sweat. In superficial miliaria, the sweat becomes trapped under layers of the thick stratum corneum to produce a crystalline miliaria. Sterile pustules may form in the deep form of miliaria, miliaria pustulosus. Staphylococcal folliculitis has an identical appearance, but the pustules are, of course, not sterile.

Cholinergic Urticaria

Acetylcholine is important in sweating, and the hot, sweating athlete may develop a cholinergic urticaria. When the skin is stroked, histamine is sometimes relased, resulting in dermatographism. These urticarial lesions at the stroked area are sometimes seen in caddies, where the golf bag strap rests over the shoulder.

Cold Urticaria

Cold urticaria may occur when a swimmer jumps into cold water. Histamine is released in reaction to the cold, hives develop, and the histamine may even cause anaphylaxis. History of sudden exposure to cold is important for diagnosis, along with an "ice-cube test," in which an ice cube is placed on the flexor part

of the forearm for 2 minutes and the area observed for urticaria for 15 minutes. Affected swimmers may sometimes be desensitized with cold showers, but this treatment must be carefully monitored, with all of the equipment available that may be needed to control a possible anaphylactic reaction.

Equestrian Cold Panniculitis

Young, healthy women who ride horses for at least 2 consecutive hours a day throughout the winter may develop cold panniculitis.[6] They frequently ride in temperatures near or below freezing, and the horses often trot or gallop into heavy winds. As a result, the lateral part of the rider's thighs becomes chilled, and tight-fitting, uninsulated riding pants may slow the blood flow through the skin, further reducing tissue temperature.

Initially, the rider notices several small, erythematous, pruritic papules on the superior-lateral part of one or both thighs. After a week, the lesions progress to indurated, red-to-violaceous tender plaques and nodules. Histologically, there is a panniculitis with very inflamed veins, particularly at the dermal-subcutaneous fat junction.

The rider who must ride in the winter should be advised to ride for shorter periods and to wear looser, insulated, warmer pants.

Frostbite and Frostnip

Frostbite may affect an athlete who is skiing, tobogganing, snowshoeing, ice sailing, ice skating, mountain climbing, or snowmobiling.[23, 24, 62]

"Frostnip" is a mild blanching of the skin that may occur after a downhill ski run. Frostbite may be superficial or deep. Superficial frostbite involves the skin and the subcutaneous tissue, giving a whiteness or a "waxy" appearance to the skin; blisters may appear after 24 to 36 hours. In deep frostbite, the skin, subcutaneous tissue, and deeper tissues, even the bone, are affected, and as these tissues cool, the blood vessels constrict to conserve body heat. When body tissue temperature drops to 15° C, erythema, burning, and hypoesthesia occur. At 10° C, numbness, redness, and, sometimes, white, patchy areas appear. At −2° C, cellular metabolism stops. Then, as the area begins to thaw, blood vessels dilate, and with this engorgement the capillaries become more permeable. The swelling of the tissues that results may produce gangrene by interfering with the circulation. Moreover, direct cold injury to the cell denatures its proteins and enzymes, and large extracellular ice crystals form, drawing water from the cell.[18]

Peripheral areas such as the earlobes, nose, cheeks, hands, and feet are most frequently frostbitten. Incipient frostbite of the fingers or toes may be recognized by a sudden cessation of cold or discomfort in the injurted part, often followed by a pleasant warm feeling. Deep frostbite, however, may occur without this preliminary period of anesthesia.

Wetness, wind, and exercise increase the chance of frostbite. Clothing has an insulating effect, but when the clothing is wet, its insulating properties are reduced. The chilling effect increases with wind; thus, the chilling effect of −6° C with a 40-mile-per-hour wind is the same as −40° C with a breeze of 2 miles per hour. This effect is slightly less at high altitude because of reduced air density.[23, 24, 62] If the person exercises too much, he will pant, allowing cold air to enter his lungs and chill his whole body. Similarly, a runner's hands may become frostbitten when he jogs. The reciprocal motion of his hands may produce a 15° F temperature drop. When wind is added, the temperature drops from 20° to 50° lower.

"Instantaneous frostbite" may occur if cold metal is touched with a bare hand, especially if the hand is wet or damp. The skin sticks to the metal and is torn off when the hand is removed. Contact of the skin with gasoline that has been stored outside in the cold may also cause instantaneous frostbite. The freezing point of gasoline lies near −70° F, and its rapid rate of evaporation and extreme chill make it very dangerous.

Frostbite may also result from prolonged direct contact with a synthetic gel pack. If the pack is placed in a freezer and frozen to −15° C, it will remain below freezing for about 15 min while retaining its flexibility and conforming to the skin. When used, the pack should be wrapped in a towel and never applied to the skin.

Prevention

Frostnip can be prevented by use of the buddy system, with each partner watching the other for telltale signs that cannot be felt. Bathing and shaving the face should be postponed until after the day's outing, since these practices remove protective skin oils, and a layer of sun cream should be applied for added protection.

To prevent frostbite, the athlete's body should be warm enough to supply warm blood to his peripheral areas, and perspiring should be avoided. Fishnet underwear will provide a layer of warm air insulation. Light, smooth, clean socks may be worn next to the skin, with one or two heavier socks over these; extra socks and insoles should be carried.

Mittens—not gloves—are best for the cold-weather athlete or mountain climber; if he must use one hand, he should wear a glove on it and a mitten on the other hand. If work must be done bare-handed on metal, he should wear silk or rayon gloves or cover the metal with adhesive tape. He may intermittently remove his thumb from the mitten-thumb and hold it in a fist in the palm of the mitten to regain warmth for his whole hand. Extra mittens, removable wool mitten inserts, or glove linings should always be carried.

Treatment

With fast skiing, numb white patches may appear on a skier's face. These areas may be rewarmed with steady pressure from a warm hand but should not be rubbed. Frostnipped fingers may be warmed in an armpit, whereas frostnipped toes or heels may be rewarmed by removing footgear and placing the foot on the abdomen of a friend. Dry socks plus clothing over the foot will restore warmth; when footgear is put on, laces should be loose to assure adequate circulation.

The frostbitten person must remain calm because panic increases perspiration, which evaporates to cause further chilling. The key to the treatment of frostbite is prompt and thorough rewarming. If the area is rubbed with a hand or with snow, the thawing tissue may be irreparably damaged. "Applying ice water or snow to a frostbitten limb makes about as much sense as treating a burned foot by putting it in an oven."[62] Since refreezing of the tissue results in more tissue loss, a frozen part should not be thawed if the thawing may be followed by refreezing. Thus, it is less damaging for a mountaineer to walk to shelter on frozen feet than on feet that have been thawed, and a strong athlete can walk a long way on frozen feet without further injury. A climber should stump down the mountain even if it takes many hours, for if the frozen part is rewarmed on the trail the athlete becomes a litter case who cannot assist in his own rescue, resulting in danger to other climbers.

Frostbitten persons should not be given alcohol because alcohol causes peripheral vasodilation. Although alcohol produces a temporary warm feeling, the blood becomes chilled and body temperature drops further. Marijuana has a similar effect of increasing peripheral blood flow, which then leads to further chilling. The frostbitten climber should also refrain from smoking because smoking causes peripheral vasoconstriction that further decreases blood flow. If the climber must make a long trip on a litter, dry gauze should be placed between his toes but not pulled into his webs. A fluff dressing may then be applied and lightly wrapped with gauze.

Once the base station or hospital is reached, a warm water bath should be prepared.[23, 24, 62] While the vessel is being filled, the victim's body should be kept as warm as possible with blankets and hot drinks. The water container may be a large bucket or a 19-liter (5-gallon) can that allows room for the frozen part to move without bumping the sides. It should be large enough so that the frozen part itself will not overly cool the liquid, and the affected part should be held in the middle of the fluid, not on the bottom. A duffle bag may be used to support the extremity behind the knee. The water must be kept at a temperature of 40° C to 42° C and, monitored with a heavy-duty thermometer. It must not be allowed to rise above 44° C; thus it should feel warm, but not hot, to a normal hand. The water temperature must never be tested with the frozen part because frozen tissue is insensitive, and even brief exposure to high temperature can cause serious damage. Water hotter than 46° C should never be added to the bath, and hot water must not be added too close to the injured part. No stove should be placed under the warming vessel.

If the container is not large enough to keep the part completely immersed, the part may be wrapped in towels. Water not warmer than 44°C should then be continually poured on. Dry heat is difficult to regulate and will not rewarm evenly, and for this reason the frostbitten extremity must never be exposed to an open fire or an engine's exhaust. However, if dry heat must be used for rewarming, the part may be loosely covered with sterile gauze and placed against another person's abdomen and covered with warm clothes or blankets. Warming a frostbitten part this way takes three or four times longer than warming with a liquid.

Rewarming in the liquid should be continued until a flush returns to the distal tip of the thawed part—a period of 20 to 30 minutes. There will be little discomfort initially, but pain will increase until it becomes quite intense at the end of the rewarming period. A 25-mg Demerol tablet may be given along with aspirins about 20 minutes before rewarming starts. Heavy doses of pain-killers are to be avoided, especially at high altitudes, where they may cause respiratory depression.

After rapid rewarming, the injured part should be soaked in a whirlpool at 37° C for 20 to 30 minutes twice a day until healing is complete. Hexachlorophine or an iodine prep solution may be added to the bath, and active motion of the part in the bath is allowed. After

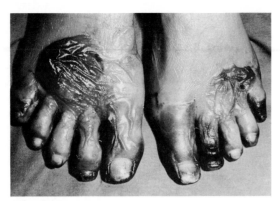

FIG. 2-5
Blisters on frostbitten feet should not be debrided.

thawing, the frostbitten area will resemble burned tissue, with blebs and blisters forming. The tissue will be very sensitive to injury and susceptible to infection, and even the slightest abrasion or irritation is dangerous; thus further cold and weightbearing must be avoided.

The subject should be kept warm at normal body temperature, with frostbitten areas uncovered. If the area must be covered, however, a soft, dry dressing that is changed infrequently is best; wet or greasy dressings should never be applied. Sterile cotton may be placed between the affected fingers or toes. A pillow under the calf will keep the heel off the sheets, but the limb should generally be kept horizontal. A box or a frame placed around the feet will protect against pressure from the sleeping bag or sheets. The frostbitten person should be encouraged to move his other joints to keep them limber.

Gangrene associated with frostbite is often a superficial dry condition that does not require emergency amputation (Fig. 2-5). Debridement and amputation are best postponed to allow a natural spontaneous debridement of the dead tissue to occur. Patience is needed because recovery takes many months. "The worst *looking* hands and feet, if treated properly and patiently, will shed their shriveled black shells painlessly like a glove, suddenly and unexpectedly revealing healthy, pink skin underneath."[62]

Shoe Boot Pernio (Chilblains)

Children who wear plastic shoe boots in a cold, wet environment may get the linings wet.[16] The waterproof outer covering prevents the evaporation of moisture that has collected. The blood vessels in the child's foot may then go into spasm, reddish-blue patches may appear on his feet, and the dorsum of his toes may turn pink. Twelve to 24 hours after exposure, the foot becomes swollen, itches, and burns, and vesicles may form. To treat this "shoe boot pernio," the foot must be rewarmed, and the subject must avoid further exposure to damp cold.

Skin Infections in Athletics

The skin may be the site of infectious diseases that can be transmitted to other athletes, especially by direct contact. Even minor infections may become major problems, ruining the season for the athlete, his opponents, or his team. The infections may be viral, such as herpes simplex and molluscum contagiosum, bacterial, such as impetigo and acne, or fungal dermatoses, including tinea versicolor, tinea cruris, and candidiasis.

Herpes Simplex

Herpes simplex is a contagious, blistering viral disorder found mostly in athletes engaged in body contact sports, sometimes referred to as "herpes gladiatorum." An infection may spread to an entire team, especially where there is close contact, as in wrestlers (Fig. 2-6A). The most frequently affected sites are the right side of the face and the forearm, which are major contact points.

A herpes lesion looks like a fever blister and usually consists of a cluster of vesicles on an erythematous base (Fig. 2-6B). The blister breaks to form an itchy, yellowish crust and is infectious during the blistering and ulceration phases, where the athlete may have tender, swollen lymph nodes.

Because some athletes are more susceptible than others to herpes infections, the team physician, the trainer, and the coach must be especially alert for such tendencies. Herpes is also more frequent in athletes who have had previous herpes infections.

Prevention requires athletes in close contact sports to shower before and after practice.[3] Exchanges of towels or clothes between players should be forbidden. All open wounds must be reported, because open skin serves as a portal for infection. Occasionally an athlete may be aware that herpes is beginning 24 hours before he has obvious skin changes. At the first sign of infection, removal from competition is obligatory. Wrestling partners should be advised to check each other for skin lesions to prevent transfer of an infection. Lesions should be caught early, the blisters broken, and a drying agent such as alcohol, silver nitrate, camphor, or alum applied. The area must also be washed frequently with Domeboro solution.

The condition is usually self-limiting, lasting about 2 weeks.

A herpes infection can be very dangerous if the athlete has underlying ectopic eczema because the herpes infection may then rapidly disseminate. This is a dermatologic emergency, and antiviral drugs may be needed.

Molluscum Contagiosum

Molluscum contagiosum is a contagious skin infection caused by a wart-like pox virus. It is characterized by umbilicated, pink papules with central gelatinous craters, and the surrounding skin is normally not inflamed (Fig. 2-6D). Lesions grow down into the dermis as multiple, closely packed, pear-shaped lobules. Removal may be done by incision of the central punctum, which extrudes the central core of viral bodies. Curretage also destroys these lesions.

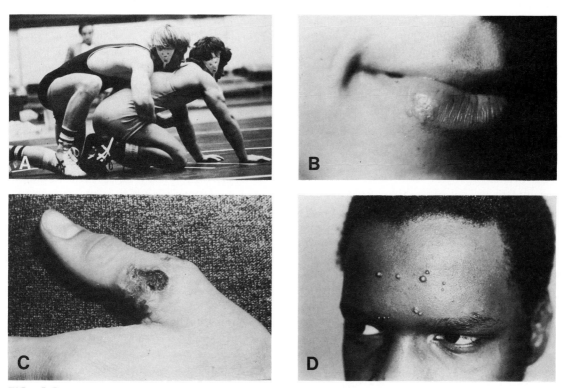

FIG. 2-6
Close contact (*A*) and skin damage may spread skin infections. Skin conditions include herpes simplex (*B*), impetigo (*C*), and molluscum contagiosum (*D*).

Impetigo

Impetigo is a skin infection most often caused by a beta-hemolytic streptococcus, although sometimes the cause may be a staphylococcus. The condition is much more contagious than viral herpes simplex. Groups of blisters are filled with clear fluid and have a similar appearance to the lesions of herpes simplex, but they evolve into sharply demarcated erosions covered with heavy, yellowish, serosanguineous crusts, and form pustules (Fig. 2-6C).

Athletes must be watched for early lesions, and if they appear the lesions should be cleaned each day with a surgical soap or with Dial soap. The athlete must take a full course of antibiotics, as glomerulonephritis will sometimes follow impetigo if it has been undertreated.

Acne

Sporting activity brings physical and emotional stress, increases sebaceous activity in the eccrine sweat glands, exposes the athlete to dirt, dust and heat, and causes him to perspire. These conditions combine with the ubiquitous *Staphylococcus albus* and *Corynebacterium acnes* to produce the pustules and small abscesses of acne.

Ambient microparticles, bacteria, and an increased production of sebaceous material block pilosebaceous follicles, setting the stage for inflammation and infection. Chemical changes in the occluded sebaceous material, such as the enzymatic release of irritating free fatty acids, also inflame the walls of the follicles. Surface frictions, as from a shoulder pad strap, may also inflame the skin and lead to an inflammatory papule that ruptures to form a pustule or a small abscess.

"Football acne" affects the skin under a tackle football player's chin strap. Even 10- to 12-year-olds who wear chin straps may suffer mild forms of football acne. The semiocclusive plastic chin strap irritates the player's skin by friction and physical pressure, blocks pores, and rubs in dirt. Patch tests for allergy to the strap in these cases are usually negative.

To treat generalized or localized "football acne," the player must gently wash his face with soap and warm water in the morning, immediately after practice or a game and at bedtime.[4] A topical cleansing agent or an astringent should be applied; drying lotions or creams may also be used. The pustules should not be squeezed because squeezing only inflames the skin and spreads the infection. If the athlete has acne on his neck, chest, and upper back, he should apply a fungistatic foot powder to absorb the perspiration and skin oils.

If an athlete has had pustules or has a strong tendency to form them, he may be started on tetracycline therapy at the beginning of the season.[5] The bacteriostatic action of low-dose tetracycline hinders the invasion of pathogens. Tetracycline also acts to reduce the hydrolysis of serum triglycerides into free fatty acids.[22]

Fungal Dermatoses

Tinea Versicolor   Tinea versicolor is a yeast infection that usually affects 18- to 20-year-olds. Its lesions may be white on black skin, black on white skin, or pink on skin of any color. Hyphae will be seen on a potassium hydroxide preparation. Selsun shampoo is applied for 10 minutes for ten nights, then once a week to treat this disorder.

Tinea Cruris ("Jock Itch")   Tinea cruris, or "jock itch," is an infectious dermatosis caused by the dermatophyte fungi *Epidermophyton floccosum, Tricophyton mentagrophytes,* and *Tricophyton rubrum.* The fungi may be passed from person to person on personal clothing or by direct contact, or it may spread from athlete's foot or fungal involvement of the athlete's nails. Skin lesions on the upper inner thighs are bilaterally symmetrical, with a clearing central area characteristic of "ringworm," and a border sharply demarcated and active. The lesions, however, seldom involve the athlete's genitalia and scrotum. A potassium hydroxide wet mount will show true hyphae in *Tinea cruris,* but if the athlete has been treating his infection the scraping may not be a good one. In these circumstances, the treatments are best stopped for a few days before scraping is repeated.

Tinea cruris may be treated with preparations such as tolnaftate (Tinactin), haloprogin (Halotex), miconazole (Mica-Tin) or clotrimazole

(Lotrimin). If *Tinea unguum* is serving as a reservoir for jock itch or athlete's foot, a 6-month or year-long course of systemic griseofulvin therapy may be needed for cure.[10]

Candidiasis Yeast may be normal flora in the athlete's groin, and they may infect chafed and eroded skin. Candida will turn an athlete's scrotum red. The yeast also produces "satellite lesions" separate from the main lesion. A potassium hydroxide wet mount will show both "pseudohyphae," which are nonseptae, nonbranching, elongated growths, and budding yeast cells. The lesions should be treated with Burrow's solution compresses for 20 minutes three times a day, until the acute phase has subsided. Medicines such as nystatin (Mycostatin), amphotericin B (Fungizone), clotrimazole, miconazole, or haloprogin are then used.

Contact Dermatitis

An athlete may come in contact with materials that cause allergic reactions or objects that rub and damage his skin, or he may be allergic to materials that contact his skin, and a dermatitis may ensue. The offending material may be a tape adhesive, a tape adherent such as benzoin, or a counterirritant used in the training room. Also, dyed clothing, or even the rubber in shoes, on balls, and on the handles of exercise equipment, may provoke an allergic response.

When an athlete develops a contact allergy, the examiner must obtain a good history from him concerning contact with substances such as those listed above. The trainer should check the materials used when he is preparing the athlete for his sport. When observing the distribution of the athlete's itchy lesions, the examiner will note whether they occupy a band area where an athletic supporter strap or the stripes on his athletic socks make contact with the subject's skin. Patch testing may be needed to locate the offending material.

The athlete may be allergic to animal dyes or the chromate used in tanning gloves and shoe leather. In such cases, the athlete may have to wear gloves and shoes that have been tanned with vegetable dyes. Because sweat in a hockey glove may also lead to a dermatitis, cotton gloves should be worn under hockey gloves to absorb moisture.

The rubber toebox of tennis shoes or all-purpose gym shoes may cause a contact dermatitis on the toes and dorsum of the foot. The condition is usually bilateral and symmetrical, and a potassium hydroxide preparation will be negative. Treatment begins with discarding the offending clothes, gloves, or shoes, and the dermatitis is then treated like poison ivy, with early skin washing, if possible, before the full reaction sets in. A steroid cream is applied after a skin reaction has appeared.

"Strawberries"

"Strawberries," also called floor burns, friction burns, and mat burns, are skin abrasions. The athlete's skin breaks from friction, rubbing off when he slides across a mat, lands on a rocky field, or slides on artificial turf.

An athlete may neglect a strawberry until an infection has set in. For this reason, such abrasions must be reported and promptly and carefully cleaned. While the area is numb, it should be thoroughly scrubbed with a soft-bristled brush that has been dipped in mild soap and water. An antibiotic ointment is then applied, and the abrasion is covered with a sterile dressing. The dressing should be changed and the wound checked each day.

Because strawberries are painful if the damaged skin is stretched or stuck, the injured athlete should wear a felt or a foam rubber protective pad over the abrasion. Soccer goalkeepers may wear football pants and hip pads to help prevent this type of injury.

"Saddle Soreness"

A novice cyclist may develop a painful bursitis over his ischial tuberosities, which rest on the bicycle saddle. He may also suffer from irritated, reddened, and itchy skin in his perineum, so-called "pruritis ani." Touring cyclists sometimes have inguinal intertrigo or "cyclist's scrotum." Moreover, friction between a cyclist's skin and his bicycle saddle may produce a panniculitis that may lead to local fat necrosis and boils. Boils may also appear on the backs of athletes doing bench presses. Such boils may be avoided if each lifter wears a shirt or by covering the bench with a towel during weight training.

The novice cyclist's ischial pain usually disappears after about 1 week of riding, and pressure can be reduced if he uses a saddle with softer padding in the ischial area. A cyclist with pruritis ani should be advised to keep the area dry, to use good toilet hygiene, and to apply a hydrocortisone cream or lotion.

Intertrigo is an inflammatory response of the skin to friction and maceration that is associated with a tight athletic supporter or tight cycling shorts. The athlete's skin becomes reddened at friction points, and the diagnosis is based on the exclusion of other groin eruptions. This condition may be prevented by avoiding tight clothes or a tight, rubbing athletic supporter. Talcum powder should be applied to the groin, and the athlete should allow air to reach the area as often as is practical. A 0.5% hydrocortisone cream will alleviate the symptoms, but the cortisone may cause skin atrophy.

The cyclist should smear petroleum jelly or sprinkle baby powder on his skin and wear cycling shorts that contain a built-in chamois to reduce friction between the saddle and his skin.

Nutrition

Poor knowledge of nutrition may contribute to unbalanced nutrition, with the athlete either underfed or overfed. A swimmer may be trying to keep her weight down, but when she goes to a party with friends, she eats cake and drinks soda pop and later attempts to compensate by omitting more nutritious foods from her diet. Youths who consume soft drinks often cut down on their milk intake. On the other hand, some athletes oversupplement diets with protein powders or tablets, raw blood, vitamins, and minerals. Heavy use of such supplements may lead to kidney trouble, hypervitaminosis, or more severe disorders.

Nutritional counseling for balanced nutrition should begin in grade school. Each young athlete should keep a record of his daily food intake and his activities for a week for review and counseling by a physician or trainer. A team nutritionist is invaluable for dietary counseling, explaining the principles of a balanced diet, and discussing dietary misconceptions and preparing meals.

The athlete should select food from each of the four basic food groups.[59] One group consists of fruits and vegetables, such as citrus fruits, carrots, and greens; another includes cereals and grains; a third is the protein group, which includes fish, meat, poultry, and legumes; and the fourth group contains milk and milk products, such as yogurt, cheese, and ice cream. About 50% of the calories the athlete ingests should come from carbohydrates, with less than 10% of these from refined sugar. About 35% should be from fat and 15% from protein, with about half of these from vegetable sources. There is no "best" diet, and variety does not necessarily mean that the diet is balanced. By careful planning to provide all of the essential amino acids, vegetarians can have a very nutritious diet, especially if beans, eggs, nuts, and milk are included to supply high-quality protein.

Athletes usually eat three meals a day, but more frequent, smaller meals eaten when hungry are probably better. The athlete should not skip meals; if he takes snacks, they should consist of fresh fruit—"nature's candy"—vegetables, or a glass of milk.

The caloric needs of an athlete will depend on his body weight and physical activity. For ordinary activity, about 3000 calories per day are needed, containing about 100 g of protein. The hard-training athlete who runs 25 to 35 km (15 to 20 miles) a day, exercises for 3 to 4 hours, or lifts heavy weights may need more than 5000 calories a day. The extra energy needs of these athletes are provided by extra calories and fats, and these and other essential elements should be contained in a balanced diet. But even an outwardly balanced diet may lack sufficient nutritional value. Food processing can destroy much nutritional value: white bread is milled and bleached, and chemicals may be added to foods that come from poor soils. Valuable nutrients may also be lost during canning, freezing, shipping, storage, and cooking.

Nutritional supplements have been decried as expensive nutritional nonsense. Although no value is gained by supplementing a nutritionally adequate diet that meets the demands of training, supplements may be needed when an athlete is training hard and his metabolic demands are high. They may also be needed when the athlete is "meeting" weight in wrestling, boxing, or weightlifting. In addition, for various reasons, some athletes are unable to eat a balanced diet and may need supplements.

Athletes often select supplements of protein, vitamins, and minerals.[63] Some weightlifters have been known to go into negative nitrogen balance during heavy training. Therefore, the growing athlete or an athlete building muscle may require as much as 2 g of protein per kilogram of body weight each day. Any excess protein intake is excreted as ammonia or converted into fat. Red meats, eggs, and dairy products are high in animal protein but are also high in saturated animal fats. Desiccated liver is a good source of animal protein, and wheat germ supplies plant protein.

Vitamins A, D, E, and K are fat soluble and can be stored in the body, whereas others such as the B-complex vitamins and vitamin C are water soluble and cannot be stored. Vitamin A is found in fish-liver oils, butter, whole milk, cheeses, dark green leafy vegetables, and yellow fruits and vegetables. Cod liver oil is high in vitamin D, as is fortified milk. Vitamin E, or alpha-tocopherol, is an antioxidant found in eggs, nuts, grains, leafy vegetables, and wheat germ oil. Spinach, cabbage, and liver provide vitamin K. The B vitamins are important for carbohydrate and fat metabolism. They are found in protein foods such as liver and whole grains, with wheat germ and brewer's yeast being excellent suppliers of these vitamins. Vitamin C is important in adrenal gland metabolism, collagen formation, and wound healing and is found especially in citrus fruits. Although the recommended minimal daily requirement for vitamin C is low, some athletes ingest 4 g a day in the belief that it diminishes soreness and speeds healing.

There are some dangers in taking vitamin supplements, as when large doses of the fat soluble vitamins are stored in the body, leading to hypervitaminosis. Also, large amounts of ascorbic acid may reduce the vitamin C in the athlete's adrenal glands.

When an athlete's vitamin intake is low, his mineral intake also may be low. The important minerals include calcium, phosphorus, magnesium, potassium, sodium, and iron. Iron deficiency is common among young women, especially those menstruating heavily; rapidly growing teenage boys, particularly those in lower income groups; those dieting to lose weight; and vegetarians. The iron-deficient athlete will lose strength and endurance and fatigue easily. A thorough dietary and menstrual history, including whether the athlete is using an intrauterine device that may increase menstrual blood loss, and a history of excess fatigue or lack of endurance may indicate an iron deficiency and the need for an iron supplement.

Intelligent food selection and preparation with an emphasis on fresh food—rather than on canned food that may be deficient—should provide the athlete with a balanced diet for optimum athletic performance. However, hard-training athletes, those meeting weight, those without access to a balanced diet, and those traveling who find it difficult to prepare meals may benefit from properly selected supplements. A blender can be invaluable in preparing nutritious shakes. For example, a combination of milk, eggs, wheat germ, powdered milk, fruit juice, yogurt, and fruit (bananas, for example) can make an excellent, nutritious shake for the athlete.

Carbohydrate Loading

Athletes in endurance events that require more than an hour of strenuous exercise can add glycogen to their muscles by carbohydrate loading. One week before a race, the athlete should train heavily for more than 2 hours to exhaust his supply of muscle glycogen. Then for 3 days, he should train regularly while on a low carbohydrate, high protein, and high fat diet consisting of meat, bacon, eggs, butter, and vegetable oils. In the final 3 days, he should train lightly while on a high carbohydrate diet of bread, spaghetti, potatoes, sugar, fruit, and fruit juices.

This carbohydrate loading results in a super compensation in the exercised muscles, sometimes almost tripling the muscle's supply of glycogen and enabling the athlete to exercise for a much longer time before muscle exhaustion. The uptake of glycogen, however, is accompanied by an uptake of water, and the muscles may feel heavy and stiff. Some athletes even develop angina, since glycogen and water are added to the heart muscle, causing electrocardiographic abnormalities to appear. If an endurance athlete decides to load with carbohydrates, he should do it only a few times a year for important contests because more frequent carbohydrate loading may disrupt the athlete's metabolic processes.

Dietary Preparation for a Match

Starting a few days before a match, the athlete should be on a balanced diet, stressing carbohydrate intake for glycogen storage. As training is reduced, the muscles recover and store the glycogen. If the athlete eats steaks, bananas, and grapefruits during the week, enough potassium for weekend athletic activity will be stored. When heavy perspiration is anticipated, he may season his food with extra salt, although highly salted foods eaten within a few days of competition may cause fluid retention and sluggishness.

The Precompetition Meal

The precompetition meal should be taken 3 to 4 hours before the match. Moderation is the rule, and the meal should not be too large. Because the athlete is usually tense, less blood will flow to his stomach and small intestine, and there is less motility of the stomach and small intestine. Digestion and gastric emptying are slowed.

The meal should be easy to digest, high in carbohydrate, but low in refined sugar, protein, and fat. Refined sugar contains only calories and is quickly absorbed to stimulate insulin secretion, which reduces blood sugar. The athlete will be hungry again in a few hours owing to the reactive hypoglycemia. For this reason, refined sugar, although a very quick source of energy, is a poor pregame food. Instead, sugar should be fructose from fruits, which converts to glucose in the liver and is available more slowly.

Before a match, the athlete should avoid foods with a high cellulose content, such as lettuce, which can induce defecation. Moreover, spiced foods may irritate the stomach, and high protein foods, such as meat, fish, and eggs, produce fixed acids that use up body water to be excreted. Fatty or fried foods slow stomach emptying. Thus, the athlete should forego whole milk, which has a high fat content, mayonnaise, and other sandwich spreads high in fat. Coffee, tea, or soft drinks that contain caffeine may increase tension in a nervous athlete. It may, however, be a person's custom to drink a cup of tea, and this psychological need should be respected. The athlete should avoid flatus-producing foods, although gas formation varies among individuals, and athletes have performed well even on pregame diets of sauerkraut.

Some champions ritualistically forego the pregame meal. The athlete who wins or performs well with a certain pregame routine is not likely to change his habit, but sound nutritional advice may have an important effect over time.

The traditional pregame football steak may impede performance. Fixed acids form and must withdraw water to be excreted, and the fat in the steak slows gastric emptying. A more proper pregame meal consists of clear soup, a lean sandwich, a noncarbonated fruit drink, or cold cereal. Commercially available liquid diets, such as Ensure, SustaCal, and Nutrument make excellent pregame meals, especially on road trips. These liquid meals are high in carbohydrates but contain some fat and enough protein to give a feeling of satiety and relieve hunger. Ordinary liquid breakfasts, however, should not be used as pregame meals because they contain too much protein. The nutritional advantages of liquid meals should be explained to athletes while emphasizing that many successful teams and individuals have benefited from their use.

The athlete should drink about 250 ml of a lightly sweetened fruit juice diluted with an equal volume of water every 15 minutes in hot and humid weather. A small increment in better performance resulting from drinking the diluted fruit juice may mean the difference between winning and losing. A solution containing more than 2.5 g of glucose per 100 ml of water will be delayed in absorption. The hyperosmolar environment in the stomach draws water into the stomach, leaving less water available for sweating, causing the athlete's exercise time to exhaustion to drop. Additives such as sugar pills, honey, or candy draw fluids into the gastrointestinal tract and cause more dehydration.

In prolonged competitions, such as tennis matches, track meets, or wrestling tournaments, the athlete should supplement his fluids with sweetened beverages during the contest. These help to maintain hydration, blood sugar, and muscle glycogen. If the competition lasts a few days, the athlete should try to eat regularly scheduled meals, each one similar to a pregame meal. After the game or match, the athlete may be keyed up or depressed and have travel deadlines. Within a few hours, a high-calorie, high-protein, high-carbohydrate meal eaten in a relaxed atmosphere—with no caffeine-containing drinks—will help to reduce tension and postgame depression.

Pharmacologic Agents

Pharmacologic agents are sometimes given to athletes to reduce pain and inflammation. Among these are nonsteroidal anti-inflammatory drugs such as aspirin, fenoprofen, ibuprofen, naproxen, indomethacin, sulindac, tolmetin, phenylbutazone, local anesthetics, and steroids.[25]

The nonsteroidal anti-inflammatory drugs can be separated into four groups based on their structure: [1] salicylates; [2] proprionic acid derivatives, including ibuprofen, fenoprofen, and naproxen; [3] indole derivatives, including indomethacin, sulindac, and, a close relative, tolmetin; and [4] others such as phenylbutazone. These agents all inhibit prostaglandin synthetase and decrease the local synthesis of prostaglandins, prostacyclins, and thromboxanes.[30] The magnitude of the prostaglandin synthetase inhibition by these drugs correlates with their anti-inflammatory potency. Both aspirin (3 g) and indomethacin (200 mg) have been shown to reduce prostaglandin excretion in humans by more than 75%.[57, 58] The blockage of the formation of these fatty acid derivatives has a widespread effect on the inflammatory sequence. There is less sensitization of pain receptors to chemical and mechanical stimuli, fewer phagocytes are attracted, and less lysozomal contents are released. Chemically induced peripheral pain is also suppressed.

Aspirin and Other Nonsteroidal Anti-Inflammatory Agents

Aspirin is frequently used in sport to treat the pain and inflammation that result from an injury and to forestall the softening of articular cartilage. It is effective against the dull, throbbing pain of inflammation, where prostaglandins sensitize the nerve endings. Aspirin is much less effective, however, against the sharp, stabbing pains from direct stimulation of sensory nerves. To forestall softening of the articular cartilage behind the kneecaps, a runner may take two aspirins about 20 minutes before a run. Aspirin may also be used after a dislocation of the patella to protect against articular cartilage softening, but the aspirin therapy must be started within a few days after the injury, for if the cartilage has already become soft and fibrillated the salicylates will not reverse the condition.

Aspirin therapy is not without dangers. The most common complication is gastrointestinal discomfort, but serious gastric erosions may develop even without symptoms.[33, 50] Although hypersensitivity is uncommon, it may be severe and include vasomotor rhinitis, urticaria, a full-blown acute asthmatic attack, or angioneurotic edema. A combination of dehydration, hyperuricemia, and high-tissue levels of aspirin may produce renal papillary damage. The aspirin may interfere with both the excretion and the reabsorption of uric acid by the renal tubules. For this reason, an older athlete prone to acute gouty attacks should not take aspirin. Further, hemolysis may occur in black athletes deficient in glucose-6-phosphate dehydrogenase. Acetaminophen may therefore be a better analgesic choice than aspirin for these athletes.

Acetaminophen (Tylenol) is effective against chronic low-grade pain but is only weakly anti-inflammatory. Because it makes some athletes relaxed and drowsy, it has a potential for abuse. Although this drug will not irritate the stomach, it may be hepatotoxic if it is used excessively and may lead to hepatic failure.[17, 45]

Other nonsteroidal anti-inflammatory drugs besides aspirin include propionic acid derivatives; indole derivatives, including fenoprofen (Nalfon), ibuprofen (Motrin), and naproxen (Naprosyn). As a group, they have fewer gastrointestinal side-effects than does aspirin. Indole derivatives include indomethacin (Indocin), sulindac (Clinoril), and tolmetin (Tolectin), a drug related to the indole derivatives. Indomethacin is a potent inhibitor of the formation of prostaglandins, but its gastrointestinal and central nervous system side-effects limit its usefulness against acute inflammation.[42] Sulindac is metabolized to a sulfide that is more active than the parent drug.

The anti-inflammatory activity of these newer drugs is about the same as that of aspirin. In the usual doses, however, they are three to five times more expensive than aspirin. Further, some of their side-effects are quite serious, including asthmatic attacks and aplastic anemia that may occur even with the usual therapeutic doses. It is thus imperative that an athlete given these agents be made aware of possible side-effects and their signs and symptoms.

Phenylbutazone

Phenylbutazone (Butazolidin) is an anti-inflammatory agent that can reduce pain and swelling in equine and human athletes. Oxyphenbutazone (Tandearil), an active metabolite of phenylbutazone, is another often-used anti-inflammatory drug. Phenylbutazone, or "bute," blocks inflammation by inhibiting the synthesis of prostaglandins. The drug is usually given in a dose of 100 mg three or four times a day with meals or milk for a maximum of 7 days.

Given its potency, phenylbutazone is too often casually prescribed. It is, for example, the most commonly prescribed drug in the National Football League.[9] In another instance of its frequent use, phenylbutazone was prescribed for 3300 courses at the United States Naval Academy during a 4-year period for conditions such as painful shoulders, tennis elbow, tenosynovitis at the wrist, inflammation, trochanteric bursitis, jumper's knee, and Achilles tendinitis.

Phenylbutazone can be a very toxic drug with reactions that include aplastic anemia, agranulocytosis, hypersensitivity reactions, and serious skin reactions. It may also limit athletic performance and mask pain, thus leading to further injury. Phenylbutazone has replaced chloramphenicol as the most common cause of drug-related aplastic anemia, in many cases a fatal disease. Although aplastic anemia may follow normal doses, large doses are most often responsible for this toxic effect.[28] Jockeys and exercise boys and girls find that it works so well for horses that they sometimes take it themselves for minor bruises and sprains. In one case, a professional jockey took horse phenylbutazone, ingesting 2 g a day for 3 days. Two weeks later he developed a severe blood dyscrasia. Despite bone marrow transplantation, he died.

Phenylbutazone is also the principal cause of fatal, drug-induced agranulocytosis, a condition in which the leukocyte count drops and the victim notices ulcers in his mouth and pharynx, a sore throat, and, often, a rash. To avoid death in such cases, the patient must have the drug withdrawn immediately and the infection aggressively treated. Thrombocytopenia is another side-effect, characterized by petachiae, ecchymoses, epistaxis, and bleeding from the mucous membranes of the mouth. A hypersensitivity reaction is of most concern with short-term use because it may produce a severe granulocytosis. When an athlete has been sensitized to phenylbutazone, a single subsequent dose may prove fatal. Because allergic reactions cannot be predicted with a routine pretreatment blood test, phenylbutazone should never be prescribed for an athlete who has had any type of previous reaction to the drug. To be safe, a physician should not give the drug to an athlete with a history of an allergy to any drug. Skin reactions to phenylbutazone, such as toxic epidermal necrolysis, may be fatal. An unfortunate athlete may also develop a peptic ulcer, hepatitis, or renal failure. Finally, phenylbutazone should not be given to a pregnant athlete, since the drug may be embryotoxic.

In view of these lethal complications, indiscriminate use of this powerful drug in the therapy of trivial, acute, or chronic musculoskeletal disorders can only be condemned. Serious complications aside, athletic performance may suffer while an athlete is using phenylbutazone. The drug blocks enzymes in the Kreb's cycle that interfere with the aerobic production of energy. The athlete also retains fluid and gains weight, and his plasma volume expands to produce a dilutional anemia.

Phenylbutazone is especially dangerous for older athletes, particularly older women, who are more susceptible to its toxic effects. Short-term use, for 1 week or less, by young athletes is said not to be particularly hazardous,[9] but the sometimes unpredictable side-effects should eliminate the drug from the physician's repertoire. If used, it should be noted that its toxicity rises if the recommended dosage is exceeded or the duration of its use is prolonged. The athlete should be made aware of the risks and possible complications and their early manifestation. The drug should be stopped immediately if a fever, sore throat, skin rash, pruritis, jaundice, or tarry stools develop.

Local Anesthetics

Local anesthetics, such as short-acting lidocaine (Xylocaine) and long-acting bupivacaine (Marcaine), are sometimes useful in sports medicine. These drugs act at the cell membrane of sensory, motor, and autonomic nerves to block both the generation and the conduction of nerve impulses. Lidocaine produces anesthesia for about an hour, with its duration depending on how long the anesthetic remains in contact with the nerve tissue. If epinephrine is also included in the injection, the duration of anesthesia almost doubles. Bupivacaine anesthesia lasts about 7 hours.

A local anesthetic may be used to block the pain from a rib fracture and may also be injected into an injured area, such as a hip pointer, to relieve acute pain. Infiltration of a trigger point with a local anesthetic can sometimes break a reverberating pain cycle and may serve to distinguish between local and referred pain. A local anesthetic can also lessen the pain of a steroid injection or joint aspiration. Most athletes will not, however, need numbing medicine.

If an anesthetic is injected, the area should first be thoroughly prepared with an iodine solution, not just wiped with an alcohol sponge. On rare occaions, an athlete may be allergic to a local anesthetic. Excessive dosages, even though given locally, may be dangerous, since the drug is eventually absorbed systemically. Numbing injections must be used discriminately, as they mask pain and thus can lead to more serious injury.

Local Steroids

Steroids, like nonsteroidal anti-inflammatory drugs, block the release of arachidonic acid from membrane phospholipids, limiting the formation of inflammatory endoperoxides, prostacyclins, and thromboxanes. Steroids reduce vascular permeability and the number of leukocytes at the inflamed site. They also seem to stabilize the lysosomal membranes of the inflammatory cells. Steroids later inhibit fibroblasts and collagen deposits, reduce capillary proliferation, and thus limit the formation of scar.

Before a steroid is injected, the injection site must be thoroughly cleaned and prepared with an iodine solution. This preparation is particularly important before injecting into periarticular structures because the needle may inadvertently enter the joint, and if the skin is incompletely prepared, bacteria may be transported into the joint.

Injecting a combination of a short-acting and a long-acting agent (Celestone, Soluspan) through a fine-gauge needle is recommended. This combination contains betamethasone sodium phosphate, a soluble ester that acts promptly, and a betamethasone acetate suspension that is only slightly soluble and affords sustained activity. The injected steroid should bathe the inflamed area, not be injected directly into the tissue. No resistance should be felt as the plunger is depressed. If only a long-acting, repository steroid is injected, it may produce a painful local reaction for the first 24 hours. When this occurs, the athlete should not apply heat, as this will increase pain and swelling; instead an ice bag should be used.

Steroid injections must be used with caution because direct injection of a steroid into an inflamed tendon may cause pressure necrosis, inhibit collagen synthesis, and degrade the collagen. The drug may diminish pain to a degree that the athlete exceeds the mechanical tolerance of the tendon, causing a rupture. The athlete who has just had a steroid injection near a weightbearing tendon, such as the quadriceps, patellar, or Achilles tendon, should be restricted from sport for 2 weeks.

Dimethyl Sulfoxide

Dimethyl sulfoxide (DMSO) is an inexpensive by-product of paper manufacturing and is used as an industrial solvent. Being highly polar, it dissolves many water-soluble and fat-soluble substances. It is also used as a preservative in the freezing and storing of human and animal tissues and cells. Because frozen DMSO does not crystallize, cells and tissues can survive freezing undamaged.

Dimethyl sulfoxide also has the remarkable property of penetrating the keratinized barrier layer of the skin and being absorbed in seconds. Through this action, it may serve as a vehicle for drugs and provide enhanced penetration of local anesthetics and steroids. Dimethyl sulfoxide also has properties of its own to reduce soft tissue swelling and inflammation in acute trauma; DMSO is therefore both a drug-carrier and a drug, although the mechanism for its biologic activity is not fully understood.

Dimethyl sulfoxide is often used by veterinarians to treat inflammatory conditions in horses, such as contusion, sprains, strains, traumatic periostitis ("bucked shin"), "shoe ball," gonitis, blisters, lacerations, hematomas, and fractures, and is used postoperatively. The drug is available as a solution and as a gel. Usually, about 100 ml is brushed on the injured area two or three times a day. The most dramatic results are obtained when the drug is applied very soon after trauma. The veterinarian should wear rubber gloves applying the medicine to prevent the drug from penetrating his skin and producing an unpleasant garliclike taste in his mouth and an oysterlike breath odor. The horse's skin should be washed, rinsed, and dried before DMSO is applied. If this is not done, the drug will carry in any chemicals that are on the skin. For this same reason, no other topical agents should be applied to the skin until the DMSO has thoroughly dried. A medical grade of DMSO is used because industrial DMSO rapidly carries impurities in through the skin. The drug is not without irritating effects: It may produce a transient erythema and local skin burning and may also be teratogenic; thus it is not recommended for horses that are intended for breeding.

Experimentation on the use of DMSO in humans was progressing until the thalidomide catastrophe, whereupon new Food and Drug Administration (FDA) guidelines and policies were instituted. Lens changes appeared in experimental animals that had been treated with DMSO, and although no eye changes had been reported in humans, the clinical investigation was abruptly discontinued. The drug has been approved by the FDA solely for use in horses as a topical treatment for acute swelling that has resulted from trauma.

The properties of DMSO as a penetrating carrier of other medicines, as a local analgesic, anti-inflammatory, and bacteriostatic agent, and as a potentiator of other compounds may someday be helpful to the injured athlete.

Oral Enzymes

Oral proteolytic enzymes are sometimes used in sports medicine in an attempt to disperse fibrin, hematomas, and inflammatory edema. These enzymes include peptidases, such as chymotrypsin and trypsin, which may be combined in tablets and taken in a dose of one or two tablets four times a day.

Although the goal of breaking up fibrin deposits that mechanically bar the resolution of edema is desirable, these enzymes only seem to work when given parenterally in large doses to experimental animals *before* the inflammation is produced. Oral enzymes have been found to be ineffective in experimentally produced ringer injuries. As proteins, they are probably denatured in the acid environment of the stomach.

Hyaluronidase hydrolyzes hyaluronic acid to decrease the viscosity of the cellular-cementing ground substance. One or two milliliters of hyaluronidase may be injected directly into the injured area, but it may produce a hypersensitivity reaction. If the enzyme is used, the athlete should first be tested for hypersensitivity to it.

These enzymes have little, if any, advantage, and because of the possibility of a hypersensitivity reaction, their use is meddlesome and dangerous.

Counterirritants

Moist heat is the rubefacient of choice for athletes. However, counterirritants are sometimes used as components of massage mixtures when the athlete is away from the training room. These rubefacients irritate the skin and, by an axonal reflex, increase the local circulation to produce warmth and comfort. Counterirritants include methyl salicylate (oil of wintergreen) and camphor, a mild local anesthetic that numbs the skin. They may cause itching and hypersensitivity reactions, and plasma may escape and collect under the epidermis to form blisters.

Drug Abuse in Athletics

Alcohol

Alcohol was formerly used as a general anesthetic until it was found to be too dangerous for that purpose. If alcohol is applied to living cells, the cells' protoplasm becomes dehydrated and precipitates. Ingested alcohol depresses the reticular activating system and the cerebral cortex, represses control mechanisms, and thus frees the brain from inhibition. This depression may cause euphoria and lessen the realization of fatigue, but alcohol does not enhance the mental or physical abilities of an athlete. The drug has been used by marksmen to ease tension and reduce tremor to produce a steady aim, but the eye then loses its alertness for tracking a target.

Although the mechanism for the effect is unknown, moderate alcohol consumption appears to increase high-density lipoprotein levels and may help to protect against coronary artery disease, as myocardial infarction rates are lower in moderate drinkers than in nondrinkers.[64] This does not, however, justify recommending that nondrinkers start drinking moderately.

Caffeine

Coffee, tea, and many soft drinks contain caffeine, a drug related to aminophylline and theophylline. Caffeine may have a direct effect on the brain or act through the reticular activating system to stimulate the cerebral cortex to wakefulness and improve psychomotor performance, unless tremors and agitation supervene.

The drug also provokes the vasomotor center in the medulla to induce peripheral vasoconstriction and a rise in blood pressure and may generate an increase in heart rate, extrasystoles, and ventricular arrhythmias.

As an endurance activity progresses, the athlete derives more and more energy from free fatty acids. If a 70-kg athlete ingests 250 mg of caffeine (equivalent to two cups of coffee) 1 hour before competition, he may stimulate the release of free fatty acids. The fatty acids may then spare glycogen, enhance endurance, and reduce the perceived level of exertion.

Most people can tolerate a moderate amount of caffeine; others are more sensitive to the drug, and it may promote cardiac arrhythmias. Caffeine is a powerful diuretic that increases the work of the heart and promotes a loss of fluid that can endanger an endurance athlete. Caffeine can also delay and lighten sleep, promote muscle tenseness, and disturb the athlete's rest periods.

Nicotine

More than one third of the adult population in the United States smokes cigarettes. As the tobacco burns, about 4000 compounds are generated, including carbon monoxide, ammonia, hydrogen cyanide, nicotine and "tar," many carcinogens, and DDT. These noxious ingredients quickly reach the brain, where they stimulate the release of norepinephrine and dopamine from the brain tissue. The heavy smoker pays a high price in toxic effects for this stimulation. The smoke has a ciliotoxic action that paralyzes the cilia in the athlete's respiratory passages, causing normal filtering to fail and the respiratory tract to become susceptible to infection. Maximum ventilatory capacity drops as carbon monoxide enters the blood, resulting in hypoxia, and the products of combustion bind hemoglobin. Along with these immediate effects, the athlete risks deadly long-term hazards from smoking cigarettes, including lung cancer, emphysema, an acceleration of atherosclerosis with coronary artery disease, cerebral vascular disease, and peripheral vascular disease.

Marijuana

Marijuana comes from the hemp plant *Cannabis sativa*. Its psychological effects depend on the compound tetrahydrocannabinol. This drug produces a sedating sense of well-being, with euphoria, relaxation, and sleepiness. The user's balance is disturbed, muscular strength drops, and he becomes less aggressive and loses his motivation to perform.

A few marijuana cigarettes a day may induce subtle personality changes and lower an athlete's interest in achievement and his pursuit of conventional goals, an amotivational state antithetical to athletics. High doses may cause hallucinations, delusions, and panic that resemble a toxic psychosis.

Cocaine

Cocaine, found in the leaves of the coca bush *Erythroxylon coca,* is a local anesthetic that blocks the initiation and conduction of nerve impulses. For recreational use, the drug is inhaled or snorted through the nose to stimulate the user's central nervous system. It potentiates the action of catecholamines in the central nervous system and, like amphetamines, elevates mood, giving an increased sense of energy.

Cocaine seems to stimulate "reward areas" in the brain. Experimental animals will select cocaine over food, lose weight, mutilate themselves, and die. The drug masks fatigue through central stimulation, but the user may become restless and excited. The price paid for the uplifted mood is a depression that follows, and some persons may become paranoid. Higher doses of cocaine produce tremors and even convulsions.

Amphetamines

In the past, some football clubs bought amphetamines in bulk to distribute to their players to allay fatigue, increase alertness, uplift mood, and increase initiative, self-confidence, and ability to concentrate. The athlete may, however, become agitated, overaggressive, hostile, and show confusion and poor judgment—a sorry state for optimal athletic performance. If the dose is high enough, he may even panic and suffer paranoid hallucinations.

The athlete pays for the relief of fatigue and the increased feeling of alertness with subsequent dizziness, mental depression, and fatigue. Further, an overaggressive, hostile athlete with poor judgment may well injure himself or his opponents. These powerful drugs mask or disguise pain and remove the normal psychological and physiologic restraints that prevent overexertion. As a result, the athlete may suffer cardiovascular collapse, arrhythmias, or musculoskeletal damage. Rapid eye movement sleep is reduced, and the athlete's sleep pattern may take awhile to return to normal. He soon feels a need for larger and larger doses to produce the euphoric feeling and to blunt pain, and for sedatives to reduce the altered state of alertness.

Anabolic Steroids

Some athletes, especially in strength sports and tackle football, take anabolic steroids to gain a competitive advantage. The athlete may feel at an unfair disadvantage if he is not taking anabolic steroids while other competitors are so doing, and he may then take them for "insurance."[54] These drugs are used almost universally at higher levels of body building and competitive weightlifting. Some athletes have, however, refused to abuse their bodies, becoming champions at the top levels of body building and weightlifting without resorting to drugs.

Do anabolic steroids work? Although many studies on animals and athletes have failed to show strength gains with these drugs, the investigators have used low doses. In reality, weightlifters take high doses of 35 to 100 mg per day, although the optimum dosage range has yet to be established. While on steroids some competitive weightlifters report increases of 9 kg (20 lb) in the maximum weight that they can lift.[61] The anabolic steroids have a euphorogenic effect that aids athletic performance by influencing the athlete's attitude to-ward training and the quality of his training. By increasing competitiveness and aggression, he can train longer, harder, and more frequently and strenuously with less fatigue. His appetite also increases, and there may be a direct action of the anabolic steroid on the muscle cell that increases the content of skeletal muscle protein by raising the activity of RNA-polymerase in skeletal muscle nuclei.[44] If a particular muscle escapes exercise during training, it will fail to show the improvement displayed by exercised muscles.

On the other hand, these extremely powerful drugs have many severe side-effects. Even though some athletes have been fortunate, taking doses up to 300 mg per day for 2 years without apparent ill effects, jaundice, raised liver enzyme levels, gastrointestinal bleeding, prostatic blockage, sex drive changes, low sperm counts, and fatal primary tumors of the liver are among the dangerous side-effects known to be associated with these drugs. They may stunt the growth of youths by prematurely closing their growth plates. Unfortunately, many female weightlifters and female athletes in strength sports are now taking anabolic steroids. These women may develop permanent vocal cord alterations as well as hirsutism and acne while risking the more serious side-effects of reproductive system dysfunction and, in cases of pregnancy, genital malformations in the developing fetus.

Test stations are set up at major competitions to detect whether athletes are using anabolic steroids. However, the drugs pose special problems because they are taken long before competition begins. Since the effect of the steroid is to increase the intensity of training, the athlete has the benefit of a strength gain that lasts through the contest, but the steroid or its metabolites are no longer detectable.

A radioimmunoassay is used to screen for anabolic steroids. If the screening test is positive, gas chromatography and mass spectrometric methods can identify the metabolites of the steroid in the athlete's urine. Some athletes stop taking anabolic steroids about 10 days before a contest and then take instead a natural testosterone to promote high-intensity training and to deceive testers.

Random testing should perhaps be done throughout the year by a detection squad traveling around the world and popping up unexpectedly to check athletes. However, even with such expensive testing as is currently done, an athlete found to be using a drug risks disqualification for only about a year, not a great blow to his career. An alternative approach would be to forego testing and spend the millions saved on educational programs.

Nonetheless, the drugs are morally and legally unacceptable, conveying an unfair advantage to the taker, who is looking for an "edge." Taking a drug that aids performance is akin to doping an opponent to diminish his performance. Determined effort, dedicated training, good coaching, and proper diet can provide the motivation to increase the athlete's intensity of training, eliminating the need for ergogenic anabolic steroids. The overwhelming majority of great athletic accomplishments reflects this combination, without the use of drugs.

Sleep

Athletic excellence and strength development rests on systematic training, good nutrition, and proper sleep. An athlete in heavy training needs a lot of sleep, as a lack of rest will show up in poor performance and a greater chance of injury. However, he may, for many reasons, be unable to sleep at night. His room may be unfamiliar, he may be suffering from jet lag, or he simply may be anxious about an upcoming contest.

Drugs are sometimes given to induce sleep. More prescriptions are written in the United States for sedative-hypnotic-antianxiety drugs than for any other class of drugs. These drugs decrease rapid eye movement sleep, disrupt dream time, and may lead to psychological dependence. If they are used the night before and after every contest, the athlete may become addicted to them. Some athletes ride a roller coaster of barbiturates to calm down and amphetamines to train.

The time that passes before the athlete falls asleep—the sleep latency—may seem long but is usually less than 1 hour. This short period of wakefulness is preferable to a dependence on hypnotics. Athletes should be advised that each person's sleep requirements differ, with some not needing the standard 8 hours. Every effort must be made to assist the athlete to meet his sleep requirements. He should avoid food or coffee near bedtime and his bedroom should be cool, with walls painted in subdued colors and the bed furnished with clean sheets and a good mattress and pillow. The worried athlete may use relaxation techniques to calm down, occupying his mind with thoughts of keeping his muscles supple. Breathing rituals and self-hypnosis may also be used.

REFERENCES

1. ADAMS R et al: Ice skating therapy. Phys Sportsmed 6(3):71–81, 1978
2. AISENSON MR: Accidental injuries in epileptic children. Pediatrics 2:85–88, 1948
3. ANDERSON S: Four tips that may save your wrestling program. First Aider, Cramer 47:11, November 1977
4. ANDREWS GC et al: Treatment of acne vulgaris. JAMA 146:1107, 1951
5. BAER RL et al: High dose tetracycline therapy in severe acne. Arch Dermatol 112:479, 1976
6. BEACHAM BE: Equestrian cold paniculitis in women. Arch Dermatol 116:1025–1027, 1980
7. BEDO AV et al: Special olympic athletes face special medical needs. Phys Sportsmed 4(9):51–56, 1976
8. BIERMANN J, TOOHEY B: The Diabetics Sports and Exercise Book. Philadelphia, JB Lippincott, 1977
9. BLACK HM et al: Use of phenylbutazone in sports medicine: understanding the risks. Am J Sports Med 8:270–273, 1980
10. BRODIN MB: Jock itch. Phys Sportsmed 8(2):102–108, 1980
11. BROGDON BG, CROW NE: Observations on the "normal" spleen. Radiology 72:412–413, 1959
12. CHANG LW, O'BRIEN TF: Australia antigen serology in the Holy Cross football team hepatitis outbreak. Lancet 2:59–61, 1970
13. CLARK MW: Competitive sports for the disabled. Am J Sports Med 8:366–369, 1980
14. CORBITT RW et al: Epilepsy and contact sports. JAMA 229:820–821, 1974
15. COSTILL DL: Energy metabolism in diabetic distance runners. Phys Sportsmed 8(10):63–71, 1980
16. COSKEY RJ, MEHREGAN AH: Shoe boot pernio. Arch Dermatol 109:56–57, 1974

17. CRAIG RM: How safe is acetaminophen? JAMA 244:272, 1980

18. D'AMBROSIA RD: Cold injuries encountered in a winter resort. Cutis 20:365–368, 1977

19. DESHAZO WF III: Case report: ruptured spleen in a college football player. Phys Sportsmed 7(10):109–111, 1979

20. DESHAZO WF III: Returning to athletic activity after infectious mononucleosis. Phys Sportsmed 8(12):71–72, 1980

21. EGGLESTON PA: Management—not avoidance—for exercise-induced asthma. J Respir Dis 1(1):25–33, 1979

22. FREINKEL RK et al: Effect of tetracycline on the composition of sebum in acne vulgaris. N Engl J Med 273:850, 1964

23. FROSTBITE. Med Lett Drugs Ther 18:25 3 December 1976

24. FROSTBITE. Med Lett Drugs Ther 22:26 26 December 1980

25. GLICK JM: Therapeutic agents in musculoskeletal injuries. J Sports Med 3(3):136–138, 1975

26. GODFREY et al: Problems of interpreting exercise-induced asthma. J Allergy Clin Immunol 52:199–209, 1973

27. HEYMSFIELD SB et al: Accurate measurements of liver, kidney, and spleen volume and mass by computerized axial tomography. Ann Intern Med 90:185–187, 1979

28. INMAN WHW: Study of fatal bone marrow depression with special reference to phenylbutazone and oxyphenbutazone. Br Med J 1:1500–1505, 1977

29. JACKSON RW, FREDRICKSON A: Sports for the physically disabled. The 1976 Olympiad (Toronto). Am J Sports Med 7:293–296, 1979

30. KATLER E, WEISSMAN G: Steroids, aspirin and inflammation. Inflammation 2:295, 1977

31. KATZ RM: Asthmatics don't have to sit out sports. A clinical review. Phys Sportsmed 4(4):45–52, 1976

32. KRIKLER PM, ZILBERG B: Activity and hepatitis. Lancet 2:1043–1047, 1966

33. LEONARDS JR et al: Gastrointestinal blood loss during prolonged aspirin administration. N Engl J Med 289:1020, 1973

34. LIVINGSTON S: Should epileptics be athletes? Phys Sportsmed 3(4):67–72, 1975

35. LIVIINGSTON S, BERMAN W: Epilepsy and athletics. JAMA 224:236–238, 1973

36. LIVINGSTON S, BERMAN W: Participation of the epileptic child in contact sports. J Sports Med 2:170–174, 1974

37. MARSHALL E: Drugging of football players curbed by central monitoring play. NFL Claims. Science 203:626–628, 1979

38. MCLAURIN RL: Epilepsy and contact sports—factors contraindicating participation. JAMA 225:285–287, 1973

39. MEISEL A: Pharmacology of anti-inflammatory drugs. Hilton Head Seminar—Resources for Basic Science Educators. Chicago, American Academy of Orthopedic Surgery, 1980

40. MORSE LJ et al: The Holy Cross college football team hepatitis outbreak. JAMA 219:706–709, 1972

41. MORTON AR et al: Physical activity and the asthmatic. Phys Sportsmed 9(3):51–59, 1981

42. O'BRIEN WM: Indomethacin: a survey of clinical trials. Clin Pharmacol Ther 9:94, 1968

43. RAMSEY R, GOLDE DW: Aplastic anemia from veterinary phenylbutazone. JAMA 236:1049, 1976

44. ROGOZKIN V: Metabolic effects of anabolic steroid on skeletal muscle. Med Sci Sports 11:160–163, 1979

45. ROSENBERG DM et al: Acetaminophen and hepatic dysfunction in infectious mononucleosis. South Med J 70:660–661, 1977

46. ROSS J: Blind break through old barriers to sports. Phys Sportsmed 5(3):98–104, 1977

47. RUTKOW IM: Rupture of the spleen in infectious mononucleosis. Arch Surg 113:718–720, 1978

48. RYAN AJ (moderator): Infectious mononucleosis in athletes. Phys Sportsmed 6(2):41–56, 1978

49. RYAN AJ (moderator): Sport and recreation for the handicapped. Phys Sportsmed 6(3):45–67, 1978

50. SAMTER J, BEERS RF: Intolerance to aspirin. Ann Intern Med 68:975, 1968

51. SHAPIRA W: Competing in a silent world of sports. Phys Sportsmed 3(11):99–105, 1975

52. SHAPIRA W: It's a new ball game for hemophiliac youngsters. Phys Sportsmed 3(12):63–64, 1975

53. SIGEL RM et al: Evaluation of spleen size during routine liver imaging with 99mTc and the scintillation camera. J Nucl Med 11:689–692, 1970

54. STACKPOLE PJ: Effects of anabolic steroids on strength development and performance. Nat Strength Coaches Assoc J 2(2):30–33, 1980

55. TAYLOR KJ, MILAN J: Differential diagnosis of chronic splenomegaly by gray-scale ultrasonography: clinical observations and digital A-scan analysis. Br J Radiol 49:519–525, 1976

56. The Athlete with Sickle Cell Trait. A Statement of the NCAA Commitee on Competitive Safeguards and Medical Aspects of sports. Athletic Training 10(1):19, 1975

57. VANE JR: Prostaglandins and the aspirin-like drugs. Hosp Prac 7:61, 1972

58. VANE JR: The mode of action of aspirin and similar compounds. J Allergy Clin Immunol 58:691, 1976

59. VAN ITALLIE TB: Nutrition and athletic performance. JAMA 160:1120–1126, 1956

60. WACKER WEC et al: The Holy Cross hepatitis outbreak. Arch Intern Med 130:357–360, 1972

61. WARD P: The effect of an anabolic steroid on strength and lean body mass. Med Sci Sports 5:277–282, 1973

62. WASHBURN B: Frostbite: what is it—how to prevent it—emergency treatment. N Engl J Med 266:974–989, 1962

63. WERBLOW JA et al: Nutrition: what's the score? Nat Strength Coaches Assoc J 2(2):20–21, 1980

64. WILLET W et al: Alcohol consumption and high-density lipoprotein cholesterol in marathon runners. N Engl J Med 303:1159–1161, 1980

Successful participation in athletic activities requires preparation. Such preparation, often called training, might be described as the systematic participation in physical exercise for the purpose of improving performance in an athletic activity. The process of training can be interpreted broadly to include learning of competitive strategies, perfection of motor skills, and establishment of a proper psychologic outlook. I shall focus here on the physical fitness aspect of athletic performance, provide guidelines for the improvement of basic fitness components in athletes, and give primary emphasis to training for improved endurance performance.

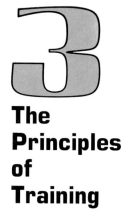

The Principles of Training

Physiologic Bases of Exercise

Metabolic Systems

Performing an athletic activity depends on the contraction of skeletal muscles, and the energy that fuels these contractions is provided through a complex series of chemical reactions localized in the individual skeletal muscle cells (fibers).[10] The single immediate source of this chemical energy is adenosine triphosphate (ATP). During contraction, ATP, a high-energy phosphate compound, is hydrolyzed to produce adenosine diphosphate (ADP) and phosphoric acid. The breakage of ATP's terminal high-energy phosphate bond releases energy used by the muscle fiber to cause contraction.

Because only a very small concentration of ATP is maintained in the muscle fiber, sustained or repetitive muscle contractions depend on rapid resynthesis of ATP. The energy to suport this resynthesis is provided through the biochemical processes of aerobic and anaerobic metabolism. Aerobic metabolism occurs in the presence of oxygen, whereas anaerobic processes function without oxygen.

Anaerobic Metabolism

At the onset of muscular work the available ATP supply is rapidly used. A small amount of ATP may be resynthesized at the expense of another high-energy phosphate source, creatine phosphate (CP), whose

RUSSELL R. PATE

role is critical because it provides a reservoir of phosphate bond energy that can be tapped immediately, thereby preventing any lag in the ATP supply. As is the case for ATP, however, only very finite amounts of CP are maintained in the fiber; indeed, at the onset of high-intensity exercise (sprinting) the available supplies of both ATP and CP could, theoretically, be depleted in a few seconds. Clearly the store of energy represented by ATP and CP is too small to support endurance exercise—that is, the *capacity* of the ATP–CP system is low. Its maximum *power* (rate of energy expenditure) is very high, however, and consequently the ATP–CP system is the predominant energy source for high-intensity, short-duration exercise.

Exercise of longer duration but lower intensity is supported, predominantly, by a second anaerobic process, *anaerobic glycolysis,* which involves the breakdown of the carbohydrate glycogen ("muscle starch") through a sequentially arranged series of 11 enzyme-catalyzed chemical reactions. Glycogen is no more than a matrix of individual glucose molecules. In glycolysis the glucose molecules are split from the glycogen matrix and enzymatically altered so as to yield two pyruvic acid molecules. Without oxygen, pyruvic acid is converted to lactic acid. The process of glycolysis releases an amount of energy from the glucose molecule sufficient to resynthesize two ATP molecules. As compared with the ATP–CP system, anaerobic glycolysis has less power but greater capacity. In anaerobic glycolysis, the rate of energy production is limited by the maximum rate of the individual chemical reactions that constitute the entire system, a rate slower than that of the ATP–CP system. The total amount of energy released, however, is limited only by the amount of glycogen available (usually plentiful) and the person's tolerance for the system's end-product, lactic acid. If lactic acid accumulates in the muscle cell, tissue acidosis and impaired functioning result, with fatigue being the outcome. Anaerobic glycolysis is a very important supplier of ATP energy during high-intensity work of moderate duration (30 seconds to 2 minutes). In such forms of work the capacity and power of the glycolytic system are well matched to the demands of the activity.

Aerobic Metabolism

The ultimate source of all energy expended by skeletal muscle, aerobic metabolism occurs primarily in the mitochondria and results in the complete oxidation of either carbohydrate or fat while producing two benign end-products, water and carbon dioxide..[7, 13]

As compared with anaerobic processes, the ATP of aerobic metabolism is characterized by a relatively low power but very great capacity. The amount of ATP energy that can be produced through aerobic metabolism is essentially infinite, being limited only by the person's store of food stuffs, such as glycogen and free fatty acids. In contrast, the power of the aerobic system is quite limited because it is restricted by the rate at which oxygen can be delivered to the active tissues by the cardiorespiratory system. The maximal aerobic power is usually expressed in terms of maximum oxygen consumption.

The aerobic metabolic system is used preferentialy during low-intensity but sustained exercise. Because the end-products of aerobic metabolism are not fatigue producing and the needed raw materials (*i.e.,* oxygen and glycogen or free fatty acids) are available, for practical purposes, in unlimited quantities, the aerobic process may continue indefinitely.

Relation Between Aerobic and Anaerobic Metabolism

Some athletic activities involve forms of muscular work that derive all the needed ATP energy from a single metabolic process. The long jump in track and field, for example, is an activity that requires a very high rate of energy expenditure for only a few seconds, and consequently the anaerobic processes provide virtually all the required ATP. In contrast, a marathon run involves moderately intense activity sustained for several hours. Many athletic activities, however, require that energy be provided through a combination of the three energy-yielding systems. During the first few seconds of the 400-meter sprint (total duration, 45 to 60 seconds), for example, most energy comes through the breakdown of available ATP and CP stores. Rapidly, though, anaerobic glycolysis begins to predominate as the provider of ATP energy. Although anaerobic glycolysis continues to function at its maximum rate throughout the run, aerobic metabolism gradually increases to provide, in total, about 25% of the ATP used. Performance in the 400-meter sprint is a function of the maximal power of the three systems in combination and the capacity of the two anaerobic systems. World-class 400-meter sprinters tend to have high anaerobic power, very high anaerobic capacity, and reasonably well-developed maximum aerobic power.

Cardiorespiratory Function

In athletic activities such as distance running and swimming, performance depends on, to a considerable extent, the maximum aerobic power ($\dot{V}O_2$max).[2] The higher the $\dot{V}O_2$max, the greater the rate at which work may be done over extended periods and the longer the work may be done at any submaximal intensity. In activities such as football, aerobic metabolism functions during recovery periods to replenish the stores of ATP and CP and to assist in clearing lactic acid. Thus the development of a high $\dot{V}O_2$max is probably beneficial in most athletic activities and critical in many.

As mentioned previously, $\dot{V}O_2$max is limited primarily by the maximum rate at which oxygen can be delivered to the active skeletal muscle tissues. The cardiorespiratory system, which transports oxygen, plays a key role in supporting skeletal muscle metabolism during exercise and comprises four functional components: lungs and respiratory tract, heart, blood vessels, and blood. During exercise the overall system responds in such a way as to increase the rate of oxygen delivery to the active skeletal muscle tissues, where the demand for oxygen increases markedly. Alterations in the functioning of each component contribute to this increased rate of oxygen transport.

Ventilation

As exercise begins, the rate and depth of breathing increase rapidly and substantially. Ventilation, regulated by both neural and hu-

moral factors, increases to a level sufficient to maintain adequate diffusion gradients across the alveolar membrane for both oxygen and carbon dioxide. At very high workloads, arterial blood is maintained at a fully oxygenated level, consequently, for most persons, ventilatory function is not considered to be a factor limiting the $\dot{V}O_2$max.

Cardiac Output

Perhaps the most important determinant of $\dot{V}O_2$max is the maximal cardiac output ($\dot{Q}$max). Cardiac output, the volume of blood pumped by the heart per minute, increases rapidly at the beginning of exercise but takes 2 to 3 minutes to reach a plateau. The level at which $\dot{Q}$ reaches a plateau is highly related to exercise intensity (and $\dot{V}O_2$) and the relation between the two variables is linear up to $\dot{Q}$max. $\dot{Q}$max is attained at the same exercise intensity as $\dot{V}O_2$max and is equal to the product of maximal heart rate and maximal stroke volume. Heart rate is linearly related to exercise intensity, $\dot{V}O_2$, and $\dot{Q}$; maximal heart rate (HR max) is age related (HR max $\approx 220 -$ age in years) but is not related to fitness level. Stroke volume, the volume of blood pumped with each beat, is a function of heart size, venous filling pressure, and myocardial contractility. Stroke volume increases with exercise but reaches a maximum at workloads requiring about 50% of the $\dot{V}O_2$max. Maximal stroke volume increases with endurance training and results in an increased $\dot{Q}$max, which in turn is reflected by a greater $\dot{V}O_2$max. Thus adaptations in myocardial function resulting in increased stroke volume represent a critical component of the body's response to endurance exercise training.

Vessels

Vasomotor function suports exercise performance by redistributing the blood flow so as to increase oxygen delivery to the active skeletal muscles. During exercise, dilation of arterioles in skeletal muscle and constriction of arterioles in nonactive tissues (particularly the digestive system) may result in tripling of the blood flow to skeletal muscle. Increased blood flow is also provided to the skin during prolonged exercise, a response that facilitates dissipation of heat to the environment and, in hot, humid conditions, may require a fraction of the cardiac output high enough to decrease significantly the fraction provided to the working muscles. With exercise, the volume of the venous system is reduced through a general vasoconstriction of venules, a response that tends to promote return of blood to the heart.

Arteriovenous Oxygen Difference

As indicated by the Fick equation, VO_2 is equal to the product of cardiac output and arteriovenous oxygen difference $(A - VO_2)$. The oxygen-carrying capacity of the blood is about 20 ml of oxygen per 100 ml of blood; however, under resting conditions only about 25% of this oxygen is removed in the tissues. With exercise, arteriovenous oxygen difference increases as the tissue's demand for oxygen increases. With high-intensity exercise, total body $A - VO_2$ (left ventricular blood versus right artrial blood) reaches values as high as 75% to 80%. Skeletal muscle tissue $A - VO_2$ may reach values aproaching 100%.

$A - VO_2$ reflects the ability of the skeletal muscle tissue to use, in aerobic metabolism, the oxygen offered to it by the cardiorespiratory system. Endurance exercise training causes profound adaptations in the skeletal muscle tissue: specifically, increases in mitochondrial density, myoglobin concentration, and aerobic enzyme activities. These changes are specific to those muscles active during training. Collectively the adaptations contribute to an increased maximal rate of aerobic metabolism in the muscle tissue and an increased whole body VO_2max.

In summary, the body's physiologic response to acute exercise includes an increased rate of aerobic metabolism in the active skeletal muscles, a metabolic response supported by the cardiorespiratory system, which in turn increases its rate of oxygen delivery to the active muscles. Cardiac, vasomotor, and ventilatory responses contribute to an increased rate of blood flow to the working muscles. The physiologic response to endurance exercise training involves both *central* (*i.e.,* cardiorespiratory) and *peripheral* (*i.e.,* muscle tissue) adaptations: Central adaptation is manifested as an increased maximal cardiac output and thus increased maximal rates of blood flow and oxygen delivery to the working muscles; peripheral adaptation allows an increased rate of oxygen use for the production of ATP energy. The outcome of these adaptations is an increase in the person's tolerance for sustained, whole-body moderately intense exercise.

Determinants of Endurance Exercise Performance

Maximal Oxygen Consumption

As mentioned previously, VO_2max (ml/kg/min) is a prime determinant of exercise endurance performance. VO_2max reflects the maximum rate at which ATP energy may be produced aerobically, and thus establishes a maximum rate at which work can be done without tapping anaerobic energy sources. The VO_2max *per se* is most important as a determinant of performance in activities that require maximal rates of energy expenditure for 4 to 10 minutes. In such activities the athlete is able to work at or near the VO_2max level throughout the competition and, although anaerobic sources do contribute to the total energy supply, the aerobic process is predominant, contributing 75% to 90% of the total energy expenditure. Clearly, in activites such as the mile run or the 100 meter swim, VO_2max should be very highly correlated with performance.

Anaerobic Threshold

In longer duration activities, other variables combine with the VO_2max to determine the maximum rate at which work can be done. One such variable is the anaerobic threshold. During a graded exercise test, individuals begin to produce and accumulate lactic acid at some characteristic intensity of work. Among different persons, this intensity varies from 50% to 90% of the VO_2max. Since lactic acid accumulation results in fatigue, exercise cannot be continued for more than a few minutes at workloads requiring oxygen to be consumed at levels above the anaerobic threshold. Thus, the higher the anaerobic threshold, the higher the $\dot{V}O_2$ and workload that can be sustained for extended periods. Conceivably, then, if two athletes have the same $\dot{V}O_2$max but different anaerobic thresholds, the one with the higher anaerobic threshold will have an advantage in any longer duration activity. The anaerobic threshold tends to increase with endurance training. In the early stages of a training program, the $\dot{V}O_2$max and the anaerobic threshold tend to increase concurrently. Later in a program and in mature athletes who have attained their ultimate $\dot{V}O_2$max, the anaerobic threshold may still be improved through appropriate training procedures.

Efficiency

Another important variable in endurance performance is efficiency. Efficiency, to the engineer, refers to the ratio of work done by a machine to energy used by it. In humans, with activites such as running or swimming, efficiency is often expressed as the rate of oxygen consumption ($\dot{V}O_2$ in ml/kg/min) needed to perform work at a given rate (*e.g.,* running at 9.6 km/h (6 miles/h) or swimming at 6.75 m/min (75 yards/min)). Individual rates of oxygen consumption needed to work at a given pace vary, due in part to differences in athletes' skill level. The significance of work efficiency is seen when it is considered in combination with the $\dot{V}O_2$max and the anaerobic threshold. The more efficient athlete needs a lower $\dot{V}O_2$ at any given work rate and therefore will work at a lower percentage of the maximal oxygen uptake at any given work rate and experience less fatigue; he also will be able to work at a higher rate before reaching the anaerobic threshold.

Muscle Fiber Types

Physiologic variables such as $\dot{V}O_2$max, efficiency, and anaerobic threshold all are subject to improvement through appropriate forms of training; however, each related variable and

overall endurance performance are related to inherited, genetic factors. In recent years, studies have shown that a person's distribution of skeletal muscle fiber types is a major determinant of performance potential in certain athletic activities.

Human skeletal muscle fibers may be categorized as either fast twitch (FT) or slow twitch (ST). Fast twitch fibers are particularly well adapted for speed and power activities because they contract rapidly and possess metabolically a high glycolytic capability. In contrast, ST fibers contract more slowly but are quite fatigue resistant because they possess a well-developed aerobic capability. Individuals vary greatly in the relative distribution of FT and ST fibers. Generally persons who inherit a high percentage of ST fibers possess greater potential for development of a high $\dot{V}O_2$max and a high anaerobic threshold, and thus greater potential for performing endurance activities. Those who inherit a high percentage of FT fibers are better adapted to high-power activities. Performance in any athletic activity, however, is multifactorial and is not determined by any single variable. Muscle fiber type is only one variable, and it alone cannot be used to derive an accurate prediction of a person's current ability or ultimate performance-potential.

Principles of Training

Typical training programs comprise numerous specific training activities and techniques. Although selecting the proper individual activities is important, combining these activities in a complementary fashion so that the result is an optimal overall training program is crucial. Adherence to the following principles should aid coaches, athletes, trainers, and team physicians in designing proper comprehensive training programs.

Overload

Perhaps the most basic principle of training is overload. Most physiologic systems can adapt to functional demands that exceed those encountered in normal, daily life. Training often systematically exposes selected physiololgic systems to intensities of work or function that exceed those to which the system is already adapted. A key, however, is to avoid excessive overload because physiologic systems are unable to adapt to stresses too extreme.

Consistency

There is no substitute for consistency in a training program. Successful athletes, almost without exception, adhere to a training regimen with extreme regularity for several years or more. Most physiologic systems require exposure to overloading activites three times a week or more. The required frequency of training, however, depends on the season, the athlete, activity, and the specific component of fitness. Thus a particular athlete might train 12 times a week during certain stages of the year and only three times a week at other stages; he might participate in endurance training six times a week and resistance training (*e.g.,* weight lifting) three times a week.

Specificity

The effects of training are highly specific to the particular physiologic system overloaded, to the particular muscle groups used, and to the particular muscle fibers performing the work. No single training technique can produce any and all desired outcomes; commercial advertising claims to that effect should be rejected.

Because athletic performance usually depends on the development of several physical fitness components, most training programs should include several training techniques and several modifications of each specific technique. The swimmer's training program, for instance, might comprise a combination of swimming activities using various strokes, intensities, and variations. In addition, the swimmer might participate in stretching exercises for flexibility and resistance exercises for muscular strength and muscular endurance.

Progression

Successful training programs plan for a steady rate of progression over a long period. If an athlete is to improve over several years of participation, his training program must progress so that the appropriate physiologic systems continue to be overloaded. At the same time, however, too rapid an increase of the training stress may lead to exhaustion and impaired performance. The job of the coach or trainer is to structure training programs that continue to challenge the athlete but avoid excessive overload.

Individuality

No two programs are exactly alike physiologically, and thus no two athletes should be expected to respond exactly the same to a particular training regimen. Factors such as age, sex, maturity, current fitness level, years of training, body size, somatotype, and psychological characteristics should be considered by the coach in designing each athlete's training regimen. In large groups in which absolute individualization of training programs may be impractical, the coach should strive for individualization by homogeneously grouping athletes. Successful teams are composed of successful individual athletes, and the optimal training program is that which best fits the needs of each team member.

Periodization

Periodization refers to the tendency for athletic performance to vary cyclically over time. Few athletes are able to sustain a peak performance level for more than a few weeks, and thus training and competitive schedules should be structured so that peak performances are attained at the desired time. Intense training and competition tends to bring the athlete to his optimal performance level. The key, of course, is to avoid attaining this level too early in the competitive season. Ideally the training program should build to maximum intensity one half to two thirds through the season so that peak performances are achieved during championship competitions at season's end.

Plateauing

In many athletes, performance tends to improve incrementally rather than in a smooth, steady fashion. An athlete may spend weeks, months, or even years on a performance plateau, leading to considerable frustration. If the athlete and trainer are certain that the training program has progressed properly, that illness is not a factor, and that the athlete has not attained his ultimate performance-potential, the athlete should persevere and maintain confidence that a substantial improvement could occur at any time.

Stress

Stress has been defined by Hans Selye, the famous stress researcher, as the body's nonspecific response to external stressors. When the body is exposed to extreme stressors for extended periods, the so-called stress syndrome is elicited, which may lead to a stage of exhaustion typified by fatigue, illness, and injury. Coaches, athletes, trainers, and team physicians must recognize that strenuous training represents a significant stressor which, if combined with other physical or psychological stressors, may lead the athlete into a stage of exhaustion. Such exhaustion, of course, is not consistent with optimal training or performance. Prevention of stress-induced exhaustion can be accomplished by designing properly individualized training programs, by carefully observing the athlete for signs of fatigue (*e.g.,* upper respiratory illness, blood shot eyes, loss of concentration), and by reducing the training load if the athlete encounters other unavoidable stressors (*e.g.,* examinations, personal conflicts, change of environment). Sensitive coaches and trainers can prevent most stress-related illnesses in their athletes. Those programs that subscribe to the "survival of the fittest" philosophy, however, can expect to lose many athletes to preventable illness and injury.

Competitive Stress

Competition is physiologically and psychologically more stressful than training, and too frequent competitions pose great risk to the athlete. Athletes who compete too frequently are particularly prone to the stress-related difficulties mentioned above. Because sporting activities vary greatly in their physical demands, drawing a generalization on the optimal frequency of competition is not possible. One may conclude, however, that the more strenuous the activity, the less frequently one should engage in competition. Contrasting examples would be golfers who compete 4 days a week over a 30- to 40-week season and marathon runners who compete at the full marathon distance only two or three times a year.

Guidelines for Training the Aerobic System

As discussed above, energy used in endurance exercise is provided primarily through aerobic muscle metabolism, which depends on the transport of oxygen by the cardiorespiratory system. Improvements in endurance performance are attained primarily through increases in VO_2max and anaerobic threshold. These increases are secondary to muscle metabolic and cardiorespiratory functional alterations, which can be generated through proper forms of exercise training. This section summarizes the procedures to be followed in designing training programs for improved performance of aerobic exercise.

Modes of Exercise

Numerous specific forms of exercise may be used to generate improvements in aerobic work capacity. All proper aerobic activities increase the body's rate of aerobic metabolism, increase the heart rate, and allow these increases to be sustained for extended periods. Primary aerobic activities include those that allow metabolic and cardiorespiratory functions to be increased to a particular predetermined level and maintained at that level throughout the activity. Secondary aerobic activities, which include many of the popular recreational games and sports, cause a more intermittent increase in cardiorespiratory functions and are less easily regulated in terms of work intensity.

Primary and Secondary Aerobic Activities

Primary	Secondary
Walking	Tennis
Jogging/running	Handball
Swimming	Racquetball
Cycling	Squash
Cross-country skiing	Basketball
Ice skating	Dance

Primary aerobic activities generate a training effect in less time than do secondary activities and are preferred for persons with impaired heart function in whom exercise intensity must be rigorously controlled. Many persons, however, find secondary aerobic activities more enjoyable, and enjoyment, of course, can promote adherance to an exercise regimen. For a given athlete, the ideal aerobic activity is that most similar to the activity for which he is training (principle of specificity) and to which he is most likely to adhere.

Frequency

Improvements in aerobic work capacity may be generated in secondary beginners with as few as two training sessions a week. Sedentary beginners, however, improve at close to the optimal rate with three sessions a week (nonconsecutive days).[1] In some athletes, daily training sessions may be needed to maintain an already high capacity for endurance work. In activities such as distance running and swimming, many athletes train twice a day. The advantages of twice a day training sessions have not been clearly documented, but apparently a high frequency of training contributes to a high-exercise caloric expenditure. The continually improving world standards in endurance activities may in part be due to the increasing amount of energy expended in training by today's world class athletes. The optimal training frequency for a given athlete is a function of his current fitness level, the relative importance of aerobic function in the particular activity for which he is training, and individual tolerance for training stress.

Duration

The average person attains an acceptable level of cardiorespiratory fitness by participating in a primary aerobic activity for a duration of 20 to 30 minutes three times a week. Sedentary beginners may need to start with intermittent exercise (e.g., alternate walking and jogging), buildiing gradually to 20 to 30 minutes of continuous activity. Endurance athletes, of course, may need much longer durations of exercise to attain full potential; marathon runners and swimmers, for example, often train for 2 to 3 hours. For most team sports, however, athletes who regularly participate in continuous aerobic activity for one-half hour will develop a cardiorespiratory fitness level consistent with championship caliber performance.

Intensity

Intensity of exercise may be quantified in several ways; perhaps most convenient is heart rate. Because heart rate and rate of aerobic energy expenditure ($\dot{V}O_2$) are linearly related and, for each person, maximal heart rate and maximal $\dot{V}O_2$ are attained at the same exercise work load, the percentage of $\dot{V}O_2$max may be accurately estimated from the percentage of maximum heart rate (see Figure 3-1). The threshold for generation of an aerobic training effect is about 60% of the $\dot{V}O_2$max, which corresponds to about 70% of the maximum heart rate.

One technique for estimating the heart rate that corresponds to the training threshold exercise intensity is provided by the following equation:

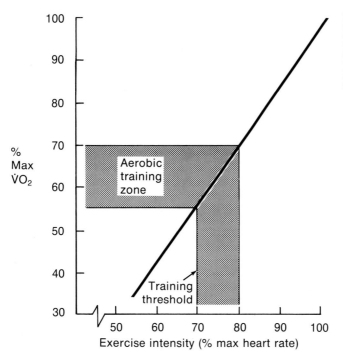

FIG. 3-1
Relation between percentage of maximal heart rate and percentage of maximal oxygen content.

THR = RHR + 0.6 (MHR − RHR), where
THR = training heart rate (beats/min),
MHR = maximum heart rate (beats/min), and
RHR = resting heart rate (beats/min).

Resting heart rate may be determined by counting the radial or carotid pulse while the individual is resting. Maximum heart rate can be estimated by the following equation:

MHR (bpm) = 220−age in years

The aforementioned technique provides a lower limit for training intensity. For trained persons, a somewhat higher intensity may be appropriate for sustained, continuous training. Very high-intensity training, at heart rates approaching maximum levels, is appropriate for some endurance athletes and for athletes striving to maximize both aerobic power and anaerobic capacity.

Specific Training Techniques

Primary aerobic activities may be used in several specific ways. Of these aerobic activities, running has spawned the greatest range of training techniques, and these methods are discussed below. Many of the techniques described are easily adapted for use by swimmers and cyclists.

Continuous Activity

Perhaps the most commonly used aerobic training technique is continuous activity. With such activity, the heart rate is increased to a predetermined level and maintained at that level for the duration of the training session. The guidelines presented in the previous section apply most directly to continuous training. The intensity of continuous activity may be varied from one training session to the next. The bulk of the training for endurance activities should consist of continuous activity of moderate intensity (70% to 80% maximum heart rate) and relatively long duration, so called long slow distance training. The endurance athlete will benefit, however, from occasional bouts of higher intensity continuous training 85% to 90% of maximum heart rate) of moderate duration.

Interval Training

Interval training involves alternating periods of very intense work with periods of active recovery. Interval training is usually done in a controlled environment (*e.g.,* a track) where the duration of work and recovery periods may be accurately timed. Interval training offers the benefit of allowing the athlete to perform, in total, a considerable volume of very high-intensity exercise in a single training session. An endurance swimmer, for instance, might perform 20 repetitions of a 50-meter sprint with 30 seconds of recovery between each sprint; altogether the swimmer will have covered 1000 meters at very high intensity. All approaches to interval training require that the following variables be designated in advance: duration and intensity of the work interval, duration and intensity of the recovery period, and the number of repetitions. Intensity of exercise may be designated in terms of heart rate. During the work interval, heart rate should increase to 75% or more of the maximum heart rate; during recovery it should fall to about 60% of the maximum heart rate.

Repetition Training

Repetition training differs from interval training only in intensity of exercise during the work and recovery phases. The work phase of repetition training should be almost exhaustive, and the recovery phase should be almost complete. For instance, in a given repetition training session, an 800-meter runner might perform two 600-meter runs at race-pace with a full recovery intervening between the two.

Fartlek Running

Fartlek running involves a combination of techniques such that continuous, interval, and repetition training are used in a single session. Fartlek is a Swedish term meaning "speed play" and denotes that the various intensities of work are selected by the athlete on an unstructured basis. A typical fartlek running session might involve an hour of continuous running during which the athlete runs, in random order, several fast sprints, interval runs, and repetition runs. Fartlek training may be conducted in an attractive environment (*e.g.,* park or golf course) and thus may be a relatively enjoyable means for the athlete to participate in high-intensity exercise.

Circuit Training, Parcours

Circuit training provides a combination of training techniques and is particularly well adapted for groups. The individual athlete rotates through a series of stations, and at each performs a different exercise. Circuit routines may include activities to improve muscular strength, muscular endurance, flexibility, and other fitness components. The training session can involve an alternation between continuous aerobic training and a series of strength and flexibility exercises.

A recently popularized modification of the circuit training concept is the parcours. A parcours is, essentially, a graded jogging trail along which exercise stations have been erected. The participant jogs from station to station, performing a different calisthenic exercise at each stop. Often attractive signs and suitable permanent equipment are provided at each exercise station.

Summary

The energy for sustained muscular work is provided through the process of aerobic metabolism. Performance of aerobic exercise depends on the cardiorespiratory system, which provides the active skeletal muscles with needed oxygen. The primary determinant of athletic performance in endurance activities is maximal oxygen uptake; however, efficiency and anaerobic threshold also affect the rate at which work is done for extended periods.

Training programs should be designed in accordance with established principles of training.

In training the aerobic system, research indicates that if a primary aerobic activity is used, 20 to 30 minutes of continuous activity three times a week at about 70% of maximum heart rate will result in the desired training effect.

Basic principles of exercise training are similar for everyone. But because each subgroup of the population possesses certain unique characteristics and needs, training programs should be tailored so as to optimize the benefits for the specific participant group. The following sections provide guidelines for the design of exercise training programs for several specific populations, including special training problems encountered by competitive athletes.

Fitness Programs for Adult Beginners

Since the early 1970s a rapidly increasing number of adult Americans have begun participating in regular, vigorous exercise. The reasons for this trend are complex, but clearly many adults have begun exercising to control body weight and to reduce the risk of coronary heart disease. Many Americans now accept regular exercise as an important aspect of a healthy lifestyle. Although a large number of adults begin exercising each year, many do not become habitual exercisers. Many drop out owing to failure to improve fitness; exercise-related injuries; or fatigue and muscle soreness after overtraining. Much of the attrition from personal fitness programs can be ascribed to improper training programs; the information that follows is intended to provide the knowledge needed to prescribe proper exercise programs for adult beginners.

Objectives and Potential Benefits

Physical fitness is the ability to perform daily tasks with vigor and alertness, without undue fatigue and with ample energy to enjoy leisure time pursuits and to meet unforeseen emergencies. This suggests that a person is physically fit if he is able to cope readily with the physical demands presented by his preferred life-style and selected environment. Of course, in our modern technological society, the life-style of the typical adult presents a few physical challenges. Thus it might seem that the average American would have no need to maintain a high level of physical fitness. Mounting evidence, however, suggests the opposite—that modern man needs, more than ever, to be concerned about his physical activity habits.

Research and clinical evidence strongly suggests that several of the more frequently observed chronic diseases are related to physical inactivity.[6] Sedentary living is itself a risk factor for developing coronary heart disease (CHD), and some studies have indicated that exercise may ameliorate other CHD risk factors, such as elevated blood lipid concentrations and hypertension. Obesity, a risk factor for CHD, hypertension, and diabetes, is clearly linked to low levels of habitual physical activity and, in most patients, is responsive to exercise therapy. Lower back pain, one of the most frequently reported health problems, is most typically due to inflexibility of the low back-hamstring region and weakness of the abdominal musculature. An accepted conservative treatment for lower back pain is exercise.

Although regular exercise may aid in the prevention and treatment of certain disease processes, it also contributes profoundly to "positive health," or "wellness." Most sedentary persons who initiate proper exercise programs report "feeling better and more energetic" within a few weeks Although this effect may be at least partially psychological, a convincing physiological explanation can be presented. With training, as a person's physical working capacity (VO_2max) increases, the percentage of his maximum working capacity required by any submaximal level of exertion decreases. Because fatigue is highly related to the percentage of VO_2max required by physical activities, the fitter person will experience less fatigue in response to standard physical work situations. Greater enjoyment of activities that require strenuous exertion results, as does less fatigue during long duration, low-intensity activity (*e.g.,* occupational endeavors).

The objectives of adult physical fitness programs should focus primarily on the health-related fitness components, including cardiorespiratory fitness, body composition, and neuromuscular function of the lower trunk region.[11, 14] Proper programs can, and should, be structured so as to develop and maintain an acceptable level of fitness in each of the health-related components. Although the designation of any specific fitness level as "acceptable" must be somewhat arbitrary, fitness levels that seem to be consistent with the avoidance of associated health problems and with maintenance of an acceptable physical working capacity may be identified.

Risks and Safety Procedures

For a small percentage of adults, the risks associated with regular exercise outweigh the potential benefits; consequently, those persons must be identified before initiation of a training program. Persons younger than 35 years of age with no history of cardiovascular disease and who show no elevation of CHD risk factors (*e.g.,* smoking, hypertension, serum cholesterol > 250 mg/dl) may safely start exercise programs without medical clearance. Persons older than 35 and sedentary should be advised to consult with a physician before initiating an exercise program. Regardless of age, those with a history of cardiovascular disease or who show significant CHD risk factors should be examined by a physician and, if feasible, complete a graded exercise stress test before beginning exercise. Among properly screened persons, the risks associated with regular exercise are minimal. Serious cardiovascular complications during exercise are exceedingly rare. Indeed, for most of the population, regular exercise is no more dangerous than any other normal activity of daily life. Some physical activities, such as jogging, involve risk of musculoskeletal injury. Mostly, these injuries can be prevented through use of proper equipment and training procedures; a small fraction of adults do, however, encounter considerable difficulties with running activities and should be encouraged to try non-weight-bearing activities such as swimming or cycling.

Principles of Adult Fitness Programs

The principles of training outlined previously apply to adult fitness programs. Research has shown that an acceptable level of cardiorespiratory fitness can be developed through participation in a primary aerobic activity three times a week for 20 to 30 minutes a session.[1] Intensity of exercise should be such as to elevate the heart rate to about 70% of maximum. Greater frequencies, durations, and intensities of activities may be safely employed by already trained participants; such training will lead to further enhancement of cardiorespiratory fitness.

All the basic tenets of training apply to adult exercisers, but two principles are of particular significance. The principle of *progression* is important for sedentary adults who seek to attain higher levels of fitness. Such persons must be convinced to begin with a very light dose of exercise and then to increase the weekly quantity of exercise very gradually. Many orthopedic injuries experienced by beginning adult exercisers are caused by a training load that increases too rapidly. Also, exercise regimens that begin at too high an intensity contribute to the high rate of recidivism in adult beginners. High-intensity exercise may contribute to muscle soreness, overuse-injuries, and long-term fatigue, all of which lead to lack of adherence to an exercise regimen.

Also of profound importance in adult fitness programs is *individuality*. Training programs for adults must be individualized according to the age, sex, current fitness level, health status, and interests of the participant. The principles of exercise prescribed above contribute to individualization by adjusting the intensity of activity to the current fitness level. Further, exercise programs should be designed so as to optimize the chances of adherence. Personal preference should carry great weight in selecting the mode of activity. The participant's health status may dictate the mode and intensity of exercise: Patients with heart disease should not exercise at intensities so high as to elicit symptoms (*e.g.,* angina pectoris, ischemic electrocardiographic changes); and exercisers with orthopedic limitations may need to use non-weight-bearing or specially modified activities.

Stretching and Strengthening Programs

While focusing on cardiorespiratory fitness, adult fitness programs should include activities that contribute to development and maintenance of adequate muscular strength and flexibility. The primary emphases should be on enhancement of flexibility in the lower back-posterior thigh region and on muscular strength and muscular endurance of the abdominal musculature. In addition, some effort should be dedicated to maintenance of adequate upper body strength.

Generally, the time required to maintain acceptable levels of strength and flexibility is less than that for cardiorespiratory fitness. Usually the use of proper activities three times a week for 10 minutes a session proves adequate. Often calisthenic exerises are used before endurance exercise (*e.g.,* jogging), thereby serving the dual purposes of contributing to warm-up while promoting strength and flexibility.

The preferred technique for improving flexibility is static stretching. First popularized by yoga enthusiasts, static stretching takes advantage of the inverse myotatic reflex that causes relaxation in a stretched muscle. With this technique, the participant stretches a particular muscle group until a moderate degree of tightness is detected (not intense pain). To be effective, the static stretch should be sustained for at least 30 seconds, or longer if tolerable. Static stretching, if used correctly, involves less risk of injury than does the more traditional ballistic stretching (*i.e.,* bouncing) and prevents postexercise muscle soreness.

Muscular strength and muscular endurance are best developed through the use of resistance exercises, which apply significant *overload* to the active muscle group(s). Although free-weights such as barbells or supported weights (*i.e.,* "exercise machines") may be used, calisthenic exercises are usually satisfactory for adult fitness programs. Worthy of particular attention is abdominal strength and endurance because weakness in the abdominal region is associated with lower back pain. Upper body strength may be increased through use of the traditional push-up exercise or modifications thereof.

Weight Control Through Exercise

Regular exercise contributes importantly to the maintenance of an acceptable body weight. *Body composition,* the percentage of total body weight that is fat tissue, is significantly correlated with habitual physical activity levels in all age and sex categories. Moderate obesity can be effectively treated by increasing the daily caloric expenditure through exercise. For most persons, such an approach to weight loss is preferable to dieting because it leads to a loss that is almost entirely fat tissue, whereas dieting alone results in a substantial loss in lean tissue. Moderate exercise combined with mild caloric restriction is most effective, since the resultant weight loss is relatively rapid and the regimen involves the adoption of habits that are quite tolerable.

Exercise programs adopted for the purpose of weight loss should adhere to all principles previously discussed. The primary focus, however, should be on expediture of calories. Thus total amount of work done rather than intensity of activity should be emphasized. In obese adults, intensity of exercise should be reduced so that duration can be increased substantially. For example, an obese person might be instructed to walk for 40 minutes at an intensity that elicits 50% of maximum heart rate. The participants should also attempt to burn additional calories whenever possible—by climbing stairs, mowing a lawn, or walking to work, for instance.

Obesity predisposes the adult exerciser to orthopedic difficulties and may require adoption of non-weight-bearing activities. Because obesity is a risk factor for hypertension, diabetes, and CHD, overweight persons should

TABLE 3-1.
Aerobics Points

Activity	Points
WALKING/RUNNING	
1 mile in 13 min 30 sec	2
1 mile in 10 min 30 sec	3
1 mile in 9 min 00 sec	7
1 mile in 8 min 00 sec	9
SWIMMING	
100 yards in 2 min 30 sec	1
300 yards in 6 min 00 sec	2.5
600 yards in 12 min 30 sec	7
1000 yards in 20 min 30 sec	9
HANDBALL	
10 min	1.5
20 min	3
30 min	4.5

be carefully screened before initiation of exercise programs.

Sample Programs

In recent years, numerous exercise and weight control programs have been promoted through the print and broadcast media. Although some of these programs are consistent with the established principles of exercise physiology, many widely advertised programs are not only ineffective but also unsafe. Before adopting or recommending any "prepackaged" exercise routine, one should evaluate a program for its consistency with the principles discussed earlier in this chapter, such as overload, consistency, specificity, and progression. Programs that offer "overnight" results, recommend crash diets, or promise maximum benefits with minimum effort should be viewed skeptically. Other programs are of excellent quality and have benefited many thousands of adult exercisers. Brief descriptions of two recommended programs follow.

Cooper's Aerobic System

In 1968, Dr. Kenneth H. Cooper, then an Air Force cardiologist, published a book entitled *Aerobics,*[3] which is credited by many as being the event that initiated a massive increase in participation in fitness activity by adult Americans. Cooper's "Aerobics System" makes two major contributions: It indicates how much exercise is enough, and it provides an easily understandable method for quantifying an exercise dose. Cooper devised a so-called "aerobic point," which is a unit of energy expenditure derived from the volume of oxygen needed to participate in physical activities. Epidemiologic and experimental studies found that about 30 aerobic points a week are needed to maintain an adequate state of cardiorespiratory fitness. Table 3-1 lists the aerobics point-values of various activities. The activities awarded the most points are those that involve maintenance of high levels of aerobic metabolism.

Another major contribution of the aerobics system has been popularization of the principle of progression. Cooper's training programs begin at a level based on the participant's state of fitness and build gradually, over 10 to 30 weeks, to a maintenance dose of 30 aerobic points a week. The aerobic system also suggests that combinations of activities (*e.g.,* handball and jogging) may be used to achieve fitness, and this approach has proved very popular among adult Americans.

Canadian 5BX Exercise Plan

One of the most popular and enduring of the prepackaged exercise regimens is that developed in the early 1960s by the Canadian Air Force.[12] The 5BX Plan consists of a combination of calisthenics and endurance exercises organized into a long-term progression. Calisthenic activities focus on abdominal, back, and upper arm strength and lower back flexibility. The prescribed endurance activities are walking, running, and running in place. The 5BX Plan has proved successful for many adults because it starts at an acceptably low level, provides a steady yet realistic rate of progression, focuses on the important health-related fitness components, and is effective in improving these components. The standard 5BX Plan has only one weakness: It calls for only 6 to 8 minutes of endurance exercise and provides no specific guidelines for setting the intensity of this exercise. By applying the guidelines presented earlier in this chapter, however, the 5BX Plan may be modified to meet accepted criteria for cardiorespiratory endurance training. An ideal approach would be to use the 5BX calisthenic routine in combination with the Aerobic System for training of the cardiorespiratory system.

Programs for the Elderly

"Aging" is a term often used to describe the biological, psychological, and sociological changes that occur in persons over time. In biology, aging has come to be associated with a gradual decline in the body's functional capacities and a reduction in the system's resistance to stress and disease. Age-related functional changes may, at least in part, be due to genetically coded phenomena, but some biological effects of aging may be due to disease processes as yet unidentified. In addition, much of the age-related decline in physiologic functioning results not from aging *per se* but from the sedentary living style that has come to be associated with advanced age in our society. This section provides insight into the relation between aging and exercise habits as well as information on the design of fitness programs for older persons.

Physiology of Aging

Cross-sectional observations of physiologic variables reveal that many exercise-related functions decline gradually with increasing chronologic age, a decline that begins at about 30 years of age. These changes, however, while consistently observed in American society, may not be "normal." Habitual physical activity often begins a gradual decline in early adulthood, and thus age-related reductions in many physiologic variables may be "abnormal" and reflective of the hypokinesis that is endemic in the older adult population of the United States.

Cardiovascular Fitness

Aging is associated with marked reductions in cardiovascular functional capacity. Maximum heart rate declines at the rate of about 1 beat a year (maximum heart rate = 220 − age), and, although data are scarce, maximum stroke volume and maximum cardiac output also probably decrease substantially. Pathologic conditions such as hypertension, CHD, and peripheral vascular disease are very common in the elderly and may combine with decreased functional capacities to reduce exercise tolerance.

Pulmonary Function

Several pulmonary function variables decline with age. Under resting conditions, vital capacity is reduced, perhaps because of decreased thoracic wall compliance. During exercise, ventilation seems to be increased at standard submaximal work loads but decreased at maximum work levels. Pulmonary diffusing capacity is reduced under both resting and exercise conditions.

Muscle Function

The body's skeletal muscle tissues reflect the aging process through decreases in muscle mass, muscular strength, and muscular endurance. After age 30, although body weight tends to increase, lean body weight decreases by about 3% a decade. This, of course, indicates that percentage of body fat increases with age, as would be expected whenever habitual physical activity decreases without a concomitant decrease in caloric intake. We do not know, at present, how aging affects the enzymatic capabilities of human muscle tissue; however, the well-documented reduction in peak blood lactate after exhaustive exercise suggests that the glycolytic enzymatic pathway may be adversely affected by aging.

Physical Working Capacity

Physical working capacity, as evaluated by maximal oxygen uptake, tends to decline with advancing years. Cross-sectional data indicate that highest mean maximal oxygen uptakes are found in the teenage years (means $\approx$ 50 ml/kg/min), with values dropping about 50% by the eighth decade of life. As mentioned above, anaerobic capacity, assessed through postexercise peak blood lactate concentration, is markedly reduced in elderly persons. These changes combine to cause a substantial reduction in the capacity for whole body, moderate- to high-intensity work in older persons.

Training

Training studies conducted by Dr. Herbert deVries of the University of Southern California have shown clearly that elderly exercisers adapt physiologically to physical training in much the same manner as their younger counterparts.[5] Significant improvement in central and peripheral cardiovascular functions and pulmonary functions have been observed. The percentage improvement in $\dot{V}O_2$max generated by aerobic training in older persons ranges from 15% to 20%, about the same as for younger adults. However, previously sedentary older adults start from a lower baseline, and thus absolute improvement in, and ultimate level for, $\dot{V}O_2$max is reduced.

Available data, although not plentiful, suggest that adults who maintain an active lifestyle through their adult years have much slower rates of decline in exercise-related functional capacities than do sedentary persons. Values of $\dot{V}O_2$max in the range of 40 to 60 ml/kg/min are often observed in habitual joggers older than age 50 years, values that compare very favorably with mean values for teenagers and young adults. Clearly high levels of physical working capacities can be maintained into later years of life.

Objectives of Exercise Programs

The objectives of exercise programs for the elderly must be established in accordance with the individual participant's age, fitness level, and health status. Each of these factors varies widely within the older population; thus one should never consider the elderly as being one homogeneous group. Although it is always important that adult fitness programs be individualized, individualization with the elderly is critical.

Nonetheless, the general goals of fitness programs for older persons are the same as those for younger adults. The focus should be on health-related fitness components: cardiorespiratory endurance, body composition, flexibility, and muscular strength and endurance. Reduced joint mobility, often secondary to arthritis, is a debilitating malady for many elderly persons, and exercise routines may be devised to aid in retention of adequate levels of static and dynamic flexibility in key joints. Accidents are a major cause of injury and death in the elderly population, and many of these tragedies can be linked to inadequate muscular strength. A strength deficiency impairs the ability to control the body weight (*e.g.,* stair climbing) and to handle external objects (*e.g.,* carrying a bag of groceries). Properly designed and graded resistance exercises can promote maintenance of acceptable levels of muscular strength.

Perhaps the most critical factor in the elderly person's ability to function independently in society is his ability to *move without assistance.*[8] Clearly, older people who maintain good levels of cardiorespiratory fitness and acceptable body composition are more likely to retain the ability to move independently longer than those who become obese or who allow their muscular and cardiorespiratory systems to degenerate. As mentioned previously, the cardiorespiratory system of the older person is trainable, and good levels of aerobic fitness may be attained. Likewise, regular exercise may lead to a loss of fat and maintenance of an acceptable percentage of body fat.

Risks and Safety Procedures

Advancing age is a highly significant risk factor for CHD and other atherosclerotic diseases. Consequently, older persons must undergo proper medical evaluation, preferably including graded exercise testing before initiating programs that involve strenuous activity. For those participants who have a history of cardiovascular disease or who manifest signs or symptoms of myocardial ischemia during exercise, intensity of activity should be rigorously controlled and scaled to a level well within personal exercise tolerance. Because many older persons have hypertension, isometric and other heavy resistance exercises should be avoided, since such activities cause elevated blood pressure, which increases the myocardial oxygen demand.

Older persons are more prone to orthopedic difficulties than younger exercisers. The various overuse syndromes, joint ailments, and musculotendonous injuries may develop rapidly in an elderly person who has been sedentary for several decades. For the most part, however, these problems can be avoided or at least minimized by designing programs that involve a very gradual rate of progression and by selecting modes of activity that avoid stressing tissues particularly vulnerable to injury in specific participants.

Ideally, elderly persons who initiate exercise programs should do so under the supervision of a competent exercise leader trained in emergency procedures such as cardiopulmonary resuscitation, knowledgeable about the characteristics and needs of the elderly, and skillful in

designing individualized exercise programs. Preferably, although not always feasible, equipment should be available to allow monitoring of physiologic variables such as the electrocardiogram during training sessions.

Sample Programs

In recent years, exercise programs for the elderly have become commonplace, and consequently several standardized programs have been developed and implemented both commercially and through nonprofit agencies.[4] The best of these programs have several characteristics in common.

All activities begin at a low level of intensity and build gradually to suitable maintenance of fitness.

Activities are incorporated that deal with cardiorespiratory fitness, flexibility, and muscular strength, including flexibility and strength exercises for all major muscle groups and joints (Fig. 3-2). The total caloric expenditure involved in each exercise session is high enough to contribute to optimal improvement of the body composition.

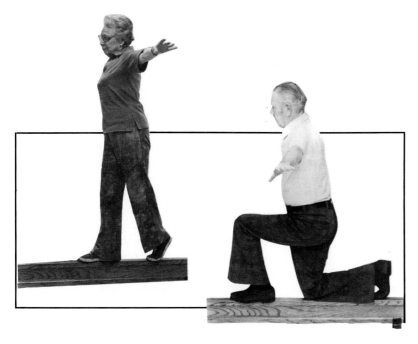

FIG. 3-2
Senior citizens can exercise on a balance beam.

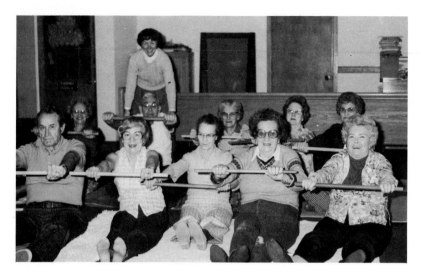

FIG. 3-3
"Gerokinesiatrics" includes flexibility training with short broomsticks.

Designated activities can easily be scaled to the fitness level and health status of each participant.

The program is easily adapted for use in a wide range of physical settings (*e.g.,* home, senior citizen centers, church halls).

The program is organized and presented in a manner that promotes enjoyment and long-term adherence. Often, background music and rhythmic activities are provided.

Brief descriptions of exercise programs designed specifically for older persons follow.

Iowa TOES Program

Developed at the University of Iowa under the direction of Dr. David K. Leslie, the TOES Program comprises a series of calisthenic activities, many of which are performed in the seated position. The exercises are arranged sequentially and are selected so as to enhance flexibility and muscular strength in all body segments.

DeVries Program

Dr. Herbert deVries of the University of Southern California has contributed greatly to our knowledge of exercise programming for older adults.[5] He has devised an exercise regimen that begins with a calisthenic routine such as the 5BX or TOES but that also focuses significantly on cardiorespiratory endurance. Us-

ing walking and jogging, the endurance phase of the program builds gradually to an acceptable maintenance level. Each exercise session concludes with a series of static stretching activities.

Gerokinesiatrics

Devised by Lawrence Frankel in Charleston, West Virginia, gerokinesiatrics, a "preventicare" program for senior citizens, comprises aerobic exercises, stretching, and general strengthening.[8] Medicine balls and short broomsticks are used for some exercises, and a subject may do these exercises even while confined to bed or while seated in a chair (Fig. 3-3).

Training the Female Athlete

An analysis of existing world record performances in various sporting activities indicates that women have not achieved the same peaks of athletic performance as have men. In track and field in 1979, for instance, world record performances by women were roughly 10% to 15% lower than those by men (*see* Table 3-2). At issue, of course, is whether the observed sex differences in athletic performance are due to genetically determined biological factors or to environmental factors such as training and societal attitudes. Available data suggest that some combination of genetic and environmen-

TABLE 3-2.

Comparison of World Track Records for Men and Women, 1979

Distance	Men	Women	Difference
m			%
100	9.95 sec	10.88 sec	9.3
200	19.83 sec	22.06 sec	11.2
400	43.86 sec	48.94 sec	11.6
800	1 min 43.4 sec	1 min 54.9 sec	11.1
1500	3 min 32.2 sec	3 min 56.0 sec	11.2
3000	7 min 32.1 sec	8 min 27.1 sec	12.2
5000	13 min 08.4 sec	15 min 08.8 sec	15.3
10000	27 min 22.5 sec	31 min 45.4 sec	16.0
Marathon	2 h 08 min 34 sec	2 h 32 min 30 sec	19.0

TABLE 3-3.

Cardiorespiratory Fitness and Body Composition in Female Distance Runners Versus Untrained Adults

	Female Distance Runners	Untrained Adult Men	Untrained Adult Women
Maximal oxygen consumption, *ml/kg/min*	60–65	36–40	30–35
Fat, %	10–14	12–16	26–30

tal factors account for these differences. Certainly society has not been totally supportive of the female athlete, and training programs for women have, in many instances, been less vigorous than those for men. In addition, a smaller percentage of women than of men have chosen to participate in athletics, and thus the process of selection has been less demanding among the women. Nonetheless, available physiologic data indicate that certain genetically determined traits do limit exercise performance in women as a group.

Characteristics

As compared with her male counterpart, the female athlete tends to be smaller, lower in metabolic capabilities, and higher in percentage of body fat. The physical performances of highly trained women, however, far exceed those of the average man (*see* Table 3-3).

The smaller stature of the female athlete has several ramifications. Obviously, performance is adversely affected in those activities in which height and body mass determine performance. In addition, the smaller body mass of the woman is composed of less lean tissue than that of the man; lower lean body mass dictates lower muscular strength because the strength of a muscle, independent of sex, is highly correlated with its gross size (cross-sectional area). A woman's lower strength-to-body weight ratio is disadvantageous in those activities that involve lifting or rapid propulsion of the body mass. The sex differences in vertical jumping and sprinting ability may primarily be due to this strength and body weight factor.

TABLE 3-4.
Maximal Oxygen Consumption*

Age	Maximal Oxygen Uptake				
	Low	Fair	Average	Good	High
Yrs	←		*ml/kg/min*		→
Women					
20–29	<24	24–30	31–37	38–48	49+
30–39	<20	20–27	28–33	34–44	45+
40–49	<17	17–23	24–30	31–41	42+
50–59	<15	15–20	21–27	28–37	38+
60–69	<13	13–17	18–23	24–34	35+
Men					
20–29	<25	25–33	34–42	43–52	53+
30–39	<23	23–30	31–38	39–48	49+
40–49	<20	20–26	27–35	36–44	45+
50–59	<18	18–24	25–33	34–42	43+
60–69	<16	16–22	23–30	31–40	41+

*Standards of the American Heart Association.

A high(er) percentage of body fat is a detriment to performance in nearly all athletic activities that involve movement of the body mass. This is particularly evident in endurance activities, such as distance running, because "excess" fat tissue adds to the mass that must be moved but does not contribute to the energy for the performance of work. The suggestion that women may actually be at an advantage in long duration activities since, in such activities, free fatty acids are an important raw material for aerobic metabolism belies an inadequate understanding of exercise biochemistry, overlooking the knowledge that use of free fatty acid is dependent not on the magnitude of the body fat store but rather on the activity of the enzymes of fat metabolism. Thus a woman's higher percentage of body fat tends to affect performance adversely in most athletic activities and accounts for many of the observed differences between men and women in sport.

Women tend to have decrements in cardiovascular function when compared with men of similar competitive standing. Heart size, stroke volume, and maximum cardiac output are smaller in women than in men even when differences in body size are controlled. In addition, hemoglobin concentration is substantially lower in women than in men, and this represents a limiting factor in a woman's oxygen transport capacity. Indeed, the differences between men and women in endurance performance may largely be accounted for by differences in hemoglobin concentration and body composition. Little is known about the biochemical characteristics of skeletal muscle in female athletes. However, available data suggest that the functional capacities of skeletal muscle are similar in the two sexes as long as muscle mass is not a factor. Muscular strength, expressed per square centimeter of muscle cross-sectional area, is similar in men and women. Maximal oxygen consumption, expressed as milliliters of oxygen consumed per kilogram of lean body weight, is only slightly lower in women than in men, a small difference probably due to cardiovascular, not muscle metabolic, limitations (*see* Table 3-4). Thus, by inference, skeletal muscle enzyme systems probably are developed about equally in female and male athletes. Likewise, no sex differences are observed in neuromuscular coordination and motor learning ability as long as muscular strength is not a significant factor in the physical skill being performed.

Trainability

At one time women were thought to be less trainable than men—that is, less improvement should be expected in women than in men in response to a training program. Available data now indicate that this premise is false.[15] Training studies have shown that, if exposed to exercise of similar frequency, intensity, and duration, women exhibit percentages of improvement similar to those observed in men. These observations have been made for strength and cardiorespiratory endurance.

Until recently, heavy resistance training for strength improvement had been rare in female athletes. Misconceptions on trainability and fear of developing masculine characteristics kept many women away from strength training. Fortunately, these reservations are gradually being laid to rest by controlled research studies that have shown women do increase muscular strength through resistance training and do so without developing the heavy musculature of men. Apparently most of a woman's strength gain occurs through neuromuscular adaptations rather than through hypertrophy of skeletal muscle fibers. Lack of hypertrophy in women may be accounted for by lower levels of testosterone, which may be an obligatory intermediate in the anabolic process of hypertrophy.

Cardiorespiratory functions in women seem to be as responsive to aerobic training as do those in men. Although the absolute pretraining and post-training levels of women are lower than those of men, the percentage of improvement tends to be similar. Of course, proper training in women results in attainment of cardiorespiratory capacities that substantially exceed those of sedentary men.

Exercise and Menstruation

The relation between exercise habits and menstruation may be studied from two perspectives: first, if exercise performance is affected in any way by the menstrual cycle. Available data indicate that it is not. Studies in which measures of performance-related physiologic variables have been repeated in the various stages of the menstrual cycle have failed to observe any consistent relationships. This conclusion is based, of course, on group findings. A particular athlete may be affected positively or negatively by the physiologic changes that accompany the stages of a menstrual cycle.

Second, interest has been expressed in the possible effects of training on menstruation. In recent years several published studies have suggested that the incidence of menstrual irregularities, such as amenorrhea and oligomenorrhea, are more common in athletes than in nonathletes. Some investigators have concluded that athletes involved in very heavy training or endurance activities are particularly prone to secondary amenorrhea. At present, the causes of so-called "athletic amenorrhea" have not been identified. One theory suggests that the reduction in body fatness that often accompanies endurance training triggers endocrinologic disturbances that result in absence of menses. Another possibility is that heavy training may be just one of many physical and psychological stressors that can disrupt endocrine functions. Although our current knowledge of athletic amenorrhea is incomplete, it appears to be reversible with reduced training.

Exercise and Pregnancy

Beliefs about exercise during pregnancy have changed markedly in recent years among both physicians and the public. At one time, pregnant athletes and fitness exercisers were advised to quit training for the duration of the pregnancy. Current thought, however, is that women should continue to be active during pregnancy unless specific medical complications are apparent. A prudent procedure is to reduce gradually the intensity of exercise as the size of the fetus increases, since the mass of the fetus contributes to the metabolic demands of any weight-bearing activity. Women also should avoid activities that are violent in nature and that may lead to fetal damage.

Maintenance of good fitness during pregnancy probably aids in preparing the prospective mother for the physical demands of delivery. In addition, women should avoid excessive weight gain during pregnancy, and continued activity contributes to control of weight.

Pregnancy, of course, need not mean the end of an athlete's competitive career. Although no extensive studies have been done in this area, a considerable volume of anecdotal information indicates that women can obtain the highest performance levels during the early stages of, and following, pregnancy.

Nutritional Considerations

The athlete's diet may affect his exercise performance. In general, the athlete's diet should be well balanced so as to prevent nutrient deficiencies, provide a caloric intake that balances caloric expenditure, and include sufficient amounts of water and electrolytes to offset the loss of these substances through sweating.

Because the caloric intake of the typical athlete is relatively high, nutrient deficiencies are quite rare in athletic populations. One apparent exception to this is iron deficiency, which, several studies have reported, is observed in 10% to 15% of female athletes. *Iron deficiency* or depletion of the body's iron stores, is best diagnosed by examination of bone marrow samples. Although iron deficiency is observed in about one tenth of female athletes, it is not clear whether this incidence of iron deficiency is higher than in nonathletic groups, as similar rates of iron deficiency have been found in randomly drawn samples of menstruating women. While iron deficiency *per se* involves no known impairment of exercise performance, it may increase the risk of developing iron deficiency anemia, a condition that does reduce endurance performance. Although the incidence of anemia in female athletes is very low, the high incidence of iron deficiency in female athletes has prompted several authors to recommend prophylactic administration of iron supplements. Existing iron supplementation studies, however, have failed to demonstrate that such a

practice increases iron storage. Thus, the most prudent course for an athlete may be ingestion of a normal balanced diet that includes adequate sources of dietary iron.

Training in Children

Sport programs for children have assumed a high profile in American society since World War II. Organized programs for boys in baseball, football, and basketball have been available for many years. But recently we have seen massive increases in participation in swimming, soccer, gymnastics, and track and field, among others. These expanded opportunities for sport participation are found in both community and school settings. Whereas the typical school system in the 1940s offered interscholastic athletic programs in only a few sports and only for secondary level boys, today many schools offer a wide range of sports activities for both boys and girls beginning at the elementary or middle school level. Clearly, sports programs for children have dramatically grown, and no plateau is yet in sight.

As the number of youthful participants in sports has increased, so has the intensity of their participation. Many of the training and competitive programs to which children are now exposed are far more intense than those designed for mature adults only a few years ago. It is not uncommon, for instance, for a young gymnast to train for 3 hours a day year-round, for a child track star to run 50 to 70 miles a week, or for a youthful football player to undergo a preseason weight training program. The intensity of athletic training programs and the competitive level in youth sports have risen in parallel, but the side-effects and long-term outcomes of high-intensity training and competition in children may not always be positive. Discussed in this section are goals for youth exercise and sports programs, physiologic trainability of children, proper training techniques for youngsters, and trends in the fields of physical education and physical fitness programming for children.

Purposes of Training Programs

Sports and exercise programs for children come in many different forms. Although the specific purposes of these programs vary according to specific circumstances, certain general goals should provide the philosophical undergirding for all exercise and sports programs for children. These goals should be considered by all persons who serve in leadership roles in youth exercise and sports programs. Such programs should do the following.

- Provide a positive experience in exercise for all children. Exercise and sports activity should be conducted in a supportive, enjoyable environment that engenders positive feelings toward exercise, sports, and physical fitness.
- Provide exposure to sports activities and training procedures. The child's sports experiences should serve to provide him with knowledge of, and basic skill in, a range of sporting activities and exercise training procedures. Acquiring such knowledge and skills is a valuable aspect of acculturation in modern American society.
- Aid in the development of acceptable levels of health-related physical fitness. Youngsters should participate in activities that promote maintenance or development of good cardio-respiratory fitness, body composition, muscular strength, and flexibility.
- Promote acquisition of basic movement skills. Later success and enjoyable participation in sports activities depends on early development of fundamental movement patterns, such as throwing, catching, striking, running, and jumping. Youth exercise and sports programs should attend to these basic skills.
- Expose children to a wide range of lifetime fitness and recreational activities. Studies show that few of the popular competitive sports for youngsters are engaged in by adults. Thus the child's experiences should include exposure to those activities that have potential lifelong usefulness and benefit.
- Provide special remedial fitness and instructional programs for youngsters who manifest fitness or movement deficiencies. Intervention programs in the areas of physical fitness and movement skills are most likely to be successful if they start early in life. Youngsters with low fitness or who fail to develop normal motor functions should be provided with appropriate special corrective programming.
- Promote enhanced athletic performance. Many youth sports programs, although focusing exclusively on this goal, fail to achieve it because of improper teaching techniques. Properly designed training and instructional programs should result in improved performance in children, and such improvements may have important, positive side-effects.

No single exercise or sports program is likely to attain all these objectives. The child's total exercise and sports experience should, however, lead to accomplishment of the stated goals. Thus the youngster's movement experiences at home and in school sports, physical education, and community-based activities should, *in toto*, provide a well-rounded and positive lead-up to an adult life characterized by vigor and enjoyable participation in physical activities.

Limits to Performance

A child's body is subject to the same primary laws of physics and chemistry that determine the movement capabilities of an adult. Basically, then, the mechanical and physiologic principles of human movement apply equally across the entire age range. Although the basic principles may be the same, however, a child's maximal performance capacities differ markedly from those of his older brothers and sisters, and these differences are important in the design of sports and exercise programs for children.

A child becomes an adult through the processes of growth and development. Growth, the gradual increase in body size that occurs during the first 15 to 20 years of life, results in marked increases in physical performance abilities. Many anatomic characteristics (*e.g.*, limb lengths, muscle mass, heart volume) can be accurately predicted from height. Likewise, numerous functional variables, such as strength, maximal cardiac output, and $\dot{V}O_2$max (liters/min), are determined largely by gross body size. In many respects, then, the performance capacity of a child is a function of his body size.

In addition, developmental processes independent of variations in body size profoundly affect the functional capacities of a child. For example, increases in certain muscle enzyme activities, hemoglobin concentration, and work efficiency accompany the aging process and serve to expand the physical working capacity at a rate exceeding that predicted from changes in size alone. In addition, muscle strength is known to be lower in younger children even when variations in body size are controlled. Thus, a child's states of growth and development are powerful determinants of his physical performance capabilities, and these factors should weigh heavily in the design of exercise programs for children.

Trainability

A fundamental belief in American society is that hard work pays off. Thus, we tend to accept as axiomatic the concept that physical training results in improved performance. For children, however, this may not always be true. As mentioned above, the primary determining factors of a child's functional capacity are his size and developmental state. Although a child's physical activity habits affect his performance capacities, these effects may be manifested only at the extremes of his physical activity range—that is, youngsters who are very sedentary tend to show physical fitness deficiencies and youngsters who are extremely active manifest higher movement capacities. It is not clear whether moderate doses of exercise generate significant physiologic adaptations in the typical youngster. Some studies of the effects of endurance training in children have reported significant gains in $\dot{V}O_2$max and related

variables; these changes, however, have been observed only with very intense and long-term training programs. Other studies have reported that children manifest little or no change in $\dot{V}O_2$max when exposed to training programs that would be expected to yield improved performance in adults. This apparent lack of responsiveness to training may indicate that the habitual physical activity level of the average child is already quite high, since mean $\dot{V}O_2$max values in children approximate 50 ml/kg/min, a value considered quite good in adults.

A well-established principle of exercise physiology is that trainability is a function of initial fitness level. A moderate dose of physical exercise may not provide a significant stimulus to the child's developmental processes, which may already be proceeding at maximal rates.

Responses to other forms of physical training largely have been unexplored in children. Some studies have shown that beneficial body composition changes occur with proper exercise programs. Little is known, however, about the trainability of children in the areas of muscular strength and flexibility.

Training Techniques

Given the dearth of training studies conducted with young subjects, extensive, specific guidelines for training procedures in children cannot be provided. In general, experience indicates that the same basic principles and techniques of training apply to both children and adults. This section emphasizes those factors that may need modification of basic training principles when working with youngsters.

Epiphyseal Injuries

The growth plates of the long bones are, of course, active in children. Until the plates ossify, they remain in a cartilaginous state that leaves them vulnerable to traumatic injury and prone to overuse. The vulnerability of the growth plates requires that training programs for children avoid activities that could traumatize these structures. Youngsters should avoid the following forms of physical activity.

- Falling, leaping or landing in the straight leg position.
- Repeated throwing movements that apply excessive stress to the shoulder and elbow joints (*e.g.,* excessive throwing in baseball or throwing implements whose weight is disproportionate to the youngster's strength).
- Extremely long-duration exercise that involves weight bearing (*e.g.,* marathon running).
- Weight training with very heavy resistances.

Sexual Maturation

Some scientific evidence suggests that heavy training may delay the onset of puberty in girls. Whether this effect, if real, is harmful in the long term is unclear, but coaches, trainers, and physicians should be aware that delayed menarche and late development of secondary sex characteristics may result from heavy training in young girls.

Psychological Burnout

Heavy training and high-pressure competition in youngsters may lead to a loss of interest in sports and exercise. Training programs for children should emphasize enjoyment, wide variation of training techniques, short competitive seasons, moderate numbers of competitions, and frequent breaks from training and competition. For most youths, early specialization in a single sport and year-round training are contraindicated by the high risks of psychological and, perhaps, physiologic burnout.

External Rewards

Most children are naturally drawn to sports, games, and exercise, thus, intrinsic motivation is usually more than sufficient to sustain a child's interest in competitive and recreational sports activities. Unfortunately, many current sports programs for children seem to assume the opposite—that numerous and elaborate external rewards (*e.g.,* trophies, uniforms) are needed. Evidence suggests that such external rewards are not only unnecessary but actually have the effect of decreasing the intrinsic motivation that initially existed. The ultimate consequence for many youngsters is failure to participate in exercise when external rewards are missing or removed, as they ultimately will be for most persons. External rewards should be used sparingly, and the highest priority should be placed on rewarding participation rather than competitive success.

Physical Fitness

Nearly everyone agrees that promotion of physical fitness in children is a worthy goal. Few have agreed, however, on how this goal can best be achieved. Indeed, there is considerable disagreement in professional circles about the basic definition of "youth fitness."

Perhaps the most traditional approach to fitness programming for children has been to emphasize *motor fitness,* a broad concept encompassing a wide range of physical fitness components (*i.e.,* movement abilities). Usually included under motor fitness are muscular strength, muscular endurance, cardiorespiratory endurance, speed, flexibility, power, agility, coordination, and balance. The concept of motor fitness is embodied in the American Alliance for Health, Physical Education, Recreation and Dance (AAHPERD Youth Fitness Test, which, since the 1950s, has been the dominant test of physical fitness in American schools and which is currently the basis for the Presidential Fitness Awards offered through the President's Council on Physical Fitness in Sports. The AAHPERD Youth Fitness Test includes the following test items.

50-yard dash
Agility run
One-minute timed sit-up test
Pull-ups or flexed-arm hang
Standing long jump
600-yard walk/run or optional distance run

An exclusive focus on motor fitness can precipitate certain problems. One problem is that many of the motor fitness components are heavily dependent on genetically determined factors. Thus it seems inappropriate to encour-

TABLE 3-5.
Health-Related Physical Fitness Components

Fitness Component	Health Factor
Cardiorespiratory endurance	Coronary heart disease risk Physical working capacity
Body composition	Diabetes Hypertension Coronary heart disease
Lower back/hamstring flexibility	Lower back pain
Strength of abdominal muscles	Lower back pain.

age youngsters to improve in areas in which training has little impact (*e.g.,* speed, anaerobic power). Moreover, motor fitness, although important for the athlete, includes several components that have little import for the typical person. Consequently, emphasizing motor fitness may result in a muddled, inappropriate definition of physical fitness. In response to these perceived problems, the concept of health-related physical fitness came into wide acceptance in the late 1970s (Table 3-5).

Health-related physical fitness is, by definition, narrower than motor fitness and includes only those fitness components significantly related to some aspect of physical health. Typically included in the health fitness category are cardiorespiratory endurance, body composition, strength and endurance of the abdominal musculature, and flexibility of the lower back and hamstring region. Each of these components of fitness has been found to play a significant role in disease prevention or health promotion.

Health-related physical fitness, long recognized as important for adults, is now receiving great attention with children, a trend manifested by the development and implementation of the AAHPERD Health-Related Physical Fitness Test (*see* Chap. 4). This new test includes the following items.

Mile or 9-minute distance run

Triceps and subscapular skinfolds
One-minute timed sit-up test
Sit-and-reach test of flexibility

In the future, motor fitness and health-related fitness should receive balanced emphasis in fitness and exercise programs for children. Motor fitness should be presented, evaluated, and interpreted for what it is: a determinant of overall physical ability particularly important in the athletic context. Health-related physical fitness should be presented as an important determinant of physical health, a matter that should concern everyone in our society.

Special Problems of Competitive Athletes

Sports medicine is rapidly being recognized as a distinct medical specialty. One reason why sports medicine has emerged as a discipline is that athletes often pose medical questions totally unique to the sports environment. This section hopes to answer at least a few problems of competitive athletes.

Long-Term Planning of Training Programs

At one time, training for athletic competition was primarily a seasonal activity. Football players, for instance, trained from August to November, basketball players from October to February, and track athletes from March to June. Now, however, attainment of championship performances requires that athletes, even at the high school level, train year-round. Further, if an athlete is to continue to improve over several years, his training and competitive program must progress in an orderly fashion from one year to the next. These factors suggest that the coach, trainer, and athlete must participate in long-term planning; no longer is it sufficient simply to plan from day to day or game to game.

Long-term planning should involve setting realistic short-, medium-, and long-term goals. Coaches should establish general competitive and training plans for each athlete on at least a yearly and seasonal basis and, in selected situations, for several years in advance. Long-term plans should include goals for training loads, training techniques, physical fitness measures, skill performance, and competitive achievements. Shorter term goals (*i.e.,* seasonal) should be established in each of these areas and should be quite specific. Monthly and weekly plans must be highly specific and individualized.

Staleness

One major reason for developing long-term training plans is to avoid staleness or overtraining. Staleness might be defined as an unexplained dropoff in performance, usually associated with overexposure to highly stressful training and competitive activities. Training plans should incorporate adequate periods of rest and other activities, mainly for psychological reasons but also for physiologic ones. Each athlete possesses a certain tolerance for sustained heavy training and competition. If this tolerance is exceeded, the athlete may lapse into physical exhaustion and psychological depression, circumstances that can be avoided by providing adequate rest periods on a weekly, seasonal, and yearly basis, by designing training programs that involve a variety of activities and

environments, and by avoiding an excessive number of competitions.

If an athlete does show signs of staleness (*e.g.,* reduced performance, illness, lack of attention, irritability), the best prescription is either reduced training or total rest. In severe cases of staleness, athletes may need a complete rest and change of environment. Under no circumstances should athletes who are stale increase their training dose. Further competition is not recommended until signs of staleness reverse.

Peaking

A major aim of the competitive athlete is attainment of optimal performances in championship competitions. This so-called "peaking" may be brought about by long-term planning and adherence to the training principle of periodization. Numerous factors combine to bring an athlete to peak performance levels, including training techniques, competitive schedule, psychological outlook, and diet. As the athlete approaches championship competitions, his training should increase in intensity but decrease in total load. Thus, as the swimmer's season progresses, his training might emphasize shorter, faster interval swims rather than total yardage.

Competitions tend to bring an athlete to peak performance; however, too many competitions may cause staleness. The optimal number and rate of competitions are quite specific to the sport and to the individual athlete. The athlete should enter championship competitions with an eager, optimistic outlook and be well rested. Before major competition in endurance activities, 2 to 3 days of significantly reduced training are recommended. During these final days before a championship, the athlete's diet should emphasize carbohydrate so as to fill the body's store of muscle glycogen. Perhaps the most important keys to successful peaking are attempting to peak only once a season and sustaining a peak for no more than a few weeks. Too many coaches and athletes meet with failure in championships because of attempts to peak too often or to sustain a peak too long.

Stitch

"Stitch" refers to pain in the upper abdominal region often reported by endurance athletes, particularly runners and joggers. No definite cause for this problem has been identified, but stitches may be due to muscle spasms in the diaphragm. Often suggested causes are engorgement of blood in the liver and trapped air in the lower sections of the lungs. Beginning exercisers are particularly prone to stitching, and in such persons progressive improvement in overall fitness and in muscular endurance of the abdominal region usually solves the problem. As might be expected, well-trained athletes tend to experience fewer stitches than beginners. Exercising on a full stomach often causes stitching, but this can be prevented by modifying the meal or the training schedule. Stitches often respond to vigorous massage of the affected region and almost always subside with cessation of exercise.

"Second Wind"

Many athletes and fitness exercisers report reduced fatigue and less ventilatory stress after the first few minutes of continuous exercise. This phenomenon, called "second wind," has not been well explained physiologically. Second wind, may, in fact, be a warm-up effect resulting from the plateauing of the oxygen consumption rate after about 3 minutes of aerobic activity. At the onset of vigorous exercise, aerobic metabolism is unable to increase rapidly enough to meet the full energy demand. Thus anaerobic metabolism must make up the difference. The lactic acid that is a byproduct of anaerobic glycolosis causes a sensation of fatigue and serves as a stress on ventilation. When aerobic metabolism reaches the requisite level, lactic acid accumulation ceases, thus allowing ventilation to readjust to a less stressful level.

Pacing

In long-duration endurance activities, one of the keys to performance is proper pacing. Research has indicated that even-pacing, perhaps with a "kick" at the end, is most effective and efficient. In moderate-duration activities, even-pacing prevents the premature accumualtion of lactic acid, which is associated with fatigue. In very long-duration events, even-pacing ensures that muscle glycogen will not be depleted earlier than necessary. Novice competitors often tend to begin races at paces significantly faster than can be sustained for the entire distance, and this always has an adverse effect on performance.

"Hitting the Wall"

"Hitting the wall," a term popularized by marathon runners, refers to the sudden onset of fatigue and depression that may be encountered in later stages of very long-duration exercise. This phenomenon is probably due to depletion of muscle glycogen and blood glucose and thus may be avoided or delayed through proper training, pacing, and nutritional practices. Highly trained athletes seldom report "hitting the wall," suggesting that experience and training adaptations may prevent the problem. Even-pacing, a high carbohydrate diet for 48 hours before competition, and ingestion of a dilute sugar solution during competition should help the endurance athlete to avoid "the wall."

REFERENCES

1. American College of Sports Medicine position statement on the recommended quantity and quality of exercise for developing and maintaining fitness in healthy adults. Med Sci Sports 10(3):7–10, 1978
2. ASTRAND PO, RODAHL K: Textbook of Work Physiology, 2nd ed. New York, McGraw-Hill, 1977
3. COOPER KH: Aerobics. New York, Bantam Books, 1968
4. CUNDIFF DE (ed): Implementation of Aerobic Programs. Washington, D.C., AAHPERD Publications, 1979
5. DEVRIES HA: Physiology of Exercise for Physical Education and Athletics, 3rd ed. Dubuque, Iowa, William C. Brown, 1980
6. Exercise Testing and Training of Apparently Healthy Individuals: A Handbook for Physicians. New York,

American Heart Association Committee on Exercise, 1972

7. FOX EL: Sport Physiology. Philadelphia, WB Saunders, 1979

8. FRANKEL LJ, RICHARD BB: Be Alive As Long As You Live. New York, Harper-Row, 1980

9. LESLIE DK, McLURE JW: Exercises for the Elderly. Iowa City, University of Iowa, 1975

10. MARGARIA R: The sources of muscular energy. Sci Am 226:84–91, 1972

11. POLLOCK ML et al: Health and Fitness Through Physical Activity. New York, John Wiley & Sons, 1978

12. Royal Canadian Air Force Exercise Plans for Physical Fitness. New York, Simon and Schuster, 1962

13. SHARKEY BJ: Physiology of Fitness. Champagne, Illinois, Human Kinetics Publishers, 1979

14. SHEPHARD RJ: The Fit Athlete. New York, Oxford University Press, 1978

15. WILMORE JH: Athletic Training and Physical Fitness. Boston, Allyn and Bacon, 1976

Today, human performances laboratories have elaborate fitness testing facilities. For practical use, however, field testing with simple, minimal equipment provides a fairly accurate estimate of fitness.

The newest American Alliance for Health, Physical Education, Recreation and Dance (AAHPERD) tests are a modern approach to measuring physical fitness.[8] The health-related tests include a skin-fold assessment of body fat, timed sit-ups for abdominal muscle endurance, a timed distance run for cardiovascular fitness, and a sit-and-reach test to measure back, hip, and hamstring flexibility. They measure a range of capacities that may be improved with appropriate physical activity and accurately reflect physical fitness status, as well as changes. Results from these four tests are also a means to an end: They are used to prescribe exercise, to identify strengths and weaknesses, to determine those needing special attention with individualized programs, and to counsel for fitness. The periodic testing emphasizes the importance of an active lifestyle. Although upper body strength and upper body endurance are important, they are not as closely related to health and thus have not, to date, been included in the modern testing.

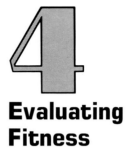

Evaluating Fitness

Somatotype Evaluation

Athletes may be classified according to physique. There is a tendency to particular somatotypes for specific athletic events, especially at the upper levels of competition.[15] A basic somatotype classification includes ectomorphs, who are frail individuals; mesomorphs, who are husky ones; endomorphs, who are soft and fat; medial, or average types; and dysplastic persons, who may be very tall and thin or have disproportionate strengths and weaknesses in their bodies. More complicated and accurate methods of evaluating somatotype have been designed but are laborious and demand high expertise. Further, most of the information obtained from somatotype assessment is redundant to that obtained by anthropometry and body composition determinations. Thus, somatotype evluation is generally employed only in research studies.

CLIFFORD E. BRUBAKER

Stature and Physique

Stature, physique, and body composition are usually important determinants of athletic performance. Taller basketball players are usually better rebounders, taller and heavier football players are often better blockers, and smaller, leaner athletes are frequently better distance runners. Occasionally an athlete is extremely successful despite being unlike the prototype, and conversely an inept performer may have ideal size. This demonstrates that other factors, such as speed, power, and agility, may be equally, or perhaps more, important to success.

Most anthropometric measurements can be taken with a flexible tape measure, but an anthropomometer gives greater accuracy for linear measurements and diameters (Fig. 4-1).[18] Anthropometric tests, however, are hampered if the precise location of anatomic landmarks is obscured by subcutaneous fat. The tester must also be certain to follow carefully a standard measurement protocol. Anthropometric data are available on the morphologic dimensions of boys and girls, and these indices have been related to athletic events.[4, 5]

Weight Loss By Wrestlers

Wrestlers often use a combination of purposeful sustained dehydration and inadequate nutrition (food deprivation) to "make weight." This practice presents a danger to the athlete's health.

The method of weight loss by a wrestler is typically chosen by consultation with his teammates or coach.[17] The largest weight reduction occurs just before the certification date, with the lightest wrestlers losing as much as 10% of their total body weight. To counter this practice and to establish healthful guidelines, investigators have studied the optimum weight and body composition of wrestlers and the effects of excessive weight loss. The percentage of body fat of average high school wrestlers in Iowa was found to be 8%, whereas that of state finalists was 5%. The finalists were older and had wider bone widths, smaller girths, and

lower skin-fold values. Assuming that the state finalists were at minimal body weight, equations have been developed to predict minimal wrestling weight from selected anthropometric measurements.[16] A regression equation with a multiple correlation coefficient of 0.93 with body weight was calculated from these selected measurements. The minimal weight could then be predicted from a short equation.

$$
\begin{aligned}
\text{Minimal weight} = \ & 2.05 \text{ height (in)} \\
& + 3.65 \text{ chest diameter (cm)} \\
& + 3.51 \text{ chest depth (cm)} \\
& + 1.96 \text{ bitrochanteric diameter (cm)} \\
& + 8.02 \text{ left ankle diameter (cm)} \\
& - 282.18
\end{aligned}
$$

R = 0.93 standard error of the estimate = 8.9 lb

This practical method of predicting minimal body weight for wrestlers eliminates the health hazards attendant in making weight in wrestling. It may be used in conjunction with the physician's judgment in questionable cases.

Body Composition

Athletes of the same apparent size may have very different body weights because muscle has a higher density than fat. Generally, an athlete with a greater percentage of muscle (and less fat) is a better athlete, especially in activities such as gymnastics or jumping, which require projection of the body against gravity.

Body Density

Body density determinations are based on Archimedes' principle, and they may be done either volumetrically or gravimetrically.[3, 19] The volumetric method measures the volume of water displaced when the body is immersed. With the gravimetric method, more widely used for determining body density, the athlete must still be immersed in water, but the tank need not be calibrated to ascertain water displacement (Fig. 4-2). The vessel is usually a

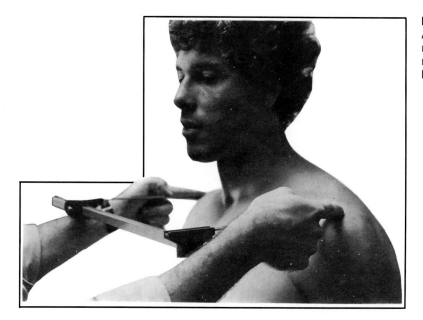

FIG. 4-1
An anthropomometer
may be used for body
measurement, such as
biacromial diameter.

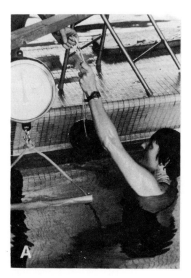
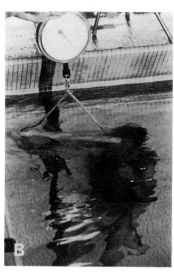

FIG. 4-2
Underwater weighing
may be done in a
swimming pool (*A*). The
subject sits on a
trapeze while a weight
plate holds her
submerged (*B*).

specially constructed tank or a swimming pool, but any vessel may be used that is large enough to accommodate the subject. The athlete is weighed in air and weighed again while submerged. He should exhale all possible air and remain motionless in quiet water and be free of adhering air bubbles. Such testing requires some learning by the subject and multiple measurements.

The athlete's body density may be calculated from the equation

$$D_b = \frac{WA}{((wa - Ww)/Dw) - Rv},$$

where D_b = body density (g/cm³); Wa = weight in air (g); Ww = weight in water (g); Dw = density of water at t degrees Celsius of water; and Rv = residual lung volume (cm³).

The residual lung volume may be approximated by multiplying the vital capacity by 0.24 for males and by 0.28 for females, or the figures of 1300 and 1000 may be used, respectively.

TABLE 4-1.
Percentage of Body Fat Among Athletes

	Men	Women
Track	4–9.6	12–18
Gymnastics	4.6	9–17
Swimming	7.9	19–26
Basketball	7.9–14.2	24
Football	7.9–14.2	
Baseball	12–14.2	

The athlete's body density may then be used to calculate the percentage of body fat according to the formula[3]

$$\% \text{ fat} = \frac{(4.570 - 4.142)}{(\text{Db})} \times 100$$

Data have been compiled on the percentage of fat of male and female athletes in various sports (see Table 4-1). The higher fat values for women reflect the basic differences in essential fat that have been determined as 3% for reference man and 12% for reference women. The fat content of average men is 15% and that of average women, 27% fat.

Skin-Fold Assessment

Skin-fold assessment is a much quicker method for estimating body composition than is direct gravimetric measurement. A satisfactory estimate of body density may be obtained from predictive equations using measurements from a few selected skin folds. With the resulting estimate of density, the percentage of fat may be ascertained from a formula. The skin folds are easy to measure and have a good test-retest validity with experienced testers. The measurements are well correlated with total body fat when the appropriate prediction equations are selected.

The tester uses a skin-fold caliper to measure the skin folds at triceps and subscapular sites in the AAHPERD test (Fig. 4-3). When a repro-

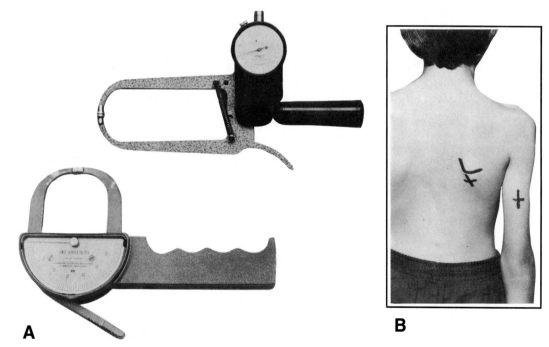

A

B

FIG. 4-3
Skin fold assessment. Skin folds are measured with calipers (*A*) at subscapular and triceps sites (*B*).

FIG. 4-4
The skin fold site is located (*A*), picked up (*B*), and pinched (*C*) between the tips of the calipers.

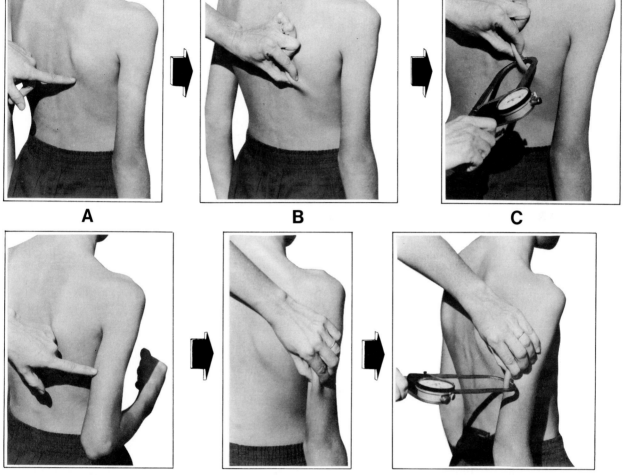

| A | B | C |

ducibility of from 1 mm to 2 mm or less is consistently achieved, the tester may begin evaluating skin folds for school children.

The triceps skin fold is taken on the right arm, halfway between the acromion and the tip of the elbow. This area is located with the youngster's elbow flexed to 90°, and the elbow is then straightened. With the arm relaxed at the youngster's side, the skin is raised parallel to the long axis of the arm. The subscapular site is on the right side, 1 cm (½ in) below the inferior angle of the scapula, in line with the natural cleavage lines of the skin (Fig. 4-4). Usually the sum of triceps and subscapular sites is recorded, but if only one site is chosen the triceps should be selected.

The tester grasps the skin fold firmly between his thumb and index finger and lifts up. The contact surfaces of the caliper are then placed 1 cm (½ in) above or below the point where the skin fold is held. If the skin fold were measured at the base, it would be too thick and not reflect the true thickness. The examiner should seek to measure a true double thickness of skin-fold fat, which lies about halfway between the crest and base of the skin fold. The grip on the calipers is slowly released, enabling the caliper to exert its full tension on the fold. After the needle stops moving, the gauge is read to the nearest 0.5 mm. Each measurement should be taken three consecutive times and the median (middle score) of the three scores recorded. If the three readings were 18, 15, and 16, for instance, the recorded score would be 16. The same tester should seek to administer the skin-fold fat test on the same subjects on each subsequent test occasion.

Convenient conversion tables are now available for the prediction of body fat from skin-fold measurements.[2, 20] But skin-fold assessments only predict and depend on the similarity of the subject to the test population. A prediction formula must be selected that is appropriate for the sex, age, and physique of the subject.

Percentile norms are available for the AAHPERD tests for boys and girls 6 to 17 years of age. The criterion for the desired degree of fatness for children is to be above the 50th percentile. The percentile ranking reflects the percentage of boys and girls in the national sample who exceed the skin-fold thickness; thus a low percentile ranking reflects a higher degree of fatness. If the child ranks below the 50th percentile but above the 25th, he should try to maintain his body weight at the same level for the current year. If the youngster is below the 25th percentile, he should be strongly encouraged to reduce his body fatness by increasing daily activity and reducing food intake. The 90th percentile is considered the ultimate level of achievement, rather than the 99th that is strived for on the other components of the AAHPERD fitness tests.

Strength

Strength is the maximum force (or tension) that the athlete can generate, but there is some confusion in defining strength. An athlete, such as a distance runner, may have a high percentage of lean body mass with a corresponding high

relative strength, and may not be regarded as having high absolute strength. High relative strength is also important in events classified according to body weight, such as boxing, weightlifting, and wrestling. Conversely, a football lineman may have high absolute strength but not as great relative strength.

A cable tensiometer may be used in the laboratory to measure strength. This technique is laborious, however, and additional equipment and expertise are needed. Alternatively, strength may be measured by using free weights or gym machines. Here, the one-repetition maximum (1-RM), the maximum weight that can be lifted once with good form, is determined by trial and error. To find the one-repetition maximum, weight is added, and the athlete is allowed an adequate recovery between trials. If he can lift the weight more than one time, more weight is added. The athlete should arrive at the one-repetition maximum within three to five trials. Norms are available for determining an athlete's ranking compared to others in a specific athletic population by the 1-RM method. Also, three or four lifts may be performed to represent the strength of different major muscle groups. Optimum values are available for the four lifts for the general population.[14]

Power

Power is the ratio of work to time and is the "bottom line" in an athletic performance. How much power the athlete can generate, or how much power he can sustain, is often the determinant of success. The vertical jump is a commonly used test. The athlete stands with his side to a wall and his feet next to the wall. He then reaches as high as possible with his feet flat on the floor. The examiner places a yardstick on the wall with the zero mark at the athlete's fingertips. The athlete next jumps as high as possible without taking steps. The difference in inches is then marked from the zero point to the highest point on the yardstick that the athlete touches, and three efforts are recorded. This test clearly measures some components related to athletic performance—but not power when the result is expressed in displacement.

A modification of the vertical jump test is the "power jump." Here, the athlete's body weight is included to calculate work performed.[7]

$$\text{Work (ft lb)} = \frac{\text{Vertical jump (ins)} \times \text{body weight (lb)}}{12}$$

Although this test does not measure power, the amount of time needed to produce the impetus for the jump does not appear to vary substantially among subjects. As a result, time may be viewed as being a constant for any particular population, and the value obtained from the above equation may be considered to reflect the "power" of the subject.

Another test for power is the timed stair climb, devised by Margaria and modified by Kalamen.[7, 11] The athlete takes a running start and runs up a series of stairs. There are switch mats on the stairs, and a timer accurate to 0.01 sec is used. Power is calculated by dividing the product of the athlete's body weight (kilograms) and the height that his body is displaced in running up the stairs by the time required to travel from the third to the ninth step.

$$\text{Power kg m/sec} = \frac{W \text{ (kg)} \times D \text{ (m)}}{t \text{ (sec)}}$$

Power may also be measured on a Cybex-II isokinetic machine. This machine can print out graphs for determining the athlete's strength, muscular endurance, total work, peak torque, time to peak torque, and relative strengths in range of motion. Work is estimated from the total area beneath the strength curve. Explosive power is the initial burst of power that initiates limb movement; it is estimated from the slope of the early part of the torque curve, and the steeper the slope, the greater the explosive power.

Endurance

Muscular

To test muscular endurance, a fixed percentage of the body weight may be used as the resistance. However, the number of repetitions that the athlete can do with 70% of the 1-RM is more often taken as the measure of muscular endurance. Usually, a recreational athlete is able to do 12 to 15 repetitions and a competitive athlete from 20 to 25 repetitions at 70% of the 1-RM.

The traditional tests of muscular endurance—push-ups, pull-ups, dips, abdominal hangs, and sit-ups—are all influenced by strength, body weight, and body proportions, and thus not always a fair measure of muscular endurance.

Sit-ups are the most common test of abdominal muscular endurance. The 30-second sit-up test has been picked as a test of muscular endurance for school children because the abdominal muscles are essential in almost every activity. The youngster tries to do as many sit-ups in good form within the 30-second period. Sometimes, a 60-second set of sit-ups is used, and the child is allowed to rest between sit-ups.

Subjects should be instructed in proper sit-up technique before beginning the sit-up test. This training will increase the reliability and validity of the test.

When performing a sit-up, the subject's heels must rest on the floor 30 cm to 40 cm (12 in to 18 in) from his buttocks, and his chin should stay tucked on his chest. His arms are both kept in contact with his chest, and the sit-up is regarded as complete when his elbows touch his thighs. The youngster then returns toward the starting position until his midback makes contact with the testing surface. A stopwatch, or a watch with a second hand, is needed, and repetitions are counted. Norms are available for the 30- and 60-second sit-up test and for the total number of push-ups done continuously.[14] Youngsters who achieve below the 50th percentile on the timed sit-up test are encouraged to improve, and those below the 25th percentile warrant an individualized remedial program.

Cardiorespiratory

Cardiorespiratory endurance, or aerobic capacity, underlies good health; it is especially important in distance running, swimming, and field sports such as soccer and lacrosse. Endurance is important even in tackle football, where the average play lasts only about 7 seconds, while the average interval between plays is about 1 minute.

Timed runs for distance are the most convenient method for assessing aerobic activity but, unfortunately, the least accurate. The athlete may be timed over a measured distance or the maximum distance that he can run in a given time may be determined. Motivation is a variable in these maximal effort tests. Youngsters may run 1 mile for time or do a 9-minute run for distance. The 1-mile run is preferable because the youngsters with all finish the run at the same place. They are scored to the nearest second, and if the 9-minute run is used they are measured to the nearest 10 yards or 10 meters. Sometimes, a 12-minute run is used for mature athletes. A distance covered of more than 1¾ miles is excellent, 1½ to 1¾ is good, and 1 to 1½ is mandatory. In all these runs, pacing is important to achieve a maximal effort. The accuracy of this test, therefore, increases with training of the subject. There is also a danger in asking certain populations—for example, older subjects with cardiovascular risk factors—to attempt maximal efforts.

Step-up tests with a measurement of heart rate response incorporate most of the advantages of submaximal testing (as with a bicycle ergometer) and the convenience of mass testing (timed runs). Because the athlete's maximal oxygen consumption is related to his submaximal heart rate, his aerobic capacity may be estimated with these tests.

The recovery index step test is a brief, simple, and practical test to evaluate cardiovascular fitness and needs little equipment or space. The athlete steps up to and down from a bench 30 times a minute for 4 minutes. The height of the bench used depends on the height of the athlete: a 12-inch bench for those athletes less than 5 feet tall; a 14-inch bench for those from 5 feet to 5 feet 3 inches; a 16-inch bench for those from 5 feet 3 inches to 5 feet 9 inches; an 18-inch bench for those from 5 feet 9 inches to 6 feet; and a 20-inch bench for athletes more than 6 feet tall.

The athlete faces the bench and, at the signal "up," places one foot on the bench and steps up so that both feet are on the bench. Then he quickly steps down again and continues the exercise at a marching count of "up, 2, 3, 4," with the signal "up" given every 2 seconds. On completing the exercise, the athlete sits quietly and his pulse is counted, beginning 1 minute after exercise for 30 seconds, then at 2 minutes after exercise for another 30 seconds, and finally at 3 minutes after exercise for 30 seconds. By referring to a table, the examiner may determine the athlete's recovery index. This step test is best used to measure a person's own progress in comparison with earlier results. Alternatively, the athlete may be observed during and after a 10-minute run, whereupon the heart rate and blood pressure are measured as above.

More recent generations of step tests are available to rate the level of cardiovascular fitness of specific populations.[2, 12, 13] Whereas the tests that measure heart rate recovery from step-ups or from a run are physiologically based, they are inferior to tests that use a steady-state heart rate to estimate aerobic capacity.[1] These more precise measurements of aerobic metabolism under stressful exercise may be performed either on a exercise bicycle or on a treadmill.

The Bicycle Ergometer

The bicycle ergometer test is a reliable submaximal test (Fig. 4-5A). Its principal value, like other predictive tests, is to determine the crude level of fitness or any changes in fitness. The subject regulates the work rate while pedaling for 6 minutes at submaximal workloads that produce heart rate responses of between 120 and 160 beats a minute. The score is determined from a table and is based on the workload and heart rate. Separate tables are available for each sex, and there is a multiplier factor for age. The athlete's score is a prediction of his maximum oxygen consumption (ml/kg/min), the highest attainable oxygen consumption that he would achieve during maximal or exhaustive exercise.[1]

To avoid an inconclusive test, the examiner

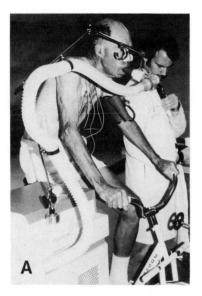 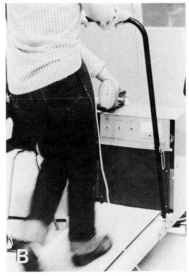

FIG. 4-5
Aerobic capacity may be measured while the subject exercises on a bicycle ergometer (*A*) or on a treadmill (*B*).

should carefully adjust the bicycle saddle before the test begins; otherwise, a person unaccustomed to cycling may have to stop in the middle of the test because of quadriceps pain. The test, though relatively simple, takes time, especially when testing an entire high school or collegiate football squad. A bicycle ergometer costs about $600.

Treadmill Testing

A motor-driven treadmill may also be used to measure aerobic capacity (Fig. 4-5B). Treadmill testing, when conducted with appropriate physiologic measurements, is the most accurate method of assessing work capacity. When used with pulse monitoring, treadmills, like other predictive tests, depend for accuracy on how similar the subject is to the test population. The speed and inclination of the machine establish and maintain the workload on the treadmill.

During a treadmill test, the athlete must be observed for shortness of breath, flushing, pallor, and, especially, chest pain. Chest pain demands immediate cessation of the test and examination of the subject.

Unfortunately, a treadmill is expensive, relatively immobile, and inefficient as to the number of tests that can be performed in a certain

time. The treadmill test is, therefore, more suited to research or clinical use than for the fitness testing of large groups.

Measuring Flexibility

Athletes differ in flexibility, and a given athlete may not necessarily have the same relative flexibility in all joints. Improved flexibility is an importannt goal for each athlete.

A simple, inexpensive flexometer can be constructed to measure joint flexibility (Fig. 4-6). A weighted 360° dial and a weighted pointer are mounted in a case. The dial and pointer move independently and are controlled by gravity. These flexometer readings are not influenced by the length of the athlete's limbs.[9]

Tests for flexibility include the back hyperextension test and the sit-and-reach test. In the back hyperextension test, the athlete lies prone and then arches his back, lifting his chest as far as possible off the floor. The distance between the floor and the sternal notch is then measured. Alternatively, the athlete may extend his back and reach up to touch a ruler as a measure of spine and shoulder flexibility. The sit-and-reach test is a component of the modern physical fitness test for school children that measures combined back, hip, and hamstring flexibility

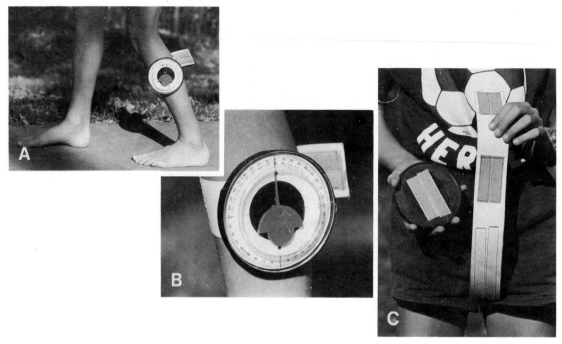

FIG. 4-6
Flexibility testing. A simple plumb dial may be used to measure joint flexibility. The subject leans forward to dorsiflex his ankle (*A*). The dial and pointer (*B*) are attached to a strap by Velcro strips (*C*).

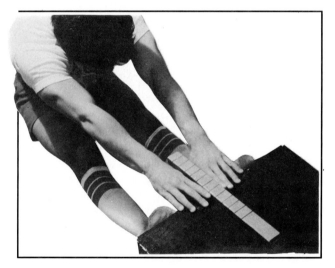

FIG. 4-7
The sit-and-reach test measures back and hip flexibility.

(Fig. 4-7). A specially constructed box is used that has a measuring scale, with the 23-cm mark at the level of the feet. The soles of the feet are scored as 23 cm, since the norm tables have been constructed on the basis of this mea-surement. The box should be placed against a wall to prevent it from sliding away. The ath-lete warms up and then removes his shoes. With his feet a shoulder width apart, and knees locked in extension, he extends his arms for-

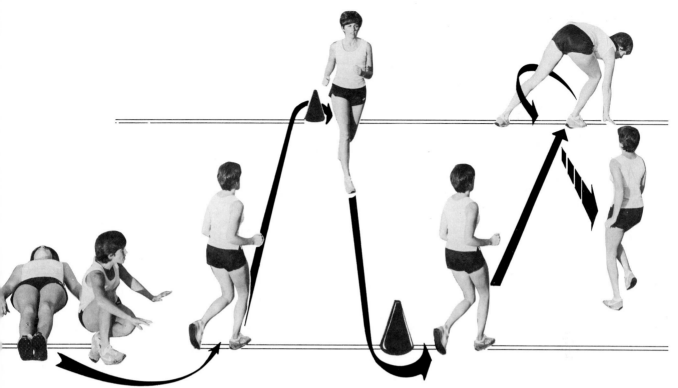

FIG. 4-8
Agility test. This one involves standing up, running forward, effecting quick turns, bending, and running backwards. The lines are 5 yards apart, and the closer pylon is 0.9 m (1 yard) further along than the opposite one.

ward with his hands placed on top of each other. The athlete reaches forward along the measuring scale four times and is scored on the distance that can be reached and held for a three-count on the fourth trial.

The percentile rank represents the percentage of students who scored at or below the test score. The larger percentiles represent higher levels of physical fitness. When a child scores above the 50th percentile, the norms can motivate this youngster by defining degree of excellence in the achievement of physical fitness.

There are some problems with this test. Long arms and short legs may give a high score on the sit-and-reach even if flexibility is low. Conversely, the child with short arms and long legs may receive a poor score. Also, many boys and girls are unable to reach the 23-cm level during a growth spurt because their legs become proportionately longer in relation to their trunk.

Agility

Agility is an athlete's ability to react quickly and shift body positions or directions rapidly while maintaining balance without losing speed. This trait requires strength, speed, balance, and coordination. Shuttle runs, purported to measure agility, are largely tests of speed.

One such "agility test" uses two lines 5 yards apart, two pylons, and a stopwatch.[5, 6] Before being tested, the athlete warms up and does some starts, stops, and cuts. The test begins with the athlete lying on his back with the top of his head on line A (Fig. 4-8). On the command "go," he gets up and runs forward as fast as he can, makes a right turn around the pylon on line B, then runs back to the second pylon on line A and makes a left turn. He then sprints forward, touches line B with his hand and races, running backwards, to the finish at line

107

A. He is scored on the time it takes to complete the drill, to the nearest tenth of a second.

REFERENCES

1. ASTRAND PO, RODAHL K: Textbook of Work Physiology. New York, McGraw–Hill, 1970
2. BAUMGARTNER TA, JACKSON AS: Measurement for Evaluation in Physical Education. Boston, Houghton-Mifflin, 1975
3. BROZEK J, et al: Densitometric analysis of body composition: revision of some quantitative assumptions. Ann NY Acad Sci 110:113–140, 1963
4. CONSOLAZIO CF, et al: Physiological Measurement of Metabolic Functions in Man. New York, McGraw–Hill, 1963
5. DUNN W: Virginia Strength and Power Manual. Charlottesville, Virginia, University of Virginia, 1980
6. EPLEY B: The Strength of Nebraska. Lincoln, Nebraska, 1980
7. GRAY EK, et al: A test of leg power. Res Q 33(1):44–50, 1962
8. LIFETIME HEALTH-RELATED PHYSICAL FITNESS TEST MANUAL. Reston, Virginia, The Amerrican Alliance for Health, Physical Education, Recreation and Dance, 1980
9. LEIGHTON J: Instrument and technique for measurement of range of joint motion. Arch Phys Med Rehabil 36:571–578, 1955
10. MARGARIA R, et al: Indirect determination of maximal O$_2$ consumption in man. J Appl Physiol 20:1070–1073, 1965
11. MARGARIA R, et al: Measurement of muscular power (anaerobic) in man. J Apl Physiol 21:1662–1664, 1966
12. MATHEWS DK: Measurement in Physical Education, 4th ed. Philadelphia, WB Saunders, 1973
13. MATHEWS DK, FOX EL: The Physiological Basis of Physical Education and Athletes, Philadelphia, WB Saunders, 1976
14. POLLOCK ML, et al: Health and Fitness Through Physical Activity. American College of Sports Medicine Series. New York, John Wiley & Sons, 1978
15. TANNER JR, et al: The Physique of the Olympic Athlete. London, George Allen, 1964
16. TCHENG TK, TIPTON CM: Iowa wrestling study: anthropometric measurement and the prediction of a "minimal" body weight for high school wrestlers. Med Sci Sports 5(1):1–10, 1973
17. TIPTON CM, TCHENG TK: Iowa wrestling study. JAMA 214:1269–1274, 1970
18. WARTENWEILER J, et al: Anthropologic measurements and performance. In Larson L (ed): Fitness, Health, and Work Capacity: International Standards for Assessment, pp 211–240. New York, Macmillan, 1974
19. WILMORE JH: The use of actual, predicted and constant residual volumes in the assessment of body composition by underwater weighing. Med Sci Sports, 1(2):87–90, 1969
20. WILMORE JH: Athletic Training and Physical Fitness. Boston, Allyn and Bacon, 1977

Cardiovascular Response to Endurance Training

To be of benefit to the cardiovascular system, exercise should be rhythmic or dynamic and involve a considerable part of the body's muscle mass. These so-called aerobic exercises including walking, jogging, running, cycling, swimming, rope-skipping, Alpine and Nordic skiing, ice skating, and roller skating. On the other hand, some exercises, such as isometric ones, may be a danger to the cardiovascular system. Isometric exercises primarily cause a marked rise in systolic blood pressure and a secondary or lesser increase in heart rate. Alone, they do not produce a cardiovascular training effect. Owing to the marked increase in arterial blood pressure and resistance with the onset and continuation of the isometric exercise, strenuous isometrics could be of some danger in patients with aortic stenosis, idiopathic hypertrophic subaortic stenosis, or severe coronary artery disease.

Maximum Oxygen Uptake

Exercise physiologists use "maximum oxygen uptake" as a measure of a person's level of physical fitness. Maximum oxygen uptake is an index of the ability of the heart to maximally eject blood to the body with systole (the maximum cardiac output), and also the ability of the body to maximally extract the oxygen delivered to it with each systolic cycle (maximum arteriovenous oxygen difference). Therefore, maximum oxygen uptake depends on the individual's maximum cardiac output and the arteriovenous oxygen difference. Maximum cardiac output is the product of the heart rate times the stroke volume (the volume of blood ejected from the left ventricle with each systole).

Heart Rate and Blood Pressure

With the onset and continuance of dynamic exercise, the heart rate increases from a resting level up to a genetically and age-determined maximum level. Physical training will not increase the maximum heart

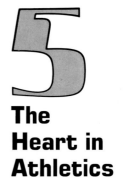

The Heart in Athletics

RANDOLPH P. MARTIN

109

rate that can be obtained with maximum exercise. For most young persons, the maximum heart rate is about 190 to 200 beats per minute. With aging, the maximum heart rate decreases. The best and simplest way to estimate a person's maximum heart rate is by subtracting the person's chronological age from the number 220. With the onset of exercise, the stroke volume, or blood pumped from the left ventricle with each systole, increases from a resting 75 to 80 ml/min to slightly more than 100 ml/min. Moreover, the extraction of oxygen by the body's cells increases with exercise, so that the difference between the arterial oxygen content and the venous oxygen content increases. Exercise normally raises the systolic blood pressure proportionally to the intensity of the exercise. The diastolic pressure generally does not rise significantly.

Coronary Artery Blood Flow

Resting skeletal muscular cells extract 25% to 35% of the oxygen delivered to them; in contrast, the myocardial cells extract 75% of the oxygen presented to them. Therefore, oxygen supply to myocardial cells is determined primarily by the blood flow through the coronary arteries, and not by increased oxygen extraction. With the onset and continuance of exercise, the cardiac muscles' demand for increased oxygen and nutrient supply must be met primarily by a fourfold to fivefold increase in flow through the coronary arteries. Hence, the coronary arterial blood flow will increase from a resting level of 75 to 80 ml/min/100 g of cardiac muscle to nearly 300 ml/min/100 g of cardiac muscle, with the onset and continuance of an exercise period. A person who has significant coronary artery disease (atherosclerosis) with narrowed coronary arteries is unable to provide an increased arterial flow through these narrowed coronary arteries at times of increased demands for oxygen. Hence, the supply of oxygen and nutrients to the heart cannot keep up with the demands that the exercise imposes.

A relative lack of oxygen and cellular nutrients to the heart cells of patients who have narrowed coronary arteries may be manifested by the symptoms of angina pectoris or chest pain. The oxygen demands of the heart are primarily determined by the heart rate, the tension developed within the cardiac chambers (this being dependent on the interventricular pressure or systemic blood pressure), and the contractile state of the heart. Although the heart rate obtained with exercise gives a good estimate of the myocardial oxygen demands, the so-called "double product" gives an even better estimate of these demands. The "double product" is the product of the systolic blood pressure times the heart rate, divided by 100. Patients with significant angina pectoris, secondary to coronary atherosclerosis, have a set double-product threshold at which angina pectoris will develop during exercise. This so-called anginal threshold has been shown to occur at the same level of systolic blood pressure and heart rate, regardless of the workload achieved during exercise or the duration of the exercise.[48]

Resting Heart Rate

Endurance training produces physiologic changes in the cardiovascular system; these changes are listed below.

Effects of Exercise Training

Increase in

Maximum oxygen uptake
Cardiac stroke volume
Arteriovenous oxygen difference
Blood volume and erythrocyte mass
High-density lipoproteins

Decrease in

Resting and submaximum heart rate
Resting and submaximum blood pressure
Resting and submaximum double product
Platelet "stickiness"
Percentage body fat

The magnitude of these changes depends on the intensity, frequency, and duration of the endurance training. The most noticeable early effect of physical training is a decrease in resting heart rate. In the early stages, this is most likely due to peripheral neurologic input to the central nervous system, whereby there is an increase in the resting parasympathetic or vagal tone to the heart. It is not uncommon for the resting heart rate to decrease from the low 70s to the low 60s with a modest level of regular physical training. More prolonged training of higher intensity can further decrease the resting heart rate to the lower 40s or even 30s.

Maximum Cardiac Output

With physical training, the plasma volume and the erythrocyte mass gradually increase. Increased plasma volume leads to increased stroke volume. Therefore, with physical training, the maximum cardiac output (heart rate times stroke volume) rises through the ability of the body to increase cardiac stroke volume—and not through an increase in the maximum heart rate obtained with exercise training, because this is a genetically and age-determined number.

Myocardial Oxygen Demands

Training also increases the ability of muscle cells to extract and use the oxygen presented to them. With training, the maximum arterial oxygen difference increases, and the myocardial demand for oxygen at any submaximum exercise load decreases. This is primarily manifested by a decrease in the submaximum heart rate and blood pressure—hence a decrease in the submaximum double product. Additionally, training enables a person to exercise at a submaximum workload for a longer period, and total myocardial oxygen consumption at this submaximum workload decreases.

With moderate endurance training, the already normotensive person does not often show a dramatic change in resting systolic and diastolic blood pressures unless he has a substantial weight loss. With long-term endurance training, however, it is not uncommon to find a fall in the resting systolic blood pressure owing to marked change in the trained person's total body fat or to alterations of dietary habits.

Myocardial Vascularity

Does physical training lead to an actual increase in the myocardial oxygen supply? Animal studies suggest that there may be an increase in actual myocardial vascularity. Tomanek[58] and Pouppa and colleagues[47] showed that training young rats on a treadmill can lead to an increase in the ratio of coronary microvessels to myocardial muscle fibers. This work suggests, but does not prove, that there is an enhanced blood supply to the individual cardiac cells after training. These changes were only seen if the training was begun in young animals and if the training was done on a regular basis. Other investigators suggest that exercise, combined with pre-existing ischemia, may increase the coronary collateral circulation of the dog.[13] Tepperman and Pearlman have shown a greater weight of the coronary arteries in the exercise-trained animal than in the nonexercised control group.[54] Therefore in the animal model, there may be an increase in the size of the microcoronary and macrocoronary circulation with exercise training if exercise is begun at a young age and done on a regular basis.

Similar findings will be difficult to show in humans. Anatomic data on the coronary circulation would be needed in a large number of persons before and after exercise training. Because this type of prospective study requiring multiple coronary angiograms on "normal" persons would be impossible, data are only available anecdotally or for low numbers of patients who have been studied by coronary angiograms. The well-known case of Clarence DeMar,[11] the famous Boston Marathon runner who died of a noncardiac cause and who, at autopsy, had very large coronary arteries, has been said by some to "prove" that exercise enlarges the size of human coronary arteries.

One can appreciate the difficulties in reliably studying the coronary arteries and cardiac performance before and after endurance training. Attempts to do this by cardiac catheterization would not only present moral and economic problems but would not allow accurate visualization of the microcirculation of the heart. Additionally, this type of study would not resolve the important question of whether the actual perfusion of blood to the myocardial cells is increased, because coronary angiography only shows the anatomy of the larger coronary arteries. Hopefully, new "noninvasive" techniques, such as thallium perfusion scans, may allow further investigation into this question of enhanced perfusion to myocardial cells. At this time, however, it remains unresolved in humans as to whether physical training actually increases the amount of blood flow to myocardial cells through an actual increase in myocardial vascularity.

Central and Peripheral Adaptations to Exercise

Claussen and colleagues have attempted to delineate the difference between central (cardiac) and peripheral (noncardiac) adaptations to training.[8] By training different extremities, they have shown that, with standard training (and not endurance-type training), maximum cardiac output and maximum full-body oxygen consumption are increased whether the trained or untrained extremities are tested. A different mechanism led to this increased maximum cardiac output after endurance training depending on whether the trained or untrained extremities were tested.

A trained limb shows neurologic, mitochondrial, and enzymatic changes. These alterations allow trained limbs to extract the oxygen presented to them better and to better regulate blood flow to them through alterations in peripheral vascular resistance. After training an extremity, it is not uncommon, especially with submaximum exercise testing, to see a decrease in the peripheral vascular resistance in that trained extremity. This means, therefore, that the heart has less vascular resistance to pump against and may be one mechanism whereby the maximum cardiac output can increase after exercise training. These peripheral adaptations appear particularly important during submaximum exercise and may be the important determinants of an enhanced submaximum exercise performance after exercise training. However, central adaptations, such as an increase in the circulating blood volume and cardiac stroke volume, may also account for the increase in cardiac output during exercise with endurance-trained muscles. When the arms are tested after training the legs, the increase in maximum body oxygen consumption is primarily achieved by an increase in the maximum cardiac output despite an increase in peripheral vascular resistance. This may be the best evidence that physical training, no matter which extremity or how many extremities are trained, produces a central improvement in cardiac performance.

Can Benefits of Endurance Training Be "Stored Up"?

Five normal persons, two of whom had previously undergone an endurance-training program, were studied at bed rest.[49] All five showed a dramatic fall in their maximum oxygen uptake, stroke volume, and cardiac output. With the resumption of exercise training after this period of bed rest, the trained persons were able to reach the same level of physical fitness (maximum oxygen uptake) that they had attained before their bed rest period. Similarly, the untrained persons who had undergone a period of bed rest showed a dramatic improvement in their maximum oxygen uptake, reaching levels much higher than their untrained or pre-bed-rest levels. The increase in both groups' maximum oxygen uptake with exercise training after bed rest was obtained primarily through an increase in the cardiac stroke volume and a widening of the arterial venous oxygen difference. From this classic study, two conclusions were reached: A trained person cannot "store up" the effect of training because there is a very rapid return to a baseline cardiovascular state if this person suddenly stops exercise; and previously sedentary persons can dramatically increase their level of physical fitness when they begin an exercise training program.

Arm Exercise, Leg Exercise, and Isometrics

For the production of an equivalent workload, the cardiac output and myocardial oxygen requirements are higher for arm work than for leg work even when both kinds of exercise require the same energy expenditure.[53] Exercise with the arms consistently produces higher heart rates and systolic blood pressures than does an equivalent load performed with the legs.[27] Similarly, exercises that are primarily isometric lead to an exaggerated systolic blood pressure response and have a higher myocardial oxygen demand than do those activities that are primarily dynamic or involve isotonic muscular contraction (if one keeps the total body oxygen requirements of the two type exercises at a similar level).[34] These differences between arm exercise as compared to leg exercise, and isometric exercise as compared to dynamic or isotonic exercise, must be remembered when evaluating a subject's exercise program.

Testing Procedures

During the past 15 years, the number of diagnostic procedures for testing the status of the cardiovascular system has grown tremendously. These tests range from invasive procedures, such as cardiac catheterization and coronary angiography, to noninvasive testing procedures, which can be done on an inpatient or outpatient basis and lend themselves to serial applications. Noninvasive methods include exercise testing, ambulatory electrocardiographic (EKG) monitoring (Fig. 5-1), echocardiography, and nuclear imaging techniques.

FIG. 5-1
Electrodes are applied to a Super Senior Tennis player (*A*), and his power pack is adjusted (*B*) for cardiac monitoring during the United States Tennis Association 75's National Clay Court Championship.

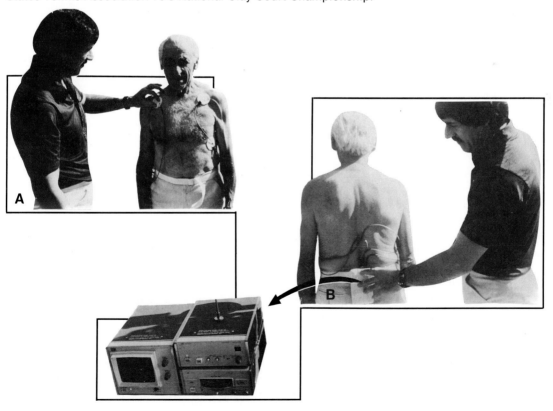

Exercise Testing

Most health-related professionals are versed in the use and role of exercise testing for evaluating physical fitness level. The level of exercise obtained during these tests—whether by bicycle or by treadmill testing—provides a good estimate of overall physical fitness level and cardiovascular health. One objective of exercise testing is to measure a person's functional capacity so that he can be cleared to participate in recreational- or rehabilitative-type exercise programs. Additionally, exercise testing has been used extensively to diagnose and to investigate coronary artery disease.

Regardless of whether a bicycle or a treadmill is used, the exercise test should monitor and measure the intensity of the subject's response through multiple workload levels. The test should begin at a low level of estimated oxygen requirement and be increased gradually through multiple stages. At each level, the workload should be maintained for a sufficient time to allow the subject's cardiovascular response to stabilize for that level of exercise. Each workload level is performed for 2 to 3 minutes during the test while subjective and objective findings are being monitored.

Subjective findings are those that the patient relates to the observer, such as shortness of breath (dyspnea), chest discomfort (typical or atypical for angina pectoris), dizziness, lightheadedness, and fatigue. Objective findings include the general appearance of the patient during the test and changes in heart rate, blood pressure, and EKG response. These last variables should be monitored not only during the test but also before the test, in both supine and standing positions and during 30 seconds of hyperventilation. Finally, in the immediate postexercise recovery period, heart rate, EKG, and blood pressure should be monitored for 6 to 10 minutes.

Exercise tests are either maximal or submaximal. A maximal test is one in which the subject has reached his maximum capacity to take up oxygen and where any increase in the intensity of exercise does not lead to additional increased oxygen uptake. The maximum oxygen uptake need not be measured; the level of exercise achieved during the test can be predicted from the exercise heart rate because an almost linear correlation exists between heart rate and oxygen consumption during an exercise test.

The systolic blood pressure normally increases as the workload increases. It is not uncommon, at maximum exercise, for the systolic blood pressure to range between 190 and 240 mm Hg. Generally the diastolic blood pressure will either remain the same or gradually fall with exercise.

Heart rate normally will increase in a stepwise fashion in response to increased external workload. When the subject has reached a maximum level of exertion, his heart rate generally will level off. Most physicians consider a target heart rate on exercise testing of at least 85% of the age-predicted maximum heart rate or of the actual maximum heart rate to indicate a maximum exercise test. Submaximum exercise tests are those in which the increased workload is stopped at a heart rate less than 85% of the maximum age-related heart rate.

The maximum heart rate obtained during an exercise test in a symptom-free person may then be used to determine the proper heart rate zone at which he should train. The best training zone for producing the beneficial physiologic effects of exercise training is determined by taking 70% to 85% of the maximum attainable heart rate during a normal maximal exercise test. Heart rates above 85% of the maximum attainable rate generally do not lead to a greater increase in overall cardiovascular fitness level. Moreover, heart rates lower than 70% will not lead to as rapid an improvement in cardiovascular fitness level unless the training periods are quite prolonged.

"Oxygen Cost" of Exercise

The "oxygen cost" associated with specific levels of exercise testing may be used to estimate exercise levels during the test. The actual level of oxygen uptake obtained during conventional, standardized exercise testing protocols has been measured; accordingly, estimates of oxygen uptake per unit of body weight per minute of workload have been obtained. In a "normal" person, the resting oxygen uptake is about 3.5 ml of oxygen per kilogram of body weight per minute of exercise (3.5 ml/kg/min)—equivalent to one MET, a unit that describes the resting oxygen uptake of a normal person. Exercise levels obtained during an exercise test are referred to as multiples of the resting oxygen consumption, or METs. Both the heart rate response and the METs obtained during an exercise test help the physician or exercise physiologist to estimate better the functional capacity of the person being tested. Generally, untrained patients limited by cardiologic symptoms are not able to perform more than 6 to 7 METs, while active but untrained healthy persons may have MET capacities of 12 or greater.

Electrocardiographic Lead Systems

Monitoring the EKG before, during, and after the exercise test serves as a screening procedure for detecting abnormalities of myocardial blood supply and cardiac rhythm. Which EKG lead system is most beneficial for monitoring the EKG response during an exercise test? The three most common lead systems are the bipolar lead system, the modified torso lead system, and the vectorcardiographic lead system. The bipolar lead system has been popular because of its ease of application and relative freedom from motion artifacts, but some examiners favor the torso-type system for its increased sensitivity in detecting EKG signs of significant narrowing of the coronary arteries. Blackburn and Katigbak studied the ability of different lead systems to detect abnormal EKG response to exercise testing in 100 cardiac patients.[3] They found that by using the modified V-5, the bipolar lead system, 89% of the abnormal responses would be detected. The additional 11% of abnormal responses would have been detected if other leads, specifically the inferior and lateral precordial leads, had been used. Just monitoring the inferior EKG leads (II, III, AVF) may produce a larger percentage of false-positive EKG responses to the exercise test.

How Safe Are Exercise Tests?

As with most testing procedures, if common sense is followed the exercise test can be safe. Obviously, those health-related professionals who are not physicians should either have extensive training in exercise testing procedures and cardiopulmonary resuscitation or have the close assistance of a physician or nurse with coronary-care-unit experience available to them during the performance of the test. If there is any question about whether a patient does have significant cardiovascular complaints, the advice of a physician should be sought before performing the exercise test. The patient population being tested will really dictate who actually performs the test. If one is dealing with a patient population in which there is a potentially high incidence of cardiovascular abnormalities, a physician or nurse practitioner should administer the test. For asymptomatic persons in whom extensive cardiac disease is unlikely, the health-related worker can safely perform the test.

Abnormal Responses During an Exercise Test

The patient must be monitored closely during the exercise test, not just during the EKG. If the patient's appearance becomes unusual, specifically if he becomes pale, or if he complains of marked shortness of breath or chest discomfort, the test should be terminated, even at a submaximum or very low heart rate level. The patient's appearance should be checked and EKG monitored during the postexercise period too. The sensitivity of the test may be increased by placing the patient in the supine position shortly after the exercise test. By so doing, the volume within the heart is increased, and this increase in the cardiac volume increases overall cardiac oxygen consumption, thereby helping to increase the sensitivity of the ST segment analysis as an indicator of the presence or absence of true coronary artery narrowing.

The person administering the exercise test must be aware of the abnormal or pathologic responses that can occur, such as abnormalities of the heart rate response, the blood pressure response, or the EKG response, Additionally, the subject may relate symptoms highly suggestive of true cardiac ischemia, specifically those types of chest discomfort characteristic of angina pectoris. Most patients will relate some fatigue during the exercise test, but a sudden onset of lightheadedness accompanied by pallor is a worrisome sign that may indicate either a sudden fall in the cardiac output owing to ventricular dysfunction or a significant ventricular arrhythmia.

Bruce has shown that an inability to elevate the systolic blood pressure to 130 mm Hg with exercise and a limited duration of the exercise test are associated with increased mortality from coronary artery disease.[6] Generally, the systolic blood pressure should rise 10 mm Hg or more with each additional stage of exercise until a maximum level of work is obtained. An inadequate systolic blood pressure rise could be due to obstruction to the egress of blood from the left ventricle (such as would occur with aortic stenosis or IHSS—conditions in which the exercise test most likely should not be performed) or due to left ventricular dysfunction with exercise. Thompson and Keleman found serious and severe coronary artery stenosis in all their patients who developed a significant fall in systolic blood pressure accompanied by chest pain typical of angina during an exercise treadmill test.[55] Therefore, with a gradual increase in exercise level during a test, a fall in systolic blood pressure of greater than 10 mm Hg and an inability of the heart rate to increase (if the patient is not on certain medication, such as beta blocking agents) are factors associated with potentially significant coronary artery disease. Although it is reassuring if a subject has an appropriate rise in his heart rate and systolic blood pressure during an exercise test and does not have chest discomfort typical of angina pectoris, this does *not* necessarily mean that the person is completely free of significant coronary artery atherosclerosis (meaning greater than 75% luminal narrowing of any of the coronary arteries).

Electrocardiographic Changes

The degree of depression or elevation of the ST segment of the EKG during and after an exercise test has been used to predict the presence or absence of significant narrowing of the coronary arteries. ST segment flattening that is equal to or greater than 0.1 mV (or 1 mm) after the J point and lasts for 0.08 seconds below the level of the preceding TP segment or PQ seg-

ment is considered electrocardiographic evidence for diagnosing ischemia. A downsloping ST segment depression appears to be a better predictor for significant coronary artery disease than is a horizontal ST segment depression. Both types seem to be more serious predictors of coronary artery disease than does an upsloping depression of the ST segment.[19] The sensitivity and specificity of the test really depends on the population being tested. In persons who are older and more likely (in this country) to have coronary artery atherosclerosis, an abnormal EKG response is more likely a true indicator of significant coronary artery disease. In an asymptomatic younger population, abnormal exercise test findings may represent a so-called false-positive response.

There is debate about whether routine exercise tests should be done in asymptomatic young persons because of the relatively high incidence of false-positive EKG responses during an exercise test. The list below relates some of the causes of false-positive exercise EKG responses.

Causes of "False-Positive" Exercise Electrocardiogram Response (Abnormal ST Segment Response Without Significant Coronary Artery Disease)

Conducting system abnormalities
    Short PR interval
        Lown-Ganong-Levine syndrome
        Wolff-Parkinson-White syndrome
    Left bundle branch block
Cardiac valve abnormalities
    Aortic stenosis/aortic insufficiency
    Mitral valve prolapse (?)
Cardiac muscle abnormalities
    Left ventricular hypertrophy
    Idiopathic hypertrophic subaortic stenosis (IHSS)
Electrolyte abnormality
    Low potassium
Anemia-hypoxia
Medication
    Digitalis
Neurocirculatory (vasoregulatory) asthenia
Women in perimenopausal years
Improper technique or criteria

One of the most well-known causes is the so-called vasoregulatory asthenia syndrome, which may be associated with an increased adrenergic state. Not uncommonly, persons with this syndrome have inverted T waves, especially when changing from a supine to an erect body position. Exaggeration of this response, along with ST segment depression, may be provoked by 30 seconds of hyperventilation. This type of patient will often have an "abnormal EKG" response early in the exercise period, which will normalize as the exercise continues. Other false-positive test findings may be seen in persons with abnormalities of the conducting system, such as the short PR interval syndrome (the Lown-Ganong-Levine syndrome); in persons taking certain medication, such as digitalis; or in persons with significant hypertrophy of the left ventricle. Some patients with the mitral valve prolapse syndrome, or deformities of the chest such as pectus excavatum, also have an increased incidence of false-positive EKG responses. Women in the perimenopausal period are well known to have a higher incidence of false-positive test responses and abnormalities of electrolyte levels (such as potassium), and anemia may be associated with false-positive test responses.

Sensitivity and Specificity of the Electrocardiographic Response

Sensitivity refers to the percentage of patients with significant angiographic evidence of disease who have an abnormal EKG response to an exercise test. The specificity of the test is the percentage of patients with normal coronary angiograms who have a normal exercise test. The sensitivity and specificity of the EKG response to exercise may be useful in determining the presence or absence of coronary artery disease. A coronary angiogram gives anatomic evidence of the presence or absence of significant obstruction, and the EKG response to exercise is an indicator of the presence or absence of myocardial ischemia. The sensitivity of the test increases as more coronary arteries are significantly involved by atherosclerosis.[10] With one-vessel coronary artery disease, the sensitivity of the test is about 40%; with two-vessel coronary artery stenosis, 67%; and, with three-vessel, 86%. The average sensitivity for the EKG response is 69%. The overall specificity of the test is about 90%.

Although the sensitivity and specificity are important for determining the value of a given procedure, the likelihood of the patient's having a disease and the test results are more important. Taking into account the odds of the patient's having a disease and the odds that the test results are true gives an estimate of the predictive accuracy of the test.

Chest pains either at rest or during exercise are generally of two types. The chest pain typical of angina pectoris is a pain or discomfort that is described as a burning or aching located behind the sternum, in the jaw, or in the arms and wrists. It is usually precipitated by exercise, emotional stress, or exposure to cold and is generally relieved within 10 to 15 minutes after cessation of the precipitating factor or by the use of nitroglycerin tablets (the relief coming within 1 to 3 minutes). Patients with typical angina pectoris are said to have about a 90% chance of having significant coronary artery disease.[10] Chest discomfort that is atypical for angina pectoris has an unusual location (over the right chest), has a prolonged duration, is not related to constant precipitating factors, and may fail to respond to medications or cessation of the precipitating activity.

Extra Heart Beats

Not uncommonly, young persons have an occasional extra heart beat. Moreover, during a maximum exercise test, premature ventricular contractions, or PVCs, may occur in as many as one third of asymptomatic men. The prevalence of PVCs appears to be related to age.[10, 22] Premature ventricular contractions are not often reproducible on repeated exercise testing. Patients with significant coronary artery disease usually will have a higher incidence of serious (multifocal or coupled) PVCs than will "normal" persons, and their PVCs usually will occur at a much lower heart rate than those found in "healthy" subjects. Premature ventricular contractions suppressed by exercise do not necessarily rule out the presence of significant coronary artery disease. Additionally, some healthy persons will have multiple runs of coupled PVCs or even a brief burst of ventricular tachycardia (three or more coupled beats of PVCs in succession) during an exercise test. This subgroup of asymptomatic persons with significant ectopic beats during exercise, although being three times more likely to develop significant coronary artery disease, does not necessarily do so, with only 10% showing symptoms of coronary artery disease.[10]

Thus the exercise test is a very useful noninvasive procedure that measures both functional capacity and cardiovascular fitness of the individual. It should be a multistage exercise test, beginning at a low level and gradually increasing to a "maximum" level in the asymptomatic individual.

With increasing levels of external work, the blood pressure and heart rate should normally rise from a resting level. Abnormal responses to an increase in the workload are indicated below.

Abnormal Responses to Increased Workloads During an Exercise Test

Symptoms
Angina
Marked shortness of breath
Confusion, lightheadedness

Signs
Pallor, cold skin
Cyanosis
Ataxia
Syncope or near syncope

Heart Rate Response
Slow or plateauing heart rate despite increasing workload

Blood Pressure
Failure of systolic blood pressure to rise
Fall in systolic blood pressure (> 10 mm Hg) with increasing workloads

Electrocardiogram
Ischemic ST depression
Arrhythmias: ventricular tachycardia (fibrillation), frequent multifocal premature ventricular contractions, high-grade atrioventricular block

Thallium Testing

Recently, the use of thallium 201, a radioactive tracer that is an analogue of potassium, has dramatically improved the sensitivity and specificity of the exercise EKG and exercise test as a predictor of significant coronary artery disease. The thallium is taken up by heart cells that have normal cardiac perfusion (*i.e.,* blood supply). In this sense, thallium testing differs from coronary angiography. For angiography, an opaque contrast agent is injected into the proximal portion of the left and right coronary arteries, outlining their internal lumens and showing the coronary artery anatomy. This technique allows for analysis of coronary artery anatomy and for detecting the presence, severity, and location of narrowing of the coronary arteries secondary to atherosclerosis. Thallium, on the other hand, does not show coronary artery anatomy but does show myocardial perfusion. Thallium exercise testing aids the cardiologist in determining the presence or absence of significant coronary artery disease. It is a test that requires highly sophisticated instrumentation but is now performed in many hospitals.

Exercise testing with thallium is performed by injecting a very small amount of this radioactive tracer into a peripheral arm vein during an exercise test. The thallium is taken up by those heart cells that have a normal blood supply. Persons with significant coronary artery narrowing will not show a uniform uptake of the thallium because the thallium will not be normally distributed to those portions of the myocardium that are "downstream" from the area of significant narrowing. At maximum exercise or at times of increased demands for blood supply to the myocardium, areas downstream from the significant narrowing do not receive an adequate blood supply. In the immediate postexercise period, the patient is placed under a special external radiographic camera, called a gamma camera, and the actual

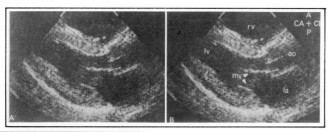

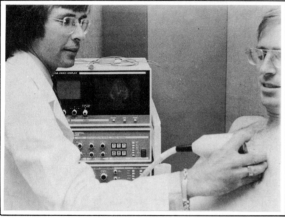

FIG. 5-2
The two-dimensional echocardiographic examination is performed by applying a transducer to the patient's chest. The echocardiographic display can be seen on the machine in the background. The top two figures are stop-frame photographs of a typical two-dimensional echocardiogram: Figure A is unlabeled, and Figure B is labeled. The images are oriented like a left lateral view of the heart. A = anterior; P = posterior; CB = cardiac base; CA = cardiac apex; AO = aorta; LA = left atrium; MV = mitral valves (with small white arrows); LV = left ventricular cavity; RV = right ventricular cavity; IVS = intervening interventricular septum.

counts of radioactive material from the heart are recorded as a picture. Those areas that have not received a normal distribution of thallium during the exercise test—meaning those areas of the heart that have had a decreased perfusion during the exercise test secondary to significant atherosclerotic narrowing of the coronary arteries—will show a dark area (defect) on the thallium scan.

Echocardiography

A different form of evaluation of the heart and its structures is obtained through the use of echocardiography. Echocardiography uses high-frequency sound waves that are emitted from a transducer placed over the chest wall near the heart (Fig. 5-2). These high-frequency sound waves pass through the chest wall and are reflected from the interfaces that compose the cardiac chambers and valves. Throughout the world, single-dimensional, or M-mode, echocardiography has become a standardized, noninvasive diagnostic procedure. The information received from the single transducer can be recorded on a strip chart or on an oscilloscope and presents a static record showing the various walls of the heart, chambers of the heart, and valvular structures. This technique has proved useful in the evaluation of certain valvular and myocardial wall abnormalities and is especially useful in detecting pericardial effusions. The single-dimensional echo may be likened to an "ice pick" or narrow beam interrogation of the heart. The information obtained from this procedure depends on which cardiac structures this narrow beam is aimed at. Because this narrow beam does not present a wide-angle view, no spatial information is gained.

Over the past 10 years, the use of echocardiography has become widespread and the technique has undergone a rapid expansion. Machinery has recently been developed that allows a so-called two-dimensional view of the heart. By using either a mechanical system, whereby multiple transducers are rapidly oscillated or rotated, or by using the principle of phased array radar, a wide-angle view of the heart through multiple tomographic planes is gained. This information is obtained in real time and recorded on videotape for playback and analysis. Wide sections of the heart may be simultaneously viewed in an anterior-to-posterior and lateral-to-medial direction. Structures such as heart valves, chambers, and walls may be imaged simultaneously in dynamic motion. The two-dimensional echo, expecially when combined with single-dimensional echo (the single-dimensional echo can be derived from one portion of the two-dimensional picture), allows the cardiologist to determine rapidly the integrity of the cardiac structures. Because this technique has no biological hazard and is totally noninvasive, it can be repeated serially or easily done on outpatients.

The Athletic Heart

Endurance-trained athletes are often referred to a cardiologist for "abnormalities," which are actually common findings in the endurance-trained athlete. There are certain cardiologic changes that occur in athletes with training, and especially with endurance training. Common findings are listed below.

Common Findings in Endurance-Trained Athletes

Auscultation
S_3 (third heart sound)
S_4 (fourth heart sound)
Systolic murmurs (grade I or II)

Chest x-ray
"Cardiomegaly"

Electrocardiogram
"Left ventricular hypertrophy" (prominent voltage, usually not meeting Estes criterion)
T-wave inversion (inferiorly)
ST-T-wave elevation (juvenile repolarization pattern)
Incomplete (or complete) right bundle branch block

Rhythm
Bradycardia (sinus)
Sinus arrhythmia
First-degree heart block
Second-degree heart block (Wenckebach)
Functional bradycardia
Premature atrial contractions
Premature ventricular contractions

Blood Chemistries
Decreased hematocrit
Increased serum glutamic oxalacetic transaminase, lactic dehydrogenase, alkaline phosphatase, blood urea nitrogen

Urine
Proteinuria
Hematuria
Casts

Auscultation commonly reveals so-called third and fourth heart sounds—sounds that may be wrongly interpreted, especially in view of the chest x-ray, as being indicative of possible cardiac enlargement or cardiac failure. If the athlete then complains of fatigue (which may be due to overtraining), the physician will continue to be concerned about possible heart failure. Many normal young persons and endurance-trained athletes will have a third and fourth heart sound, and auscultation of these sounds, even if accompanied by faint murmurs, is not considered unusual.

As many as 30% of endurance-trained athletes will have "cardiomegaly" (an enlarged cardiac silhouette) on their chest x-ray, most likely due to an increase in the end-diastolic volume of the endurance-trained heart. The M-mode echocardiogram has been used to study the morphologic changes in the heart secondary to exercise training. Morganroth and associates have studied 56 athletes, aged 18 to 24, with M-mode echocardiography.[44] Those who engaged in endurance aerobic training had increases in their left ventricular end-diastolic dimensions (i.e., volume) but not an actual increase in the thickness of their left ventricular free walls. Some of those who trained primarily with isometric strength training techniques (wrestlers) had an actual increase in the wall thickness of their left ventricle but not necessarily in their end-diastolic dimension. Perhaps, endurance training leads to volume increases in the heart and strength training to changes similar to those seen with pressure overloads on the heart. Gilbert and coworkers compared echocardiographic measurements in 20 runners with those in 26 sedentary control subjects.[17] The runners showed a modest degree of right and left ventricular chamber enlargement and possibly left ventricular function when compared to the control subjects. Perhaps, the running produced adaptive changes in ventricular volume and in ventricular mass.

DeMaria and associates investigated the effects of modest aerobic training in normal young persons by performing echocardiographic examinations before and after training.[12] These subjects developed an increase in the end-diastolic dimensions of their left ventricle, a decrease in the end-systolic dimensions of their left ventricle, and an increase in the percentage of fractional shortening, suggesting an increase in left ventricular performance after training. Additionally, they found an increased left ventricular mass after training. Interestingly, hemodynamic monitoring after training showed the same cardiac output with a reduced heart rate but an increased stroke volume secondary to the increase in left ventricular dia-

stolic volume. Thompson and colleagues did not find any changes in cardiac dimensions in subjects after 11 weeks of aerobic training.[56] Echoes were read in a double-blind fashion, and the findings of the above authors in cardiac dimensions after training were not substantial (very small millimeter differences). From my years of experience performing echocardiograms on many people, including many endurance-trained athletes, I believe that there is very little difference between the so-called untrained person's echocardiogram and that of the endurance-trained person.

Electrocardiographic Findings

As many as 60% to 70% of endurance-trained athletes will have some electrocardiographic findings suggestive of hypertrophy of the left ventricular free walls. These findings may depend on the actual increase in the circulating blood volume and cardiac mass (blood volume plus muscle) or may be due to the relative thinness of the endurance-trained athlete, and hence the closeness of the heart to the external chest leads. It is very common to see some form of T-wave abnormalities, such as T-wave inversion, especially in the inferior leads. Additionally, there is often some ST segment or J-point elevation. Obviously, these findings should not be interpreted as signs of myocardial ischemia or pericarditis. Because endurance training produces an increase in the vagal tone to the heart, the endurance-trained athlete will not only have a very slow resting heart rate, but also may have multiple sinus arrhythmias, such as marked alterations in the resting heart rate on a moment-to-moment basis, first-degree heart block (a prolongation of the PR interval), or even second-degree heart blocks of a Wenckebach nature. Similarly, there may be incomplete right bundle branch block patterns and premature atrial or even premature ventricular beats.

Because it is not uncommon for endurance-trained athletes to overtrain and complain of fatigue, the physician must be aware of certain alterations that exercise produces on blood chemistry values and blood cell variables.[37] Often, the erythrocyte count (the hematocrit) is lower than "normal." Fatigue may then be erroneously ascribed to an "anemic" state. As has been discussed previously, endurance training produces an increase in the plasma cell volume and a secondary increase in erythrocyte mass. Because the plasma volume increases to a greater degree than the lesser increase in the erythrocyte mass, there is a relative fall in the hematocrit owing to a dilutional effect. Commonly, endurance-trained athletes will have hematocrit percentages in the low 40s, whereas the untrained person at sea level will usually have a hematocrit percentage in the high 40s.

Certain blood enzymatic biproduct levels, such as serum glutamic oxalacetic transaminase, lactic dehydrogenase, and alkaline phosphatase, are higher in trained persons than in untrained ones. The reason for these elevated levels is unclear, but they do not necessarily reflect abnormalities of hepatic function. The blood urea nitrogen, may be slightly higher in a trained person secondary to a possible dehydrated condition.

Finally, active runners commonly have urinary "abnormalities." These runners may spill a small amount of protein in the urine that is detected on a urinalysis. Additionally, there may be microscopic amounts of erythrocytes. Sometimes, painless, asymptomatic gross hematuria (bright red blood) may occur in an athlete after an especially long run. This disquieting occurrence is not necessarily a predictor of significant renal or bladder disease.

Sudden Death in Athletes

Thompson and associates have shown that sudden coronary artery deaths can occur in endurance-trained runners.[57] Early statistics from Kuller suggested that coronary artery disease accounted for 75% of the deaths in unconditioned joggers.[32] Although unsuspected coronary artery disease often is the culprit in sudden death during running, this does not necessarily mean that myocardial infarctions always occur. People with occult but significant coronary artery disease may die from a ventricular arrhythmia while running. Also, heat prostration or heat stroke may account for sudden death in runners during a run. All cardiologic sudden death events that occur in runners are not necessarily secondary to pure coronary artery disease.

Maron and coworkers investigated the cause of 23 sudden deaths in young, nonrunning, active athletes, including football players, basketball players, tennis players, and swimmers.[36] The cause was hypertrophic cardiomyopathy in 3 athletes, silent coronary atherosclerosis in 3, anomalous origin of the left coronary artery system in 3, and Marfan's disease in 2. Silent coronary artery atherosclerosis (meaning no symptoms of angina pectoris) and an anomalous takeoff of the left coronary system are impossible to predict. Although it is unfortunate that children and young adults cannot be screened for anomalous takeoff or development of their coronary artery system, clearly a certain number of deaths in young persons with this genetic developmental abnormality of coronary artery diseases will occur while these persons are exercising. This abnormality cannot be reliably predicted unless there are symptoms suggestive of angina pectoris.

Contraindications to Exercise Testing and Training

Coronary Artery Atherosclerosis

Young or old, people with definite symptoms of coronary artery atherosclerosis or ischemia should be referred to a cardiologist before engaging in an exercise program. Further, the new onset of classic angina pectoris or a change in a stable pattern of angina pectoris to a crescendo-type pattern or an unstable (meaning multiple bouts of angina pectoris at rest or with minimal exercise) pattern should be a firm contraindication to beginning or to further participation in exercise programs until the patient is evaluated by a cardiologist. Other abnormalities that might restrict or prohibit a person from engaging in an exercise program are listed below.

Contraindications to Exercise Training and Testing

Absolute

Recent myocardial infarction (< 5 days old)
Recent aortic dissection
Massive ventricular aneurysm
Uncontrolled ventricular tachycardia
Atrial fibrillation with uncontrolled rapid ventricular response
Uncontrolled congestive heart failure
Acute myocarditis
Recent pulmonary embolus
Unstable or crescendo angina pectoris
Severe triple vessel or left main coronary stenosis (> 55% stenosis)
Uncontrolled hypertension
Severe pulmonary hypertension
Certain cyanotic congenital heart disease
Severe aortic stenosis
Severe subaortic stenosis (IHSS)
Severe thrombophlebitis
Acute febrile illness (rheumatic fever)
Severe anemia
Uncontrolled diabetes mellitus, thyroid disorders, renal or liver failure

Relative

Cardiomegaly
Complete heart block
Fixed-rate ventricular pacemaker
Electrolyte disorders

Valvular Heart Disease

The many forms of acquired and congenital valvular heart disease can become clinically significant at any age. The type and severity should be carefully assessed in those patients known to have valvular abnormalities. No proven evidence exists that exercise improves the function of the affected valves themselves. Because there can be all types of severity of valvular abnormalities, some valvular abnormalities might allow exercise more easily than others. In fact, an exercise program may actually assist the heart in adapting to the mechanical limitations imposed by the valvular lesion. A specific example is the slowing of the heart rate at submaximum levels of exercise, which might allow a more efficient filling of the left ventricle in those patients with mild rheumatic mitral stenosis. This more efficient filling could theoretically improve the total cardiac output at rest and at submaximum exercise levels.

A patient with severe mitral stenosis would most likely be unable to train because of marked shortness of wind. Additionally, the rapid heart rate that would ensue with exercise in a patient with severe mitral stenosis could impair the filling of the left ventricle and the cardiac output during the exercise and could lead to elevated pressure in the pulmonary vascular bed. Hence, patients with severe tight mitral stenosis should refrain from exercise training and testing. Other valvular abnormalities that could contraindicate exercise testing or exercise training include moderate to severe aortic stenosis and subvalvular aortic stenosis, especially the subaortic hypertrophic type, such as IHSS. Severe aortic stenosis may lead to sudden death during exertion, but more often the patient with severe aortic stenosis has symptoms of near syncope with exertion, chest pain, or bouts of congestive heart failure. Patients with moderate to severe aortic stenosis should definitely not undergo vigorous physical exercise training or testing. In contrast, patients with isolated aortic insufficiency appear to tolerate exercise testing and training for many years; in fact, many marathon runners have moderate aortic insufficiency. When a patient with aortic insufficiency becomes symptomatic, he should be evaluated by a cardiologist. A cardiologic evaluation is especially necessary for the symptomatic patient with aortic insufficiency who is considering beginning an exercise program; for those symptomatic persons already engaged in an exercise program, the feasibility of continuance in this program must be determined.

Exercise training or testing may be harmful to persons with Marfan's syndrome, a genetically inherited abnormality of the connective tissues throughout the body. People with Marfan's syndrome are extremely tall and have very long arms and very flexible joints. They also have an increased incidence of dilatation of their aorta and often develop aortic aneurysms or rupture. These patients often have associated abnormalities of the aortic valve, leading to aortic insufficiency, and of the mitral valve, leading to mitral valve prolapse. Although all these patients should not be totally prohibited from engaging in exercise, they should gain cardiologic clearance before engaging in vigorous exercise programs. If they have a significant amount of aortic insufficiency and a markedly dilated aortic root, they must choose their exercise activity very carefully. Some physicians have advocated treating these patients with beta blocking agents, hoping to reduce the forcefulness of systolic contraction and, hence, impairing further dilatation of the aorta.

A final area that has gained notoriety over the past 10 to 15 years is the mitral valve prolapse syndrome. The true incidence of the syndrome is unknown, as is its exact spectrum. It does appear, however, to be relatively common in females and not rare in males. In its full-blown state, mitral valve prolapse syndrome is manifested by a systolic prolapse of one or both of the mitral valve leaflets into the left atrium. This may be associated with systolic regurgitation of blood from the left ventricle to the left atrium. These patients often have chest discomfort that is atypical for true angina pectoris. They may also have atrial and ventricular ectopic beats. Only a very small subset of patients with the full-blown syndrome have significant ventricular arrhythmias that would necessitate medication. At physical examination, these patients may have a click or an isolated murmur.

Echocardiography has been used to substantiate the diagnosis of mitral valve prolapse, but debate continues as to what constitutes "borderline" mitral valve prolapse on the two-dimensional or single-dimensional echo. Most patients with the mitral valve prolapse syndrome do not have marked mitral regurgitation. Patients with minimal symptoms or minimal findings of mitral valve prolapse may participate in any level of physical activity that they desire. Obviously, patients with marked mitral regurgitation and chamber enlargement should not train vigorously unless cleared by their physician.

Exercise testing and training can be done easily in patients who have undergone valvular replacement and whose overall cardiac function is intact (Fig. 5-3). A supervised cardiac rehabilitation program is, in fact, recommended for patients after an uncomplicated postoperative recovery from valvular replacement. Obviously if the patient's valvular disease or coronary artery disease has damaged the myocardium either before or after the valvular replacement, exercise testing and training could be dangerous, depending on the severity of the left ventricular dysfunction. This type of left ventricular dysfunction is generally associated with symptoms that would bring the patient to his physician's attention.

Septal Defects

Those subjects or patients with the common congenital abnormalities of atrial septal defect or ventricular septal defect may successfully undergo exercise training and testing if they have normal pulmonary artery pressure and resistance. Congenital abnormalities that could be dangerous to the patient if he were to be exercise-trained or tested include severe coarctation of the aorta, severe congenital aortic or pulmonic valvular stenosis, and certain cyanotic abnormalities, such as Ebstein's anomaly or tetralogy of Fallot. Young people with congenital abnormalities should be evaluated by their physician and undergo tests to determine their level of physical capacity in order to avoid unnecessary restrictions in their activity. The exercise test also serves as a baseline to follow improvement or deterioration with physical training.

Cardiomyopathies

Congestive cardiomyopathies, especially if uncontrolled, are a frank contraindication to exercise training or testing. This condition is characterized by a very large dilated left ventricle, which has a global severe impairment in left ventricular function characterized by an inability to empty itself adequately—a very low ejection fraction. If there is any question as to whether a patient has congestive heart failure or a cardiomyopathy, the opinion of a cardiol-

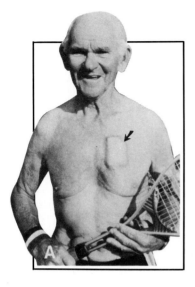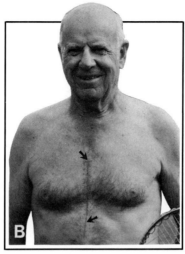

FIG. 5-3
A United States Tennis Association National 85's champion (*A*) competes wearing a pacemaker. A 75's player (*B*) competed successfully at the National Clay Court Championship 2 months after he had undergone a heart valve replacement.

ogist should be obtained before exercise testing or training.

Persons with an active myocarditis (meaning an active inflammation of the myocardium) should not be allowed to engage in exercise during the period of active inflammation. Experimental studies have suggested that exercise can definitely be harmful in patients with acute viral myocarditis.[33] Typically, the young patient who contracts a viral myocarditis will have been healthy before getting an influenza (flu)-like syndrome, followed within a few weeks by a noticeable decrease in his exercise tolerance. Many persons with the flu or a cold will not feel quite up to par for a week to 10 days, but this does not mean that they have a myocarditis. If, however, the patient is known to have had a recent myocarditis, a cardiologist or pediatric cardiologist should "clear" the patient before the patient engages in any active exercise program.

A form of cardiomyopathy called hypertrophic cardiomyopathy is characterized by excessive thickening of part of the muscular walls that compose the left ventricle. The classic type of hypertrophic myopathy is the so-called idiopathic hypertrophic subaortic stenosis (IHSS). Patients with IHSS may have associated obstruction of the left ventricular outflow tract. These patients with hypertrophic myopathies have a relative restriction to adequate diastolic filling of the left ventricle owing to abnormal stiffness or loss of compliance of their left ventricles. Episodes of sudden death may occur with exercise testing or exercise training in patients with obstructive IHSS. If there is any question as to the patient's having a hypertrophic cardiomyopathy, exercise test or training procedures should not be done without previous consultation with a cardiologist.

Hypertension

Long-standing uncontrolled hypertension may result in a uniformly thickened but dilated left ventricle. Similarly, long-standing uncontrolled hypertension may affect certain target organs, such as the kidney. Patients with severe uncontrolled hypertension should not undergo exercise testing or training until their hypertension is adequately evaluated.

Other Contraindications

Other absolute contraindications to exercise testing or training outside a supervised cardiac rehabilitation program or cardiology-supervised laboratory include recent myocardial infarction, recent massive pulmonary emboli, severe pulmonary hypertension, uncontrolled diabetes mellitus, or thyrotoxicosis. In addition, persons with abnormalities of cardiac rhythm, such as complete heart block or a fixed-rate ventricular pacemaker, should consult with a cardiologist before beginning exercise testing and training.

Patients with severe varicose veins or acute thrombophlebitis (an inflammation of the vein) should certainly not undergo exercise testing or training until they are cleared by their physician. Clinical observations suggest that regular physical activity may lead to a diminution in the size of superficial varicose veins. An increase in venoconstrictor tone could explain this finding, but to date there is no substantiation of this clinical finding. Similarly, there have been no adequate studies showing a decrease in the rate of thrombophlebitis in patients with varicose veins after the institution of regular exercise training. The Committee on Exercise of the American Heart Association does not believe there is any justification for the fear that an increase in physical activity would cause the onset of thrombophlebitis in patients with varicose veins. This committee suggests that regular exercise considered valuable for other health reasons would most likely prevent thrombophlebitis.

Persons with atherosclerotic lesions involving the large and small arteries of the lower extremities who have claudication (pain in the calves on exertion) show a delay in the onset of their symptoms after exercise training. They are also able to exercise longer once the discomfort occurs before it becomes unbearable. Both of these effects suggest an improvement in arterial circulation or venous circulation to the lower extremities with exercise training.

Coronary Artery Disease

Can exercise prevent the development, or mitigate the effects, of coronary artery disease? To investigate the possible role of exercise in the primary or secondary prevention of coronary artery disease manifestation, the known risk factors for developing coronary artery disease should be reviewed. Recently there has been a change to a more active life-style among the American populace[59] a change seemingly coincident with decreased mortality from, but not the incidence of, coronary artery disease. Coronary artery disease still remains a major adult health problem and a primary cause of premature death among persons in industrialized nations.

Risk Factors

Of all known risk factors, the genetic makeup of the individuals plays the key role in predisposing or protecting a person from developing coronary artery disease. A strong history of coronary artery disease manifestations (angina pectoris, myocardial infarction, sudden death) at an early age in a close family member is one of the best markers of the potential of any person to develop significant coronary artery disease. Data from the Framingham study have shown that, besides genetics, the three major risk factors for developing significant coronary artery disease and its manifestations are elevated cholesterol levels, elevated systolic blood pressure, and a high consumption of cigarettes. Other less well-delineated risk factors include obesity, diabetes mellitus, glucose intolerance, physical inactivity, and stress. In any given person, certain risk factors may be more important than others. Just as the development of coronary artery disease is a multifactorial process, so the effects of exercise may be multifactorial and may alter or mitigate risk factors in any given person in many ways.

Prevention Through Exercise: Possible? Probable? Impossible?

Because of the multifactorial nature of risk factors involved in atherogenesis, the influence of physical activity on the primary or secondary prevention of coronary artery disease and its manifestations is a very complex question to resolve. Extravagant claims have centered around the beneficial effects of exercise on cardiovascular health. Some advocates say that either the physical conditioning needed to run a marathon or the life-style of a marathon runner provides nearly certain yearly immunity from the coronary artery disease manifestations of heart attack or sudden death.[2] Others have stated that no level of exercise or physical fitness will protect and it is solely the genetic set that one inherits that determines whether the manifestations of coronary artery disease will develop.

Pathologic studies from the Korean and Vietnam wars and autopsies done on young persons dying of other causes have shown that, in this country and probably in other industrial countries, there is a high incidence of atherosclerosis in all major blood vessels of the body at an early age. Can exercise help in the primary prevention of this coronary artery disease and its manifestations? We know that endurance training reduces the heart rate and the blood pressure at any submaximum exercise level, reduces the myocardial oxygen requirement at any given submaximum level, increases the cardiac stroke volume at any submaximum level, raises the plasma volume, and increases the maximum oxygen uptake with total exhaustive exercise. Primary prevention means modification of the risk factors that may lead to the development of coronary artery atherosclerosis.

Effects of Exercise on Risk Factors

Exercise training affects the three major risk factors (hypertension, cigarette smoking, and elevated cholesterol). The effect of exercise on resting blood pressure is interesting: The mean arterial pressure of endurance-trained athletes is not significantly different from the "normal" blood pressures of sedentary persons. The question of whether exercise training will significantly lower the blood pressure, then, really depends on whether the blood pressure, both systolic and diastolic, is elevated before the start of an exercise program. Those persons who appear to have a higher than normal, or upper limits of normal, systolic and diastolic blood pressure at the beginning of an exercise training program will often show a decrease in both their systolic and diastolic blood pressures after an exercise program.

Evidence suggests that regular exercise, especially in the early stages of hypertension, may lower the resting blood pressure.[5, 31] Whether the changes in the resting systolic and diastolic blood pressures are due to exercise training *per se* or to a loss of body fat and a decrease in sodium intake is not totally resolved. Middle-aged hypertensive men, when kept on the same diet and medication, have a significant drop in both the systolic and diastolic blood pressures when the only change in their management is the institution of an exercise training program.[26] Therefore exercise training of a modest level, when combined with loss of body fat and a restriction of excessive sodium intake, may be a beneficial first step in the early management of patients with essential hypertension.

Many epidemiologic studies have shown that, with the onset of physical training, cigarette consumption tends to decrease. Whether the individual stays at that lower consumption level or remains totally abstinent from cigarettes may depend on whether he continues his exercise program.

The literature on the effects of exercise on cholesterol levels has been extensive but, at times, confusing, especially reported changes in total serum cholesterol.[9, 16, 18, 28] These studies have been criticized because the subjects had an associated decrease in body weight or body fat. Two reports, however, show a significant decrease in serum cholesterol despite no significant changes in body fat.[43, 52] An equal number of investigators have shown no significant decrease in serum cholesterol levels with exercise training.[4, 14, 29, 35]

There have been good data on the effects of exercise on the various lipoprotein particles that make up the total cholesterol level. In humans, total cholesterol is carried in three major lipoprotein groups. Large, very low-density lipoprotein particles (VLDL) primarily carry serum triglyceride and only a small portion of total body cholesterol. Low-density lipoproteins (LDL-beta particles) carry a major portion of the total serum cholesterol. Finally, high-density, or alpha, lipoproteins (HDL) carry only a small portion of total serum cholesterol and a larger proportion of phospholipids and proteins. Miller and Miller[39] have suggested that the serum concentration of LDL is the best determinant of the rate at which cholesterol particulate matter is deposited within the arterial walls, and the LDL level appears to be linearly related to the incidence of coronary heart disease in a population. Studies that have shown a linear relation between the incidence of coronary heart disease and total serum cholesterol levels most likely reflect increases in low-density cholesterol levels.

Interestingly, as the level of HDL cholesterol increases in a population, the incidence of coronary artery disease is inversely related to the level of HDL cholesterol. The HDL cholesterol may determine the rate at which cholesterol particles are actually removed from the arterial walls. Perhaps the plasma level of HDL lipoproteins is increased with exercise training.

Work by Martin and by Wood and others have shown the effects of habitual vigorous exercise on the lipoprotein fractions.[37, 61] Although the serum concentration of total cholesterol was not dramatically different between untrained and trained persons, there was a dramatic difference in the level of HDL, LDL, and triglycerides. These changes did not seem to depend on abstinence from alcohol. From these data, it appears that endurance-trained athletes have a higher level of HDL proteins than do untrained control subjects. Body fat reduction and modest alcohol intake will also produce an increase in HDL. Work from lipid research clinics has shown that the effect of exercise in increasing HDL seems to be independent of weight loss or alcohol intake.[24] Whether this increase in HDL, secondary to exercise training, will offer primary protection from developing atherogenesis is unclear.

After each episode of physical exertion, the serum triglyceride level is reduced, and those people who regularly exercise will often have a much lower triglyceride level than will nonexercising control subjects. The triglyceride level *per se* may not, however, be an independent risk factor for developing coronary artery disease. Cooper and associates have studied the effects of the physical fitness level, as measured by total time on a graduated treadmill stress test, on serum cholesterol, triglycerides, blood pressure, blood glucose, blood uric acid, and percentage of body fat.[9] All of these factors were significantly higher in the men with poor exercise performance than in those in the excellent fitness group. These fit persons appear to have a lower fasting blood sugar and uric acid level than do the untrained. The regular exercise produces an increased cellular sensitivity to insulin, a decreased level of circulating blood glucose, and decreased requirements for exogenous insulin. Consequently, regular exercise is now recommended as a way to decrease both the circulating blood sugars and the dosage of hypoglycemic agents that are required to manage the diabetic patient.

Trained persons who exercise regularly appear to have decreased "stickiness" of the blood platelets and a significantly higher fibrinolytic activity than do nontrained persons.[60] Because platelets play an integral part in the atherosclerotic process, the decrease in the clotting process that occurs through decreased platelet stickiness or increased fibrinolytic activity of the blood may be an important effect of exercise in decreasing the development of an atherosclerotic lesion.

Exercise has psychological effects, too. People who exercise gain an improved self-image, an improved sense of well-being, and a reduction in anxiety levels, especially in the hours after they exercise. These psychological benefits may motivate a person to improve other potentially harmful health habits. He may, for example, stop smoking cigarettes. Clearly, regular exercise encourages a life-style (either through modification of risk factors or through some inherent protection of the exercise) that appears to be associated with a low risk for developing coronary artery disease.

Alterations in risk factors may interact with the incidence of coronary artery disease in either of two ways: They may either delay the development of atherosclerosis or an atheromatous lesion, or they may mitigate its effects once it is established. The question of a delay in the development of an atherosclerotic lesion by exercise training is a difficult one to resolve. A large number of pathologic examinations and postmortem studies have not provided convincing evidence that atherosclerotic lesions are definitely less evident in a more active person. Selvester and coworkers have shown in a large prospective study that patients with documented coronary artery disease (by coronary angiography) who then engage in a regular exercise program appear to have less progression of their coronary artery atherosclerotic lesions than do those who do not engage in regular exercise programs;[50] however, the group involved Selvester's study who engaged in regular exercise training also underwent modification of their cigarette smoking habits and other risk factors. If it cannot be conclusively proved that exercise can delay the development of atherosclerotic lesions, can exercise mitigate the effects of atherosclerosis once it has appeared?

Myocardial oxygen supply could, theoretically, be improved by increased collateral coronary circulation or increased coronary capillary development. Coronary collaterals have been developed in endurance-trained animals, but this has not been consistently confirmed in humans. In humans, however, myocardial oxygen demands have been shown to be reduced at submaximum levels of exercise, a reduction perhaps due to metabolic alterations in the heart cells themselves, making them more efficient users of oxygen, or to decreased heart rate and blood pressure that occur after physical training at any given level of submaximum exercise. Thallium-201 exercise scintigraphy, a technique that shows the actual perfusion of blood to the myocardial cells, may answer the question of whether endurance training actually increases myocardial blood supply, and hence perfusion.

Epidemiologic Studies

Those interested in support for their decision to promote exercise as a primary or secondary prevention method have turned to the epide-miologist for data. If the postulated preventive and protective mechanisms of exercise are in effect in those persons who are physically active, population studies should show that the more physically active persons have a lower incidence of coronary artery disease and its manifestations. To date, epidemiologic studies have been of a retrospective and prospective nature. Retrospective studies evaluate populations after the development of significant coronary artery disease to analyze those factors that may have predisposed the population to the disease. Unfortunately, retrospective studies often analyze populations where the data were obtained in the past without attention having been focused on the epidemiologic question, which is asked later.

Retrospective Studies

The classic retrospective study on exercise and coronary artery disease was done by Morris and coworkers.[42] They reviewed the records of London Transport employees and found a 1.5 times higher incidence of coronary artery disease in sedentary bus drivers than in the more active ticket takers and conductors. The sudden death rate and the death rate during the first 2 months after a myocardial infarction were twice as high in sedentary bus drivers. Many thought these were unequivocal epidemiologic data supporting the effect of regular exercise on preventing or mitigating the manifestations of coronary artery disease. This study did not attempt, however, to substantiate the total activity levels of these two groups, particularly in reference to their leisure-time activities. It also did not consider that a selection process may have been involved. Perhaps the bus drivers chose sedentary jobs because they were sedentary in their leisure-time activities. A subsequent review of Morris' data has shown that, even at the time of their job applications, the drivers had higher blood pressures and cholesterol levels than did the conductors. Further epidemiologic data come from a study comparing blacks and whites in Evans County, Georgia.[22, 38] The higher physical activity levels and lower social standards among the blacks in this county seemed to account for a much lower incidence of coronary artery disease manifestations than occurred in the more affluent, less active, white age-matched control subjects.

Prospective Studies

Prospective studies are used to evaluate populations and groups and then to follow them over time to determine the effects of various risk-factor modifications on the development of a disease process. The most widely quoted prospective study on coronary artery disease is the Framingham study.[30] This study showed that persons with a sedentary life-style had significantly more coronary artery disease than did the more active age-matched control subjects. Paffenbarger and Hale have recently reported on a long-term follow-up of longshoremen in the San Francisco Bay area.[46] The longshoremen who did heavy work and expended high levels of energy had a lower mortality rate from coronary artery disease than did age-matched control subjects who expended light to medium levels of energy. There was no difference in the lesiure-time activity levels of these groups. During the 16-year follow-up, the less active group had a one-third higher incidence of coronary artery disease deaths than did their more active colleagues. This significant difference held even when blood pressure and smoking habits were taken into consideration.

More recently, college men and alumni were examined to determine the level of energy expenditure that offers some protection from the manifestations of coronary artery disease.[45] Results show that the heart attack rate declines with increasing activity in persons of all ages and for both nonfatal and fatal heart attacks. There appears to be a clear division as to the level of energy expenditure required. Energy expenditures of more than 2000 kilocalories a week have a strong inverse relation to heart attack risk. Casual sports activities offer no modification of the risks from developing a myocardial infarction.

From these epidemiologic studies, there seems to be an inverse relation between a high level of physical activity and coronary artery disease manifestations. Active persons appear to have at least one half the incidence of coronary artery disease manifestations and one third the mortality from coronary artery disease when compared to less active persons. But is the activity selective or protective in its effect? Do people who exercise regularly make up a self-selected group in whom the initial risks for developing coronary artery disease are quite low, or does the exercise training itself produce a protective effect against coronary artery disease manifestations? Perhaps, a selective mechanism is involved.[51]

Siegel and coworkers questioned marathon runners who reported a less frequent paternal history of coronary artery disease than did their age-matched nonrunning controls. These observations suggest that the reduced rates of coronary heart disease among subjects who exercise regularly may, in part, be due to a decreased familial predisposition to the disease. Whether this is a genetically transcribed protective factor or an environmental factor is unclear. Although Siegel reported a 40% lower incidence of heart attacks in the fathers of marathon runners, the fathers themselves were physically active. Perhaps their marathon-running offspring had an environmental interest in physical activity and not necessarily a selected genetic difference. Paffenbarger and others have shown that, at any given level of risk, physically active persons seem to have fewer manifestations of coronary artery disease than do inactive persons. Thus high levels of exercise done regularly may offer some protection against developing manifestations of coronary artery disease.

What amount of exercise is needed to protect against coronary artery disease manifestations? Whereas some early investigators suggested that a regular expenditure of low levels of calories might offer some protection, Paffenbarger and associates suggest that a regular high-energy expenditure (greater than 2000 kilocalories a week above resting caloric expenditure) may be needed to lead to a protective effect.

Regular physical activity of a moderate to

high level (meaning job-related plus leisure-time physical activity) may decrease one's risk for developing the manifestations of coronary artery disease. Unquestionably, regular physical activity programs improve the quality of life. Although it is unclear whether regular exercise increases a person's life span, some experts argue that even if the quantity is increased, the extra years gained would be spent only in the actual performance of the exercise. The debate goes on.

A high level of daily physical energy expenditure (meaning the activity, and the lifestyle, of a marathon runner) has not been proved to offer complete immunity from coronary artery disease manifestations in any given individual. Recent work by Thompson and associates[57] and Noakes and colleagues[44] has unequivocally, through postmortem examinations, shown that marathon runners and distance endurance runners can develop symptomatic coronary artery disease. Autopsy studies have also shown that there may be an increased risk of sudden death associated with atherosclerotic coronary artery disease lesions during, or immediately after, each period of physical activity. Obviously, it is impossible to know, without a coronary angiogram, whether a person does have a significant coronary artery atherosclerotic lesion.

No evidence suggests that running *per se* is more dangerous than other activities, including sleep. What minimal evidence there is does incriminate intermittent sudden bursts of activity, such as weekend racquetball or touch football games, as possibly worse culprits for inducing a sudden death as compared to more sustained activities, such as running. Thompson's study clearly shows that neither superior athletic performance nor habitual exercise will guarantee protection against the manifestations of coronary artery disease or exercise-related coronary artery deaths.[57] Even those persons who have engaged in a high level of exercise for years will often disregard the warning symptoms of coronary artery disease. Those who die suddenly while running might have been able to prevent their sudden death if they had sought proper medical attention.

Cardiac Rehabilitation and Secondary Prevention

Outpatient cardiac rehabilitation exercise programs have become a widespread way of treating patients with coronary artery disease. The principles of exercise training apply to patients with cardiovascular disease as well as to "normal" persons. The aim of the cardiac rehabilitation program, or judiciously prescribed exercise, is to enhance overall cardiovascular performance, to improve the patient's sense of well-being and psychological confidence in his ability to return to a useful life-style, and to attempt secondary prevention of coronary artery disease manifestations. Secondary prevention means a modification of risk factors associated with coronary artery disease after a coronary artery disease manifestation or even has appeared (*i.e.,* after the onset of angina pectoris, myocardial infarction, or cardiovascular surgery).

Inpatient and Outpatient Rehabilitation

Cardiac rehabilitation, as applied to patients hospitalized for myocardial infarction or cardiovascular surgery, begins during the hospitalization. In those patients without contraindications for early low-level exercise testing or exercise training, cardiac rehabilitation may begin very early in their hospitalization. Obviously this form of exercise conditioning and training is only done in the hospital under the direct supervision of a cardiologist and other health-related persons well-versed in the application and safety of low-level exercise testing and training to this patient population. Most cardiac rehabilitation programs are done on an outpatient basis.

The basic principles of exercise training are the same for cardiac patients and "normal" persons, except that patients with increased risk for cardiac events initially should be doing exercise training under direct supervision. Before starting an outpatient cardiac rehabilitation program, those patients who have recently been hospitalized for cardiac events should undergo an exercise stress test to clear the patient for participation in the program, to determine the appropriate heart rate level of training for the patient, and to be aware of any serious and previously undiagnosed subclinical myocardial ischemia or significant arrhythmias. Patients with unstable angina pectoris, uncontrolled ventricular arrhythmia, or congestive heart failure are obviously not candidates for low-level exercise testing or cardiac rehabilitation programs. Thus exercise therapy is obviously not appropriate or useful for all patients with coronary artery disease. Patients recovering from a myocardial infarction that was uncomplicated, patients with stable angina pectoris, and patients who have had coronary artery bypass surgery are ideal subjects for cardiac rehabilitation programs.

Benefits

Those patients who engage in regular aerobic exercises in a cardiac rehabilitation program show changes physiologically similar to those observed in so-called "normal" persons. Within a relatively short time after the start of a regular exercise program (3 to 8 weeks), these patients have an increased overall work capacity and a decreased resting heart rate and heart rate with submaximal exercise. Moreover, blood pressure at submaximal exercise levels is decreased. With continuation of the training program, the cardiac patient may have fewer manifestations of myocardial ischemia, or the manifestations may appear only at higher workload levels than they did before the cardiac rehabilitation program was initiated. As mentioned previously, every patient with angina pectoris will develop pain at the same double-product level.

The beneficial effects of exercise training in lowering the resting heart rate and the heart rate and blood pressure (and the double-product) at any submaxium workload means that the cardiac patient may exercise for a longer period or to a more intense level of exercise before reaching his preset anginal threshold. Such an effect is not too dissimilar from that seen when beta blocking agents are used for the medical therapy of angina pectoris. The ability

to perform more exercise before the onset of symptoms is obviously a physiologic and psychologic improvement for the patient. Additionally, the frequency of ectopic heart beats may be reduced, and those patients with previous systolic hypertension may actually have a decreased resting blood pressure level. (This might be secondary to alterations in other risk factors for hypertension and not due solely to the training.)

Morbidity and Mortality

Over the past 15 years, many investigators have stressed the benefits that patients with angina pectoris or postmyocardial infarction states derive from an increased overall activity level achieved through cardiac rehabilitation programs. Gottheiner reported on a 5-year follow-up study of more than 1000 male patients with coronary artery disease.[20] When a 5-year comparison was made between those patients engaged in a regular exercise training program and a similar nonexercising group with previous myocardial infarction, there was a marked difference in mortality from secondary coronary artery events. Patients who engaged in a regular exercise program had a 3.6% mortality in the 5-year period, compared to a 12% mortality in the nonexercising group. Patients in the cardiac rehabilitation program also had reduced resting heart rate and resting and exercise blood pressure levels.

Hellerstein reported on the results of exercise training in more than 600 middle-aged men.[25] The death rate for those cardiac patients who engaged in exercise training was less than one half of the expected rate. Kentala randomly assigned postmyocardial infarction patients into either control or exercise groups.[31] These two groups were matched for age, severity of myocardial infarction, serum cholesterol levels, smoking habits, and premyocardial infarction activity levels. Although there was no difference between the exercising and nonexercising groups in mortality from a second coronary event or in morbidity (meaning nonfatal coronary artery events), these results may be explained by the fact that only 13% of the exercise-trained group regularly attended their exercise sessions and 14% of the nonexercising control group engaged in regular physical training programs on their own.

Bruce and colleagues analyzed the morbidity and mortality figures of patients in an exercise training program, depending on whether the patient remained in the program or became a "drop-out."[6] More than one half of the active participants in the exercise program were working, whereas only one third of the drop-outs were engaged in useful work. There also was a difference in total mortality figures between the active participants and the drop-outs. From these data, it appears that those who engage in a regular exercise training program not only have an enhanced level of physical conditioning, but also a decreased morbidity and mortality when compared to nonactive control subjects. Obviously patients should be matched not only for risk factors, but also for the same extent of coronary artery disease. This matching would necessitate knowledge of the exact size of a patient's myocardial infarction, the location of the infarction, and the severity of the coronary artery disease (as determined by coronary angiography). This, however, is a difficult, if not impossible, amount of information to be obtained on a population that would then be randomized to either nonexercise or exercise. Regardless of whether this type of study will ever be done, exercise training for patients with myocardial infarction appears to be beneficial physiologically and psychologically.

Many studies have shown that patients who engage in a regular exercise program after myocardial event or cardiovascular surgery are more likely to return to work. In a 6-year survey of patients engaged in a cardiac rehabilitation program, Fletcher reported that 58.9% of his actively exercising group returned to full-time employment.[15] Subtracting the retired group from this figure, nearly 90% of the patients who had engaged in regular exercise training achieved full-time employment. Only 16% of the patients who had dropped out of an exercise program were fully employed. Patients who have had successful coronary artery bypass surgery also benefit from an exercise program. Work by Ahmadpour and associates suggests that the improved physical work capacity seen after surgery is superior to medical therapy only if exercise training or conditioning is incorporated into the postsurgical rehabilitation of the patient.

Safety

With increased use of exercise training as part of the management of patients with coronary artery disease, the safety of cardiac rehabilitative training programs must be studied. The absolute incidence of mortality during a supervised cardiac rehabilitation program is very low. Haskell has reported a 3.3% mortality per year for current programs in the United States, an average of one death per 268,922 man-hours of participation, a very low number.[23] I have supervised a large cardiac rehabilitation program and believe that persons can safely participate in a supervised cardiac rehabilitation program, even if they have had severe triple-vessel coronary artery disease. There have been two successful resuscitations over a 2-year period in our cardiac rehabilitation program and no unsuccessful resuscitations. Both of the resuscitations were done by nurses with coronary care unit experience and by physical fitness leaders.

Exercise Prescription

Exercise training may be used as a therapeutic modality designed to promote beneficial clinical effects in patients with coronary artery disease. When exercise is used therapeutically, the same principles apply to its application as apply to the prescription of a drug. Consequently, the prescriber of exercise must know the specific indications and contraindications and possible adverse side-effects of exercise training.

Individualization

The exercise prescription is individualized for each patient and updated periodically. It incorporates general knowledge about the patient plus the results of the exercise test evaluation.

The exercise stress test provides information, such as the maximum heart rate obtained during the test, and reveals the limiting symptoms of the patient. The prescribed exercise should be substantially below the level of exercise that precipitated these symptoms. Moreover, the test may uncover any asymptomatic ischemic EKG changes, blood pressure changes, or arrhythmias.

In developing an exercise prescription, one should find out the previous exercise level of the patient, the type of exercise he prefers, and whether he prefers a group or individual exercise program. His motivation must also be assessed, and the amount of time he has to devote to exercise training because of other time commitments must be ascertained. When this information is available, the exercise prescription may be written in terms of intensity, frequency, duration, and type of exercise activity.

Target Heart Rate

The easiest measurement to use in developing an exercise prescription is the maximum heart rate that the patient attains during the exercise test. A target heart rate for training should be between 70% and 85% of the maximum obtainable heart rate and should be one that did not produce marked ST segment displacement or an excessive blood pressure rise or symptoms. Therefore the maximum obtainable heart rate from which the target heart rate zone is calculated should be one relatively free of signs and symptoms of significant myocardial ischemia.

Exercises

The exercises used in cardiac rehabilitation should be primarily isotonic, rhythmic, aerobic ones. The training period is preceded by a warm-up and is followed by cooling-down. The warm-up period lasts for 5 to 10 minutes and comprises simple, rhythmic, and repetitive light activities that slowly bring the heart rate up into the conditioning zone. The dynamic training period in the target heart rate zone follows the warm-up and lasts from 20 to 40 minutes. The exercise session ends with a 5-minute cool-down period of gradually decreasing exercise levels. To be effective, the physical conditioning must be done three or four times a week.

Supervision

Close contact must be maintained with the patient during the exercise program. The patient's awareness of special or new types of discomfort should be closely monitored. Each patient should be taught to obtain an accurate heart rate count by palpating a radial pulse or a carotid pulse before, during, and after each exercise period. An accurate heart rate may be obtained by this method during exercise by stopping the exercise and counting the heart rate for 10 seconds. I know of no symptoms that have occurred by allowing patients to palpate a carotid artery to obtain an accurate heart rate.

Return to Work

To evaluate the ability of any patient to return to useful employment, one should match the physical demands that will be placed on the patient during the job to the patient's physical capacity. Most "normal" persons can sustain a work output through an 8-hour period in the range of 25% to 40% of their maximum aerobic capacity, but different types of work demands may have different types of cardiac demands for oxygen supply. Because there are different myocardial oxygen demands for arm-work than for legwork, and for isometric exercises as compared to isotonic ones, the type of exercise that the patient will have to do during his work activities might lead to alteration in the type of exercise stress testing that is done.

REFERENCES

1. AHMADPOUR H, et al: Long-term effects of coronary surgery vs exercise training on physical work capacity. Circulation 58:140, 1978
2. BASSLER TJ, SCAFF JH: Exercise, running and the heart. N Engl J Med 292:1302, 1975
3. BLACKBURN J, KATIGBAK R: What electrocardiographic leads to take after exercise? Am Heart J 67:184, 1963
4. BONNANO JA, LIES JE: Effect of physical training on coronary risk factors. Am J Cardiol 33:760, 1973

5. Boyer JL, Kasch FW: Exercise therapy in hypertensive men. JAMA 211:1668, 1970

6. Bruce EH, et al: Comparison of active participants and dropouts in CAPRI cardiopulmonary rehabilitation programs. Am J Cardiol 37:53, 1976

7. Bruce RA: Exercise testing for evaluation of ventricular function. N Eng J Med 296:671, 1977

8. Claussen JP: Effect of physical training on cardiovascular adjustments to exercise in men. Physiol Rev 57:779, 1977

9. Cooper KH, et al: Fitness levels vs selected coronary risk factors. JAMA 336:116, 1976

10. Coppes G, et al: Treadmill exercise testing: Part II. In Harvey WP (ed): Current Problems in Cardiology, vol 7, 8, 9. Chicago, Year Book Publishers, 1977

11. Currens JH, White PD: Half a century of running: clinical, physiological and autopsy findings in the case of Clarence DeMar ("Mr. Marathon"). N Engl J Med 265:988, 1961

12. Demaria AN, et al: Alterations in ventricular mass and performance induced by exercise training in man evaluated by echocardiography. Circulation 57:237, 1978

13. Eckstein RW: Effect of exercise and coronary artery narrowing on coronary collateral circulation. Circ Res 5:230, 1957

14. Fitzgerald O, et al: Serum lipids and physical activity in normal subjects. Clin Sci 28:83, 1965

15. Fletcher GF: Exercise and the coronary patient. In Harvey WP (ed): Current Problems in Cardiology, vol. IV(3), p 46. Chicago, Year Book Publishers, 1979

16. Garret HL, et al: Physical conditioning and coronary risk factors. J Chronic Dis 19:189, 1966

17. Gilbert CA, et al: Echocardiographic study of cardiac dimensions and function in the endurance-training athlete. Am J Cardiol 40:528, 1977

18. Golding LA: Effects of physical training upon total serum cholesterol levels. Res Q 32:499, 1961

19. Goldschlager N, et al: Treadmill stress tests as indicators of presence and severity of coronary artery disease. Ann Intern Med 85:277, 1976

20. Gottheiner V: Long-range strenuous sports training for cardiac reconditioning and rehabilitation. Am J Cardiol 22:426, 1968

21. Guidelines for Graded Exercise Testing and Exercise Prescription. American College of Sports Medicine. Philadelphia, Lea and Febiger, 1975

22. Hames CG: Evans County cardiovascular and cerebrovascular epidemiology study (introduction). Arch Intern Med 128:883, 1971

23. Haskell WL: Cardiovascular complications during medically supervised exercise training of cardiacs. Circulation 51 and 52 (suppl 11):118, 1975

24. Haskell WL, et al: Strenuous physical activity, treadmill exercise test performance, and high-density lipoprotein cholesterol. Circulation 62:53, 1980

25. Hellerstein HK: The effects of physical activity: patients and normal coronary prone subjects. Minn Med 52:1335, 1969

26. Hellerstein HK, et al: Exercise and hypertension. Phys Sportsmed 4(12):34, 1976

27. Herschfield S, et al: Relative effects on the heart by muscular work in the upper and lower extremities. Arch Phys Med 49:249, 1968

28. Hoffman AA, et al: Effects of exercise program on plasma lipids in senior Air Force officers. Am J Cardiol 20:516, 1967

29. Hollszy JO, et al: Effects of a 6-month program of endurance exercise on serum lipids of middle-aged men. Am J Cardiol 14:753, 1964

30. Kannel WB: Habitual level of physical activity and risk of coronary heart disease: the Framingham study. Can Med Assoc J 96:811, 1967

31. Kentala E: Physical fitness and feasibility of rehabilitation after myocardial infarctions in men of working age. Ann Clin Res 4(suppl 9):1, 1972

32. Kuller L: Sudden death in arteriosclerotic heart disease. Am J Cardiol 24:617, 1969

33. Lerner AM, et al: Enteroviruses in the heart. Mod Concepts Cardiovasc Dis 44:7, 1975

34. Lind AR, McNicol GW: Muscular factors which determine the cardiovascular responses to sustained and rhythmic exercises. Proceedings of the International Symposium on Physical Activity and Cardiovascular Health, Toronto, October 11–13, 1966. Can Med Assoc J 96:12

35. Mann GV, et al: Exercise to prevent coronary heart disease. Am J Med 26:12, 1969

36. Maron BJ, et al: Etiology of sudden death in athletes (abst). Circulation 58:II-236, 1978

37. Martin RP, et al: Blood chemistry and lipid profiles of elite distance runners. In Milvy P (ed): The Marathon: Physiological, Medical, Epidemiological, and Psychological Studies, vol 301, p 347. New York, New York Academy of Sciences, 1977

38. McDonough JR, et al: Coronary heart disease among Negroes and whites in Evans County, Georgia. J Chronic Dis 18:443, 1965

39. Miller GJ, Miller NE: Plasma high-density lipoprotein concentration and development of ischaemic heart disease. Lancet 1:16, 1975

40. Montoye HT, et al: The effects of exercise on blood cholesterol in middle-aged men. Am J Clin Nutr 7:139, 1959

41. Morganroth J, et al: Comparative left ventricular dimensions in training athletes. Ann Intern Med 82:521, 1975

42. Morris JN, et al: Incidence and prediction of ischaemic disease in London bus men. Lancet 2:553, 1966

43. Naughton J, McCoy JF: Observations on the relationship of physical activity to the serum cholesterol concentration of healthy men and cardiac patients. J Chronic Dis 19:727, 1966

44. Noakes T, et al: Coronary heart disease in marathon runners. Ann NY Acad Sci 301:593, 1977

45. Paffenbarger RS Jr, et al: Physical activity as an index of heart attack risks in college alumni. Am J Epidemiol 108:161, 1978

46. PAFFENBARGER RS JR, HALE WE: Work activity and coronary heart mortality. N Engl J Med 292:545, 1975

47. POUPA O, et al: The effect of physical activity upon the heart of vertebrates. In Brunner (ed): Physical Activity and Aging. Medicine and Sports, vol IV, p 202. Baltimore, University Park Press, 1970

48. ROBINSON BF: Relation of heart rate and systolic blood pressure to the onset of pain in angina pectoris. Circulation 35:1073, 1967

49. SALTIN B, et al: Response to exercise after bedrest and training. Circulation 38 (suppl 7):1, 1968

50. SELVESTER R, et al: Effects of exercise training on progression of documented coronary arteriosclerosis in men. Ann NY Acad Sci 301:495, 1977

51. SIEGEL AJ, et al: Paternal history of coronary heart disease reported by marathon runners. N Engl J Med 301:90, 1979

52. SIEGEL W, et al: Effects of a quantitated physical training program on middle-aged sedentary men. Circulation 41:19, 1970

53. STENBERG J, et al: Hemodynamic response to work with different muscle groups, sitting and supine. J Appl Physiol 22:61, 1967

54. TEPPERMAN J, PEARLMAN D: Effects of exercise and anemia on coronary arteries of small animals as revealed by the corrosion cast technique. Circ Res 9:576, 1961

55. THOMPSON PD, KELEMAN MH: Hypotension accompanying the onset of exertional angina. Circulation 52:28, 1975

56. THOMPSON PD, et al: Generalized training effects without changes in cardiac performance. Med Sci Sport 10:1, 1978

57. THOMPSON PD, et al: Death during jogging or running: a study of 18 cases. JAMA 242:1265, 1979

58. TOMANEK RJ: Effects of age and exercise on the extent of myocardial capillary bed. Anat Rec 167:55, 1970

59. WALKER WJ: Changing United States lifestyle and declining vascular mortality: cause or coincidence? N Engl J Med 297:163, 1977

60. WILLIAMS RS, et al: Effects of physical conditioning on stimulated fibrinolytic activity in healthy adults (abst). Clin Res 27:216A, 1979

61. WOOD PD, et al: Plasma lipoprotein distributions in male and female runners. Ann NY Acad Sci 301:348, 1977

Strength is the ability of an athlete to do work against resistance. It is the force that a muscle group can exert against resistance in a single maximum effort, or the maximum weight that an athlete can lift one time through a full range of motion.

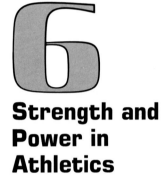

Strength and Power in Athletics

Strength and Muscle

An athlete develops strength by working against workloads greater than he normally encounters, responding to the stress of an overload resistance by becoming stronger.

Overload is the basis for progressive resistance exercises (PRE) in which the athlete becomes stronger as the resistance against which he works increases. The PRE principle was demonstrated in 6 B.C. by Mylo of Crotona, who is said to have carried a bull calf every day from its birth to its maturity, when he carried it around the stadium at the Olympic games. Progressive resistance exercises are also used to improve muscular endurance, since prolonged repetitions by underloaded muscles have little effect on this factor.[51]

Muscular contractions may be static, concentric, or eccentric. In a static or isometric contraction, the muscle does not shorten. With concentric contraction, the muscle does shorten, as in a biceps curl with a dumbbell. In eccentric contractions, the muscle lengthens while it is contracting, as when lowering a weight during a bench press or while losing at arm wrestling. An eccentric contraction allows the handling of heavier weight.

Muscular strength is a consequence of individual muscle fiber tentanization and the recruitment of a number of muscle fibers that act to lift, maintain, or lower a weight. An athlete may increase his strength by stretching a muscle just before he works with it. Prestretching may be seen in a golfer's backswing, the cocking phase of throwing, and the take-off in jumping and in a sprint start, where the quadriceps muscle is stretched just before the knee is extended. Such prestretching activates a stretch reflex that summons an added volley of impulses and recruits fibers to supplement the muscular contraction.

Muscles exercised against overload resistance will hypertrophy because of increased cross-sectional diameter of the muscle fibers.[28] Shortening of a muscle is a consequence of interdigitation of actin and myosin protein filaments contained within the membrane of the muscle fiber, the sarcolemma. As more myofibrils form per fiber, the total amount of protein increases, especially in the myosin filaments. Some of the gain in the number of fibers may even result from longitudinal fiber splitting. Such splitting may be found in muscles after prolonged weight lifting;[27] the amount of connective tissue and the capillary density in such muscles also increase. Endurance training causes more capillaries to form, improving the blood supply to the active muscles, and decreasing the distance over which molecules must diffuse from the blood to the mitochondria.

In addition to the muscular effect of training, there is a neuromuscular effect. Training increases the ease of transmission of nerve impulses across the motor end plates. This is important because the application of force in athletics demands fine neuromuscular control.

Weight lifters have a higher degree of motor unit synchronization than do nonathletic control subjects.[42, 66] Motor unit synchronization would provide a very rapid rate of maximum tension generation per cross-sectional area per unit of time for a given muscle. To vary the degree of force the athlete applies, he may change the number of motor units that contract together, or he may establish a summation wave by varying the frequency of impulses sent to the muscles. The neuromuscular system probably is inhibited by means of complex nervous system controls, and release of this inhibition may account for extraordinary feats of strength. "Shot and shout" stimuli overcome the inhibition, leading to a stronger contraction.

Strength helps to prevent injury by promoting increased stability of joints and by enabling the athlete to move faster to avoid injury. The muscle bulk itself protects underlying structures. Strength may be measured with a dynamometer or a cable tensiometer, by the maximal amount of weight an athlete can lift, or on a Cybex-II machine.

An athlete's strength reaches its maximum at 25 years of age, dropping at the rate of 1% per year thereafter. At 65 years of age, the athlete has lost about one third of the strength he had when he was 25 years old. Developing strength is hard work, but once gained it is relatively easy to retain. If the athlete stops training, he will lose strength at about one third the rate at which it was gained, but as little as one session a week of maximum contractions will prevent such strength loss.

Ligaments and Tendons

Exercise strengthens ligaments and tendons, in addition to muscles. Thus when rats are placed on a systematic running program, the strength of their medial collateral ligament attachments to bone increases. Rabbits trained on a running machine will develop significantly increased strength in their anterior cruciates.

Running on an uneven surface promotes a significantly greater increase in ligament strength than does running on a smooth surface. Thus when an athlete runs on an uneven surface, as in a cross-country race, he enhances his proprioception while increasing his ligament strength to a greater extent than when running on a track.

Exercise also strengthens tendons. When young animals are trained, the cross-sectional area of their Achilles tendon increases; in older animals, however, only the muscle hypertrophies. The tendons become stronger with training, but no quantitative compositional changes occur.

Strength Training Methods

Methods for building strength include gymnastic exercises, isometrics, isotonic weight lifting, intermedialis and isokinetic exercise, isodynamics, and plyometrics.

In *gymnastics,* the athlete's own body provides the resistance for strength development, whereas *isometrics* are static contractions—"dynamic tension"—performed against a fixed resistance. *Isotonic* exercises include conventional weight lifting or use machines with guided weight stacks. In *intermedialis* exercises, the athlete works against a partner's resistance. Throughout the range of motion in the latter exercise, the athlete momentarily stops the movement and starts again. This method builds functional strength, enhances proprioception, and prevents athletic injury. In *isokinetic* strength training, the athlete works against a hydraulic mechanism or a moving lever and gears, with the resistance he meets accommodating to the force he applies. An athlete may also perform the motions of his sport using weights or with overweight implements. A boxer, for example, may use heavy dumbbells to imitate his moves for related power and light weights for specific, imitative power. Some athletes use ankle weights, but these may overburden the legs and cause shin splints. Other weighted implements include heavy baseballs, weighted footballs, leather medicine balls, weighted bats, or an overweight shot, discus, or javelin. All of these devices build strength but may disturb the athlete's coordination. In *isodynamic* strength training, a rubber strap, surgical tubing, or a lightweight bicycle inner tube provides elastic resistance as the athlete mimics the moves used in his event. *Plyometrics* include hops, bounds, and depth jumps that develop power.

Which of these methods may be best for strength development will be determined by the athlete's specific needs and how the method affects his performance.[11]

Free Exercise

In strengthening by free exercise, the athlete's own body provides the needed resistance. These exercises include push-ups, chin-ups, pull-ups, dips, sit-ups, leg-raises, and abdominal hangs. The degree of difficulty of the exercises may be increased by adding weights or by modifying the exercise; for example, the difficulty of push-ups may be increased if the athlete places his legs on a stall bar or on a bench, or if he places a weight on his back or has a partner lie on his back. A woman beginning a strength program should start with modified push-ups that allow her knees to rest on the ground.

In chin-ups, the athlete's palms face him, and in pull-ups his palms face away. Dips on the parallel bars or on dip bars will strengthen the athlete's triceps as he lowers himself to the point where his elbows are bent 90° or more before pushing back up. In chin-ups, pull-ups, and dips, the athlete may strap a weight around his waist or hold a medicine ball between his legs to add resistance.

Sit-Ups

Strong abdominal muscles make breathing easier and give power to the midsection. These muscles include the rectus abdominus, external obliques, and internal obliques and are strengthened by sit-ups, twists, and leg raises. To do a sit-up, the athlete crosses his arms on his chest or holds his hands behind his head.[49] He begins by contracting his abdominal muscles to tilt his pelvis posteriorly, thus flattening his lumbar spine against the floor. He then raises his head and follows this cervical spine flexion with flexion of his thoracic spine. Next, the flexed spine is raised, maintaining the curl throughout the exercise. He uncurls as the trunk descends, with the lower back touching first, then the thorax, the cervical spine, and finally the head. The last step is relaxation of the pelvic tilt. Sit-ups should be done slowly to provide a maximum abdominal muscle contraction and to maintain the pelvic tilt and curl throughout the sit-up.

The trunk curl should be emphasized rather than the achievement of a full sit-up because electromyography has shown that abdominal muscles are vigorously active only during the first 30° to 45° of a sit-up. This is near the time when the scapulae leave the supporting surface. At about 30°, the trunk is already fixed, and for the rest of the sit-up the hip flexors, which are many times more powerful than the abdominal muscles, flex the trunk on the thighs.

An athlete is sometimes told to flex his hips and knees during a sit-up to put the hip flexors "on slack." Electromyograms show, however, that in the bent knee position, even more iliopsoas activity is needed to maintain the hip flexion.

The athlete should avoid arching his back, as arching puts undue stress on the lumbar spine. If his abdominal muscles are not strong enough to maintain the pelvic tilt, the sit-up position should be modified to the easier flexed-hip and flexed-knee style, where the pelvis is posteriorly tilted from the beginning.

Should an athlete's legs be held during sit-ups? An athlete's center of gravity moves toward his feet during a sit-up; thus a long-legged person's feet need not be held, but the athlete with a heavy trunk and short legs may need this assistance. The sit-up should not be started too quickly by snapping up, and the athlete should not rock on his buttocks or kick his legs down in an attempt to move his center of gravity distally to counterbalance his trunk. The athlete can hold a weight plate over his chest or above his head to make the sit-up more difficult.

Sit-ups may also be done on an inclined bench, or the athlete can do twisting sit-ups, "V-ups," and twists that are done with his body extended over the edge of a table or platform (Fig. 6-1). Whereas sit-ups work mainly on the upper abdominal muscles, leg-raises are a companion exercise that work the lower abdominals. With the sit-up board set at about a 30° slant, the athlete grasps the board behind his head, then bends his knees and lifts his feet to a vertical position. Keeping constant tension on his abdominal muscles, he slowly lowers his feet but does not allow them to rest on the floor. This exercise may also be done on the floor.

Abdominal Hangs

Abdominal hangs especially strengthen the athlete's lower abdominal muscles, lower back, hips, and upper thighs. To perform these, he hangs from a bar while a partner steadies him by pushing in on his lower back, or the athlete hangs from a wall bar (Fig. 6-2). As he squeezes the bar tightly, he raises his legs as high as possible, keeping his legs straight and holding this position for a count of 7 seconds. He then lowers his legs very slowly and raises them again, concentrating every second. Three sets of hangs are done with the legs straight ahead and then one set to each side. For added resistance, he may hold a medicine ball between his legs.

Plyometrics

Plyometrics are vigorous drills for developing power that can be used in running, jumping,

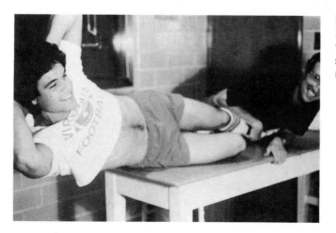

FIG. 6-1
Side sit-ups and twisting sit-ups strengthen the athlete's midsection.

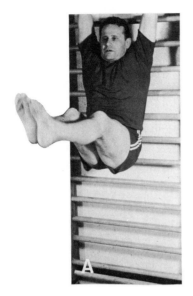
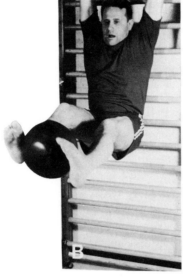

FIG. 6-2
Abdominal hangs may be done on the stall bars (*A*) with a medicine ball (*B*) for added resistance.

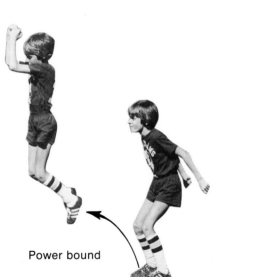
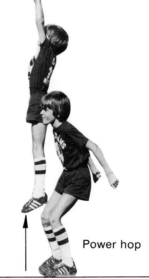

Power bound

Power hop

FIG. 6-3
Plyometric drills, like power bounds and power hops, develop power.

and throwing. The drills include hops and bounds (Fig. 6-3), depth jumps, jumping with weights, and medicine ball techniques.[20, 41, 54] Plyometrics are based on the stretch reflex that occurs when a muscle contracts more forcefully and quickly from a prestretched position than from a relaxed state. The faster a muscle is forced into an eccentric prestretch, the more tension is created during the concentric contraction, producing a more explosive effort. The rate at which the prestretch occurs is more critical than the physical length of the stretch.

The critical factors in explosive activities is the ability of the athlete's nervous system to switch muscular contractions from eccentric to concentric. Neuromuscular efficiency is needed, in contrast to strength movements, which depend mainly on the number of fibers innervated and how well developed they are. Plyometrics train the neuromuscular mechanism for switching the momentum of the lengthening phase to the contracting, working phase.

Hops develop neuromuscular links and may improve jumps and a sprinter's speed from the starting blocks.[41] The athlete begins each hop from a partial squat, then explodes upwards as high as possible without making a conscious effort to attain forward speed. Bounds stimulate the stretch reflex response and improve jumps and a sprinter's maximum running speed. They are even more physically demanding than hops. The athlete begins each bound from a partial squat, then jumps as high and as far as possible.

Hops may be done one day and bounds the next. Each hop or bound is part of a continuous sequence with maximum effort. The athlete may start his plyometric program over a 50-yard course, then add 5 yards a week until he reaches 100 yards, continuing to train at this distance. Plyometrics are done in two sets, each comprising double-leg, right-leg, and left-leg hops or bounds, with a 10-minute rest between each set.

Depth jumps are plyometric drills where the athlete steps off a bench, falls freely, and then rebounds up off the ground onto another bench to repeat the exercise.

Plyometric upper body drills use medicine balls and sandbags. Basketball players catch and pass the medicine ball. As the ball is caught, eccentric contractions occur that quickly switch to concentric ones as the ball is passed.

Olympic-style weight lifters have the highest power outputs and best vertical jumps in athletics, feats attributed to the plyometric nature of the double knee-bend technique in the snatch and the clean-and-jerk. Other athletes may train with these moves or perform high pulls, power cleans, and power presses (jerks).

Plyometrics may be applied to all sports that demand speed and power, with innovations limited only by the imagination and ingenuity of the athlete and his coach. Flights of hurdles may be arranged for high jumpers, long jumpers, and basketball players to clear plyometrically.[20] Skiers may jump plyometrically back and forth, sideways, and obliquely over obstacles, such as narrow 18-inch high benches or pipes.

Because plyometrics are so demanding, they should not be done every day. The athlete must develop basic leg strength amounting to about two times his body weight before these exercises are added to his training program. The exercises should be done on turf or mats to prevent heel bruises and shin splints. The very young athlete may not be ready for plyometric exercises.

Isometrics

In an isometric contraction, the muscle contracts without shortening because the external force that the muscle contracts against is greater than the force that the muscle can generate, resulting in a "static contraction." During an isometric contraction of more than 60% of maximum strength, blood flow to the muscle is temporarily occluded, producing an oxygen deficit in the muscle. Isometric strength increases may be related to the amount of oxygen deficit in the muscle during contraction.

The athlete may perform isometrics against his own hand or leg, a medicine ball, or an immovable object or do paired isometrics. In the last-mentioned exercise, a partner provides the resistance, a system especially good for neck strengthening.

Five to 10 static contractions of two thirds of maximum for 2 seconds each result in a 5% strength gain each week. It is difficult to judge, however, what two thirds of maximum is; thus the athlete is best advised to do a near maximum contraction.[47, 55] A 3-day-a-week training program may include, for example, five to eight repetitions of 6-second maximum contractions at three joint angles per joint.

Isometrics take little time and can be done almost anywhere. Because the strength gained is very specific to the joint angle at which the contractions are done, the athlete should train at several joint angles.[4, 57] Isometrics have the disadvantage of lacking carry-over to motor performance, and static contractions actually reduce maximal limb movement speed.[3, 61] Because isometrics lack feedback movement, athletes on this type of program may lose motivation.

Isotonic Strengthening

Although isotonic means equal or constant tension, the word is a misnomer because the tension in a muscle undergoing an isotonic contraction varies while lifting a constant load. Barbell programs are isotonic. In an isotonic *concentric* contraction, the muscle shortens as it contracts, whereas during an isotonic *eccentric* contraction, the muscle lengthens as it contracts.

Initially, isotonic strength training programs contained 70 to 100 repetitions, with 7 to 10 repetitions per set. Later programs dropped to three sets of 10 repetitions every other day. The repetition maximum (RM) is the maximum load that the athlete can lift for a given number of repetitions before his muscles show fatigue. The first and second set of lifts are warm-up sets, with the former entailing 10 repetitions at a load one half of the 10 RM, and the latter requiring 10 repetitions of a load three fourths of the 10 RM. The third is the overload set, in which the overload stress principle applies, consisting of 10 repetitions at the 10 RM. Because the athlete may be quite tired during this last set, variations in the program have been devised; for example, the athlete may perform the first set at 85% of the 10 RM and the third at 75% of the 10 RM.

Although isotonic training increases strength, lean body mass, and motor performance,[5–8, 58] training with free weights has some disadvantages, including a "sticking point," inertia, poor accommodation to fatigue, both limbs often being used against the same resistance, and eccentric contractions. The "sticking point" is the weakest point in a joint's range of motion, and the weight that an athlete can lift is limited by what he can handle at this point. Maximum resistance is met here, not at other joint angles. Momentum develops during isotonic exercise, and the movements become ballistic. Once inertia is overcome, little added work is needed to move the weight. Even though the athlete fatigues and weakens, the resistance he meets remains the same. With a barbell and on most isotonic machines, both of the athlete's arms and both legs must be used together, although in actual athletic activities, each body part would be working independently. One arm or a leg, however, may be weaker than the other.

Heavily loaded eccentric contractions may cause muscle soreness,[52] but these contractions can be eliminated. After the athlete concentrically pushes the weight up in the bench press, for example, spotters can remove the weight and replace it on his chest, and he can press it up again. The heavy weights used for eccentric repetitions can also be a safety problem, as when a lifter suffers a pectoralis muscle rupture and the weight abruptly crashes down too fast for the spotter to stop it. An eccentric training session may also require more time than does other training.

Variable Resistance Machines

Many athletes train on a Universal Gym or Nautilus machine. Some of the Universal stations have a weight stack with a lever arm that changes its length to provide "dynamic variable resistance." This machine is good for circuit training (Fig. 6-4).

Nautilus machines use a cam shaped like a nautilus shell for variable resistance. The cam changes the machine's moment arm—and hence the resistance—to compensate for variations in the athlete's muscle force at different joint angles. The machine is planned on an average force-angle curve, but because of differences in limb lengths, the greatest resistance may not be where the athlete has the greatest strength.[62] The athlete's head is supported, and there is no need for him to use energy-sapping,

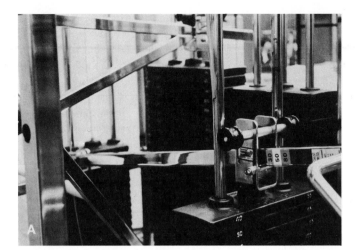

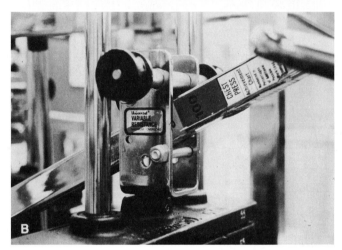

FIG. 6-4
The Universal Gym
provides variable
resistance as the lever
arm length changes
from "30" (*A*) to "100"
(*B*).

blood-pressure-raising isometric contractions to grip a bar. Some machines allow a compound exercise immediately after an isolation exercise.

The Nautilus pullover machine is often used by swimmers, who benefit especially from its prestretch feature (Fig. 6-5). Some swimmers, however, may sublux their shoulders or overstretch muscles on this machine, especially if the resistance is not carefully regulated. The Nautilus machines may help the athlete build a strong base of strength, and when this is established, he can advance to free weights for power training and a more direct application to the playing field. The machines, however, are expensive and take up a lot of floor space.

Intensity Of Effort

An athlete can best increase strength and muscle mass by training hard. Increasing the intensity of effort is achieved by lifting heavier weights, doing the work in less time, and, through sheer determination, carrying each exercise set to the point where another repetition is not possible. The athlete must strain his capacity to do the last, seemingly impossible, repetition. The athlete's motivation, a coach's or partner's encouragement, or startle procedures such as noises may induce greater effort in those who believe they have reached the limit of their strength. An athlete's perception of his effort exerts an important effect on realization of his potential, and this aspect of training needs as much attention as do other aspects to achieve optimal results. Obviously, psychological preparedness in sport is equal in importance to physical, technical, and tactical training to attain satisfactory integration of mind and body.

"Prefatigue"

In some instances, it is not possible to overload or to fatigue fully a muscle with a single exercise. Compound exercises such as dips or bench presses, for example, work both the pectoralis major and triceps, but the pectoralis major is not totally worked because the weaker triceps muscle gives out before the stronger pectoralis. To work the pectoralis muscles more com-

FIG. 6-5
The Nautilus pullover machine provides a prestretch that recruits muscle fibers.

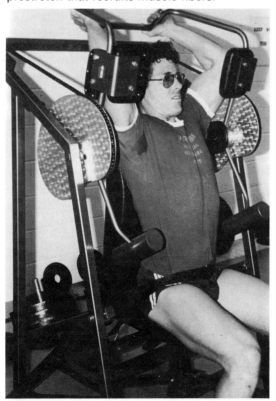

pletely, the athlete should "prefatigue" them in an isolation exercise such as dumbbell flies or on the Nautilus chest machine. This fatigues the pectoralis major but preserves the triceps. The athlete immediately does dips or bench presses. With these exercises, the triceps will have a temporary advantage over the exhausted pectoralis major, resulting in more work for the pectoralis major and greater strength and bulk gains.

Negative Resistance

The three levels of strength include concentric or positive strength, as in raising a weight by shortening of a muscle; static or isometric strength, as in holding a weight steady; and eccentric or negative strength, as in lengthening a muscle as it contracts by controlled lowering of a weight.

To work a muscle totally, the athlete must exhaust both concentric and eccentric strength.[37] This is done by training to total muscular fatigue with strict (good form) positive repetitions, with the athlete lifting until he cannot do any more repetitions (usually six repetitions). The training partner then helps him do some forced repetitions. The partner does not support the weight sufficiently to make these repetitions easy but gives just enough help to allow the athlete to complete the repetitions. The partner then lifts the weight for the athlete to lower, and the athlete does negative repetitions until total fatigue is almost reached.

Strength Gains

No single combination of sets and repetitions gives maximal strength gains for everyone; therefore the program designed will depend on the athlete's needs and level of skill. For any of the combinations of sets and repetitions, the key is to overload and to lift with intensity to fatigue. The athlete may perform three sets and choose from three to eight repetitions maximum (RM); 5 RM, for example, means lifting a weight five times with good form to fatigue.

The load is increased as the lifting improves. Weight is added if the athlete has had three good workouts in a row and is increasing his repetitions. The amount of weight added depends on the particular lift and is usually in increments of 5 to 10 pounds.

Strength is gained quickly during the first weeks or month of training as the athlete learns the lifting skills. If the training load is monotonous and frequently applied, however, he becomes accustomed to it. As he follows the same routine, fatigue and boredom set in, his nervous system becomes deadened, and his strength gains stop.[63] To avoid this stagnation, exercises should be varied. Different exercises may be used to develop the same muscles, or machines and then free weights may be used. The athlete's training load can be varied by changing the volume, intensity, number, and sequence of exercises, the number of repetitions per set, or the tempo (slow, moderate, or fast speed) at which the exercise is done.[63] Because each type of strength exercise will produce results in the early stages of strength development, the method used is not important. Instead, during this early period the novice can become familiar with many forms of strength training.

Strength Training Errors

Strength training errors include irregular training, gross overtraining, using the wrong sequence of exercises, employing a loose, jerky style, and not carrying each set to a point of fatigue.

Although regular workouts have a good cumulative effect, strength training sessions should not be held more often than 4 days a week (usually 3), with each session lasting no longer than an hour. The athlete must recognize the importance of following a correct sequence of exercises for maximal strength gain. An isolation exercise might be done first, for example, with a compound exercise immediately following, and each set should be carried to the point of fatigue for maximum gains in strength and bulk.

Isokinetics

Isokinetic means constant speed. Isokinetic training provides an accommodating resistance that allows the athlete to maximally load his dynamically contracting muscles at each point of a joint's range of motion, thus enabling him to do more work than is possible with either constant or variable resistance. Skilled trainers have used the isokinetic concept for years, applying manual resistance. Intermedialis exercises are isokinetic, and, today, isokinetic machines may be used to condition, rehabilitate, screen, and test athletes.

When an athlete trains on an isokinetic machine, the machine automatically adjusts to, and matches, the force that he applies,[43–45] causing his muscular contractions to remain constant. The harder he pushes, the harder it gets; it should therefore be possible to do voluntary maximal contractions on each repetition, with resulting maximal strength gains. To achieve this accommodation, some machines use hydraulics (Orthotron, Hydra-Gym), and others have a motor, gear box, and clutches (Cybex-II). There is no "sticking point" with isokinetics because the tension developed by the muscle as it shortens is maximum at all joint angles. More motor units are thus activated to provide a maximum contraction for each repetition.

Strength gained at slow speeds does not carry over to fast speeds. Strength gained at high speeds, however, converts to fast movement on the playing field and carries over to a strength gain at slower speeds. A variable adjustment allows the speed of the machine to be preset at slow, intermediate, or fast, and the velocity of movement may be varied from 0°/sec (isometrics) to 300°/sec.

Isokinetic machines allow the athlete to work on quickness and power, and he is less likely to be injured on them because inertia is eliminated. Further, he will not meet more resistance than he can handle. As he tires, he applies less force, and the machine matches this reduced force with less resistance. His angular velocity, however, remains constant, and his joint range of motion stays the same. This contrasts with isotonic work, where inertia is brought in and the resistance is fixed, with the last repetition being as heavy as the first. In isotonics, the speed is variable and unknown, and as the athlete tires, he slows down and his range of motion lessens. Another advantage of isokinetic machines is that the athlete uses his limbs independently against their own maximum resistance, with less soreness resulting because only concentric contractions are used. A disadvantage of the machines is that the athlete might not be sufficiently motivated because he is unable to perceive movement of a weight.

The Orthotron device is a hydraulic machine with a variable speed adjustment (Fig. 6-6). It has two gauges, one to record flexion torque and the other to record extension torque. The machine is most useful in the rehabilitation of the knee, ankle, and shoulder, and like other isokinetic devices, accommodates for pain and fatigue. If isokinetics are begun too early in knee rehabilitation, however, soreness may be produced as the athlete kicks out. Isotonic work thus remains the best way to gain important terminal extension of the knee.

The Cybex-II isokinetic machine may be used for the screening, rehabilitation, and testing of athletes (Fig. 6-7) and will isolate and test joints and muscle groups at many speeds.

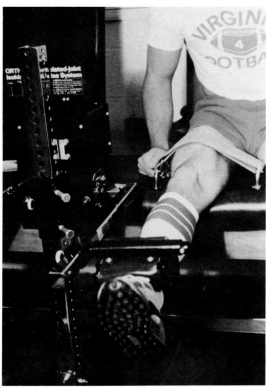

FIG. 6-6
The Orthotron system allows isokinetic rehabilitation and training at many speeds.

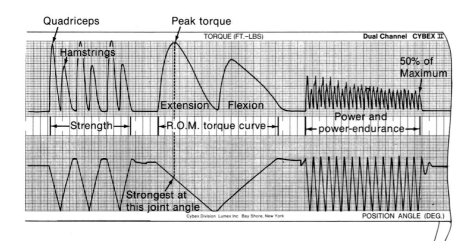

FIG. 6-7
The Cybex recorder prints out valuable data.

Like other isokinetic devices, it accommodates for pain and fatigue. The Cybex-II contains a motor, gear box, and two clutches (one for each direction). The athlete moves a lever to engage the clutches, and as he tries to increase speed, resistance increases. The trainer can speed up the motor to allow the clutch to go faster.

The Cybex-II provides a graphic read-out of key measurements, including peak torque that the athlete can generate at speeds ranging from 60°/sec to 300°/sec, peak torque at various joint angles, the speed at which the athlete can develop peak torque, and his endurance, total work, and joint range of motion. The examiner may also locate and analyze variations in torque at specific points in the range of motion caused by pain, weakness, or instability. The balance between muscle groups and both sides of the body can also be tested at various speeds.

Some isokinetic devices are especially useful for conditioning an athlete. The isokinetic swim bench allows a swimmer to lie prone and duplicate his swim strokes (Fig. 6-8). A strong swimmer, however, may overpower the machine and must do hundreds of repetitions for a good workout.

The Hydra-Gym is a conditioning system especially suited for the training of high school athletes. This device has durable pistons, similar to those used on trucks and airplanes, at each station (Fig. 6-9), and the system is compact and arranged to accommodate many athletes on a circuit. Athletes work at high intensity and only concentrically, never meeting more resistance than they can handle. They are never "defeated." The machines also eliminate inertia and accommodate to fatigue, thus reducing the chance of injury. The athlete may perform 20 repetitions in 20 seconds at a selected station, rest 40 seconds, and move to the next station. The difficulty of the workout may be varied by presetting a dial on the pistons.

Machines Versus Free Weights

When an athlete steadies, controls, and balances an Olympic barbell, his ligaments are strengthened and his proprioception enhanced. In addition, the strength gained from training with these free weights converts well to work on machines and the playing field.[50] Concentration is important for an athlete, and free weights

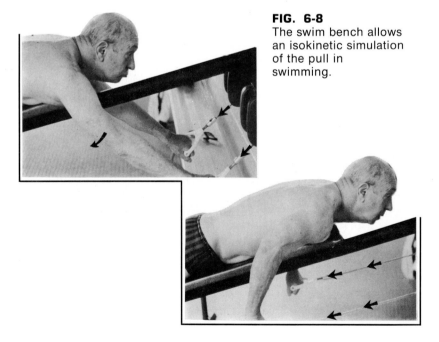

FIG. 6-8
The swim bench allows an isokinetic simulation of the pull in swimming.

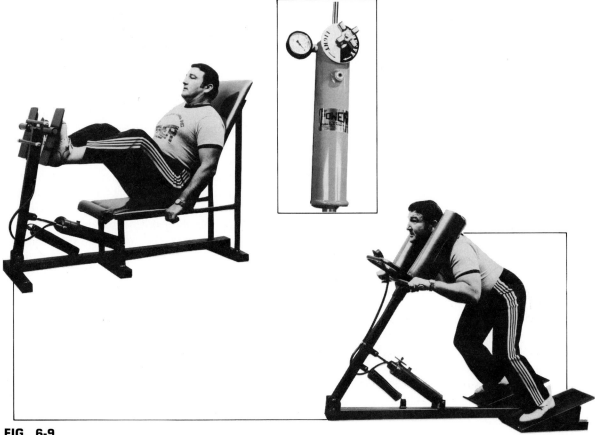

FIG. 6-9
The heart of the Hydra-Gym equipment is the durable piston (center). A Hydra-Gym circuit allows athletes to work isokinetically and safely.

help develop this faculty, as the athlete must be attentive when he "grabs the iron." The value of free weights is demonstrated by the fact that Olympic-style weight lifters and power lifters train with free weights.

Unlike free weights, strength-building machines are set in a constant movement pattern. Because the athlete need not balance the resistance, he reaps less ligament strengthening and less proprioceptive gain. Prime moving muscles are strengthened but not the synergistic muscles. Machine-gained strength does not convert well to free weight lifting or to whole body activity. In practice, a combination of machines and free weights is usually favored for optimum strength and power training. The

athlete may use the machines to develop a strength base and the free weights to develop power. If the athlete does not have a coach to supervise and teach him proper technique, however, he may be safer using the guided weights.

A strength coach is valuable for a conditioning program, as shown by the growth of the National Strength and Conditioning Association over the past 3 years from 200 to more than 4000 members. The association provides for an exchange of ideas through meetings and through their publication, *The National Strength and Conditioning Association Journal*. Hopefully, strength coaches will soon be certified to assure quality conditioning for athletes in all sports.

Returning to Weight Training After an Injury

Athletes who return to major lifts too soon after an injury risk further injury. For this reason, they should follow a systematic program of associated exercises to determine readiness for return to full training. A typical case might involve an athlete with an acromioclavicular sprain who wishes to return to bench presses. He must first begin his resistance exercises with shoulder flexion, extension, and abduction while holding a 1-lb weight. When he is able to perform painlessly 20 repetitions of these exercises with a 10-lb dumbbell, he can return to the bench, selecting a weight he can bench press for 10 repetitions without pain. From this point, he gradually increases to his previous level.

A mild injury may become more severe if it causes the athlete to change his lifting technique. To avoid this, the athlete can substitute exercises that involve little technique—for example, vertical leg presses on a weight sled rather than squats—until the injury has healed. Power cleans should not be done if an athlete has a back problem.

Sport-Specific Strength Training

Each sport has specific strength needs, and a skilled coach must be able to design programs that meet these needs. The following sections introduce some of the training programs for various sports.

Basketball

Basketball is a game in which the athlete needs power to jump for rebounds, to take jump shots, and to block shots, in addition to strength to hold position under the backboard. The strength program should be set up before the season starts and take into account the number of games to be played and the need for recovery.

Jumping employs the same plyometic moves used by Olympic-style weight lifters in high pulls and power cleans. Because these lifters develop great vertical jumping ability, basketball players profit from adopting some of the lifters' training techniques, including the snatch high pull, power cleans, and squats. In addition, the power press involves jumping with the weight,[32] working hip and knee extension and the calf. Players are taught to perform skillfully the rotary hip jerk, starting with the bar in the catch position, rising on the toes, and then dipping about 15 cm (6 in).[39, 40] As their legs push off, the weight goes up.

Other plyometric drills include depth jumps, hops, and bounds. In depth jumps, the athlete steps off a box and falls freely to the ground before rebounding onto another box. He usually does three boxes and then sprints back to the start. This activity is similar to rebounding. Other lifts include latissimus pulls for rebounding, bent-over rowing for grabbing the ball off the floor, and triceps extensions and wrist curls for increasing the shooting range.

The basketball player needs strong wrists and hands for shooting, dribbling, passing, and rebounding. This strength is gained by rope climbing, finger-tip push-ups, and passing and catching a medicine ball. With a medicine ball, an eccentric contraction occurs during the catch and becomes a concentric one during the pass.

Trunk curls and back hyperextensions with weights are very important because they tie the upper and lower body together.

To improve agility, the athlete may perform bench jumps, jumping back and forth sideways over a narrow 45-cm (18 in)-high bench for 30 seconds, do forward and backward runs, cuts, and shuffle drills, or jump rope.

Gymnastics

A gymnast may use free weights to develop strength, but his coach may also weave strengthening exercises into his practice sessions. This approach develops coordination and agility along with strength.[9]

The gymnast first establishes a standard routine. Then, to tax him, the coach may increase the number of skills in his routine, increase the number of times the routine is executed, decrease the rest interval time, or speed up the routine. If the coach detects a specific weakness,

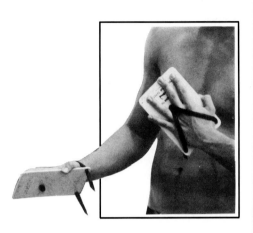

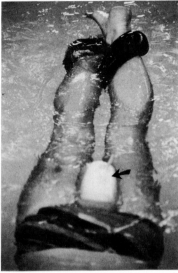

FIG. 6-10
A swimmer can use hand paddles, a tube, and a float (*arrow*) to tax his arms.

that area in the routine may be isolated for strength work. For example, if a gymnast lacks the strength to press into a handstand on the parallel bars, he may increase his strength by an assisted swing or by handstand push-ups.

Swimming

A swimmer pulls himself through the water, doing 90% of the work with his arms. He may use aids such as hand paddles, tubes, and floats to improve his upper body strength (Fig. 6-10). Hand paddles add more resistance to the pull, and a tube and float restrict the swimmer's leg motion, requiring that his arms take up the slack.

Latissimus pull-downs and a back program are important for swimmers. Some swimmers enjoy the Nautilus pull-over machine that features a prestretch although a swimmer may sublux his shoulders on this machine. A swimmer may also train on an isokinetic swim bench to develop powerful starts and push-offs, duplicating strokes in a horizontal position. Strong swimmers, however, usually overpower these machines and need too many repetitions for a good workout.

A strong swimmer may duplicate the pull of the stroke on a Total Gym, an exercise apparatus comprising a rolling platform that moves

FIG. 6-11
The Total Gym is especially useful for a home exercise program.

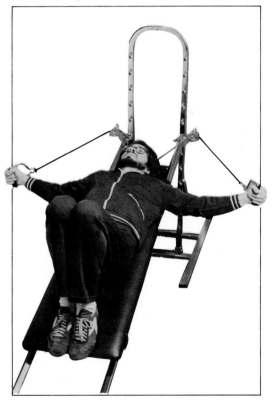

up and down on an adjustable incline plane (Fig. 6-11). A number of exercises are possible on this apparatus, using the rolling sled with or without a cable and pulley assembly. Twelve incline positions provide a variety of work loads, with the athlete's body and the rolling sled becoming a moving weight stack. This apparatus is particularly good for a general conditioning program and allows an athlete with a lower extremity injury to maintain or to improve his cardiovascular condition.

Circuit training is used by swimmers and wrestlers during the season and by other athletes in off-season conditioning programs to develop muscular strength, power, and muscular and cardiovascular endurance. A circuit may consist of six to ten exercise stations set up so that the same group of muscles is not exercised at two consecutive stations; thus one muscle group will be recovering while another muscle group is being exercised. An athlete should do as many repetitions as possible with good form at 50% of one-repetition maximum in 30 seconds. He then should rest for 15 seconds to recover partially before advancing to the next station. With ten stations, the total time needed to perform three full sets will be just over 20 minutes.

A swimmer can also have an intensive iso-dynamic workout by swimming against the resistance of flexible tubing, tied around him and around the starting platform. Special tanks have been developed to allow a swimmer to swim against a current, much as a salmon swims upstream.

Football

The tackle football player needs leg strength, a strong lower back, and shoulder and arm strength. Leg strength is needed to run, drive, hit, and jump, lower back strength to deliver the rising blow, and shoulder and arm strength to deliver and to absorb blows without sustaining injury.[19, 25] Free weight lifting is used to achieve these goals because this type of program will increase total body strength better than any other method, and the strength obtained may be used immediately on the football field.[50] Muscle bulk is gained by slow, heavy

repetitions and power by high-intensity explosive movements of the large muscle groups. Before training with explosive exercises, however, the player needs to build a strength base with a program lasting 3 to 4 months.

The three major lifts are the bench press, power clean, and full squat (Fig. 6-12). The bench press strengthens the pectorals, deltoids, and triceps; power cleans work the arms, forearms, back, hips, thighs, and legs; and full squats work the lower back, gluteus maximus, hips, thighs, and calves. These lifts are supplemented by chin-ups, dips, sit-ups, pull-downs, upright-rows, and other exercises as needed. To avoid bouncing, jerking, or throwing the weight, the athlete must know proper technique.

Each player follows an off-season program based on the three major lifts and comprising three high-intensity workouts a week to increase his strength and power. During the season, players work out twice a week for shorter periods to retain the strength built in the off-season, conserving energy by reducing the duration of the training sessions while doing sufficient work to stimulate muscle growth.

At each training session, the player readies himself by warming up with a jump rope, twisting with a bar, and stretching and performing sit-ups. Three players are involved in each exercise, one lifting while the others are loading and spotting. At each station, the lifter approaches the bar and assumes a stable position before attacking the weights in an explosive, all-out effort. The player must concentrate his mental and his physical energies to train with the required intensity. Although explosive training may cause an injury in the untrained, a well-conditioned athlete who has been on a good strength program need not fear injury. Explosive training is needed for sports that require power, and every set in each exercise must be done with the purest possible form. An athlete should never cheat on a movement because this will bring other muscles into play and lessen the effect of the exercise.

Bench Press

To begin a bench press, the athlete lies flat on the bench with his feet flat on the floor, his

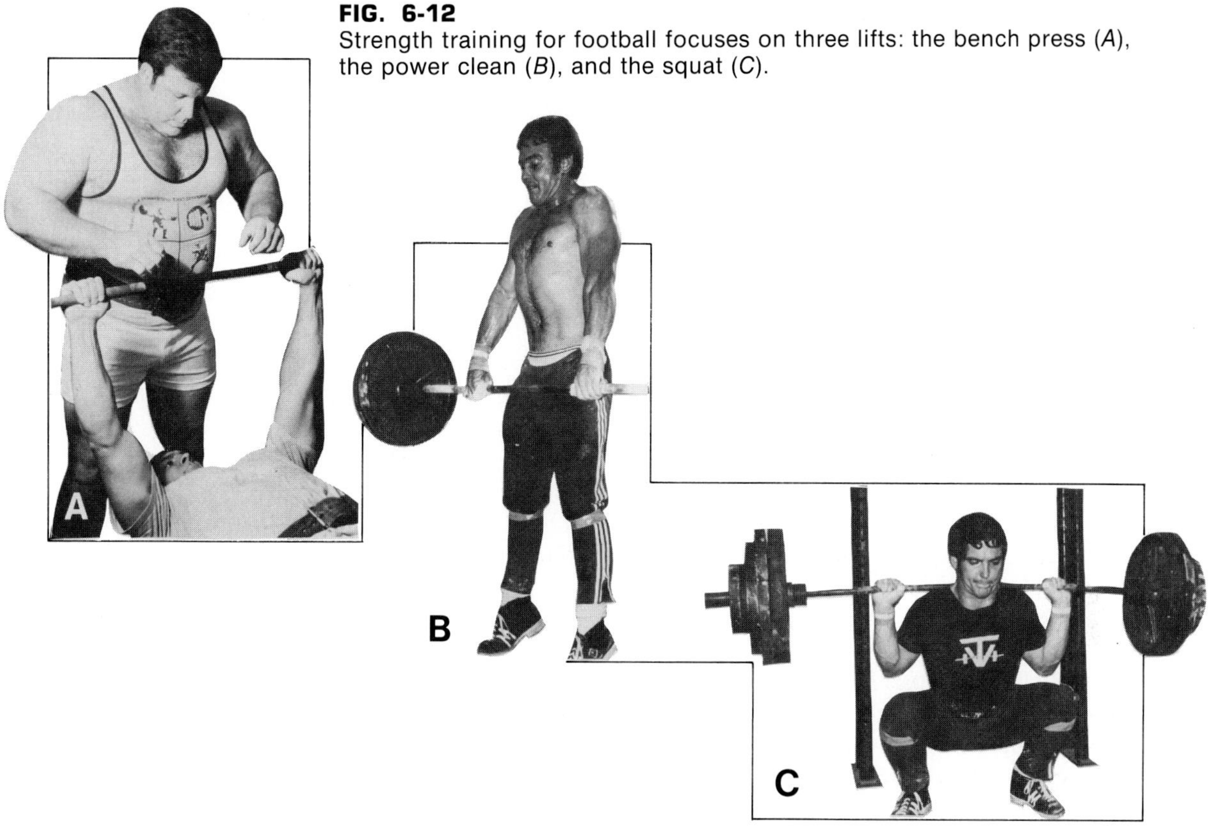

FIG. 6-12
Strength training for football focuses on three lifts: the bench press (*A*), the power clean (*B*), and the squat (*C*).

hips positioned securely on the bench, and his lower back flattened to the bench.[19, 25] His shoulder blades are pulled together, pushing his chest as high as possible, and his chin is pulled down to his neck. His hands are positioned on the bar so that his arms are tucked in to his sides during the lift to make the bench press resemble the movement of delivering a blow to an opponent. The player takes the bar off the rack and inhales deeply before lowering the bar in a controlled manner to his chest. The bar should touch the highest point on his chest. The athlete then drives the bar up to arm's length in an explosive movement that conditions the muscles to react quickly, and he exhales as his elbows lock out. On maximal exertions, he may want to hold his breath before resuming breathing the moment the bar is securely past the sticking point. The lifter should avoid bridging his back, or raising or shifting his head, shoulders, buttocks, and feet. A cambered bar may be used for the bench press, as it allows the player to start his press from a more retracted position of the shoulders.

The incline press is a variant of the bench press with a slightly different angle, giving a measure of rest to muscles used in the bench press. The bar is gripped at points slightly wider than shoulder width with the bar directly above the chest, near the neck, and driven out to arm's length.

A lifter must always be spotted while performing a bench press, although even with the best spotters he can be seriously injured if he suffers a pectoralis major tear. The heavy weight may drop onto his chest or face; to avoid such a problem, the heavy-training athlete should train on a Maxi-Rack.

Power Clean

To begin a power clean, the player takes a stance with his feet at shoulder width and the bar lined up over the balls of his feet.[19, 25] His grip should be slightly wider than his shoulders. With his lower back flat and his arms straight, he starts the lift by straightening his legs. He must do this part of the lift slowly. As the bar passes his knees, his shoulders are out in front of the bar and his knees slightly bent. This position puts a stretch on the hamstrings, which, combined with an awareness of scooping or rotating, brings the hips down and forward and the athlete's body to the bar.[38, 39] The dip is 5 to 10 cm (2 to 4 in). The downward action is needed to ensure adequate knee bending to gain the strongest leverage for lifting, jumping, or charging. The hips and legs stop rotating when the shoulders come to a position slightly ahead of the bar, and the feet remain flat on the ground. This is the "strong position" of the hips and legs, and from here the legs and hips forcefully extend until the athlete goes up and straight over onto his toes. As he fully extends onto his toes, he shrugs his shoulders to initiate the arm-pull. His elbows lift directly to his sides, and the athlete should feel as if he is jumping straight up with the bar. The bar is kept close to the body during the entire pull and rested on the upper chest by slipping the elbows under it. The athlete then carefully lowers the bar, keeping his back flat. It is best to work power cleans easily at first while concentrating on technique and speed. This will allow the athlete later to pull heavy weights that cannot be pulled if his technique is poor. The player may use straps that will aid him in concentrating on speed or heavy weight rather than on grip.

Full Squat

The squat is the best exercise for adding muscular strength and body weight. The athlete wears a weightlifter's belt and starts the squat with his feet shoulder width apart and with his toes pointing outward 5° to 15°.[19, 25] His head is up, and he keeps an arch in his lower back, with the bar supported on the trapezius, not on the neck. If there is neck discomfort, he may wrap a towel around the bar. The athlete slowly goes down to the lowest position possible with his back remaining flat. If his back rounds over, he should stop at this point. With practice, the athlete will be able to do deeper squats with his back absolutely flat. He should

always be spotted when doing heavy squats unless he uses a power rack or a Maxi-Rack. The power rack is a good safety device in the early stages, as its pins are a safeguard that may be set at the exact lower position for each athlete. If a lifter is caught under the weight, he can let the bar settle on the pins.

As the athlete reaches the bottom of his squat, he pauses momentarily. This is important to avoid rebounding. However, he should stay tight at the bottom without relaxing because relaxing will round his back, putting extra stress on it and breaking his position. After the pause, he drives explosively upward with the plates rattling at the top of the thrust, a movement that builds a quick start off the line. The lifter breathes only at the standing position, first inhaling and then holding his breath throughout the movement, exhaling only as he comes back erect. The bar is carried on the trapezius, and the athlete's head is lifted as he comes out of the bottom position. This straightens the lower back and keeps the lifter from rounding over. If he cannot hold his balance because of ankle inflexibility, he should place a block under his heel until he is more flexible. The squats will stretch the calves, and then the block will not be needed. The athlete can also practice squats with a broomstick if he lacks flexibility. An ankle board for calf stretching should be placed by every squat rack to be used between squat sets. To teach balance in the squat, a balance board may be placed under the lifter's feet.

Testing

Athletes should be tested several times each year for maximum single efforts in the bench press, power clean, full squat, chin-ups, dips, vertical jump, and flexibility.[19, 25] Known as "maxing out," or trying for a personal record, maximum lifts are recorded only on testing days, as the weight room is primarily a place for building strength and power, not for demonstrating it. If a 1-RM is used and the weight is too high, the athlete may sustain an injury. As an alternative to a 1-RM, a 2-RM may be used, or the athlete may do repetitions until his technique gives out.

College freshmen usually improve the most

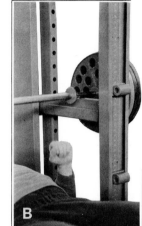

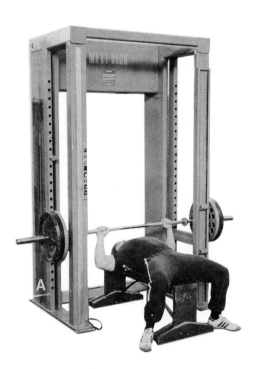

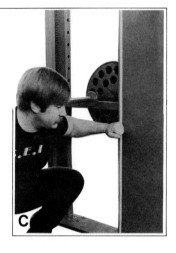

FIG. 6-13
The Maxi-Rack (*A*) has safety features for hard-training athletes. If the lifter cannot raise the weight, the machine will (*B*). The lifter can then lower the weight eccentrically, taxing his muscles to the ultimate. If a lifter is caught under a weight, he can tap a switch on the machine (*C*), or depress a foot switch, and the machine will raise the weight.

dramatically in a weight training program, possibly because they have never before trained in a weight program or because they are using free weights for the first time. Testing is usually conducted at the beginning of fall practice in mid–August, at the start of winter workouts in early December, just before spring practice, and before leaving school for the summer.[25] Each player is put on an individualized program for the summer months. How strong a player may be compared to his teammates is much less important than that athlete's growing stronger week by week.

Maxi-Rack

When an athlete is pushed to his limits in a barbell exercise, especially in power move-

ments, his safety is compromised. Muscular failure, sudden fatigue, momentary loss of consciousness, or an injury during a heavy lift may cause a serious injury. Such injuries are most likely to occur in the bench press, inclined bench press, and squat, where the lifter can be trapped under the weight. Even though spotters are attentive, they may be asked to catch weights that they are at a mechanical disadvantage even to hold.

The Maxi-Rack allows the use of free weights to the limits of their potential while stressing safety for the lifter. Although the barbell is unencumbered, it is confined within the structural framework of the Maxi-Rack (Fig. 6-13). This confinement protects the lifter and others in the area from possible injury from a runaway weight. The heart of the Maxi-Rack is a hydraulically operated lifting mechanism that catches and raises a weight that the athlete has dropped or is unable to lift. Its hydraulic cylinders can be operated automatically or manually: In the automatic mode, the cylinders will actuate and raise the barbell when it makes contact with the lifting crossbars attached to the cylinders; in the manual mode, the cylinders can be activated by a foot switch (lying or sitting position), by a tape switch that runs along the rear upright of the unit (for the squats), or by an emergency raise button on the control panel.

Two positioners on the front of the Maxi-Rack set the upper and lower limits within which the lifting crossbars operate. Each athlete can adjust the movement of the crossbar to his specific body dimensions for all exercises. Upper and lower limits can be positioned to fractions of an inch so that safety is not compromised, as when a lifter's chest does not conform to a machine's established settings. The positioners may be adjusted to allow the crossbars to operate through a full range of motion, from the floor to 2.4 m (8 ft) high, or they can be set to operate through limits as close as 5 cm (2 in) at any point within this range. By adjusting the crossbar, the athlete can perform partial movements to help overcome "sticking points."

The Maxi-Rack allows athletes to train intensively beyond their former limits in an eccentric (negative) fashion by lowering the weight from lock-out to any predetermined point. When the barbell touches the lower limit set by the athlete, the Maxi-Rack returns the bar to the lock-out position. The athlete can "rep-out" (lift to fatigue), with confidence that the Maxi-Rack will remove the weight from him whenever he fails to complete a movement.

Track

In addition to superior leg strength, a runner works to develop torso and upper body strength, employing many repetitions with a light weight to avoid bulk. Good flexibility is also needed for injury prevention and to make the running stride more efficient.

Plyometric drills include depth jumps, hops, bounds, and running up stadium steps to develop a runner's leg power. Frontal and lateral dumbbell raises help the intercostals and, together with abdominal work, make breathing easier. To strengthen his midsection, the runner does sit-ups, twisting sit-ups, leg raises, twists with a barbell, and back extensions. He also performs the running arm action while holding dumbbells for the time it takes him to run his event.

Sprinters may train with uphill and downhill runs. Running up a 10° grade makes the runner lift his legs higher, whereas running downhill on a 5° grade increases the frequency of foot strikes and the stride length, a combination that increases the runner's speed. The neuromuscular effect is retained on flat surfaces. The runner may also do harness running, do isodynamic running, and pull a weighted sled.

Field Events

The shot put, discus, hammer, and javelin events require great body control, as the athlete must throw with his whole body.

The shot putter strengthens his trunk rotators and abdominal muscles by means of twisting sit-ups and twists with a loaded bar. Rotational training is important for the throwing sports and for the rotational and lateral movements needed in most other sports.[34] Explosive one-arm jerk presses help the athlete develop power, and incline presses serve his needs better than standard bench presses. Finger push-ups strengthen his hands.

A strong midsection is especially important for the discus thrower, and for this reason trunk exercises compose nearly half of his strength workout. Trunk curls and back hyperextensions "tie" his upper and lower body together, and twists help to develop his midsection. The athlete lies supine with his upper body and midsection extending over the edge of a high platform while a partner holds his legs down. The athlete holds a weight plate that simulates the discus, and twists, reaching his throwing arm down toward the floor, then twists up again, doing maximal repetitions in good form. The discus thrower also does flies and works with pulleys. As he simulates the throw, his hip must always lead.

Hammer throwers use pulleys, and javelin throwers do pull-overs on the Nautilus and with pulleys and surgical tubing. The field event athlete also benefits from trampoline work that teaches him how to handle his body in space. "Gaming," or free play in basketball, soccer, or racquetball, gives practice with starts, stops, jumps, and lateral movements.[10]

Wrestling

Wrestling is explosive work in all directions against resistance. A wrestler pushes, pulls, lifts, and uses leg action; thus the muscles involved in these movements are worked during a weight program.[21, 22] Strength training for wrestling should be explosive and of high intensity. In the off-season, the wrestler works for strength and power, and in the preseason and in-season, he works with more repetitions for muscular stamina. Strength, however, is often lost over a wrestling season because workouts are continuous for 5 or 6 days a week and the wrestler is on weight control. The strength decline is tempered by two-man resistive drills, chinning, rope climbing, and specific wrestling exercises, such as body lifts. Because strength can be increased only by overload, a wrestler must work with weights at least two times a week during the season to maintain his strength. Hands can be strengthened by climbing a rope, doing finger-tip push-ups, and by throwing and catching a medicine ball.

The wrestler should establish an aerobic base with distance runs before the season; during the season, he may sprint, run stairs, and run short hills. Circuit weight training also helps to provide needed endurance. "Burnouts," or high-intensity weight-training workouts until exhaustion, are excellent but may be too grueling for most wrestlers. Burnouts bring out a wrestler's competitive instincts much as a match does and may give him a psychological edge, especially in the final period of a match. They should not, however, be done more often than once every few weeks.

A wrestler can perform isodynamically some of the moves normally used in a match by practicing against the resistance of surgical tubing. A Greco-Roman wrestler can practice his throws on a dummy usually 25% lighter than his weight class. With this preparation, the wrestler enters the match fully warmed up and ready to use all his moves right from the start, thus lowering his chance of injury.

Weight Lifting

How do weight lifting and weight training differ? Weight lifting is a competitive sport, whereas weight training is part of the preparation for sports. The yearly workload of weight lifters has increased sharply, with some men lifting 2000 to 2500 *tons* per year. For a lifter to train at this level, his coach must adjust the training program and make changes at optimal times to produce the best results.[63] Sound recovery methods for repair and recuperation, such as good food, adequate rest, and skilled massage, are equally important.

The lifter trains year-round, and his training cycle is divided into three periods: preparatory, competitive, and transitional.[63] At the start of the preparatory period, he works on general conditioning to develop his strength, speed, endurance, agility, flexibility, and motor skills. He thus creates and improves the foundation on which to develop competitive form. His volume and intensity are gradually increased, with volume emphasized more. Later during this preparatory period, the lifter works proportionally more on competitive lifts and hones his technical skills in simulated practice competitions. Microcycles of heavier and lighter work, the "lead-up phase," bring the lifter to competition in optimal form.

During the competitive period, the lifter's objective is to achieve his best performance. He polishes his technique and mobilizes his physical and mental powers maximally. A postcom-

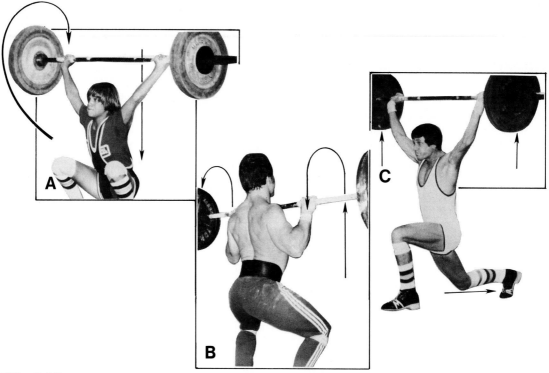

FIG. 6-14
Olympic lifting includes the snatch and the clean-and-jerk. The snatch (*A*) is an especially quick lift, while the clean-and-jerk (*B, C*) is slower, but more weight is lifted.

petitive microcycle follows immediately after competition for up to a week. During this time, he can rest and correct technical errors.

Weight lifting includes Olympic-style weightlifting, power lifting, and body building. The Olympic-style lifts are the snatch and clean-and-jerk (Fig. 6-14). Power lifters perform the bench press, dead lift, and squat. Body builders "pump iron" to define and to proportion their muscles in preparation for posing.

Olympic-Style Weight Lifting

In the snatch, the weight lifter lifts the barbell, with his arms locked, from a position in front of his legs to above his head in a single, uninterrupted motion. He must then hold the bar-

bell overhead for 2 seconds to receive the referee's signal of approval.

The clean-and-jerk consists of two distinct moves, one to the chest and the second over the head. The pull from the floor places the barbell at the lifter's shoulders (the clean), and from this point he must lift it to an overhead, locked-arms position (the jerk).

Injuries to Olympic-style weight lifters may include fractures, dislocated elbows, forearm tendon strains and forearm fractures, slipped distal radial epiphyses in young lifters, blisters, spondylolysis and spondylolisthesis, quadriceps or patella tendon ruptures, and knee problems, such as chondromalacia and meniscal tears.[36]

As a heavy barbell is pressed overhead, the lifter's serratus anterior contracts to protract his scapula and hold it against the chest wall. The upper slip of the serratus anterior jerks on the first rib, and the rib cracks in its weak part at the subclavian groove. During the snatch, the weight lifter may dislocate his elbow, since the elbow is hyperextended when he holds a heavy weight. If his elbow strikes his thigh, his forearm tendons may be strained, or both bones of his forearm may break. A youth with poor lifting technique may slip his distal radial epiphysis as he catches the weight during the clean. Weight lifters often compete with painful blisters caused by calluses being ripped by the knurling on the bar. These may be prevented by good hand care and the use of hand wraps while training.

Hyperextension of the weight lifter's spine may lead to spondylolysis and spondylolisthesis. The main offender, the Olympic press, is no longer included in weight lifting competitions. Olympic-style weight lifters may also suffer quadriceps and patella tendon ruptures. In one case of rupture, the force on the lifter's patella tendon was calculated to be more than 17 times his body weight with his knee flexed to 90°.[64] If a lifter has soreness in a major weightbearing muscle group or tendon, he should refrain from training and from competing until the soreness has been alleviated through hot and cold applications and stretching in order to avoid a major rupture. Weight lifters develop knee problems from ballistic movements, such as squat snatches and the split in the clean-and-jerk. Barbell plates are 45 cm (18 in) in diameter; thus the bar is about 22.5 cm (9 in) above the platform. If a lifter slips under the bar, his raised knee may be caught and injured. Although Olympic lifters handle heavy loads, their injury rate is low because they train hard to develop technique and their flexibility is exceptionally high.[36]

Preventing Injuries

Because there is a shortage of Olympic-style weight lifting coaches in the United States, the American lifter must often rely on literature such as translated Bulgarian notes for training tips. Ideally, a coach should observe and critique every lift, but if a lifter lacks a coach, fellow lifters can be enlisted to observe and comment on his technique.

Improper technique and inflexibility account for most of the injuries in Olympic-style weight lifting. A lifter needs full shoulder flexibility to "rotate out," that is, rotate his shoulders behind his back if the weight gets behind him. He may practice shoulder "dislocates" with a broomstick, starting with his hands out comfortably on the stick and moving them in a bit each week until the snatch grip is comfortable.

Weight lifting should be done only on a lifting platform. The area on and around the platform should be cleaned to give the lifter a clear area in which to bail out from an unsuccessful lift. In gymnasiums that lack a platform, mats are sometimes placed under the weights, but these may encourage a conscientious young lifter to fight the weight in an attempt to place it down properly, and he may injure himself.

A lifter is well advised not to perform maximum squats without a safety rack or spotters because he may fall forward and be badly injured. He should also wear weight lifter's shoes with good midfoot support and a heel that aids his balance.

Weight Lifter's Blackout

A weightlifter may become dizzy and confused and suddenly fall to the floor while lifting a heavy barbell. This occurs most commonly after a hard stand-up while cleaning a weight in the clean-and-jerk. Such blackouts are caused by a combination of events that lead to a fall in cerebral blood flow, including hyperventilation, squatting, and lifting the weight and holding it while breathing again.[14]

Many competitors overbreathe just before lifting in the belief that this will help to produce a maximum effort. Such hyperventilation, however, reduces a lifter's cerebral blood flow by dilating muscle vessels while constricting cerebral vessels. If the lifter remains in a squatting position for a long time while preparing for the stand-up that must follow, he may suffer peripheral vasodilation, and he may become dizzy as both his peripheral resistance and the venous return to his heart drop.

Esophageal pressure balloons record that the lifter's thoracic pressure rises greatly when weight is lifted (in the range of 60 mm Hg). Without this climb in intratruncal pressure and added pneumatic support, the forces on the lifter's spine would exceed his capacity to resist them. Raised intrathoracic pressure is initially transmitted to central vessels and to the arterial pulse. The high pressure, however, also obstructs venous return so that the cardiac volume, stroke volume, and pulse pressure soon begin to fall. If the lift takes a long time to perform, even more time is available for reflex vasodilatation in response to the initial rise in arterial pressure. Cineradiography shows that the heart size becomes greatly reduced during the lifting phase, and the pulsations of the heart, pulmonary artery, and aorta are barely visible.

At the end of the clean, the lifter holds the weight and catches his breath in preparation for the jerk, causing the intrathoracic pressure to drop acutely. The arterial blood pressure falls steeply to as little as 50 mm Hg. Simultaneously, the great veins and splanchnic vessels expand, and the filling of these expanded vessels causes a lag in blood reaching the left ventricle. Three or four electrocardiographic complexes go by unaccompanied by an arterial pressure wave, suggesting the absence of ventricular ejection. Cineradiography shows that the pulmonary artery pulsates almost immediately but aortic pulsation is delayed. The lifter's heart has "pumped dry," and he faints from cerebral ischemia.

Spirits of ammonia will usually be helpful in reviving an unconscious lifter. Inhalation of the irritating vapor reflexly stimulates his medullary centers by way of the trigeminal, and perhaps the olfactory, nerves.[65] Resistance blood vessels in his limbs constrict, his systemic blood pressure rises, and his capacitance vessels reflexly constrict, all serving to raise his cardiac filling pressure and to revive him.

A lifter is less likely to "black out" if he avoids hyperventilation. Squatting should be as brief as possible, with the weight quickly raised and normal breathing resumed. When a lifter feels that he is losing the weight, he can back out from under it by pushing the bar. Experienced lifters know when a lift is lost, whereas a novice may fight the weight and be injured.

A competitive lifter must occasionally fight lifts that are not in perfect balance, but he is aware when he is going to lose the lift.

Power Lifting

Power lifters compete in three lifts: the bench press, the dead lift, and the squat (Fig. 6-15). In the dead lift, the lifter stands up while holding the weight, using a combination overhand and underhand grip to keep the bar from rotating. A super heavyweight can deadlift more than 405 kg (900 lb). In the bench press, the lifter lowers the bar to his chest before pressing it up. Although super heavyweight power lifters can bench press more than 225 kg (500 lb), their pectoralis major sometimes tears. If the tear is in the muscle mass, it is not repaired; if the strong tendon of the pectoralis major rips, however, it should be repaired. In squats, the loaded bar is on the lifter's shoulders, and he must bend his knees to more than 90°, then stand up. Power lifters take a deep breath and execute through the highest intensity part of the lift before breathing again.

Body Building

Body builders lift weights to develop all of their muscle groups to definition in proper proportion and symmetry.[46] They assess their development with mirrors, like sculptors observing the progress of their work.

A body builder enters a contest shaved, oiled, and "pumped," and his definition, proportion, symmetry, and posing determine his score. He must be flexible because he needs a good range of motion for posing. These athletes are strong, but the strongest body builder is not necessarily the most successful. They sustain few musculoskeletal injuries in competition but do strain muscles when training, and their low endurance capacity is similar to that of healthy sedentary subjects. If a body builder stops training, his muscles will shrink about 50%, but if he maintains only a light training schedule, good musculature will remain.

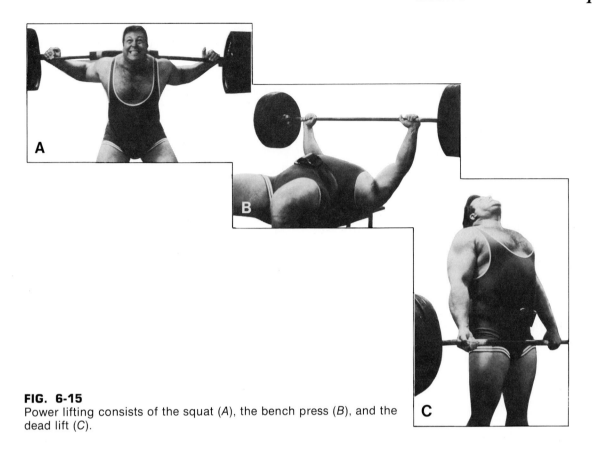

FIG. 6-15
Power lifting consists of the squat (*A*), the bench press (*B*), and the dead lift (*C*).

Many body builders take anabolic steroids despite the dangers of liver cancer and shrunken testes. Some athletes, however, reach the highest levels of body building without using these drugs. Female body builders tone up and develop bulk that is dependent on their testosterone level, and those who take anabolic steroids risk damage to complex hormonal mechanisms.

Weight Lifting for Women

A woman's absolute strength is about two thirds that of a man, but when strength is related to body weight, the difference decreases. In fact, when strength is related to lean body weight—that is, total weight minus fat weight—women are actually slightly stronger than men.[12] A woman's upper body strength is only 30% to 50% that of a man's, but the leg strength differences are minimal. When leg strength is related to body size, a woman's leg strength is nearly the same as a man's. A woman's legs are slightly stronger than a man's when leg strength is related to lean body mass.

Strength differences between men and women probably are related to differences in normal body proportions and the daily activity patterns of men and women. Muscle quality is the same in both men and women in its contractile properties and its ability to exert force.

The female athlete can double her strength over a 10-week period without muscle hypertrophy,[58, 59] a rapid development that is more of a neuromuscular than a purely muscular process. Strength training is a new experience for women, and they start far from their potential development.

When a woman follows the same strength training program as a man, she can make the same percentage gains in strength that a man can. Low testosterone levels keep her from becoming overmuscled, and subcutaneous tissue conceals muscle definition. Women who do become excessively muscular probably have higher testosterone levels.

Weight Lifting for Youths

Because most youths are strangers to hard work, they are generally weak, but weight lifting will improve their strength and help prevent injury. However, uncoached weight lifting before their growth plates have fused may cause permanent injury.

When young men train in Olympic-style weight lifting, they work on speed and technique; such technique can be taught even to 8-year-olds. Some countries hold competitions for youths in which technique is judged. When a youth reaches 12 to 13 years of age, weight can be added, but occasionally a young man is only lifting the bar without plates. A young lifter may suffer a slip of his distal radial epiphysis, dislocate his elbow, or develop spondylolysis even with good coaching. Expert coaching is nontheless imperative, although youths should avoid power lifting, especially the dead lift, because power lifting emphasizes heavy weights.

Weight Lifting for Older Athletes

An athlete reaches maximum strength at about 25 years of age. Thereafter, he loses about 1% of strength per year; thus, at age 65, the athlete is about 65% as strong as he was when he was 25 years old.

The older athlete's goal should be total conditioning. He should seek to gain and to maintain his strength with lighter loads, on a Hydra-Gym circuit, or isodynamically against the resistance of surgical tubing. Heavier training loads may lead to rupture of a tendon, such as the biceps, quadriceps, or patellar tendon. Isometric exercises are dangerous for a hypertensive person but are probably less hazardous to a normal older person's cardiovascular system than has been presumed.

Muscle Soreness

Acute muscle soreness starts during or immediately after exercise and may persist for a few hours.[1] Stress-induced ischemia impairs the muscle's ability to remove quickly metabolic waste products, such as lactic acid and potassium, and these accumulate to cause pain. When the athlete stops exercising, blood flow increases, and his pain soon disappears.

Delayed soreness appears from 8 to 48 hours after exercise[33] and may result from tears of tissue, tissue irritation, local muscle spasm, or eccentric work. Violent exercise may tear muscular or tendinous tissue. High hydroxyproline levels are found when there is delayed soreness; thus connective tissue irritation may be a factor. During less vigorous exercise, local muscle spasm will produce ischemia, releasing pain substances that stimulate pain endings and provoke further local muscle spasm. Finally, heavy eccentric work may generate a diffuse, delayed soreness.

A full warm-up will help the athlete prevent soreness. He should follow the training principle of *progression,* with gradual increases in his workload and its duration. Athletes are also advised to warm down to dissipate waste. Ice can be applied to exercised areas to lessen muscle spasm, followed by massage to rid the area of wastes and a pneumatic, intermittent pressure device to press out edema.

The athlete with muscular soreness should stretch statically to the point of pain onset and hold the stretch there. If the soreness is severe, he may be given cryotherapy with ice massage or ice packs. When ice is applied, he will first feel coldness and then aching. The area soon becomes numb, and he may then begin stretching, performing 1-minute stretches in sets of three, separated by 5 minutes of ice massage.

Muscle Cramps

Muscle cramps may be due to electrolyte depletion or to fatigue where partial relaxation causes spasm. When an athlete changes from everyday walking shoes with heels to sports shoes with no heels, running on soft ground may cause increased tension in his calf muscles, generating fatigue and cramps. Athletes salt their food or eat potato chips during two-a-day workout periods to replace the salt that they have lost through sweating and to prevent muscle cramps. Moreover, they should follow a good stretching program and avoid fashionable high-heeled footwear to help keep cramps to a minimum.

When a cramp occurs, the athlete should lie down while the examiner grasps the affected muscle and squeezes it firmly from the sides. When the spasm stops, the muscle should be stretched through its normal range of motion and massaged to help restore circulation. An athlete may stop his own cramps by squeezing the muscle firmly or, in the case of calf cramps, by grabbing his toes and pulling them toward him, then releasing and repeating this procedure. An unusual but often effective method for relieving a cramp is to pinch the athlete's upper lip.[2]

REFERENCES

1. ABRAHAM WM: Exercise-induced muscle soreness. Phys Sportsmed 7(10):57–60, 1979
2. ALLEN MF: Acupinch. First Aider, Cramer 50(4):11, 1980
3. BALL JR et al: Effects of isometric training on vertical jumping. Res Q 35:231–235, 1964
4. BEKA D: Comparison of dynamic static and combination training on dominant wrist flexor muscles. Res Q 39:244–250, 1968
5. BERGER R: Effect of varied weight training programs on strength. Res Q 33:168–181, 1962
6. BERGER R: Optimum repetitions for the development of strength. Res Q 33:334–338, 1962
7. BERGER R: Comparative effects of three weight-training programs. Res Q 34:396–398, 1963
8. BERGER R: Effects of dynamic and static training on vertical jumping ability. Res Q 34:419–424, 1963
9. BOONE T: Muscle strength and gymnastics. Athletic J 56(3):68–69, 1975
10. BURTON R: The Oregon weightmen: a power philosophy. Natl Strength Conditioning Assoc J 2(5):19–20, 1980
11. CALDWELL F: The search for strength. Phys Sportsmed 6(1):83–88, 1978
12. CHRISTENSEN C: Relative strength in males and females. Athletic Training 10(4):189–192, 1975
13. COE S, GANDY G: Seb Coe's secret, circuit training: the technique of the future. Runner's World 15(1):45–49, January 1980
14. COMPTON D et al: Weight-lifter's blackout. Lancet 2:1234–1237, 1973
15. COUSILMAN JE: The importance of speed in exercise. Scholastic Coach 46:94–99, October 1976
16. DELLINGER W: Oregon track: Part II. Strength and conditioning for middle distance runners. Natl Strength Conditioning Assoc J 2(4):22–23, 1980
17. DELORME T, WATKINS A: Techniques of PRE. Arch Phys Med Rehabil 29:263–273, 1948
18. DeVRIES HA: Quantitative electro-myographic investigation of the spasm theory of muscle pain. Am J Phys Med 45:119–134, 1966
19. DUNN W: Virginia Strength and Power Manual. Charlottesville, Virginia, University of Virginia, 1980
20. DYATCHKOV VM: "High jumping" track technique. J Technical Track Field Athletics 36:1123–1158, 1969
21. DZIEDZIC S, FARRELL W: USA National Weight Training and Conditioning Program for wrestlers: Part II. Natl Strength Conditioning Assoc J 1(5): 14–17, 1979
22. DZIEDZIC S, FARRELL W: USA National Training and Conditioning for Wrestling: Part III. Natl Strength Conditioning Assoc J 1(6):16–19, 1979
23. ELLIOTT J: Assessing muscle strength isokinetically. JAMA 240:2408–2409, 1978
24. ENOKA RM: The pull in olympic weightlifting. Med Sci Sports 11(2):131–137, 1979
25. EPLEY B: The Strength of Nebraska 1980. Lincoln, Nebraska, University of Nebraska, 1980
26. FOX E, MATTHEWS D: Interval Training: Conditioning for Sports and General Fitness. Philadelphia, WB Saunders, 1974
27. GONYEA WJ et al: Skeletal muscle fiber splitting induced by weight-lifting exercise in cats. Acta Physiol Scand 99:105–109, 1977
28. GONYEA WJ: The role of exercise in inducing increases in skeletal muscle fiber number. J Appl Physiol 48:421–426, 1980
29. HALLING AH, DOOLEY JN: The importance of isokinetic power and its specificity to athletic conditions. Athletic Training 83–86, Summer 1979
30. HISLOP H, PERRINE J: The isokinetic concept of exercise. Phys Ther 47:114–117, 1967

31. HOFFMAN T et al: Sex difference in strength. Am J Sports Med 7:265–267, 1979
32. HOOLAHAN P: Strength and conditioning for basketball. Natl Strength Conditioning Assoc J 2(5):32–34, 1980
33. HOUGH T: Ergographic studies in muscular soreness. Am J Physiol 7:76–92, 1902
34. JESSE JP: Misuse of strength development programs in athletic training. Phys Sportsmed 7(10):45–66, 1979
35. JESSE JP: Olympic lifting movements endanger adolescents. Phys Sportsmed 5(9):61–67, 1977
36. KULUND DN et al: Olympic weight-lifting injuries. Phys Sportsmed 6:11, November 1978
37. MENTZER M: Heavy Duty. Marina Del Ray, California, Dingman's Company, 1978
38. MILLER C: Bulgaria: Part I. Selection, a key to success. Personal notes
39. MILLER C: Rotary action of leg and hips common to many sports. Natl Strength Conditioning Assoc J 1(6):20–22, 1979
40. MILLER C: Sequence exercise to learn the rotary action of the legs and hips common to many sports. Natl Strength Conditioning Assoc J 2(3):38–39, 1980
41. MILLER J: Plyometric training for speed. Natl Strength Conditioning Assoc J 2(3):20–22, 1980
42. MILNER-BROWN HS et al: Synchronization of human motor units: possible roles of exercise and supraspinal reflexes. Electroencephalogr Clin Neurophysiol 38:245–254, 1975
43. PIPES TV, WILMORE JH: Isokinetic vs. isotonic strength training in adult men. Med Sci Sport 7:262–274, 1975
44. IPES TV: The acquisition of muscular strength through constant and variable resistance strength training. Athletic Training 12(3):146–151, 1977
45. PIPES TV, WILMORE JH: Strength training modes: What's the difference? Scholastic Coach 46:36–37, 1977
46. PIPES TV: Physiologic characteristics of elite body builders. Phys Sportsmed 7(3):116–121, 1979
47. RASCH PJ, MOREHOUSE LE: Effect of static and dynamic exercises on muscular strength and hypertrophy. J Appl Physiol 11:29, 1957
48. ROSENTSWEIG J, HINSON M: Comparison of isometric, isotonic and isokinetic exercises by electromyography. Arch Phys Med Rehabil 53:249–252, 1972
49. SIMMONS WK: The sit-up. Natl Strength Conditioning Assoc J 2(3):42–43, 1980
50. STARR W: The Strongest Shall Survive: Strength Training for Football. Annapolis, Maryland, Fitness Products, 1976
51. STULL GA, CLARKE DH: High-resistance, low-repetition training as a determiner of strength and fatigability. Res Q 41:189–193, 1970
52. TALAG TS: Residual muscle soreness as influenced by concentric, eccentric and static contractions. Res Q 44:458–461, 1973
53. THOMPSON H, STULL G: Effects of various training programs on speed of swimming. Res Q 30:479, 1959
54. VERKHOSHANSKI UV: Perspectives in the improvement of speed-strength preparation of jumpers. Track Field 9:11–12, 28–34, 1966
55. WALTERS L et al: Effect of short bouts of isometric and isotonic contractions on muscular strength and endurance. Am J Physiol Med 39:131–141, 1960
56. WHITBY D: Oregon track strength and conditioning for sprinting. Natl Strength Conditioning Assoc J 2(3):18–19, 1980
57. WILLIAMS M, STUTZMAN L: Strength variation throughout the range of joint motion. Phys Ther Rev 39:145–152, 1959
58. WILMORE JH: Alterations in strength, body composition and anthropometric measurements consequent to a ten-week weight training program. Med Sci Sports 6:133–138, 1974
59. WILMORE JH: Exploding the myth of female inferiority. Phys Sportsmed 2:54–58, 1974
60. WITHERS R: Effect of varied weight-training loads on the strength of university freshmen. Res Q 41:110–114, 1970
61. WOLBERS CP, SILLS FP: Development of strength in high school boys by static muscle contractions. Res Q 27:446–450, 1956
62. YESSIS M: Viewpoint: a response to nautilus. Natl Strength Conditioning Assoc J 2(3):42–43, 1980
63. YESSIS M: The key to strength development: variety. Natl Strength Conditioning Assoc J 3(3):32–34, 1981
64. ZERNIKE RF et al: Human patellar tendon rupture. A kinetic analysis. J Bone Joint Surg [Am] 59:179–183, 1977
65. ZITNIK RS et al: Hemodynamic effects of inhalation of ammonia in man. Am J Cardiol 24:187–190, 1969
66. ZORBAS W, KARPOVICH P: The effect of weightlifting upon the speed of muscular contractions. Res Q 22:145–148, 1951

A warm-up is an activity that mentally and physically mobilizes the athlete for athletic activity. The usual and most effective warm-up is an active one, consisting of general and specific exercises. A passive warm-up, such as a shower or a massage, is less effective.

A general warm-up comprises jogging, stretching, calisthenics, and some resistive exercises. The sport-specific part of the warm-up includes specific stretches and the movements that the athlete will use in the sport, but not at maximum intensity.

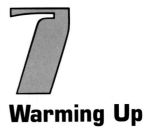

Warming Up

Effects of Warm-Up

The warm-up, with its psychological, cardiovascular, and muscular effects, has become an accepted way of preparing for athletic activity. Psychologically, it relieves tenseness and tightness and relaxes the athlete so that he is calm and can concentrate. Physiologically, the warm-up increases circulation and respiration.[3, 4, 6] Oxygen becomes more accessible to the cells because the vascular resistance is lower and hemogloblin gives off oxygen quicker. Warm-up also reduces the chances of developing myocardial ischemia at the onset of vigorous exercise.

The warm-up literally warms up the muscles, producing faster and more forceful contractions. The metabolic processes involved in contraction and relaxation progress quicker. Muscle viscosity drops, making contractions easier and smoother. The heating of the muscles reduces the activity of gamma nerve fibers and lessens the sensitivity of the muscle spindle to stretch, relaxing the muscle.

Muscle soreness may well be avoided by a proper warm-up. The warm-up will also promote agility and alertness and decrease movement time. The range of motion of joints increases, allowing better technique, new skill acquisition, and a reduction in injuries.

Warm-Up Process

The athlete jogs to the warm-up area. The nature of the warm-up will depend on the athlete's needs, his sport, his present disposition, and any

MIKLÓS TÖTTÖSSY

tight areas; it should be intense enough to increase the athlete's body temperature and cause some sweating but not so intense as to cause fatigue.[5] The eyes are exercised first, by moving them to all quadrants, for they are the master sense, so important for competition. Players, such as lacrosse goalies, who must shout instructions to their teammates, should warm up their temperomandibular joint muscles, too. Next, neck and shoulder exercises will decrease tension in these areas. Inverted postures, such as shoulder stands and head stands, are done early to energize the legs, relieving leg tension and tiredness. They should not, however, be done by persons with high blood pressure. Torso exercises are very important because they involve the largest muscle groups, which are the seat of power around the athlete's center of gravity, linking the upper and lower extremities.

Calisthenics have come to mean short, jerky movements with shallow mouth breathing in a frenetic atmosphere that detracts from concentration.[2] An example of these calisthenics is the jumping jack done by tackle football players while wearing shoulder pads that restrict the arm motion. Much more appropriate stretching exercises have evolved over some 5000 years from Hatha yoga, the branch of yoga that deals with the physical body.[2]

Stretching

Stretching is part of the warm-up, but stretching in itself does not comprise a complete warm-up.[1] The stretching is slow and graceful, since bouncing would set off a stretch reflex, and the part would then become tighter. An easy, relaxed stretch is held for 30 seconds and should produce a good feeling of mild tension. After 30 seconds, the athlete stretches a little further for another 30 seconds; he generally keeps his eyes closed because stretching is an indrawn process. He breathes deeply through his nose and concentrates on the part that he is stretching; he should not rush or skip steps.

If a specific area is tight, the athlete should focus on loosening this area. He may have slept in an unusual position. Through stretching, the athlete gets to know his own body and its needs. He should stretch within his limits, remembering that stretching is not competitive. All athletes cannot stretch to the same degree: An athlete may even have some tight joints and others that are loose. If the stretching is painful the athlete is overstretching, and this will produce tightness or an injury.

Breathing

Short and shallow mouth breathing is associated with excitement and a loss of emotional control. This panting only uses the upper sections of the lungs and may reduce the deliberateness of the athlete's actions. Abdominal breathing through the nose is a key element for relaxation and concentration, both of which are needed for good exercise and competition.[2] A person normally breathes through his nose when calm. Moreover, the air is filtered and warmed. The athlete breathes slowly and steadily in through the nose only, allowing the stomach to come out with each breath. Then, as inhalation continues, the stomach is pulled in toward the spine and the chest is filled. Finally, while still breathing in, the athlete raises his shoulders to fill the top of his lungs. He holds his breath for 5 to 10 seconds and then exhales slowly and steadily through the nose. The athlete concentrates on the feeling and sound of his breathing.

These slow, deep breaths slow the heart rate, provide extra oxygen, and put less strain on the cardiovascular system. The athlete can breathe in this manner while he is waiting to perform in practice and during time-outs and breaks in the action. This breathing is a part of relaxation techniques used as preparation for sporting activity. The athlete lies on his back, breathes through his nose, and concentrates on the techniques that he will use and the assignments he will have in the upcoming event or contest. He mentally rehearses the upcoming activity, imagining a perfectly executed, skilled performance.[7]

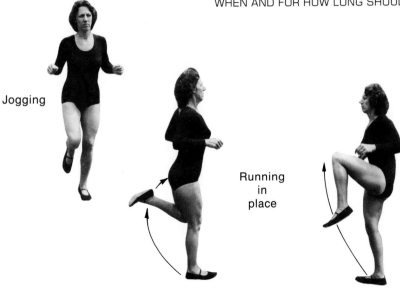

Jogging

Running in place

FIG. 7-1
The athlete begins warming up by jogging. Running in place can be done with a back kick or leg lifts.

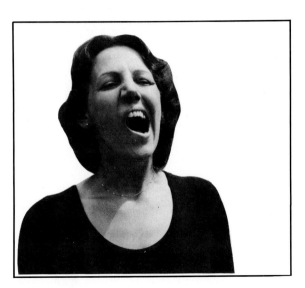

FIG. 7-2
Mandibular exercises prepare the temperomandibular joint. They are especially important for goalkeepers and goaltenders who must shout instructions to teammates.

When and For How Long Should the Athlete Warm Up?

An athlete should warm up in a warm-up suit each day before practice and after breaks in practice, before the start of a game, and before the second half begins. Substitutes should, of course, warm up before entering a game. The warm-up usually begins 30 to 40 minutes before a contest, tapers off from 10 to 15 minutes before competition, and ends about 5 minutes before a contest.[5] This allows recovery from any slight and temporary fatigue without the loss of the warm-up effects.

The athlete should also warm down after each practice or competition. The warm-down includes light jogging and stretching that relaxes the athlete, breaks down muscle spasm, and removes the waste products of exercise. Soreness will thus be reduced, and the athlete will feel good when he leaves the field.

The following exercises may be used during a warm-up (Figs. 7-1 through 7-17). Specific exercises would be chosen for the individual and for the sport.

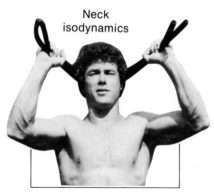

Neck isodynamics

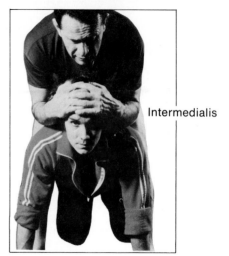

Intermedialis

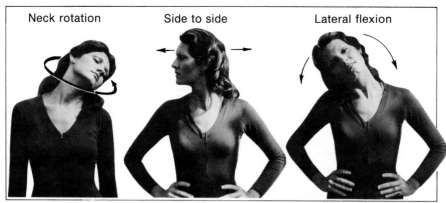

Neck rotation

Side to side

Lateral flexion

Fig. 7-3

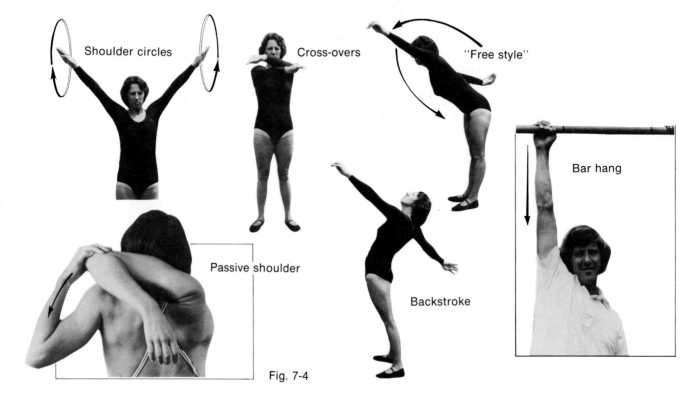

Shoulder circles

Cross-overs

"Free style"

Bar hang

Passive shoulder

Backstroke

Fig. 7-4

◀ **FIG. 7-3**
The neck is readied for activity by movements
and strengthened isodynamically or against a
partner's resistance.

◀ **FIG. 7-4**
Active and passive movements warm up the
shoulders. The shoulder capsule is stretched
by hanging from a bar.

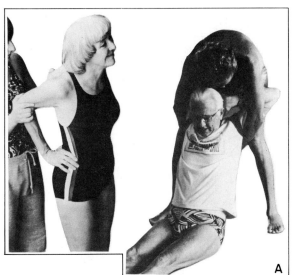

FIG. 7-5
Stretching with a skilled partner can produce
great gains in flexibility. These stretches are
done slowly in a controlled manner. An
external rotation stretch of the shoulder by a
partner is particularly important to throwers.

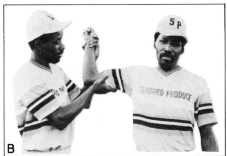

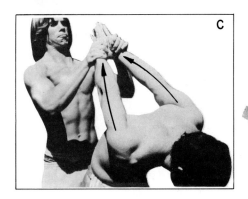

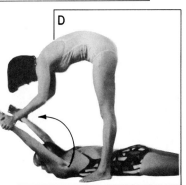

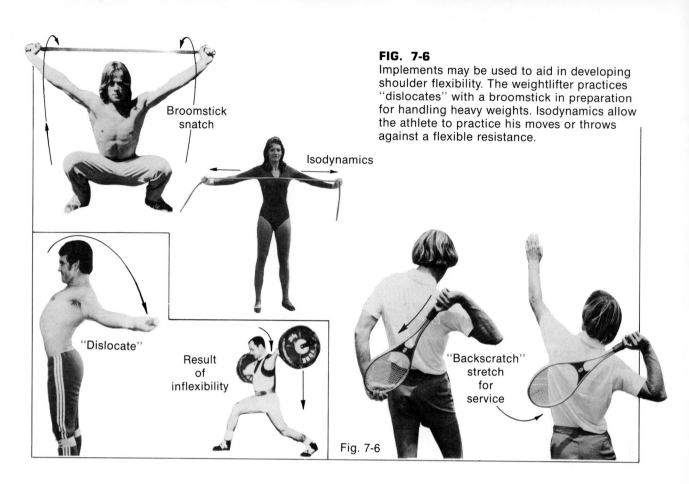

Broomstick snatch

Isodynamics

FIG. 7-6
Implements may be used to aid in developing shoulder flexibility. The weightlifter practices "dislocates" with a broomstick in preparation for handling heavy weights. Isodynamics allow the athlete to practice his moves or throws against a flexible resistance.

"Dislocate"

Result of inflexibility

"Backscratch" stretch for service

Fig. 7-6

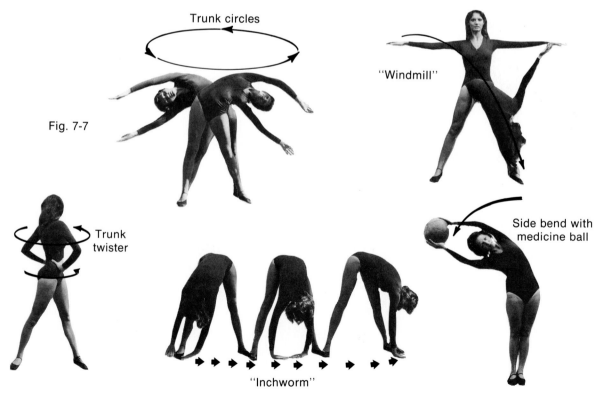

Trunk circles

"Windmill"

Fig. 7-7

Trunk twister

"Inchworm"

Side bend with medicine ball

Fig. 7-8

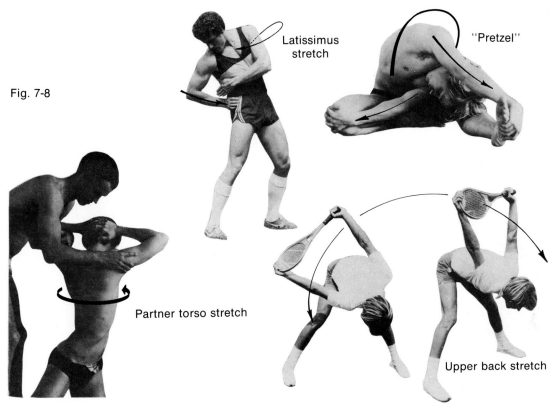

Latissimus stretch

"Pretzel"

Partner torso stretch

Upper back stretch

FIG. 7-8
Trunk twisting may be done freely, with help from a skilled partner, or
with an implement.

FIG. 7-7
Preliminary twisting and bending movements
of the trunk are an important way to prevent
back strains.

FIG. 7-9
Back flexion may be done freely or with a medicine ball.

FIG. 7-10
Back extensions may be done freely or with help from a partner.

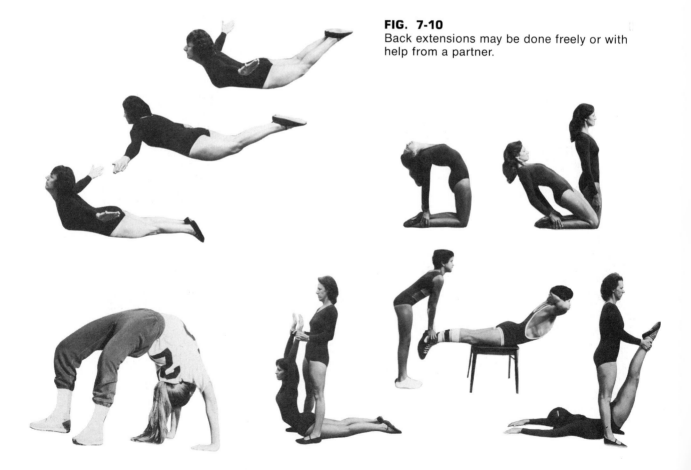

Fig. 7-11

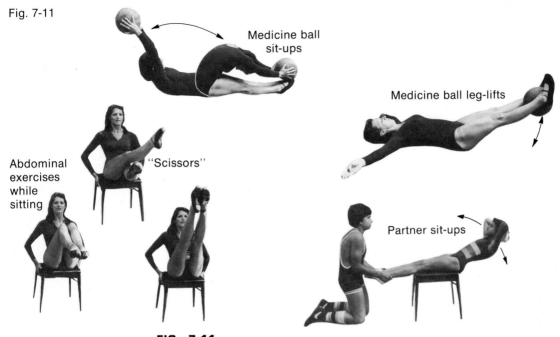

Medicine ball
sit-ups

Medicine ball leg-lifts

"Scissors"

Abdominal
exercises
while
sitting

Partner sit-ups

FIG. 7-11
The athlete may strengthen her abdomen with sit-ups, weighted sit-ups,
leg raises, or assisted sit-ups.

FIG. 7-12
The athlete may strengthen his abductors and adductors against the
resistance of a partner. The gluteal stretch is important for runners.
Flexible tubing may be used for isodynamic strengthening.

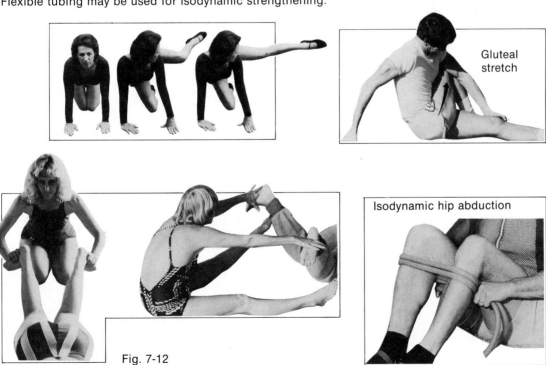

Gluteal
stretch

Isodynamic hip abduction

Fig. 7-12

174

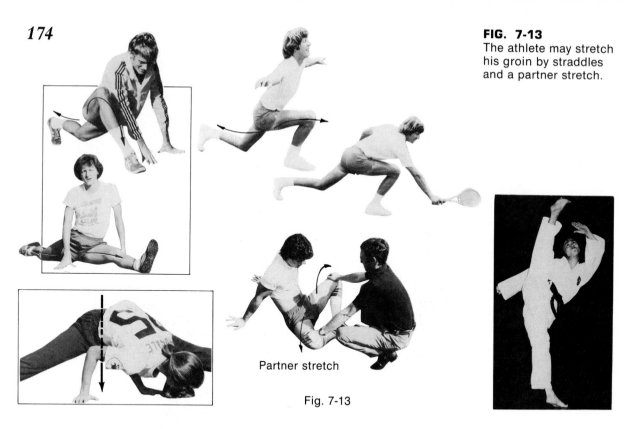

FIG. 7-13
The athlete may stretch
his groin by straddles
and a partner stretch.

Partner stretch

Fig. 7-13

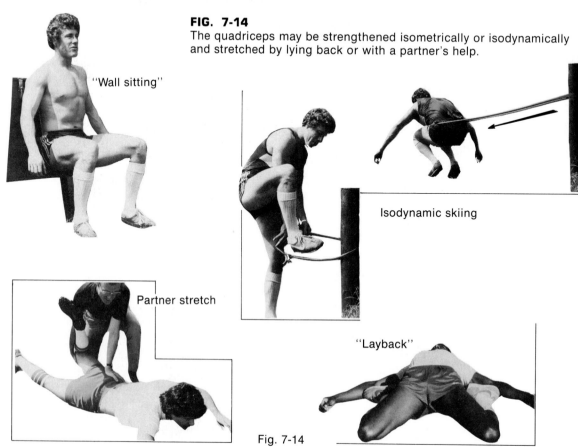

FIG. 7-14
The quadriceps may be strengthened isometrically or isodynamically
and stretched by lying back or with a partner's help.

"Wall sitting"

Isodynamic skiing

Partner stretch

"Layback"

Fig. 7-14

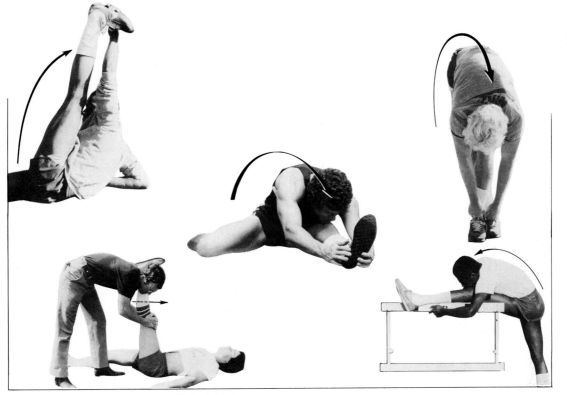

FIG. 7-15
Hamstring stretching is an important part of the warm-up. It is most effective with a partner by the "contract-relax" technique.

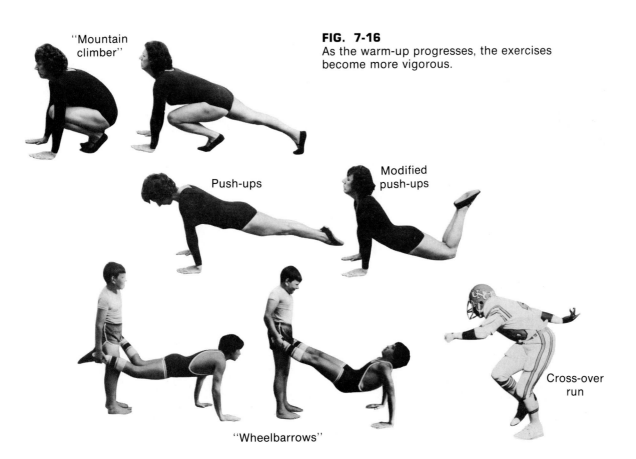

"Mountain climber"

FIG. 7-16
As the warm-up progresses, the exercises become more vigorous.

Push-ups

Modified push-ups

"Wheelbarrows"

Cross-over run

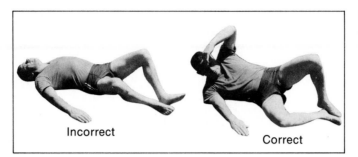

FIG. 7-17
Athletes can avoid injury by practicing how to fall correctly.

Incorrect

Correct

REFERENCES

1. ANDERSON B: Stretching. Bolinas, California, Shelter Publications Random House, 1980
2. COLLETTO J, SLOAN JL: Yoga Conditioning and Football. Millbrae, California, Celestial Arts, 1975
3. DE BRUYN/PROVOST P: The effects of various warming up intensities and durations upon some physiological variables. Eur J Appl Phys 43:93–100, 1980
4. KARPOVICH PV, HALE C: Effect of warming-up upon physical performance. JAMA 162:1117–1119, 1956
5. JENSEN C: Pertinent facts about warm-up. Athletic J 56(2):72–75, 1975
6. MARTIN BJ: Effect of warm-up on metabolic responses to strenuous exercise. Med Sci Sports 7:146–149, 1975
7. TSCHUDI O: See yourself ski: technique of relaxation and visualization. Ski 44(3):155, 1979

Sports, by their very nature, invite injury. Each year, millions of injuries occur to the more than 4 million boys and almost 1½ million girls who participate in interscholastic and intercollegiate athletics. More than 1 million boys at 14,000 high schools participate in football alone. Yearly, these players sustain over 110,000 major injuries that result in 3 weeks or more of inactivity. Most of these injured athletes never see a physician.

Some high schools have a physician in attendance at games, but more than 65% of athletic injuries occur in practice. Who will aid these athletes? Good medical care is especially important in high schools because these youths are often uncoordinated and only beginning to mature physically and mentally. Moreover, only 5% of high school health care personnel are certified athletic trainers. About 75% of health care is given by coaches, and more than 80% of these coaches do not meet any standards for health care personnel. At 2-year colleges, 7% of health care personnel are certified athletic trainers, and at 4-year colleges 28% are certified trainers.

The overworked coach assigned the duties of an athletic trainer may lack knowledge of emergency first aid, cardiopulmonary resuscitation (CPR), and transportation procedures. The coach is also placed in a conflict-of-interest situation where he must decide when a young athlete may return to competition. Some high schools have student trainers, but these students lack supervision and often overstep their abilities. The student trainer may lack sports medicine knowledge and jeopardize the athlete by not referring him to a doctor. Obviously, optimal health care is not provided by coaches or rendered by student trainers who lack first aid skills; thus negligence is likely to occur. Although the blame lies with the school system, the coach often ends up in court. Athletes should not participate in interscholastic or intercollegiate sports without optimum health care. Without a certified athletic trainer, optimum health care is impossible.

To assure basic competency and the finest health care for athletes, some states now require that athletic trainers be licensed. Certification is another answer. One possible route to certification is through a National Athletic Trainers Association (NATA)-approved undergraduate or graduate program. Another is through an apprenticeship. Also, phys-

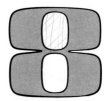

The Athletic Trainer and Rehabilitation

JOE H. GIECK

177

ical therapists and trainers actively engaged in the field may supplement their training and be eligible for certfication.

All applicants for certification must possess at least a bachelor's degree, have a current CPR and first-aid card, be a NATA member, be recommended by a certified athletic trainer (ATC), and pass the written and oral tests developed and administered by the NATA. The candidate must also successfully complete a competency evaluation by a certified athletic trainer, a test that includes injury evaluation (including heat illness), first aid, strapping, and the rehabilitation (including therapeutic modalities) of all types of athletic injuries.

Curriculums approved by the NATA provide 1 to 4 years of experience with a certified athletic trainer. The candidate must have a minimum of 800 hours of practical experience with a certified trainer. Required courses are anatomy, physiology, physiology of exercise, kinesiology, psychology, first aid and safety, nutrition, remedial or adapted exercise, personal, community and school health, and techniques of athletic training.

Serving an apprenticeship requires 2 to 4 years of work under a certified athletic trainer and the amassing of more than 1800 hours of clinical work. Physical therapists may also qualify to take the examination if they have worked 2 years with a certified athletic trainer for a minimum of 800 hours. Eligible too are active trainers currently practicing in the field who have amassed more than 1800 hours under a certified athletic trainer, supplemented with certain academic courses or a faculty-trainer program.

The University of Virginia, Northwestern University, and the State Department of North Carolina now educate secondary school faculty members to become athletic trainers. The NATA has also adopted a continuing education policy. A trainer must gain six continuing education units in 3 years (one unit per 10 contact hours) to maintain certification.

Duties

The athletic trainer sees to it that athletes in his trust receive excellent health care. The trainer not only works with members of athletic teams, but also may provide medical emergency care in physical education and school situations. A student who falls down a flight of stairs, for example, or is otherwise injured benefits from the emergency medical skills of the athletic trainer. The trainer administers first aid ranging from the treatment of simple abrasions to splinting, CPR, and other life-saving techniques.

The athletic trainer is charged with the prevention, treatment, and rehabilitation of athletes in his athletic setting. Preventive measures are taught for avoiding injury. If injury has occurred, however, proper care reduces recovery time, and the athlete may enjoy a quicker return to competition. The athlete is rehabilitated for a return to competition, not just back to the activities of daily life; this requires greater levels of strength, flexibility, power, endurance, speed, and skill. The trainer uses heat and cold but employs exercise as the major modality (Fig. 8-1). Under the care of an athletic trainer, an athlete is less likely to return to action before being ready, thereby reducing the chance for reinjury.

The trainer is a link between the team physician and coach, the athlete and coach, and others. He is responsible administratively to the athletic director for policies and budget items and medically to the team physician. The team physician cannot be at all practices and games; thus the athletic trainer refers the athletes to the doctor as necessary. The trainer is also responsible for carrying out the team physician's instructions.

The athletic trainer sets up and directs conditioning programs for flexibility, strength, and endurance that will help prevent injury. He also may advise coaches as to the safety of their practice procedures, inspect playing facilities for safety, and fit and check protective equipment. He serves too as a health counselor to athletes, especially those who lack family health care. Counseling is also an important role of the athletic trainer.

In addition to health care duties, the trainer is the administrator of the health care facilities and personnel and is involved in purchasing. Some trainers are faculty members who work

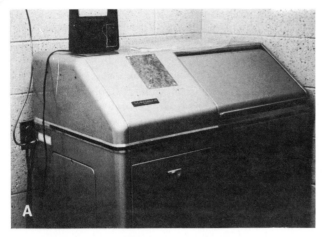
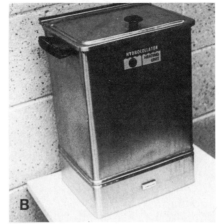
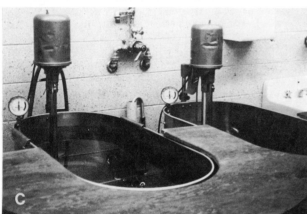
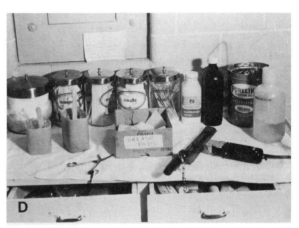

FIG. 8-1
The training room should contain an ice box (*A*), heating unit (*B*),
whirlpool (*C*), and training table (*D*).

mornings in the school's student-health physical-therapy department or teach courses.

When school administrators are asked why their high school does not employ a certified athletic trainer, the reply is often, "We cannot afford one," or, "We haven't had one before, so why do we need one now?" Granted, many schools cannot afford a full-time athletic trainer, but the trainer can be a full-time faculty member with training in the principles of athletic training, CPR, first-aid, and transportation of the injured. Such a faculty member could receive a supplement, like a coach's supplement, for athletic training. The prevention of even one serious injury because of the presence of a trainer would justify allocating the necessary funds.

Athletic Activity in the Heat

Control of Body Heat, Water, and Salt Balance

The athlete's body heat is regulated by the hypothalamus, where sensitive heat receptors respond to the temperature of blood that courses from the periphery.[14] Afferent nerve impulses also affect the heat receptors. The hypothalamus can then directly affect peripheral vessels, or act through the pituitary, which secretes antidiuretic hormone (ADH). This hormone decreases urine flow by influencing the amount of water reabsorbed in the kidney tubules. To maintain a normal plasma water content, body fluid is drawn into the plasma from the interstitial fluid. Adrenocortical activity provides for reabsorption of salt in the kidney.[17] This sodium conservation and potassium loss may produce a potassium deficit.

Heat Exchange

Heat may be exchanged through conduction, radiation, convection, and evaporation.[6, 9, 41] Conduction of heat from a hot helmet and pads will raise a football player's body heat. If the athlete drinks cool water, his body loses heat by conduction because the water must be warmed to body temperature. Radiation of heat from solid surroundings may also increase the athlete's body heat, but this gain may be reduced by about one-half if the athlete wears white clothes. Heat gains by convection may be controlled by ventilation, shade, and insulation.

When the environmental temperature is less than skin temperature, which is 32° C (87° F), 70% of body heat is lost through conduction, radiation, and convection and 30% through evaporation. Ventilation with cool air will increase the elimination of heat by convection and evaporation. Once the temperature rises above 32° C, however, heat is added to the athlete's body. With a high environmental temperature, heat may be supplied faster than the athlete's body can eliminate it by evaporation or by perspiration, which is normally the primary protective mechanism of the body against overheating.

Classes of Heat Disorders

Heat disorders include circulatory instability, water and electrolyte balance disorders, heat stroke, and heat hyperpyrexia.[11] Circulatory instability may be characterized by *heat syncope*. The athlete may feel lightheaded or dizzy, nauseated, and weak during periods of prolonged standing, postural change, or exercise. A weak, fast pulse and a decreased blood pressure reflect peripheral vasodilation, venous pooling, and hypotension. Recovery is rapid if the athlete reclines for a few minutes.

Disorders of water and electrolytes lead to heat edema, water-depletion heat exhaustion, salt-depletion heat exhaustion, and heat cramps. *Heat edema* is swelling of the ankles and feet during early exposure to heat and is probably due to pooling of blood in the legs. Heat disorders have their most profound effects on the cardiovascular system, especially in unacclimatized persons. Heat stroke may result as the cardiovascular system is overloaded from having to pump more blood to cool the body. For each degree rise in body temperature, the athlete needs 7% more oxygen to maintain body processes, and the heart must also increase its blood supply to the lungs.

Salt-Depletion Heat Exhaustion

Salt-depletion heat exhaustion may follow large intakes of unsalted fluid, vomiting, and diarrhea. Along with salt depletion is a secondary water depletion, as less water is reabsorbed from the renal tubules. Salt-depletion heat exhaustion generally progresses over 3 to 5 days. The athlete may have a normal or slightly elevated temperature. Symptoms include weariness, headache, nausea, vomiting, diarrhea or constipation, and muscle cramps. Some athletes seem more susceptible to these cramps, which are caused by water intoxication as water enters the intracellular fluid and dilutes the sodium chloride. Normal saline solution is given for the prevention and treatment of salt-depletion heat exhaustion. Enteric salt may be used for prevention, but plain salt, one teaspoon of salt in each pint of water, is used for treatment. The athlete may use beef tea, consommé, or tomato juice to mask the salty taste of this fluid.

Water-Depletion Heat Exhaustion

Water-depletion heat exhaustion is caused by sweating and by loss of fluid from diarrhea. The athlete's rectal temperature rises, and his pulse and breathing become rapid. His skin is inelastic, cheeks are hollow, and eyes sunken. The athlete notes a tingling and numbness in his limbs and may become restless, hysterical, and uncoordinated. Water-depletion heat exhaustion may progress to hypotension, circulatory and kidney failure, cyanosis, heat stroke,

TABLE 8-1.
Differences Between Water-Depletion and Salt-Depletion Heat Exhaustion

Water Depletion	Salt Depletion
High intake of salt without water dangerous	High intake of water without salt dangerous
May occur immediately	Generally progresses over 3 to 5 days
Urgent thirst	Slight or no thirst
Fatigue less prominent	Fatigue prominent
Usually no vomiting	Vomiting
No muscle cramps	Muscle cramps
Skin inelastic and usually dry	Skin clammy and moist
Temperature high	Temperature near normal
Predisposes to heat stroke	Does not predispose to heat stroke
Treat by cooling and rehydration	Treat by cooling and saline drinks
If death occurs, it is generally from heat stroke	Death rare

coma, and death. A severe drop in an athlete's body weight on the weight chart forewarns of this disorder. Athletes with water-depletion heat exhaustion should be rehydrated in a cool area. Salt- and water-depletion heat exhaustion may coexist. (Differences between the two types of heat exhaustion are shown in Table 8-1.) The danger of progressing to heat stroke should be utmost in the minds of those treating heat exhaustion.

Heat Stroke

Heat stroke results from a thermoregulatory failure in the body's response to heat stress. The combination of water depletion and high-output cardiac failure may lead to a complete failure of sweat production. The environmental temperature need not be very high for heat stroke to occur; in fact, fatal heat stroke has occurred at 18° C (64° F) and high humidity.

The athlete with heat stroke will usually have a pulse rate of about 130 beats/min and rapid, labored, gasping respirations of about 35/min. His skin is usually hot and dry but may sometimes be cool and pale. The athlete may suddenly become irrational and disoriented, become incontinent, convulse, and lose consciousness. Renal failure and shock may de-

velop. A temperature of about 43° C (110° F) in heat stroke can damage the hypothalamus; if the athlete survives, he will be more susceptible to heat disorders. Heat stroke is fatal in about one half of cases. In contrast to an athlete with heat stroke, an athlete with heat hyperpyrexia is conscious and rational, and his body temperature rises to only about 40° C (105° F). Untreated cases of either heat hyperpyrexia or heat stroke are fatal.

The athlete with heat stroke must be rapidly cooled.[4] Cooling is usually life-saving if the body temperature can be reduced to 39° C (102° F) within an hour. The cooling methods include a slatted table designed to spray cool water, at about 7° C (44° F), on all sides of the victim. Other effective cooling methods are wet sheets, submersion in cold water, and cold blankets, used in heart surgery. One of the most practical methods is to let a fan blow across the victim while his extremities are being massaged vigorously with cool, wet towels to promote circulation. If the athlete is over-chilled, however, vasoconstriction may cause shock or shivering. The physician may give chlorpromazine to help prevent shivering, a drug that depresses the hypothalamic heat center and promotes vasodilation.

TABLE 8-2.
Practice in the Heat*

Attire	Length of Exercise	Wet-Bulb-Glog Thermometer		Length of Water Break
	min	°C (°F)		*min*
Full pads	45	28.8 (84) or below		5
Full pads	45	28.8–29.5 84–85	to	10
Full pads	30	29.5–31.1 85–88	to	10
Helmet, shoulder pads, shorts, shoes	30	29.5–31.1 85–88	to	5

*The above is for a 2-hour practice session once daily. No more than one 2-hour practice session a day should be undertaken in the heat. Ideally, managers give each group continuous and unlimited fluids.

The weather during early fall and late spring football practice sometimes produces high heat stress, and artificial turf compounds the problem. The athletes most susceptible to heat disorders are older, obese, unacclimatized, physically unfit persons with cardiovascular disorders, those just recovering from febrile illness, and those with a history of heat illness. A sound approach to acclimatization and the prevention of heat illness, however, allows athletes to compete safely in the heat.

Acclimatization to the Heat Athletes must exercise in the heat to adapt fully to it (Table 8-2). Most acclimatization occurs during the first 4 to 7 days and is usually complete in 12 to 14 days. Initially, the athlete's sweat rate may increase to 3 liters an hour to provide improved cooling. After about 2 weeks, however, the sweat rate returns to near normal, and, with acclimatization, the sweat is less salty.

The acclimatized athlete tolerates dehydration better than does the unacclimatized. Although the heart rate initially increases during heat stress, as acclimatization progresses the athlete's rectal temperature and heart rate drop to near normal. Acclimatization allows the athlete to work effectively in 27° C (80° F) heat, whereas physically unfit persons cannot perform in environments where the temperature is much above 18° to 24° C (65° to 75° F). Experienced athletes usually learn to pace themselves to avoid the effects of the heat suffered by inexperienced athletes.

Two 2-hour practices each day provide optimal acclimatization to the heat. Longer sessions only put an extra strain on the athlete. One of these practice sessions should be held during the hot part of the day, and one when it is cool. Readings from a wet-bulb-globe thermometer, or sling psychrometer, provide a useful index as to the number of salt and fluid breaks and the length of practice. The wet-bulb-globe thermometer is especially useful in southern climates, where the humidity must be considered. The athlete's clothing should be light, loose, and white, whenever possible. Mesh or net jerseys allow body cooling, and the athlete should certainly not wear a rubber sweat suit for weight reduction.

Athletes must be motivated to report to preseason practice in good condition. At the beginning of hot weather training, fitness tests indicate who is in poor condition. These athletes should be especially observed for heat illness. The endurance test may be a series of 300-

yard sprints, with a 90-second rest in between, or 300-yard shuttle runs.

A common conditioning error in early practice is to overwork the athletes who have reported in poor physical condition. These unfit, unacclimatized, obese athletes cannot tolerate as much work as fit ones but are often pushed harder. This overwork, along with a restricted diet, makes unfit athletes prime targets for heat illness. These athletes should be worked by themselves or in selected drills until they are ready to participate with the rest of the squad. Other athletes who should be watched carefully during periods of heat stress are the highly competitive, overenthusiastic ones. These persons are often doing more than the rest of the team and may have a dry uniform at the end of practice because their perspiration has been exhausted.

Overtraining, beyond the point of fatigue, will actually decondition athletes. Once liver and muscle glycogen stores are exhausted, usually at about the third or fourth day of two-a-day practices, an athlete's work capacity will drop rapidly. After overtraining, the question often is not who is in the best shape for the first game but who is the least tired and worn out.

Prevention of Heat Stroke The major way to prevent heat stroke is to allow the players unlimited access to water. The purpose of a replacement fluid is to maintain blood volume, and water does this best. During exercise, fluid is lost more rapidly than it can be taken in, and satiating thirst will account for only 50% of the body needs. To meet an athlete's fluid needs, he should ingest several glasses of fluid just before competition and drink water during breaks, even if he may not be particularly thirsty. Also, he may need 5 to 15 g of salt a day at the start of the acclimatization process. Potassium, calcium, and vitamin C are important in the athlete's diet at this time. Tablets are available that contain salt, potassium, calcium, vitamin C, and dextrose (Thermotabs). The high sugar content of some commercial electrolyte solutions interferes with gastrointestinal tract emptying. A 10% glucose solution, for

example, will slow gastric emptying by one half.

An athlete working in the heat should maintain a normal caloric intake. The best diet for him contains many carbohydrates because carbohydrates have a high water content. Proteins, on the other hand, need large amounts of water for digestion and thus add to fluid imbalance. A large fluid intake before or during a meal will lead to loss of appetite and may cause vomiting and diarrhea. Before eating, then, an athlete working in the heat should drink just enough fluid to quench his thirst. After eating a good meal, he may then drink extra fluids. Heavy meals should be avoided before exercise so that the blood may be used for cooling. A cold shower taken before competition will also increase the body's tolerance to heat.

If heat stroke occurs, it is usually during the first 3 to 5 days of practice in dehydrated persons. Players should be weighed in and weighed out for each practice. The weight charts should then be checked to find those athletes who have lost 0.9 kg to 2.3 kg (2 to 5 lb) in 24 hours: These are the candidates for heat illness. Ideally, they should be excluded from practice for 24 hours. Moreover, any athlete who has signs and symptoms of heat illness should be withdrawn immediately from activity, and those players with minor heat problems should be excluded for 24 hours. Vomiting and diarrhea will further dehydrate the athlete's body and are contraindications for heavy workouts in the heat.

Athletes should avoid drinking alcohol during periods of heat stress because this drug promotes dehydration and increases the metabolic load. Belladonna and antihistamines inhibit sweating and should not be taken by athletes who will be training in the heat. Athletes taking diuretics to control high blood pressure should be closely observed when they participate under stressful heat conditions.

During off-practice hours, air conditioning benefits an athlete by conserving the energy his body would have to expend to cool itself. Because sweating is reduced, dehydration is not as much of a problem. Air conditioning also helps to prevent skin disorders that accompany chronic wetness. The athlete can rest easier in a cool environment, and this rest serves to diminish fatigue.

Fitting of Protective Equipment

Helmets and shoulder pads are the primary pieces of protective equipment in tackle football and are worn by more than 1 million high school players. Today's football equipment provides adequate protection for these players. With all of the contact in high school and college football, professional ranks, and assorted leagues, it is amazing that there are not more serious injuries. The equipment so fully protects the wearer, however, that he plays with much more abandon, making it more likely that he or an opponent will be injured.

Even with excellent protective equipment, an improper fit is dangerous. The equipment may then cause injury or increase the severity of an injury. To assure that the equipment will provide the optimum protection for which it was designed, all personnel who fit protective equipment must be extremely knowledgeable in fitting. Improper fitting is especially a problem at the high school level, where coaches, managers, and student trainers often lack proper knowledge of fitting. Sometimes, the first string is given the best equipment, although it is not necessarily properly fitted, and the rest of the squad takes what is left. Not only do all of these athletes need the best equipment, but players must be fitted individually for each piece of equipment. A player should not be given a medium fit because he is of medium size.

Football Helmet

The football helmet distributes and attenuates shocks and recovers rapidly. Shock reduction is only optimal when the helmet is properly fitted.[10] All football helmets bearing the National Operating Committee on Standards for Athletic Equipment (NOCSAE) seal provide adequate protection if they are properly fitted. When a school purchases a particular brand of helmet, the sales representative should demonstrate proper fitting technique to those persons charged with fitting the helmets.

Basic Guidelines

Short hair allows a better fit of the football helmet.[18] If an athlete has long hair, he should wet his hair before trying on the helmet. The fit will then be a proper one for sweaty competition. The helmet should fit snugly on the athlete's head and not slide excessively from side to side, forward or backward. To check for excess motion, the fitter should grasp the face mask, with the chin strap fastened, and apply pressure while the player holds his neck stiff (Fig. 8-2). If the helmet slides excessively, it is improperly fitted, regardless of whether the size corresponds to the player's head size. A special fitting will usually be needed to ensure a proper fit in an athlete with a long, oval head. Jaw pads should be of the proper size— for example, thick pads for a thin-faced player.

The frontal crown of the helmet should be one or two finger breadths above the eyebrows. This position should remain the same when the player overlaps his fingers on top of the helmet and presses down (Fig. 8-3). If the helmet descends over his eyebrows, spacers or a custom-cut closed-cell foam crownpiece (Ensolite) may be inserted.

The padding on the front lip of the helmet reduces lacerations and abrasions of the nose. If, however, the posterior tails of the chin straps are loose, the helmet may still slide forward over the player's nose. Proper tension on the anterior straps keeps the helmet from sliding backward during contact (Fig. 8-4). The back edge of the helmet should not impinge on the player's neck when he extends it.

Players should be advised that a properly fitted helmet may feel slightly tight for the first few days of practice, especially if the helmet is new. If a player feels that the fit of his helmet is unsatisfactory, he should report back promptly to the person in charge of fitting. All

FIG. 8-2
To check for excess motion of the helmet, the face mask is grasped with the chin strap fastened, and pressure is applied while the player holds his neck stiff.

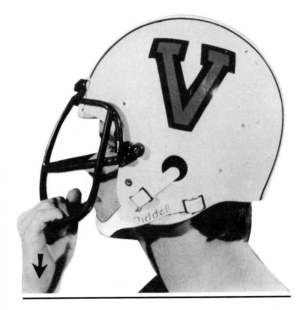

players should be shown how to put on a helmet correctly. First, the player puts his thumbs in the earholes, with the helmet tilted back. He then rolls the helmet forward onto his head and removes it in the reverse order. The helmet must not be jammed onto the head or jerked off, as this only causes discomfort and external ear damage. Each player's number should be marked inside his helmet, and players should never swap helmets.

A player should never wear a cracked helmet. Cracks may appear in the helmet at areas of stress where facemask hardware has been attached. The helmets should be checked for soundness during and after the season and after reconditioning. The examiner looks for cracks in the shell, loose rivets, and loose or bent facemasks. During the season, padded suspensions tend to bottom out, and air pads and fluid pads may leak.

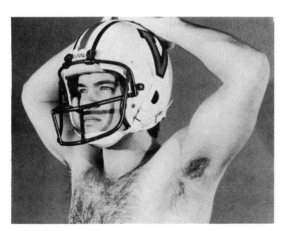

FIG. 8-3
The helmet should not slip down when the player overlaps his fingers on top of the helmet and presses down.

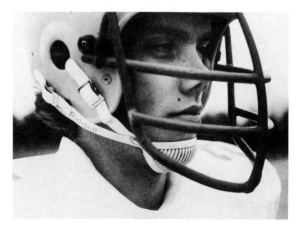

FIG. 8-4
Anterior and posterior chin straps (a four-way chin strap) keep the helmet from shifting forward or backward.

Shoulder Pads

The two basic types of shoulder pads are flat pads and cantilever pads.[10] Flat pads are worn by those players in limited contact positions who need more glenohumeral motion—for example, quarterbacks and receivers. Cantilever pads are named for the bridge that extends over the shoulder and are worn by players who are in constant contact. Most flat pads are less protective than cantilever pads, but, when properly constructed, can afford excellent protection for linemen and linebackers. Of the cantilever pads, the inside cantilever is the most common. The outside cantilever affords somewhat more protection with a larger blocking surface and is the most popular for offensive linemen. The pads for linebackers and for players receiving blows in a standing position are larger anteriorly and slanted forward.

The neck opening of shoulder pads should have enough room for the player to extend his arm overhead without the pad's impinging on his neck. However, the neck opening should not be so large as to allow excessive sliding around on the shoulders, as in the case of oversized pads. A pad too large will slide to one side and invite neck injury, and an improperly fitted shoulder pad may allow injury to the player's acromioclavicular joint.

The tip of the shoulder pad should reach just to the lateral edge of the shoulder, and the flaps, or epaulets, should cover the deltoid area (Fig. 8-5). A pair of calipers may be used to speed proper fitting (Fig. 8-6). The fitter should measure from the edge of one shoulder across to the other shoulder.

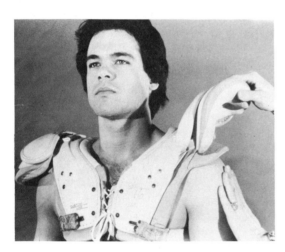

FIG. 8-5
The shoulder pad should extend to the tip of the shoulder.

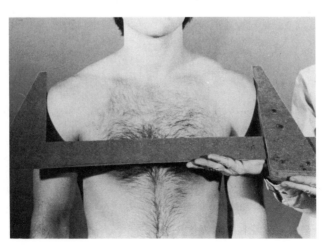

FIG. 8-6
Calipers help in the proper fitting of shoulder pads.

The elastic axilla straps that hold the pads to the chest and to the back must be tight but comfortable. These straps allow the impact of a blow to be distributed onto the chest and back. If the straps are loose, the pad may flatten out and press over the acromioclavicular joint.

Shoulder pads should be inspected constantly for cracks, frayed straps and strings, loose rivets, and other failures. At the end of the season, all equipment must be inspected. Defective equipment should be discarded, but if the equipment is salvageable it may be sent to a reputable athletic equipment reconditioner. When the equipment is returned from the reconditioner, it must again be inspected carefully.

Physiologic Response to Injury

When tissue is damaged by being crushed, stretched, or torn, an inflammatory response occurs. This is a normal response to injury whereby active peptides, histamine, prostaglandins, lytic enzymes, blood cells, and plasma all enter the injured region. The active polypeptides are kallidin and bradykinin, vasodilators that produce edema and evoke pain by acting on nerve endings. Histamine is released from mast cells and relaxes fine blood vessels, increasing their permeability.

Prostaglandins are synthesized locally in the tissues from a fatty acid precursor, arachidonic acid. The major biosynthetic pathway involves activation of the enzyme cyclo-oxygenase with the formation of intermediate endoperoxides. Prostaglandins act synergistically with bradykinin to amplify pain by sensitizing the afferent nerve endings to chemical and mechanical stimulation. They are also potent vasodilators, less so than bradykinin but more potent than histamine. They induce erythema, increase the leakage of plasma from vessels, and attract leukocytes to the injured area.

Polymorphonuclear leukocytes migrate to the site of the injury and release lysozymes from lysosomes (packets of proteolytic enzymes) to digest the proteins that accumulate as cells are destroyed. Hemorrhage and swelling occur, which, along with the direct effect of the inflammatory products on nerve endings, produce pain and spasm. The spasm not only splints the damaged tissue, but also compresses pain fibers. Moreover, it lessens the efficiency of the vascular system and can result in ischemia at the injured area. The pain fiber compression and ischemia establish a vicious pain-spasm cycle. As a result, more cells are eventually injured than were initially injured.

A hematoma forms when blood vessels are torn. Plasma also leaks into the damaged area to produce brawny edema. The fibrinogen in the plasma causes the extracellular fluid to clot, and fibrous tissue grows to produce adhesions and tissue thickening. The damaged area, with its inflammatory products, edema, hemorrhage, blood stasis, and debris of dead and damaged cells, becomes walled off from the surrounding tissue by a fibrin network. Sometimes there are calcium deposits and mucoid degeneration in the tender scar, and bone may even form if there has been periosteal stripping.

Swelling is the greatest enemy of healing. The goal of early treatment is to delay or minimize swelling. By limiting the swelling, pain and muscle spasm decrease and the magnitude of the injured is reduced. Early motion is also important; otherwise, if the athlete avoids using the part, his muscles will atrophy in a few days. The joint will then be less stable and reinjury more likely.

Types of Injuries

Contusions

A blow to an athlete's body may damage tissue and cause swelling, bleeding, and pain. These bruises are especially painful at the shoulder and iliac crest where large muscles arise. Blows to the front of the arm or front of the thigh may result in myositis ossificans traumatica. Initial treatment is ice, compression, and elevation. If the injured area is very fluctuant, the team physician may decide to aspirate it. Once the reaction has died down, cryotherapy is used, and when the danger of further hemor-

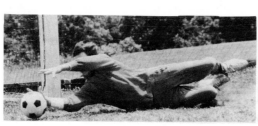

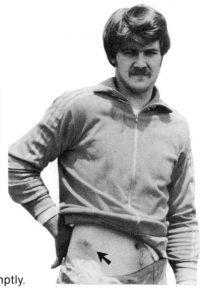

FIG. 8-7
A goalkeeper's abrasion should be treated promptly.

rhage is over the region may be massaged. The area is taped to reduce abnormal motion and a protective pad applied.

Abrasions

If an abrasion is considered trivial, it is sometimes treated inadequately. These wounds should be treated promptly, and if suturing is needed it should be done before swelling occurs. After an athlete sustains an abrasion (Fig. 8-7), such as a slide burn, he should scour all dirt from the wound with soap and water during his shower and then scrub the wound with sterile gauze pads. The wound should be covered with a protective dressing; a 3 mm-thick hydrogel sheeting may, for example, be used as the dressing. This viscoelastic material is backed on both sides with an inert, low-density, polyethylene film that controls water vapor and gas transmission. It absorbs friction and pressure and can imbibe its own weight in blood, serum, or perspiration. An infection may set in if the wound is inadequately cleaned. There is no such thing as a "mild" infection. Signs of infection may include soreness and redness around the wound, red streaks, and swollen lymph nodes.

Sprains and Strains

A sprain refers to a damaged ligament and a strain to a damaged muscle or tendon. Sprains and strains are graded as either first, second, or third degree or mild, moderate, or severe. A mild sprain or strain is damage to the tissue but no loss of continuity of the fibers. The area will be tender and may be swollen. These mild sprains are treated by cryotherapy, and the athlete may experience an early return to athletics.

A moderate injury, a partial tear that allows increased laxity with some "give" on testing, is treated with ice, rest, and crutches to prevent extension to a complete tear. A severe sprain or strain is a complete tear, producing instability and necessitating surgical repair.

Fractures

Fractures are immobilized to prevent further damage and compounding of the injury. The joints above and below the fracture are splinted. Early treatment of a fracture also includes ice, compression, and elevation. The ice is left on until after x-rays have been taken. An open fracture should be covered with a sterile dressing.

Treatment of Injury

Ice

Ice, by delaying or minimizing swelling, decreases pain and muscle spasm and limits the magnitude of an injury. The lower tissue temperature induces local vasoconstriction, which lessens capillary permeability, making the blood more viscous. Less blood flows into the injured area, and the hematoma is smaller.

The ice dulls peripheral pain by interfering locally with nerve impulses and decreasing nerve conduction velocity. It relieves spasm by decreasing muscle activity, muscle spindle firing, and acetylcholine levels so that ischemia is prevented. Ice limits the magnitude of an injury by lowering metabolism in peripheral, uninjured cells. By decreasing the cellular demand for oxygen, cells are put in partial hibernation, and thus extension of the injury is avoided. Otherwise cells that have survived the initial trauma may not be able to withstand the lack of oxygen imposed by the disruption of local circulation.

Initial treatment of an injury follows the acronym *ICE,* meaning *Ice, Compression,* and *Elevation.* The injured part should also be protected from painful stimuli. Ice may be applied initially for 30 minutes. The athlete may then shower before receiving another 30-minute icing. If a fracture is suspected, ice is left in place until x-rays are taken. Ice keeps the swelling down so that a better-fitting cast may be applied.

If ice is applied for more than 20 to 30 minutes, reflex vasodilation may increase the swelling and prevent lowering of the skin temperature. To reduce the effects of this reflex, ice should be applied for only 30 minutes and then removed for 10 minutes two times. This sequence should be repeated several times during the first 24 to 48 hours.

There are many ways to apply ice, including ice wraps, icepacks, ice slush, or a cold whirlpool. Elastic wraps are kept in a water bucket, and the bucket is placed in an ice chest. After injury, a cold, wet ice wrap should be applied right away. (If the wrap were dry, it would act as an insulator.) When ice is not available immediately, the cold water from a groundskeeper's hose may be run over the injured area, with care taken not to spray the water directly onto the wound and produce a massage effect. The "magic sponge," a sponge dipped in ice water, is also an effective initial treatment.

An icepack should be placed over the ice wrap. Chipped or crushed ice conforms better than do cubes. The ice may be put in a plastic bag to prevent dripping or be placed in a towel that is moistened only on the skin side. The dry side acts as an insulator over the ice. Chemical ice packs are expensive and can only be used once; ethyl chloride and other cold sprays are expensive, too, and may cause skin reactions, but all are useful until something better is available. The spray may temporarily relieve the pain from a hard blow by superficially cooling the skin. It does little, however, to control internal bleeding. Synthetic gel packs stay below freezing for about 15 minutes but remain flexible and conform to the injured area. These reusable frozen gels are dangerous because they may cause frostbite. If one is used, it should be wrapped in a towel and not applied directly to the skin.

Ice slush is made by mixing chips or flakes of ice in water to produce a temperature of 12.8° C to 18.3° C (55° F to 65° F). Because the limb hangs down into the slush, it should be wrapped with a wet elastic wrap. To provide some comfort, the athlete may wear a neoprene toe cap over his toes.[38]

The water temperature in a cold whirlpool is kept in the 13° C to 18° C range (55° F to 65° F). This range does not induce as much cold vasodilation as a lower temperature would; thus hemorrhage and edema are minimized. Cold treatments at temperatures below 13° C (55° F) have no beneficial physiologic effects and are uncomfortable.

Sprained ankles are almost always placed in an ice whirlpool after 24 hours. The ankle is positioned off to the side in the whirlpool, out of the direct flow of the water. A cold elastic wrap may be applied before the limb is placed in the whirlpool. Besides the beneficial effects of the cold, the whirlpool provides buoyancy, and the athlete can move the injured part through a range of motion.

Cold

Physiologic Effects

Vasoconstriction for 20 minutes, followed by vasodilation for 5 minutes
Decreased local temperature to a depth of up to 10 cm
Less blood flow to the area and less edema
Less venous and lymphatic drainage
Slowing of nerve conduction and muscle depolarization
Less muscular excitability and spasm
Breaking of pain cycle by analgesia
Reduced cellular metabolism
Increased muscle viscosity

Methods of Application

Ice bags
Ice slush in a bucket
Cold sprays
Ice massage
Contrast treatments (iced whirlpool)

Indications in Athletes

Prevention of swelling after acute injury
Reduction of muscle spasm and pain
Reduction of inflammation
Treatment of heat illness, minor burns, and blisters

Pre-exercise to allow exercise and increased range of motion (cryotherapy)

Contraindications

Circulatory insufficiency
Hypersensitivity to cold
Hyposensitivity to cold

Compression

A cold, wet elastic wrap provides comfort and stops swelling and hemorrhage mechanically. Elastic wraps work best on cylinders, and because the wrap will not compress in hollows, a felt horseshoe or foam rubber pad should be placed in these areas. For an ankle sprain, an open basket-weave taping is applied to prevent limping. Straight strips will support and approximate the stretched or torn ends of the ligament, and elastic tape may be wrapped around the strapping to add compression. Some areas, such as where the trunk muscles insert into the iliac crest, are harder to compress than others. In the case of a thigh bruise, an elastic thigh sleeve provides even compression. In the case of a knee injury, the limb may be wrapped with an elastic wrap from the toes to the upper thigh.

Intermittent compression serves as a valuable adjunct to cold in reducing edema (Fig. 8-8). Some of these units even combine a refrigerant

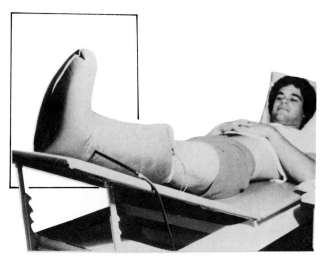

FIG. 8-8
An intermittent compression device is combined with elevation to treat an ankle sprain.

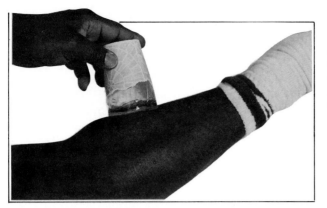

FIG. 8-9
For ice massage, a paper cup is filled with water and then frozen. When the ice has formed, the cup is partly peeled back and the injured area gently massaged.

fluid with the compression. The extremity is encased in an air-filled glove. Pressure is then alternately applied and released to force edema from the limb. Whenever a snug wrap has been applied or when an intermittent compression device is being used, the limb should be elevated, which decreases blood flow to the limb, limits venous pooling, and encourages and assists venous return to the heart. An elevation block should support the entire limb. The commonly used smaller blocks or pillows placed under the distal part of a limb are uncomfortable and place a strain on the knee.

Ice is well accepted for first aid but is still not well accepted for later treatment. For years, ankles have even been plunged into hot whirlpools. A much better approach is headlined by the acronym *ISE,* meaning *Ice, Stretching* (or range of motion), and *Exercise.* The exercise begins 1 day after a mild or moderate injury and is the most important modality. Light exercise increases range of motion and prevents disuse atrophy. Ice allows the athlete to exercise pain-free because muscles relax and the ice blocks painful nerve impulses. With less pain and muscle spasm, the athlete exercises better, which in turn improves the circulation. When in doubt, ice should be used rather than heat. Ice lessens the chance of aggravating the inflammatory response.

Cryotherapy, a combination of ice and exercise, starts with an ice application. The athlete first feels coldness, then burning, aching, and tingling, and finally numbness. The numbness stage is reached in 7 to 10 minutes; during the icing period, the athlete should begin gentle, pain-free range of motion exercises. When the area is numb, the athlete may perform 10 to 20 repetitions of pain-free resistance exercises. If the lower extremity is involved, he may also walk, if he has no limp. The athlete should resume the ice and range of motion program as the analgesia wears off. Each cryotherapy session lasts for 20 to 30 minutes three or four times a day. If the resistive exercises are uncomfortable, isometrics may be substituted provided they are pain-free. The athlete should be advised that he may feel some slight discomfort as the blood flows back rapidly into the injured area when he returns his foot to a dependent position.

At home, the athlete may conveniently use cryokinetics (ice massage) to increase his tolerance for exercise. A water-filled paper cup should be placed in the freezer. Once the water has frozen, the paper cup should be stripped back to expose the ice (Fig. 8-9). The injured area is massaged until it feels numb and the skin has turned a bright red. The injured part is then brought through a normal range of motion, and pain-free resistive exercises are performed after 7 to 10 minutes, as in cryotherapy. The use of crutches is far better than to allow limping. Often, ice can be used throughout the entire treatment program until the athlete returns to competition. The only time that cryokinetics should not be used is for acute injury, because it does not include compression or elevation and the motion may promote further bleeding.

Ice should be used until there is no further hemorrhage or edema, range of motion is full and pain-free, no more hyperthermia of the skin occurs, and as long as progress is being made with cryotherapy. At this time heat may be used.

Contrast

Contrast treatments may be started when the athlete no longer achieves progressive good results with cold treatments. Contrast treatments provide an alternating vasodilation-vasoconstriction effect that mobilizes edema. First, the injured part is placed in a 40° C (104° F) tub or whirlpool for 4 minutes. Then, the part is placed into a cold ice slush tub or a cold whirlpool at 13° C to 18° C (55° F to 65° F) for 1 minute. Each phase is repeated four times, always starting with hot and ending with cold. The last treatment with cold prevents edematous effects from the heat and allows pain-free exercise. Contrast treatments are given three or four times daily.

Heat

Heat is used only in rehabilitation, whereas ice may be used to treat acute injuries and in rehabilitation. Some athletes are averse and sensitive to cold. The choice of heat for rehabilitation, then, may be based on the athlete's comfort; the athlete's cooperation may be hard to obtain if comfort is not considered. Both ice and heat are analgesic and reduce muscle spasm, but in most cases heat produces more comfort as a result of its sedating properties. Heat induces vasodilation and increases blood flow, resulting in an influx of oxygen and nutrients to the injured area and waste products being carried away. Cellular metabolism increases, leading to rapid repair and healing. Regardless of whether heat or cold is used, however, it still takes time for an injury to heal.

After acute symptoms have subsided, the recovery rate with heat or cold is about the same.

The modality of prime importance is exercise. Cold or heat allows exercise to be more pain-free.

The many methods of applying heat include whirlpools, hot packs, heating pads, and analgesic balms. The injured part may be placed in a warm, soothing whirlpool for 20 minutes. The water temperature may range from 37° C (98° F) for subacute injuries to 41° C (106° F) for chronic injuries. Heat packs are segmented canvas bags filled with a heat-absorbing silicone gel. These packs are stored in a water-filled stainless steel container and wrapped in moist towels for use. Waterproof heating pads are especially good for home contests. A moist towel is placed underneath the pad against the skin to provide moist heat. Analgesic packs that contain an analgesic balm are sometimes used for away contests. The analgesic balm may be an external analgesic, such as methylsalicylate. The analgesic is usually applied to the skin and covered with an insulating cover, such as an old towel. Only mild surface analgesics should be used, as the stronger ones may be dangerously irritative.

Heat

Physiologic Effects

Vasodilation and increased blood flow
Increased local temperature
Increased swelling
Rise in influx of oxygen and nutrients; also in venous and lymphatic drainage
Increased local metabolism
More permeable capillaries to leukocytes
Sedative effect
Less pain and muscle spasm
More elasticity of muscles, tendons, and ligaments

Methods of Application

Heating pad
Moist hot packs
Whirlpool
Ultrasound
Infrared lamp
Counterirritants

Indications in Athletes

Reduction of muscle spasm and pain after acute phase of injury

Pre-exercise, allowance of increased range of motion

Increase in local blood flow

Facilitation of wound healing

Contraindications

Acute injury

Diminished sensation

Circulatory problems

Hypersensitivity to heat

Hyposensitivity to heat

Febrile conditions

No diathermy if athlete has metal implant

Rehabilitation of the Injured Athlete

The team physician can do only a limited amount; the remainder, in the form of rehabilitation, must be done by the athlete. The athlete must not just be given a list of exercises and sent away. The best effects are achieved when the trainer shows concern and gives individual attention to the athlete from the time of injury to his return to practice and competition.

Each injury to an athlete has both physical and emotional effects, and emotional conflicts may undercut rehabilitation (*see* Chap. 10). Thus the athlete must be both physiologically and psychologically rehabilitated. There are four mental phases in the response to injury: denial, anger, depression, and acceptance. At first, the athlete will not accept the diagnosis. "It can't happen to me." He then becomes angry: "Why did this happen to me?" This anger may be vented on the athletic trainer. The trainer should hold back because anger cannot be reasoned with and should listen and avoid being easily offended. If the trainer were to react defensively, the trainer–athlete relationship would be strained, making successful rehabilitation a trying experience. In the depression phase, the athlete surmises, "I'll never be able to play again." However, in the acceptance

phase, which is the final and desirable phase, the athlete decides that "I accept what I've been dealt, but I shall overcome the effects."

During the first three phases, the athlete may not listen to or believe what the trainer says. Repetition, patience, and reinforcement are important. The athletic trainer seeks to guide the athlete into the final acceptance phase as rapidly as possible, and his interest helps to heal the athlete's shattered sense of worth. The trainer should be nonjudgmental, show empathy, concern, and understanding, and give encouragement. Lack of interest and beratement results in mutual frustration and paranoia for the athlete. If the trainer fails to be positive, the athlete may never emerge from one of the first three phases and never reach full potential.

The athletic trainer should not make too many promises. He should not, for example, give a specific time for healing. His goal is to return the athlete to the same activity level as before the injury in the shortest possible time.

Objectives

The objectives of rehabilitation are to regain range of motion, strength, flexibility, muscular endurance, power, cardiovascular endurance, speed, balance, agility, and skills. The rehabilitation process comprises many steps, and each one must be successfully completed, pain-free, before the athlete returns to competition. Criteria for return are established for each injury in terms of skills and abilities that the athlete will need to regain before returning to his sport. He may return only when near-normal strength, flexibility, speed, power, endurance, and agility have been regained. The athlete must be told what these criteria are so that he can strive for concrete goals. Return to competition will demand agreement from team physician, athletic trainer, coach, and athlete. The athlete must be involved in this decision so that maximum performance can be achieved; otherwise, he may lack confidence and aggressiveness, which will result in subpar performances and possible reinjury.

Healing and rehabilitation take time. When mild or moderate injuries are properly treated, the athlete may lose up to 3 weeks from competition. Reinjury and possible early joint deterioration may result if the athlete returns to competition too early. Further, if rehabilitative procedures are inadequate, reinjury is more likely to occur.

Exercise

Rehabilitation is tied closely to the modalities of cold and heat. The most important modality, however, is exercise, which does more than ice or heat to restore muscle and joint function and prevent fibrosis. The formula ISE (*I*ce, *S*tretching, and *E*xercise) is used from the second day after injury for mild to moderate musculoskeletal injuries. Exercise progresses as long as the athlete has no undue pain and swelling after each session or upon awakening the next morning. Ice is applied after exercise to reduce pain and swelling, and heat treatment is not begun until the criteria for using heat are met.

In all exercises, the athlete works to just below the point of pain and without limping. Even a minor limp lengthens rehabilitation time. In a lower extremity injury, then, the athlete should always use a cane or crutch if he has a limp. When using a cane or crutch, the athlete should bear as much weight as possible. The cane or crutch is kept on the side opposite the injury, and pressure is applied on the hand grip to prevent a limp.

The two early goals of rehabilitation are to regain strength and to regain flexibility, and thus prevent degenerative changes associated with early muscle weakness. Swimming and other water activities and cycling are also started early to increase endurance.

Strength

Isometrics are the exercise of choice early in rehabilitation, when joint movement may be undesirable. Strength, however, is gained only at the angles at which the athlete exercises. Initially, the athlete needs to hold only a 40% to 50% contraction for a few seconds to gain strength. As his strength increases, however, he needs more forceful contractions to further his strength development. He should hold these maximal contractions for 6 seconds.

Isotonic exercise with free weights is started as soon as possible to strengthen gaps left by isometric exercise. In regular strength training, repetitions are usually done with maximum weight. In rehabilitation, however, the athlete should go through a range of motion with submaximal weight to prevent the edema and soreness that would develop with three sets of maximum lifts. The muscles to be exercised should be isolated to prevent accessory muscles from doing the work of the desired muscle group. Momentum and inertia are minimized by doing the exercises slowly during the early phases.

Early in rehabilitation, strength is gained from daily work efforts. As strength-gains peak, weight training should be done every other day. Three sets of repetitions are needed for good strength and bulk gains. The repetitions are done slowly with a two or three count through a range of pain-free motion and a two or three count while returning the weight to the starting position. Four sets of ten repetitions are generally the rule for rehabilitative strength-gain. The athlete's ten-repetition maximum (10-RM) is determined by the maximal amount that he can lift through a complete range of motion ten times. The athlete first performs ten repetitions at one half of the 10-RM, then does ten repetitions at three quarters of the 10-RM, and ends with ten repetitions at the 10-RM. A fourth set comprises ten repetitions at the 10-RM plus 1.1 kg to 2.3 kg (2.5 lb to 5 lb). When this new weight is achieved, it becomes the 10-RM.

Flexibility

Joint degeneration can be halted if the athlete regains strength and flexibility early. Slow, static stretching, proprioceptive neuromuscular facilitation, and joint mobilization techniques are methods that may be used to help gain flexibility. The goal is a normal joint, not a hypermobile one. A corresponding gain in strength provides joint stability so that a normal range of motion may be achieved without producing abnormal motion.

Power

An athlete must regain power before returning to competition. If he trains only with slow repetitions, he will gain strength but will not be ready for the rapid speeds of competition. The athlete should start high-speed power training as soon as his strength is adequately developed. For power training, a weekly one-repetition maximum (1-RM) should be determined first. Then, the athlete should train three times a week with three sets of 30-second repetitions with one half of this 1-RM, and rest for 20 seconds between sets. These sets are done explosively with proper technique.

Isokinetic machinery may be used for rehabilitation of the injured athlete. With isokinetics, the speed of muscle contraction remains constant as the load changes throughout to accommodate to different strength levels at each point in the range of motion. Isokinetics may also be used for "cross training," wherein exercise of the sound limb helps to maintain strength in the injured limb. Unfortunately, early isokinetic exercise for weakened structures often results in edema and soreness and delays recovery, especially in knee rehabilitation. Moreover, knee extension slows down as the knee reaches terminal extension; thus the stimulus is least where it is needed most. Strength-gain is lacking in terminal motion because resistance is not provided once the joint is "locked out."

Endurance

Muscular

Rehabilitation for muscular endurance should not be neglected, although it takes time and can be monotonous. Endurance training may be done during the intermediate phases of rehabilitation in the intervals between strength exercises. Underwater exercises in a pool are one way to regain both strength and endurance early. The athlete can usually begin these exercises as soon as his cast is removed. The buoyancy of the water allows him to perform exercises that would otherwise be painful. These exercises are especially beneficial in the rehabilitation of injuries to weight-bearing joints.

Pool Rehabilitation for Knees

	Water Depth
Walk	
10 laps, down and back	Waist to neck
Front-back kick	Waist
30, rest, 30	
Flutter kick	On back
2 min, rest, 2 min	
Scissors	On back
35, rest, 35	
High step	Armpit
8 laps	
Walk–run	Waist to neck
10 laps	
Tucks	6 ft
10, rest, 20	
Sitting kick	N/A
1 min, rest, 1 min	
Body lifts	8–10 ft
15	
Squats	Waist
15, rest, 15	

Cardiovascular

An injured athlete should strive to have better cardiovascular endurance upon return to competition than he had at the time of injury. If the athlete were just to rest or if he performed specific exercises without regard to cardiovascular endurance, he would be more likely to be reinjured as a result of fatigue.

Agility, speed, and skills are regained in the final phases of rehabilitation as the athlete performs the activities involved in his specific sport. These activities are begun at a low level and are gradually sped up to a competitive level. The injured athlete is considered successfully rehabilitated only after he has competed for at least one season in his sport.

Massage

Massage, a manipulation of soft tissue that can benefit an athlete mechanically, physiologically, and psychologically, may be used before competition as part of the warm-up, during breaks, during time-outs, or at halftime, after a workout, for rehabilitation from an injury, and after a cast has been removed.

Before competition, a pitcher's arm or a runner's or cyclist's legs are massaged to produce the peripheral vasodilatation that warms up these parts. During breaks in competition, such as between periods in a Greco–Roman wrestling match, a wrestler's arms are massaged and shaken to break muscle spasm and remove waste products.[16] After a race, a runner's or cyclist's legs are massaged to break spasm, remove wastes, and reduce swelling. As a substitute for massage, inflatable boots can be used for the athlete's legs. The intermittent pneumatic compression unit will reduce swelling and the fatigued feeling in the athlete's legs and feet (see Fig. 8-8). After a day of activity, all athletes benefit from automassage of their feet. The long arches of the feet should be massaged at bedtime, too. Circular motions up and down the long arch will relax the feet. A massage after exercise is restorative in that it promotes relaxation,[13] reduces muscle tension, relieves swelling, and helps prevent soreness. Massage is especially useful in rehabilitation after sprains, strains, or fractures, stimulating both the arterial and venous circulation, accelerating the flow of lymph, reducing edema, breaking up undesirable fibrosis, relaxing muscle spasm, and relieving discomfort by increasing the pain threshold.[35]

Muscles thrive on all forms of massage: friction, stroking, kneading, percussion, and shaking (Fig. 8-10). A friction massage is done with circular motions of the fingers or thumb and is especially useful over joints, where there is not much soft tissue. The circular motions loosen scars and adhesions and can break muscle spasm. A stroking massage has a sedative effect, relieves pain and swelling, and diminishes muscular tension. Both friction and stroking massages are useful after a cast has been removed. This combination breaks adhesions and reduces swelling. Kneading massage relieves cramps and keeps tissues supple. Skin and muscles are lifted, rolled, squeezed, and twisted. Percussion is a technique of hacking, cupping, or slapping that is invigorating and stimulating before a competition.

Massage is an art that demands a confident approach. The athlete should take a shower beforehand or otherwise clean the area to be massaged. He should rest in a comfortable position, with the area accessible and relaxed. The trainer stands with his knees bent, back straight, and legs turned out to allow him to swing up and down the length of the training table by shifting his weight from one foot to the other.

The trainer applies a generous amount of lubricant to his hands and to the athlete's skin; otherwise, the skin will become irritated. The lubricant can be a liniment, any petroleum-based material, vegetable oil, or a powder. A favorite massage mixture is a combination of olive oil and methyl salicylate (oil of wintergreen). The ratio of these two ingredients depends on the purpose of the massage and the size of the area to be massaged. The ratio is generally one to one. For a pitcher's warm-up massage, however, it is three parts methyl salicylate to one part olive oil. For massage of very large areas, the ratio is three parts olive oil to one part methyl salicylate.

The trainer directs all his attention to the massage. Talking, which detracts from the athlete's relaxation, is kept to a minimum. Flowing music may assist the rhythm of the strokes and add to the relaxation. All movements are centripetal, following the course of the lymphatics to the heart. The trainer notes any knots, nodules, or tender areas and focuses attention on those areas.

Massage is contraindicated directly over a new injury because it may create additional

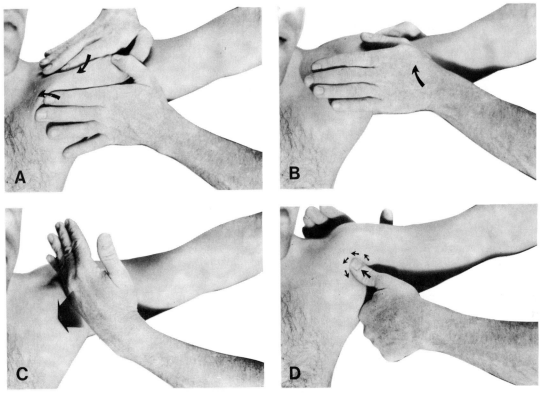

FIG. 8-10
Massage techniques include stroking (*A*), kneading (*B*), percussion (*C*),
and friction (*D*).

hemorrhage. The area around an injury, however, can be stroked to eliminate some of the swelling. The trainer should record the presence of any skin lesions, moles, or lumps. Massage is not done in the presence of skin rashes, eczema, herpes, or other skin infections.

Massage is a very effective modality, but its use has generally been supplanted by machinery, such as ultrasound, transcutaneous electrical nerve stimulators (TENS), and whirlpools, mainly because of time constraints on athletic trainers. However, once an athlete experiences an effective massage, he will always want one. To satisfy this demand, athletes can be taught automassage and partner-massage. In addition, a professionally trained massage specialist can be an invaluable member of the sports medicine team.

Hyperstimulation Analgesia

An athlete's pain may be relieved by stimulating a trigger point. Trigger points and acupuncture points often correspond;[22] both were probably derived from the empirical observations that pressure at certain points produced a particular pain pattern and that brief, intense stimulation at these points sometimes resulted in prolonged pain relief. A trigger point is a tender site that may contain a tender nodule. Acupuncture points are based on ancient conceptual systems of meridians.

Pain may be relieved by numbing a trigger point with a local anesthetic or by stimulating it at low intensity with a TENS unit. Astonishingly, pain may also be relieved by applying a painful stimulus at the trigger point.[42] Some of this pain relief may be explained by the power of suggestion, distraction of attention, and release of the body's own morphinelike painkillers (endorphins); however, the degree and the long duration of the pain relief are as yet unexplained.

The midbrain receives input from widespread parts of the body and communicates with all levels of the brain and spinal cord.[31] There is some degree of anatomic organization in the midbrain. If certain sites are stimulated experimentally, gradients of analgesia are produced wherein the maximum analgesia is felt in a relatively small part of the body, such as in a foot or part of a leg.[3, 19, 28] Integrating mechanisms in the central nervous system may allow an interaction of inputs from widespread parts of the body. Then, a "central biasing network" (CBN) may exert inhibitory control in the pain-signaling system.[20] This type of system would explain some of the complex, spatial-somatic interactions of painful areas and trigger–acupuncture points that otherwise cannot be explained from current understanding of the traditional organization of the peripheral nervous system.

Stimulation of a trigger point may also relieve chronic pain. The chronic pain may be produced by abnormally firing neuron pools, self-exciting neuron chains, and prolonged reverberatory activity. These memorylike processes are initiated and maintained in the spinal cord by abnormalities at distant sites. A brief, intense input of pain may disrupt these abnormal intraspinal activities and produce a descending inhibition from the CBN. As a result of these neurologic changes, centrally projected volleys evoke less pain. The combination of less pain and more normally patterned activities might then gradually lower the number of abnormally firing neuron pools that gave rise to the pain.

Many types of hyperstimulation have been used effectively to relieve pain. Among these techniques are "dry needling," the injection of normal saline, TENS, acupuncture, acupressure, and osteopressure. In *"dry needling,"* a sterile needle is simply moved in and out of the trigger area without injecting any material.[39]

The injection of normal saline will produce an intense pain, but this may be followed by pain relief. A TENS unit may be used to produce an intense but tolerable stimulation. The voltage should be raised slowly until the person feels pain, whereupon it should be lowered slightly and left on for 20 minutes.[24] Acupuncture produces brief, intense pain from rotation of the needles or by passing an electric current through them.[1] The deep ache may be due to a local reflex that causes the muscle to grip the needle below the acupuncture point. Firm pressure on a trigger point from the ball of a thumb or finger pulp is called *acupressure*.[26, 27] This hyperstimulation technique, like the above methods, can be used to relieve pain. By so doing, the athlete gains further control over his pain. Acupressure may also be used to relieve menstrual cramps.[30] The primary trigger point for this purpose lies about 2.5 cm (1 in) to the right of the spinous process of the third lumbar vertebra. If this area is not tender and cramps persist, additional points should be pressed. In *osteopressure,* firm pressure is applied over bony prominences with the thumbs.[29] Acupressure and osteopressure both raise the pain threshold at other sites and may be used to blunt the pain of an injury or the pain that attends a procedure, such as the placing of sutures.

Electricity

Electrical devices may aid in the rehabilitation of an athlete's injury. These devices include diathermy, low-frequency muscle stimulators, ultrasound, galvanic stimulators, and TENS (Fig. 8-11).

Diathermy

Diathermy uses a high-frequency alternating current of more than 10,000 cycles/sec. The athlete's body provides a resistance to an electrostatic current that produces heat as it passes through the tissues. Diathermy can produce an internal temperature of 41° C (106° F) at a 5-cm (2-in) depth. Moisture will concentrate the electrical energy; thus one must be careful when using diathermy. A burn may occur if the athlete merely changes position during a treatment. Applications should be restricted in edematous areas, and strict supervision is important to prevent burns. Diathermy should not be used in athletes with metal implants because metal selectively picks up the current. In fact, diathermy may start fires in metal surroundings. Because superficial applications of heat or cold have proved so successful in acute and subacute injury, diathermy has been relegated to use only in some chronic injuries.

Alternating Low-Frequency Current

Alternating low-frequency currents stimulate contractions in innervated muscle. The current may be interrupted in a pulsing or surging manner, causing it to rhythmically rise and fall, or a continuous or tetanizing current may be maintained. The alternating low-frequency current is usually applied over the length of the muscle. When low-frequency alternating current is desired for prevention of disuse atrophy, however, a small electrode can be placed over the neuromuscular junction. In combination with ultrasound, low-frequency alternating current may relieve the pain and discomfort of injuries such as cervical strain, lower back strain, or the pain from throwing injuries of the shoulder.

Ultrasound

Ultrasound is a frequently used electrical modality in the rehabilitation of athletic injuries. A quartz, lithium sulfate or other type of

FIG. 8-11
The athlete can often administer his own electrical modalities (*A*). A cream is used to conduct ultrasound (*B*), or underwater treatments are given (*C*). Sterile electrodes allow transcutaneous electrical nerve stimulation to begin immediately after an operation (*D*).

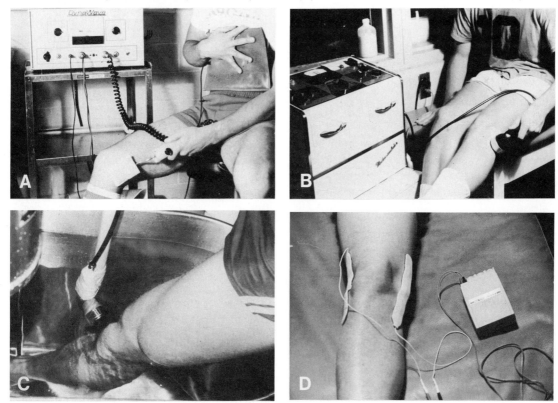

crystal in the sound head converts electrical energy into high-frequency ultrasound by a piezoelectric effect. This energy then creates heat as it passes through body tissue. Ultrasound easily penetrates fat to allow selective absorption of its energy in muscular structures. The micromassage effect within the cells penetrates from 4 cm to 8 cm.

Continuous ultrasound may be used over large muscular areas. A conducting medium is needed, since ultrasound is not transmitted through air. An ultrasound cream is preferred as the conducting medium, but mineral oil may also be used. Ultrasound may also be delivered in pulsed form at 0.1 to 1 w/cm². Pulsed ultrasound is preferred in instances where continuous ultrasound causes pain or when the heating effects of ultrasound are not desired, such as in the treatment of an acute injury.

Ultrasound can relieve the acute pain of a sprain, a strain, and a contusion and its associated muscle spasm. It raises the athlete's pain threshhold and helps break the pain cycle. Ultrasound may also be effective in treating tendinitis and bursitis, and sometimes it dissolves small mature calcific deposits and breaks down scar tissue. To enhance its benefits, ultrasound may be used over nerve roots that correspond to a painful dermatome. Trigger points may be located with either continuous or pulsed ultrasound. Unlike diathermy, ultrasound may be used over areas of edema and over metal implants. Muscle stimulation is an option with some units. A cream must be used for this application of ultrasound, as mineral oil will not conduct the current needed for muscle contraction.

Ultrasound is applied in a circular motion, as a stationary application may cause periosteal pain from reflection of sound waves back and forth from bony surfaces to the sound head. The absorption of ultrasound in superficial tissues is enhanced by preheating, but deep absorption improves after precooling the part. Treatments usually last about 5 minutes, although longer treatments may be desired over large areas. Where bony irregularities prevent maximum contact by the sound head, ultrasound is administered under water. Ultrasound should not be used directly over an athlete's spinal column, eyes, epiphyses, active myositis ossificans, or reproductive organs.

Direct Current

Low-frequency direct current modalities, such as galvanic stimulation and TENS, break the pain-spasm cycle that often follows injury.

Galvanic Stimulation

The main value of galvanic stimulation is to relieve pain and thus allow the athlete to exercise more safely and more intensely for a rapid return to activity. The direct current electrochemically mobilizes edema and increases blood flow. Galvanic stimulation is most effective in relieving the pain and spasm of lower back strain and the pain and swelling of an acute ankle injury or a hip pointer. With lower back pain, moist heat is used in conjunction with the galvanic stimulator, and the athlete is then able to perform the lower back exercise routine more effectively. After an acute ankle injury, the injured ankle may be placed into a tub of cold water. Electrodes are then put into this conducting medium, and the athlete can exercise the ankle in the tub. Galvanic stimulation may also be used to stimulate either innervated muscle or denervated muscle, as in an anterior tibial compartment syndrome.

Transcutaneous Electrical Nerve Stimulators

Transcutaneous nerve stimulation activates sensory nerves to produce low-grade noxious stimuli that block the more severe pain of an injury or operation. A stimulator may be used after an injury and right after surgery. After surgery, sterile electrodes are placed against the athlete's skin under his cast or wrap. He then may begin quadriceps setting and straight-leg raises faster and more effectively without excess pain, swelling, and inflammation. The use of TENS after surgery, or after an injury, often will reduce dramatically the athlete's need for analgesic medication. In addition, the same electrodes may be used for muscle stimulation postoperatively without having to remove the cast or bandage. In knee surgery, for example, the electrode is placed over the vastus medialis.

Transcutaneous nerve stimulation may allow an athlete to perform an exercise program without resultant pain or edema, thus facilitating heavier progressive resistance exercise. He also will be able to perform his normal daily activities more comfortably. Sometimes, the units have even been used during competition, without apparent harm.

Playing Field Surfaces

Artificial Turf

Artificial turf initially was designed for indoor use. It provides a uniform playing surface for athletic contests under many playing conditions and allows intensive and varied use of the stadium.[40] Artificial turf has its critics, however; one has said that "the only good thing about artificial turf is that it keeps uniforms clean."[7]

Not all artificial turfs are the same; they have different types of pile fibers, backing fibers, and pads.[37] Astroturf, for example, has 1.3-cm (0.5-in) nylon pile on a polyester nylon mat bonded to a 1.6-cm (0.63 in) closed-cell, nitrile rubber and polyvinyl chloride pad. The pad rests on an asphalt base. Just as brands differ, old artificial turf differs from new artificial turf.[5] As the pad wears out, the aging turf has a diminished impact-absorbing capacity and different traction qualities.

Are these surfaces as safe as, or safer than, natural grass? The Stanford Research Institute (SRI) study compared injuries on artificial surfaces and natural grass in the National Football League.[12] More major ligamentous injuries occurred on artificial surfaces than on natural grass. The investigators concluded that generally natural grass is safer and recommended a return to natural grass in all undomed stadiums. However, a study by the National Athletic Injury/Illness Reporting System (NAIRS), a computerized data-gathering system located at Pennsylvania State University, concluded that no surface is an inherent hazard to the athlete and that "artificial turf did not constitute an imminent hazard to the college tackle football and soccer football teams using it in 1975."[40]

Further, in a study at the University of Wisconsin that compared Tartan-Turf to natural grass, more serious sprains occurred on the natural surface, and investigators concluded that this specific brand of turf may be a good surface.[15]

There are many disadvantages to the use of artificial turf. Purists, for example, are often unhappy about the changes that occur in their sport because of the artificial surfaces. In baseball, the ball travels dangerously fast and bounces high on artificial turf, sometimes making a mockery of a great game. Soccer football on artificial turf differs markedly from the same game on natural grass; on artificial surfaces, the athletes refuse to risk the "turf burns" from sliding tackles. With the exception of the goalkeeper, referees will not allow the players to wear "long johns" on this surface. Moreover, the touch line is often dangerously close to the asphalt.

An artificial surface allows increased running speed. Perhaps the "uniformity of these synthetic surfaces accounts in part for the increase in speeds, since no adjustment is needed to compensate for perturbations on the playing surfaces."[37] This increased speed results in increased collision forces, which cause more serious injuries. The SRI study showed 33% more concussions on synthetic turf than on natural grass, and these concussions may be fatal.

"Turf burns" are the common abrasions from artificial turf; "green dust" is ground into the wounds and may become secondarily infected. Turf burns are often over joints, where bending causes the wound to stay open. A physician cannot aspirate or operate on the joint through or near the damaged skin. Thus a turf burn may ruin the chance for early repair of a torn ligament. Many turf burns can be prevented with extra pads, and some athletes smear petrolatum on their legs so that they can, for example, tackle in soccer.

Leg fatigue and shin splints are common problems on artificial surfaces. Traction is greater, and if the player's feet slide in his shoes, blisters will form. Many players wear shoes that are too light and too flexible, and they may sprain the matatarsal-phalangeal joint of the great toe when it is hyperextended or hyperflexed. This debilitating sprain may be avoided by wearing a protective stainless steel or orthoplast splint inserted between the midsole and the insole of the shoe. Many players prefer a soccer-style shoe with molded cleats when they play on artificial turf, but a basketball-type shoe with a ribbed, elastomeric sole has as much traction as the cleated shoe.

Heat builds up tremendously on artificial turf, especially near the surface, and in the summer months heat exhaustion is a constant danger. The players fatigue more easily, reducing their coordination and increasing the chance of injury. The heat that builds up on a synthetic field is related to a lack of moisture. Natural grass absorbs moisture from its roots and evaporates it into the air, cooling down the field. If artificial turf is wetted down, the surface will cool, and the coefficient of friction decreases. If the wetting is not uniform, however, the resultant wet and dry areas may increase the chance of injury. Moreover, tackle football fields are built over a crown, and it takes longer for the edges to dry out than the center. In areas of the country with high humidity, wetting the field may increase the incidence of heat illness.

Natural Grass

Just as the brands of artificial turfs differ, the quality of grass field varies. A natural grass field is only as good as its groundskeeper, and even parts of the same field may vary. Some "grass" fields are in fact grass, others are grass and dirt, some are dirt or clay, and some are rocky. Many fields are poorly maintained. When the top layer of dirt becomes maximally compacted, water is unable to go down through this layer.

Durable, fast-draining natural grass surfaces are now available. They have the safety advantages and aesthetic qualities of grass and a cumulative cost less than the artificial surfaces. A good strain of natural grass is used with a 2.5-cm (1-in) layer of topsoil. Underlying this soil is a deep, sandy, porous base for deep root development. Pumps work through perforated

pipes to irrigate or, by suction, to dry the field through the roots. Subterranean heating cables may be used in colder climates to prevent the field from freezing.

The well-being of the athlete should come first, and an excellent natural surface is the best surface to spare them injuries. An artificial surface has a place indoors, where grass will not grow, and outdoors when extremely heavy use under poor weather conditions would quickly ruin a natural field.

Playgrounds

Virtually every child is exposed to playground equipment. Public playground-equipment-related injuries have been tabulated by the National Electronic Injury Surveillance System (NEISS). Lightweight home equipment, however, has somehow not yet come under the NEISS reporting system. The NEISS is a computer-based network of 119 selected emergency rooms located throughout the United States. The system collects two levels of injury data: surveillance and investigation. In-depth investigations are done if the hazard pattern reveals contact with a protruding sharp edge or impact with the equipment or if the equipment had already been broken at the time of the accident.

Public playground injuries resulted in 93,000 emergency room visits in the United States in 1977.[32] Falls were the most common cause of injury, totaling about 66,000, 55,000 of which were falls to the surface. Falls to paved surfaces produced a disproportionately high number of severe injuries compared to falls to protective surfaces, such as sand or wood chips.

Climbing apparatus accounted for more injuries than did any other type of playground equipment, totaling 38,650 injuries, more than half of these from falls. Twenty-two percent of the youngsters struck another part of the apparatus; 15% fell against, or ran into, the apparatus while they were on the ground; and about 3% were injured by protrusions, pinch-points, sharp edges, or sharp points.

Swings accounted for 21,300 injuries in 1977; more than two thirds of these were from falls or jumps to the surface. One fourth came from moving impact, and four of five of all the moving impact injuries in the survey involved swings. Almost one half of all injuries to children younger than 5 years of age were related to swings, and deaths resulted from hanging by the chains and equipment failure. The impact from a heavy, hard-cornered, chairlike infant swing is especially dangerous.

Slides accounted for 15,000 injuries; 12,000 of these involved falls. Falls from most types of playground equipment were from less than 1.8 m (6 ft), but most falls from slides were from higher than 1.8 m (6 ft). All of the deaths from slides were from head or neck injuries; sometimes clothing was entrapped and ropes were involved. Merry-go-rounds caused 7300 injuries in 1977, mostly from falls. See-saws accounted for 4400 injuries, with many large splinters from worn-out or poorly maintained see-saws.

About 55,000 of the 93,000 injuries were perhaps preventable through modifications of playground equipment layout, spacing, and design. The United States Consumer Product Safety Commission (CPSC) and the Product Safety Division of the National Bureau of Standards are now developing a set of technical requirements for playground equipment. Suggestions for safety on the playground include well-designed and well-spaced equipment, sand or wood chip surfaces, routine inspections, and regular maintenance.

Planning an Athletic Contest

Track Meet

Advanced planning is the key to a safe athletic contest for athletes and spectators. Planning for a track meet, for example, includes space allotments, scheduling, and safety instructions. The field-event danger zones must be roped off and must not overlap when one station is in use. Field-event warm-ups are especially dangerous because the athletes may not be fully ready or concentrating. Concurrent activities, moreover, may cause crowding.

At all-comers meets, athletes of different skill levels compete. Each athlete, however, should have a skill level that enables him to keep the discus or javelin, for instance, within the competitive corridors. In a poorly run track meet, a javelin may land on the timer's table or on the pole vault cushion. If an athlete lacks skill in the discus, for example, he should practice by throwing a rubber discus into a net or canvas.

Dangers in the vaulting area are reduced by good spotting and proper care of the landing cushion and poles. Spotters should be alert to break the fall of a vaulter if he misses the landing area and keep the crossbar from landing on the athlete. Another spotter catches the vaulting pole so that it is not scratched or otherwise damaged. If the air cushion has separate side cushions, the athlete may catch his leg or arm in one of the gaps. On hot days, the cushion may actually burn the athlete; thus water should sometimes be splashed on it.

The overloading of a fiberglass vaulting pole may cause it to break and to impale the vaulter. Safe force limits for the vaulting pole are determined by the weight of an athlete, the speed of his run, and his hand-hold position. Each pole has a definite weight limit usually specified for the vaulter's weight. The faster athlete has a greater plant force, and the pole should be correctly placed in the emplacing box. Proper hand position is crucial to achieve a maximum safe bend of the pole. An unsafe position of the hands may cause an awkward vault and a loss of control.

There should be at least one trained person whose only duty at the meet is safety. All athletes must completely understand and respect the safety regulations. If an accident does occur, a causal analysis should be done.

Rebound Tumbling

Rebound tumbling is the most likely sports activity to produce a spinal cord injury. Most injuries occur on the trampoline bed, even when spotters are in proper position and alert.

A trampoline should never be used in a routine physical education class; there are many less dangerous things for youngsters to learn. With proper coaching and spotting, however, the trampoline may be used as an integral part of the training and conditioning of some athletes. Divers, for example, may practice flips and twists on it. Safety belts may be used for difficult or new stunts. The tumbling belt has rings, and the twisting safety belt has slots for twisting.

To increase safety in rebound tumbling, the trampoline must have safety side pads or frame pads and safety spotting decks on the ends. The rebound tumbler should master the basic landing positions and progress systematically. If the trampoline is used in a physical education class, no somersaults or tricks with inversion of the head should be allowed, and only basic skills and twisting routines should be done. Somersaulting is only for the advanced athlete who uses overhead spotting devices, except in elite performances.

Exercise programs should be brief because fatigue increases injury potential. Two-and-three-quarter forward and two-and-three-quarter backward somersaults should be banned, except in elite performances. In these somersaults, a gymnast may not see his position until it is too late to correct a wrong landing. Rebound tumbling should be judged as an art form.

Rebound tumbling requires great concentration; therefore, no children should be allowed near the apparatus to distract the gymnast, and there should never be more than one person on the trampoline. "Minitramps" should not be used for complicated tricks. The trampoline must always be folded and locked when not in use.

If an athlete's neck is injured and he is lying on the trampoline, the elastic trampoline bed may cause movement of his head and neck if standard methods of removal are used. To prevent excessive movement, a plank and plywood rescue method should be used.[2] This framing technique uses four wooden planks and a sheet of plywood. The wood should be stored near the trampoline along with a scoop stretcher.

To facilitate a rescue, the boards should be placed on the bed, extending a foot beyond each side of the trampoline. These boards form a frame around the athlete, and the rescuers support the injured athlete on the trampoline by holding the plywood under him with their upper backs or legs. While the athlete's head is being held steady, the trainer directs four assistants to place the athlete on the scoop stretcher. Head straps are then applied, the athlete's wrists are secured, and he is transferred from the trampoline without commotion.

REFERENCES

1. ANDERSON DG et al: Analgesic effects of acupuncture on the pain of ice-water: a double-blind study. Can J Psychiatry 28:239–244, 1974
2. BAGGETT R et al: Successful trampoline extrication. Athletic Training 14(2):74–76, Summer 1979
3. BALAGURA S, RALPH T: The analgesic effect of electrical stimulation of the diencephalon and mesencephalon. Brain Res 60:369–379, 1973
4. BONAME JR, WILHITE WC: The acute treatment of heat stroke. South Med J 60:885–887, 1967
5. BOWERS KD, MARTIN RB: Aging astroturf: a threat to safety and performance. Phys Sportsmed 3(10):65–67, 1975
6. CONSOLAZIO CF et al: Environmental temperature and energy expenditures. J Appl Physiol 18:65, 1963
7. EPSTEIN RK: The case against artificial turf. Trial 13(1):42–45, January 1977
8. FOX RJ, MELZACK R: Transcutaneous electrical stimulation and acupuncture: comparison of treatment for low-back pain. Pain 2:357–373, 1976
9. GIECK JH: Influence of environmental factors: temperature. Encyclopedia of Sports Medicine, pp 1120–1123. New York, Macmillan, 1971
10. GIECK JH, McCUE FC III: Fitting of protective football equipment. Am J Sports Med 8(3):192–196, 1980
11. GOLD J: Development of heat pyrexia. JAMA 173:1175–1182, 1980
12. GRIPPO A: NFL Injury Study 1969–1972. Final Project Report (SRI-MSD 1961). Menlo Park, California, Stanford Research Institute, 1973
13. HALL D: A practical guide to the art of massage: anyone can administer a good massage that will give relief to a tired body. Runner's World 14(10):85–89, 1979
14. HARDY JD: Physiology of temperature regulation. Physiol Rev 41:521–606, 1961
15. KEENE JS et al: Tartan Turf[R] on trial. Am J Sports Med 8(1):43–47, 1980

16. KOPYSOV VS: Use of vibrational massage in regulating the pre-competition condition of weightlifters. Sov Sports Rev 14(2):82–84, 1979

17. KNOCHEL JP et al: The renal, cardiovascular, hematologic and serum electrolyte abnormalities of heat stroke. Am J Med 30:299–309, 1961

18. MALACREA R: Protective Equipment Fit. Proceedings of the NATA Professional Preparation Conference. Nashville, NATA Professional Education Committee, 1978

19. MAYER DJ, LIEBESKIND JC: Pain reduction by focal electrical stimulation of the brain: an anatomical and behavioral analysis. Brain Res 68:73–93, 1974

20. MELZACK R, WALL PD: Pain mechanisms: a new theory. Science 150:971–979, 1965

21. MELZACK R: Phantom limb pain: implications for treatment of pathologic pain. Anesthesiology 35:409–419, 1971

22. MELZACK R: The Puzzle of Pain. New York, Basic Books, 1973

23. MELZACK R, MELINDOFF DF: Analgesia produced by brain stimulation: evidence of a prolonged onset period. Exp Neurol 43:369–374, 1974

24. MELZACK R: Prolonged relief of pain by brief, intense transcutaneous somatic stimulation. Pain 1:357–373, 1975

25. MELZACK R et al: Trigger points and acupuncture points for pain: correlations and implications. Pain 3:3–23, 1977

26. MONKERUD D: Put your health in your hands. Runner's World 11(12):32–37, 1976

27. MONKERUD D: Putting your finger on the source of pain: the solution to many of the pains running cause may already be at your fingertips. Runner's World 14(8):59–61, 1979

28. OLIVERAS JL: Behavioral and electrophysiological evidence of pain inhibition from midbrain stimulation. Exp Brain Res 20:32–44, 1974

29. PARSONS CM, GOETZL FR: Effect of induced pain on pain threshhold. Proc Soc Exp Biol (NY) 60:327–329, 1945

30. PRENTICE BE: Acupressure massage to relieve menstrual cramps. Trainer's corner. Phys Sportsmed 9(3):171, 1981

31. ROSSI GF, ZANCHETTI A: The brainstem reticular formation. Arch Ital Biol XCV (Fasc 3–4):199–435, 1957

32. RUTHERFORD GW JR: Injuries Associated with Public Playground Equipment. HIA Hazard Analysis Report. Washington, D.C., U.S. Consumer Product Safety Commission, 1979

33. RYAN R (moderator): Artificial turf: pros and cons. Phys Sportsmed 3(2):41–50, 1975

34. RYAN R (moderator): Artificial vs. natural turf. Phys Sportsmed 7(5):41–53, 1979

35. RYAN J: The neglected art of massage. Phys Sportsmed 8(12):25, 1980

36. SOLA AE, WILLIAMS RL: Myofascial pain syndromes. Neurology 6:91–95, 1956

37. STANITSKI CL et al: Synthetic turf and grass: a comparative study. J Sports Med 2(1):22–26, 1974

38. TOVELL J: Ice immersion toe cap. Athletic Training 15(1):33, Spring, 1980

39. TRAVELL J, RINZLER SH: The myofascial genesis of pain. Postgrad Med 11:425–434, 1952

40. TROY FE: In defense of synthetic turf. Trial 13(1):46–47, 1977

41. VEGHTE JH, WEBB P: Body cooling and response to heat. J Appl Physiol 16:235–238, 1962

42. WAND-TETLEY JI: Historical methods of counter-irritation. Ann Phys Med 3:98, 1956

Adhesive Tape

Adhesive tape may be used to prevent excessive motion in injured and normal joints. The tape relieves pain by splinting injured soft tissue and aids healing by approximating torn tissue. In some fractures, taping is preferable to a cast because the tape may be removed to allow applications of cold or heat and exercise of the limb. Tape may be used to cover blisters, wrap around shoes as an augmentation or "spat" taping, identify travel bags, and label jars in the training room.

Adhesive tape varies in color, width, strength, and the nature of the backing to the adhesive material. The tape must be strong enough to withstand the rigors of athletics. Its strength is determined by the thread count (the number of threads per inch). Cotton- or cloth-backed, rubber-based white adhesive tape is the most commonly used tape in athletics and is available in speed packs or tubes. A speed pack is wound looser, and the roll is bigger than a tube; it bruises easily, however, and may dent while traveling. The cost of adhesive tape has nearly doubled in the last few years. Generally, 3.8-cm (1.5-in)-wide white cloth-backed adhesive tape, although inelastic, meets most needs at a school with a low budget. If more funds are available, elastic tapes may be considered.

Elastic tape stretches and may be used where gentle compression, which reduces muscle spasm and the sensation of instability, is required. The elastic tape may also be used to support damaged tissue, such as strained muscles. More rugged elastic tapes are needed for shoulder and hip injuries. Elastic tape is also used to secure protective pads, especially in areas such as the shoulder, upper humerus, forearm, hand, thigh, and shin. A gymnast may use elastic tape for hand taping: His fingers are passed through holes cut in the tape, and the tape is then pulled down and secured at the wrist with white adhesive tape. The weaker elastic tapes are preferred when tissue must be protected, but free movement is needed. A waterproof, hypoallergenic, plastic-backed tape may be used to secure bandages and dressings and to approximate wound edges, but this tape is not as durable as cloth tape. Moleskin tape is designed with a soft, thick-napped, cotton cloth for cushioning.

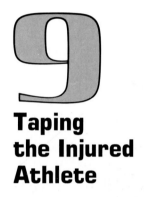

9

Taping the Injured Athlete

THOMAS H. SOOS

Taping Technique

Taping is an art, and the trainer must be proficient at preparing and protecting the athlete's skin, applying the tape properly, and removing the tape with care. The tape job must be effective and comfortable and should conform with consistent pressure. For taping to be effective, the trainer must know which motions should be limited to reduce the stress on the injured body part. The function of taping should be explained to the athlete, along with how it should feel.

The athlete is positioned for taping with the injured part at a comfortable working level. For a knee taping, for example, the athlete stands up on the trainer's table with his heel raised and his knee slightly flexed. A band of hair should be shaved at either end of the area to be taped to serve as an anchoring base. The anchor area should be wide so that the anchoring point may be moved each day. Otherwise, if the same anchoring point were used for consecutive tapings, the skin might become irritated, eroded, and infected. An electric clipper is preferable to a razor for shaving, as the razor may cause cuts. If a razor must be used, the shaving should be done the night before.

The skin in the taped area should be carefully cared for, as the athlete may have to be taped two or three times a day. Sweaty and dirty feet should be cleaned and dried before being taped. The skin should not be prepped with irritating organic solvents that remove all of its natural oils, but it must be free of oily contamination before taping, as the tape will not adhere well

FIG. 9-1
The athlete's ankle is shaved at the anchoring area (*left*) a foam prewrap applied (*right, top*) followed by anchor strips (*bottom*).

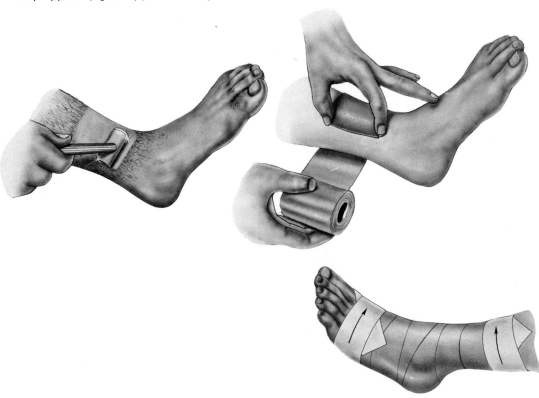

to skin to which ointments have been applied. If the skin is sweaty or if an athlete must be taped in the midst of competition, a tape adherent may be needed to prevent slippage and to help prevent mechanical erosion. Tincture of benzoin, or Friar's balsam, will improve adhesiveness; however, it is not generally necessary to use it with the more adhesive modern tapes, and the benzoin itself may cause irritation. If a skin preparation is needed, a fast-drying, less irritating, non-benzoin-containing material may be used.

Adhesive tape should be applied only to skin that is at room temperature. If placed on skin too hot or too cold after a treatment, the skin may be damaged as the tape is removed. To protect the skin, the tape may be placed over an underwrap or prewrap, which is a thin, porous, polyurethane foam wrap (Fig. 9-1). The prewrap may, however, limit the supportiveness of the tape, and, in some cases where more support is needed, it may be necessary to shave the entire area and apply the tape directly to the skin.

After an ankle sprain, an open basket-weave taping (a "Gibney wrap") may be applied over a foam prewrap, and an elastic wrap is then wound over the basket weave. A preventive taping for an ankle may include two stirrups and two heel locks (one in each direction) and a figure-of-eight (Fig. 9-2). The components of a preventive ankle taping vary from school to school and from trainer to trainer. The order of application of the specific features is not important as long as the preventive taping limits only inversion, and not plantar flexion, dorsiflexion, or eversion.[1] To help achieve this goal, the tape is applied with the ankle at 90° and slightly everted.

The first straps of a taping are applied parallel to the injured muscle, tendons, or ligaments, and no more than a few inches of the tape are pulled from the roll at a time while the tape is being applied. The continuous wrapping of a part is not the most effective way to support the underlying tissue, and the tape may cause constriction. If the part must be encircled, the tape is applied in single strips, with each strip circling the injured part just once. This method produces uniform pressure and avoids constriction.

Adhesive tape is torn by rapidly twisting the tape as it is held tightly between the thumb and index finger. The right and left hands twist quickly in opposite directions. Another useful tearing method is to lay the thumb of one hand firmly across the tape as it lies in position on the body part being taped. The roll of tape is then rapidly rotated with the other hand. Beginners learn how to tear tape by tearing it into very small pieces.

Gaps and Wrinkles

The trainer must avoid gaps between strips of tape or wrinkles in the tape that may cause blisters and new areas of discomfort. Gaps are avoided if each strip overlaps the preceding strip by about one third (Fig. 9-3). Gaps are most common in the Achilles tendon region; thus this area should always be inspected before the athlete leaves the taping table. Wrinkles generally result from carelessness. All layers of tape, especially the innermost, should be made neat and free of wrinkles by applying it with smooth, even tension. The site of application may itself, of course, favor wrinkles because most body parts are not cylindrical but conical.

To avoid wrinkles when tape is being applied to these curved surfaces, the trainer may use several narrow strips instead of one wide strip. Sometimes a wide strip may be torn at either end to make several narrow tabs, which unite at the middle of the strip. Wrinkles normally occur in places such as in front of the ankle or behind the heel where the skin itself must wrinkle to allow movement. These areas may be protected with a cushioning pad of gauze, cotton, felt, or foam that has been covered with a skin lubricant. To prevent tape from splitting at bending areas, such as near the kneecap, the edges of the tape may be rolled.

A taping should be comfortable. If it aggravates pain, then it has been improperly applied or not indicated. If the strapping itself produces

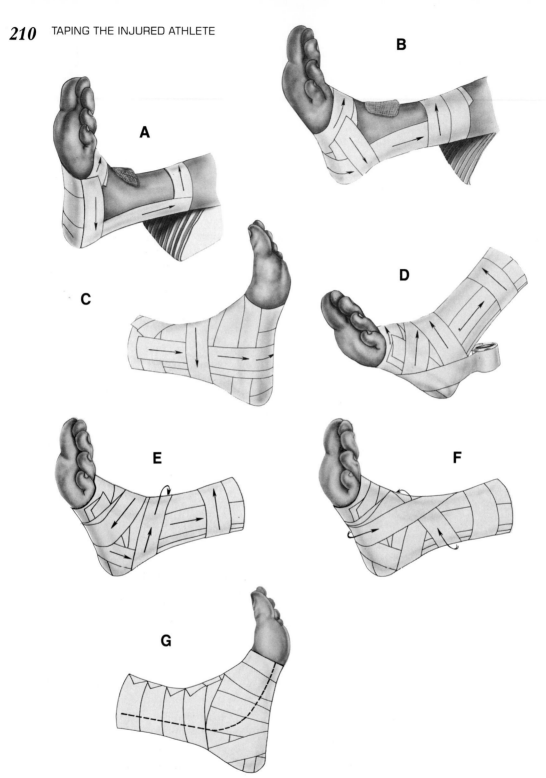

FIG. 9-2
Ankle taping starts with ''stirrups'' and ''horseshoes'' (*A, B*). The trainer
then applies a figure-of-eight, two heel locks, another figure-of-eight
(*C–F*), and closes the tape job with separate strips (*G*).

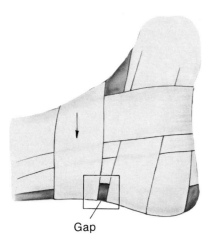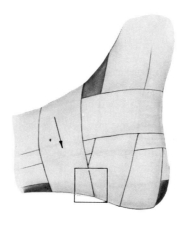

Gap

FIG. 9-3
Gaps may occur, especially in the Achilles tendon area, causing blisters and new areas of discomfort. Gaps may be avoided if each strip overlaps the preceding strip by about one third the width of the tape. Tape job should be checked for gaps and wrinkles before the athlete leaves the taping table.

undue tension and pain, numbness, or pinching, then the tape must be reapplied.

Removal of Tape

Just as there is a proper way to apply tape, there is a proper way to remove it. "If you don't want it to hurt, rip if off," is bad advice. As much care should be taken in removing tape as in applying it. Tape is best removed by gently pulling along the long axis of the strapping, not across it. It is usually easier to push the skin away from the tape than to rip or pull the tape away from the skin. A solvent, such as ether, may make removal easier. If tape has been applied to an area where there is still some hair, the tape should be removed in the direction of the hair growth; it should not be jerked or yanked, as this method would increase the amount of hair removed and mechanically irritate the skin.

Most tapings will develop a natural crease while being worn. These creases are convenient places to cut through for removal of the tape. A sharp-tipped implement should never be used to remove tape. Instead, the trainer should use bandage scissors or a special commercial tape cutter. He may dip the scissors into skin lubricant, which will allow them to slide. The tape is then cut away from the injury site. In removing an ankle strapping, vertical and horizontal cuts may be made with the bandage scissors. Once the tape has been cut, it is gently removed from the skin, and after the athlete has showered, he should rub massage lotion into his skin to restore its moisture.

Tape Rash

Tape rash occurs most commonly right after summer, when the player's skin is not ready for two-a-day tapings. Most reactions to tape come from mechanical irritation and, to a lesser degree, from chemical irritation. Daily tapings especially cause moisture to build up under these occlusive tapings, which softens the stratum corneum and reduces cohesion between cells. When the tape is removed, the soft stratum corneum is stripped away with the adhesive tape mass. This separation does not occur at the skin-adhesive interface but deeper, to cause irregular delamination of the stratum corneum.[2] The more adhesive the tape, the more cells are removed. After the tape is removed, the adhesive surface of the tape may be covered with a film of desquamated epidermis. In this case, the skin should be cleansed with a neutral soap and thoroughly dried before the tape is reapplied. If hair follicles and the skin that surrounds them have been irritated from the tape being pulled away from the skin, the irritated area is treated like an abrasion, and the part is not taped for a few days. The tape also blocks sweat pores, and, within 3 days, explosive bacterial growth will occur under occlusive tape and an infection may start. Fortunately, tape is usually worn only for a short time in athletic activities.

Acrylate tapes allow for long-term adhesion. Their molecular structure permits water vapor to pass through so that the stratum corneum is not overhydrated from perspiration.[1] With these tapes, only a small amount of stratum corneum is lost during tape removal. The plane of separation develops near the surface of the stratum corneum in the region of the naturally desquamating cells. Thus, these tapes may be used repeatedly with only minimal skin damage. Itching may be from mechanical or chemical factors, or both. There seems to be little correlation between the presence of visible skin lesions and itching. The athlete may have bad lesions without itching or may itch without a single visible lesion.

Only infrequently are athletes truly allergic to adhesive tape. An allergic reaction includes erythema, edema, papules, vesicles, and, in severe cases, desquamation. The response becomes more severe the longer the tape is left on and usually intensifies for some time even after the tape has been removed, requiring days to subside completely.

The allergic athlete may react to an individual ingredient of the tape or to the component mass. If an athlete is allergic, he should be patch-tested with different brands of tape. Conventional rubber-based adhesives have many ingredients, including elastomers, plasticizers, tackifiers, pigments, and stabilizers.[2] There may be source variation and the potential for introducing irritants and sensitizing agents. Acrylate adhesives do not have as many components, and thus are hypoallergenic.

REFERENCES

1. EMERICK CE: Ankle taping: prevention of injury or waste of time? Athletic Training 14:186–188, 1979
2. Professional Uses of Adhesive Tapes, 3rd ed. New Brunswick, New Jersey, Johnson and Johnson Company, 1975

After an injury, an athlete typically undergoes a sequence of predictable psychological reactions similar to those of a person facing death.[16]

1. Disbelief, denial, and isolation
2. Anger
3. Bargaining
4. Depression
5. Acceptance and resignation while continuing to remain hopeful

An athlete initially responds to an injury by saying that there is no damage, that the injury is less severe than originally thought, or that it will probably be better tomorrow. When tomorrow comes and the injury remains, the athlete feels isolated and lonely. Once the athlete begins attending to the injury, he commonly becomes irritated with himself and others. Anger is followed by a true sense of loss. With his arm in a sling or his leg in a cast, he lacks his ordinary comfort and freedom. He is well aware that the injured limb makes the difference between actually competing and merely watching from the sidelines. Ideally, this depression stage should be followed by that of acceptance and hope, but various factors may intervene to delay or prevent this from happening.

An Athlete's Perception of Injury

Athletes perceive injuries in different ways. One may perceive the injury as a disaster, another may see it as an opportunity to show courage, and yet another may find it a welcome relief from the embarrassment of poor performance, lack of playing time, or a losing season. The injured athlete may wonder whether he will completely recover. He must be prepared for the end of participation and yet remain positive and enthusiastic about the prospect for total recovery. Because of his injury, his self-image is attacked, and he loses the opportunity to display prowess. If the injury should end his athletic career, he may suffer an "identity crisis."

Emotional and irrational thinking may take over. The injured athlete may then become lost in "the work of worry," excuse his own mistakes

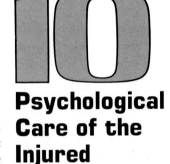

Psychological Care of the Injured Athlete

ROBERT J. ROTELLA

213

and responsibilities, and be overwhelmed by anxiety. These self-defeating thought patterns may interfere in his recovery.

When an athlete is thinking irrationally, he might exaggerate the meaning of an event, disregard important aspects of a situation, oversimplify events as good or bad, right or wrong, overgeneralize from a single event, or draw unwarranted conclusions, even though evidence is lacking or contradictory.[3] He may, for example, decide that the trainer is giving preferential treatment to "major-sport" athletes over "minor-sport" ones. He may exaggerate the meaning of an event, thinking his athletic career has been ended by the injury. He may disregard important aspects of a situation and become terribly discouraged after, for example, 10 days of therapy, even though he was told it would take at least 2 or 3 weeks to complete. The injured athlete may oversimplify events or overgeneralize from a single event. He may, for instance, know of another athlete who had a similar injury and, despite intensive rehabilitation, failed to recover. Because of this, he may believe that nothing can help him to recover. Moreover, an athlete who is injured once may decide that he is "injury prone." This thought may cause him to be more anxious, and as a result he may well become more frequently injured.

Coping with Injury

When injury occurs, the athlete should be encouraged to view it in a rational, self-enhancing way rather than from a self-defeating perspective. He should understand that when an injury blocks the attainment of important goals, it is reasonable and appropriate to think that the injury is unfortunate, untimely, and inconvenient and to feel irritated, frustrated, and sad. It is unreasonable, however, for an athlete to convince himself that the situation is hopeless, that the injury should be hidden from his coach or trainer, that the season or his career has ended, and that he will never again be able to perform effectively.

An athlete with emotional self-control will be able to cope with his injury by responding rationally to it, and not being overwhelmed by it. He can best exert self-control if he has knowledge of his injury and the rehabilitation process. He cannot be positive and relaxed if he is unknowledgeable, anxious, and wondering. Much of an injured athlete's anxiety results from uncertainty, misconceptions, or inaccurate information. If uncertainty persists, he may have trouble getting through the denial and isolation stages. Honest and accurate information, padded with hope, helps him move into the acceptance stage.[15] Further, the athlete who understands what he is doing in rehabilitation, and why, is more likely to work hard and be able to provide useful information to the trainer about his progress.

What an athlete says to himself and imagines after an injury has occurred helps to determine his behavior. Fortunately, he can learn coping skills to control his thoughts and what he says to himself. When he notices faulty or self-defeating internal dialogues, he can use his coping strategies to change his thinking.[3, 20-23] He may use an intervention strategy such as "thought stoppage."

Controlling Inner Dialogue with Thought Stoppage

Injury-related situation (potential source of stress): The extent of the injury is explained to the athlete and a rehabilitation program outlined.

Self-defeating inner dialogue: The athlete worries about the injury and feels sorry for himself. "I'll never play again this year, if ever." "There's no sense listening to this; it will heal itself eventually anyway. I know others who went to therapy, and it didn't help them." The athlete is so preoccupied with self-defeating thoughts that he does not even hear the rationale for rehabilitation or the program outlined. He gives himself excuses for missing treatments.

Self-enhancing inner dialogue: The athlete recognizes that worrying and feeling sorry for himself have no value. He stops thinking negatively and redirects his thoughts to listening closely to the rehabilitation program outlined. He asks questions about the exercises he is unsure of. He directs his thoughts to preparation for tomorrow's first treatment session. He plans his schedule for tomorrow and looks forward to rehabilitation in a positive manner.

Controlling Dialogue with Thought Stoppage (Continued)

7:30 A.M.

Injury-related situation: The athlete gets up and limps to the training room for rehabilitation exercises, but the training room is locked with no trainer in sight.

Self-defeating inner dialogue: The athlete gets mad at the trainer for not showing up for the therapy session. "This is typical. He never shows up. He gives me a big talk on the importance of rehabilitation and then he doesn't show up. To hell with him! I won't show up anymore either until he comes and apologizes to me." The athlete, seeing only the negative side, accepts no responsibility for himself. He fails to realize that he will be the one who will suffer by not getting therapy.

Self-enhancing inner dialogue: The athlete gets mad but then recognizes that this is self-defeating. He relaxes, takes a deep breath, and stops his thoughts and thinks: "I wonder what happened. He never misses a treatment. Something important must have happened. I know he wants me to get better, and if I'm going to get better, I will need my treatments. If I don't get them, I will be the loser. I'll wait or stop by later to get another meeting time for my treatment." The athlete attempts to understand why the trainer did not show up. He recognizes the importance of taking responsibility for therapy and makes sure that he gets it, so that he can return to action sooner.

10:30 A.M.

Injury-related situation: In class, the athlete is getting constant attention from his classmates about his injury.

Self-defeating inner dialogue: The athlete enjoys the attention. "This is nice. I enjoy the attention. I feel like someone special. Gosh, many people who never recognized me before now know who I am." The athlete begins to enjoy the attention of others that comes from being injured. Consciously or unconsciously, he may begin to like being injured and to question the value of a speedy rehabilitation.

Controlling Dialogue with Thought Stoppage (Continued)

Self-enhancing inner dialogue: The athlete enjoys the attention but recognizes that this may work to his disadvantage by decreasing his motivation to get better. The athlete thinks, "It's nice to know that others care, but I don't want their sympathy; I want their respect as an athlete. The best way to get it is to rehabilitate myself and get back into competition." The athlete feels good that others care about him and uses these thoughts to motivate himself to return quickly to competition.

2:30 P.M.

Injury-related situation: The athlete is in the training room receiving treatment and going through rehabilitation exercises while experiencing a great amount of pain and little apparent improvement in the injured part.

Self-defeating inner dialogue: The athlete worries and questions the benefit of treatment and exercise. "This is awful. This hurts too much to be beneficial. These exercises will probably cause me more harm. Besides, I've been doing this for 3 days now, and I can't see any progress. It would be a lot easier to just let it heal on its own. I don't think I'll come in tomorrow. If it's really important, the trainer will call me. If he doesn't, it will mean I was right. It really doesn't matter if I get treatment." The athlete does not get as much out of today's treatment and begins to develop excuses for not continuing therapy.

Self-enhancing inner dialogue: The athlete worries and questions the benefits of treatment and exercise. He thinks, "STOP. These exercises hurt, but it's OK—they'll pay off. I'm lucky to have knowledgeable prople helping me. I'll be competing soon, because I'm doing these exercises. I must not let the pain bother me. If the pain gets too severe, I'll speak up and tell the trainer. He'll want to know. Otherwise, I'll live with it and think about how happy I'll be to be competing again." The athlete has a good treatment session and prepares himself to continue for as long as necessary. He develops rapport with the trainer, who feels good about the athlete.

4:00 P.M.

Injury-related situation: The athlete watches the practice session.

Self-defeating inner dialogue: The athlete sees other athletes practicing and feels sorry for himself. "Why me? Why am I the one who has to be injured? I was in better shape than anyone. I'll probably lose my position on the team by the time I'm healthy again. I hope the team doesn't play too well without me. I hope I'm missed." The athlete gets more discouraged with himself. He is seen by his teammates negatively. He is obviously more concerned with himself than with the team.

Self-enhancing inner dialogue: The athlete observes others practicing. He starts to feel sorry for himself but recognizes these inappropriate thoughts and stops and redirects them. "I wish I hadn't been injured. The fact that I'm in really good shape will help me get back on the field a lot faster. I hope everyone plays well without me so we can still go to the tournament. I'm going to do everything I can to help. I'll go to practice and help out and cheer for my teammates. I'll make sure I know what's going on, so that when I'm healthy again, I'll be ready to return." The athlete feels good as a result of enthusiasm during practice. Teammates are happy to see him and encourage him to stick with his treatments and to get back soon because the team needs him.

When his faulty thinking is recognized, the athlete says "STOP," and then repeats self-enhancing thoughts. A sports psychologist can help him recognize faulty thought patterns and anticipate destructive thoughts and can "inoculate" the athlete with coping strategies. Team physicians and trainers can also learn to teach these strategies that may shorten the time the injured athlete needs to progress from disbelief to acceptance, to productive rehabilitation, and to a safe, successful return to competition.

In addition to coping with faulty thinking, the injured athlete will have to cope with the conditions of the hospital and training room and the stress of special treatment procedures. He is encouraged to express his feelings, to establish rapport with hospital and training room staffs, and to balance accepting help from others and retaining independence. With safety considered, the athlete will gain confidence by mastering skills such as ice massage, ultrasound, and crutch-walking.

Visual Imagery as a Coping Skill

The athlete's imagination can greatly influence his response to an injury. Often he imagines the worst thing that could happen. Athletes can be taught to control their visual images and to direct them productively to reduce anxiety and to aid in rehabilitation. Visual imagery strategies include emotive imagery, body rehearsal, mastery rehearsal, and coping rehearsal.

Emotive Imagery

In *emotive imagery,* a technique that helps the athlete to feel secure and confident that his rehabilitation will be successful, scenes are imagined that produce positive, self-enhancing feelings, such as enthusiasm, self-pride, and confidence. Some athletes, for example, can recall success in recovering from an earlier injury and returning to competition. Others may think of the admiration that coaches, teammates, and friends will have for them when they have overcome the injury. The athlete is instructed to think of other athletes like himself who have overcome the same injury and to generate other scenes that produce positive feelings.

Body Rehearsal

In *body rehearsal,* a mental rehearsal technique now being investigated, the athlete is given a detailed explanation of his injury. Whenever possible, colored pictures are used to help him develop a mental picture of the injury. The healing process and the purpose of the rehabilitation techniques are then explained to him so that he can envision what is happening internally to the injured part during the rehabilitation process. After the athlete has clearly visualized the healing process, he is asked to imagine it occurring in color during his treatments and at intervals throughout the day. Body rehearsal may become a way of influencing healing.

Mastery Rehearsal for Knee Surgery

> "I'm looking forward to surgery and feel great about the upcoming operation and rehabilitation. I'm glad I'll no longer be bothered by my knee. I have a well-qualified surgeon who'll do a successful operation. I'll begin rehabilitation shortly afterwards with a caring and talented athletic trainer. Rehabilitation will be short and successful. Each day, I'll make progress. In a few weeks, I'll be training again. I'll feel good and be excited. I know I'll be successful."

Coping Rehearsal for Knee Surgery

> "I'm looking forward to surgery, but I'm anxious. I'm likely to become even more anxious as the day of surgery approaches. Whenever I realize that my mind is running wild with anxiety, I'll 'STOP' and replace these thoughts with helpful thoughts and 'let go' and relax.
>
> "Rehabilitation will be long and demanding, challenging my self-discipline and willpower. But if I want to reach the goals I've outlined for myself, I can't let the injury stand in my way. I must have confidence in my ability to overcome this challenge.
>
> "What must I do? I'll work out a plan that will prepare me for successful rehabilitation. I must keep cool and not respond emotionally. If I find myself responding emotionally, I'll relax and become more aware of my self-statements. If I'm thinking self-defeating thoughts, I'll 'STOP' them and repeat helpful thoughts to myself. If I become discouraged, I'll think of athletes who have overcome far worse injuries than mine. An injury such as mine has ruined some athletes' careers, but successful athletes realize that successful management of injuries and rehabilitation is part of becoming a successful athlete.
>
> "There will be many excuses for not going to therapy: 'I can't find time,' 'I'm too busy,' 'I have a test tomorrow,' 'the training room hours are ridiculous.' I will make sure that I'm ready for these excuses and realize that they will only work against me. I will always find a way to get my treatments.
>
> "There will be days when I'll see little or no progress in therapy. I will also probably experience pain that is likely to make me tense, irritable, and frustrated. When this occurs, I must remember to stay calm and positive and to keep my sense of humor. Then the trainer will enjoy helping me more, and I'll feel better about myself. Think how good I'll feel when my rehabilitation is successful."

Mastery Rehearsal and Coping Rehearsal

Mastery rehearsal and coping rehearsal are used to prepare the athlete for difficult situations and to achieve important goals. *Mastery rehearsal* is a positive imagery technique that builds confidence and provides a motivational framework for the athlete's rehabilitation. In mastery rehearsal, the athlete only imagines the successful completion of tasks, whereas in *coping rehearsal* he actively anticipates potential problems. By using his imagination to anticipate problems and appropriate responses to these problems, he can plan effective measures to cope with the difficulties. Coping rehearsal is the more realistic of the two rehearsal methods and prepares the athlete for difficulties that might realistically occur. Coping rehearsal does induce some anxiety itself, however, and in some cases may overwhelm an injured athlete.

Self-Control of Pain

Pain is influenced by motivational and cognitive factors. The athlete can be taught non-imagery and imagery strategies to control or to eliminate pain.[22, 23] He must be careful, of course, not to completely block out pain signals that could otherwise warn him of danger.

Pain has three dimensions: the sensory-discriminative, motivational-affective, and cognitive-evaluative. Different coping skills are needed for each of these dimensions. For the sensory-discriminative dimension, relaxation techniques can control the sensory input of pain and reduce the tension that otherwise magnifies the intensity of the pain. Other strategies include attention diversion, somatization, imaginative inattention, and transformation of context.

The athlete can exclude the sensation of pain by diverting his attention to other stimuli in the external environment. He can, for example, do mental arithmetic, count ceiling tiles, or plan his daily schedule. Another nonimagery strategy is somatization. Here the athlete focuses directly on the pain at the injured area and ignores other sensations. When, for example, his foot is placed into ice water, he focuses on a feeling of pleasant dampness and numbness.[6] Imaginative inattention requires the athlete to imagine "goal-directed fantasies" that are usually pleasant and allow him to ignore the pain. The athlete becomes totally absorbed in the guided fantasy, such as a perfect performance in an upcoming contest.[5] He may also imagine the injured or painful part to be numb or minimize the pain as being insignificant or unreal.[4, 8]

The athlete may also imaginatively transform the context in which he is feeling the pain. He acknowledges the pain and includes it in a fantasy, transferring the context or the setting in which the pain occurs. He may, for instance, imagine himself to be a spy who has been shot and is now in a car that is being chased down a winding mountain road by enemy agents. The car chase should require more attention than the pain. Relaxation can also reduce the sensation of pain. The athlete imagines that it is a summer day and he is relaxing in a rowboat on a calm pond, or that the injured part is warm and heavy.[6, 14]

A second dimension of pain is the motivational-affective. Negative feelings of anxiety and helplessness may increase the perception of pain, whereas positive feelings of confidence and control decrease it. Thought stoppage techniques and positive self-statements may help.

The third dimension is the cognitive-evaluative. How bad the athlete expects the pain to be will usually influence how much pain he will report. Thought stoppage and self-instruction statements are valuable.

Biofeedback is another way to gain control over pain.[27] The athlete's awareness is raised and his self-control is improved by listening to recordings of psychophysiologic processes. Biofeedback may also be used to show the athlete the effectiveness of his self-control strategies.

Relaxation Training

The injured athlete may use relaxation training to help manage stress and anxiety and to control pain. The relaxation techniques allow him to develop more vivid and productive visual images. The athlete learns how to relax deeply by systematically tensing and releasing muscle groups and by learning to differentiate between the tense and relaxed feelings.[11, 12] Progressive relaxation techniques may not, however, be equally effective for all athletes. Those who tend to be anxious about an injury or who have insomnia, tension headaches, or general tightness benefit most. Many other athletes have learned on their own how to cope with stress and have been coping well for years. They should not be forced to spend extra time on relaxation training.

Introducing the Athlete to Relaxation Training

At the beginning of the relaxation training session, the sports psychologist explains the reasons for, and benefits of, relaxation training and conveys his enthusiasm for the technique. Then he answers any questions that the athlete may have. Relaxation training takes place in a quiet, calm, comfortably warm, and dimly lit area. The sports psychologist will need some light to ascertain that the athlete is following directions correctly and relaxing his body properly. The athlete should wear loose, comfortable clothing and unbutton his collar and loosen his belt. Female athletes should wear a shirt or blouse and slacks. Contact lenses, eyeglasses, and watches should be removed.

The athlete's body should be completely supported in a recliner chair that has well-padded head, arm, and leg rests. Pillows are placed under the athlete's head and behind his knees to further relax these areas. Some athletes prefer to recline on a wide couch or on a carpeted floor; others lie in a position that appears to be quite uncomfortable but may be the athlete's most comfortable position.

As the athlete reclines in the chair, the therapist stands nearby and gives directions. For the first few exercises, the therapist speaks in a conversational tone. As relaxation progresses, his voice becomes softer, and he speaks slower. When the athlete is instructed to tense his muscles, the therapist speaks louder and faster. He might say the following to the athlete.

"Focus your attention on the way your body feels. If your mind wanders onto other things, calmly tell yourself 'STOP,' push those thoughts away, and concentrate on your body's feelings. These exercises will teach you to recognize muscle tension and muscle relaxation so that you will become more aware of it. You will then be able to eliminate muscle tension once you recognize it, and so be able to relax.

"Close your eyes, but do not force them shut. Hold them comfortably closed. With your heels about 6 inches apart, point your toes away from your body and tighten the muscles in your calves, thighs, and buttocks. Feel the tension as you hold it. Remember this feeling. 1 . . . , 2 . . . , 3 . . . , 4 . . . . Repeat the words 'let go' to yourself, and slowly let the tension flow out of your body. Again concentrate on your calves,

thighs, and buttocks. Let your toes point upward and flop to the outside. Feel the relaxation. Remember how good it feels. Feel the heaviness and the warmth flowing through your lower body. Let it feel good. If you have any tension anywhere in your lower body, 'let go.'*

"Now, concentrate on your stomach. Tighten your stomach muscles as much as you can. Feel the tension as you hold the tightened position. Remember the feeling. 1 . . . , 2 . . . , 3 . . . , 4 . . . . Repeat the words 'let go' to yourself, and slowly let the tension flow out of your body. Again concentrate on your stomach muscles. Feel the relaxation and remember how good it feels. Let it feel good for a moment. If there is any tension anywhere in your body, let it go.

"Now concentrate on your chest muscles. Tighten them as much as you can. Take a deep breath through your mouth, and then hold it. As you hold it, you may feel tension spots in your chest. Remember where they are—they may surface when you are stressed. Now, slowly 'let go'— very slowly. Breathe normally and comfortably as if you were sleeping or resting. Make sure you have eliminated the tension spots. Completely relax your entire body.

"Tighten all of the muscles from the tips of your fingers to your shoulders in both arms as much as you can. Raise your arms about one foot off the floor. Clench your fists. Feel the tension in your fingers, hands, arms, and shoulders. Hold it. 1 . . . , 2 . . . , 3 . . . , 4 . . . , and feel the tension. Slowly 'let go.' Let your arms drop and your fingers spread, and completely relax. Concentrate on how your hands and arms feel. If there is any remaining tension, remember where it is. You are likely to have tension there when you are in a stressful situation. Now, 'let go,' and completely relax. Once again, concentrate on just your fingers. Relax them completely. Feel how warm and heavy they are. Relax your upper arms completely. Eliminate any excess tension.

"Now concentrate on the muscles of your upper back—the muscles between the shoulder blades and the neck. These muscles are very sensitive to tension. You may have often experienced soreness here. Tighten these muscles as much as possible.

Feel the tension and hold it. 1 . . . , 2 . . . , 3 . . . , 4 . . . . Slowly 'let go.' Dwell on the feelings of relaxation as you so do. Concentrate on these relaxed feelings, and remember them.

"Now, tighten your entire body as much as you can from the tips of your fingers to the top of your toes. Hold it. 1 . . . , 2 . . . , 3 . . . , 4 . . . . Slowly 'let go,' and completely relax your entire body. If you have any tension remaining anywhere in your body, let it go.

"Imagine a pleasant scene, such as walking on a beach or lying in a rowboat on a calm pond—any place that you feel completely relaxed. Let your whole body feel calm and relaxed. Enjoy the feeling. Take a couple of very deep, slow breaths. Inhale deeply into your stomach: 1 . . . , 2 . . . , 3 . . . , 4 . . . ; then exhale slowly: 1 . . . , 2 . . . , 3 . . . , 4 . . . . Feel your body become more and more relaxed. Breathe normally, smoothly, and calmly. Continue to feel your body, and let go of any remaining tension."[11]

After the first relaxation session, athletes have generally related positive experiences. Some problems, however, have arisen during relaxation training.

Anticipating and Solving Problems

Some problems that may arise while relaxation skills are being taught are laughter, falling asleep, muscle cramps, and mental distractions.

Laughter Younger athletes may think that relaxation training is humorous and begin laughing. The laughter may be due to something that the therapist said or did, a distracting thought that crossed the athlete's mind, or to self-consciousness. If the athlete is self-conscious, let him know that he is doing the exercises right. Encouraging statements give him comfort and confidence.

Falling Asleep An athlete sometimes falls asleep during relaxation training. Unfortunately, he cannot practice the skills while asleep. There may be some difficulty in determining whether an athlete is practicing relaxation techniques or is sleeping. The therapist must watch closely to see if his directions are being followed. An athlete who tends to fall asleep may be asked to give a signal to indicate whether a particular muscle group is relaxed or not. If there is no signal, the athlete may be asleep.

Failure to Relax Certain Muscle Groups An athlete may have difficulty in completely relaxing an area, such as his shoulders, hamstrings, or jaw muscles. Clearly, extreme tension in any of these areas will affect performance adversely. He should spend extra time learning to relax these muscles.

Muscle Cramps Relaxation training is sometimes interrupted by muscle cramps, particularly in the calves and feet. These cramps can usually be eliminated if the athlete tenses less during the tensing phase of each exercise. If this strategy does not prevent cramping, the athlete may massage the cramped muscle. While he massages, he should keep his eyes closed and remain as relaxed as possible. The interruption is followed by a review of the last few exercises and extra work on relaxation. With practice, the athlete will learn to tense just below the level that causes cramps. Occasionally, however, the athlete will have to skip the tensing phase for a particularly troublesome muscle group.

Mental Distractions An athlete may have trouble paying attention to the skills being presented to him. Perhaps he is distracted by a fear of forgetting, anxious thoughts, overanalysis, or sexual arousal. The athlete may be worried that he will not remember the exercises when he is home alone. To relieve this fear of forgetting, the relaxation training session may be taped for the athlete to take home.

Some athletes are distracted by anxious thoughts related to the injury or to some aspect of their athletic performance. Athletes should be reminded before and after each relaxation session that the relaxation exercises they are learning will facilitate a successful rehabilitation and return to sports participation. Other athletes overanalyze or worry about whether they are doing the exercises correctly. The therapist must be certain that he is giving clear and consistent directions to the athlete. The athlete should be reminded to focus on the body parts being tensed or relaxed. Encouraging and supportive feedback is helpful.

An athlete may question the value of relaxation training before giving it a chance. As a result, his mind may wander to other activities that he finds more enjoyable. Sometimes an athlete becomes sexually aroused during a relaxation training session. Certain aspects of the environment may have to be changed. The athlete can be shown thought stoppage techniques to redirect thoughts in a more appropriate direction. If the problem persists, the only solution is to find another therapist.

Home Practice

The athlete should leave the relaxation training session with a well-thought-out plan, enthusiastic about practicing and using the relaxation skills. Athletes usually learn the skills quite easily, as sport has given them good control of their bodies and minds. Whenever possible, the athlete should take a tape recording or a written copy of the exercises home. His room should be free of distractions from other people or sounds. This may take some planning: The telephone may have to be taken off the hook, a "quiet please" sign put on the door, or relaxing music played to help block out noise.

Relaxation skills are practiced twice a day for about 20 minutes each time. Usually, one session is in the middle of the day and the other late at night. The night session may help the athlete get to sleep, especially when pain is associated with the injury. (Later, relaxation skills may be used to enable the athlete to fall asleep before an important contest.) If, however, the athlete has homework due or a test to take the next morning and he does not wish to fall asleep, an alarm clock should be set for ½ hour.

Returning to Competition

Despite the great advances in physically preparing an athlete for a return to sport after an injury or surgery, little use has been made of systematic psychological rehabilitation. As a result, psychological scars may be overlooked. These "scars" may be rational or irrational anxieties that cause him to lose his ability to concentrate and may lead to reinjury or to an injury of another area. It also may take a long time for the athlete to regain his confidence for peak performance.

Football Running Back's Fear Hierarchy for a Shoulder Injury*

1. You are told by the trainer that you are ready to return to practice.
2. In the huddle for the first time after return to practice and you must block.
3. In the huddle for the first time after return to practice and you must carry the ball on a sweep play.
4. In the huddle for the first time after return to practice and you must carry the ball on a dive play.
5. You must jump high in the air to catch a pass with a defender about to tackle you on the side of the injured shoulder.
6. You must jump high in the air to catch a pass with a defender about to tackle you on the side opposite the injured shoulder and you are about to land on the injured shoulder on a turf field.
7. Imagine successfully running the ball on various plays and avoiding or breaking tackles. (This was the state of the athlete's mental process before his injury.)

* The athlete imagines doing each step successfully over and over while maintaining a relaxed state before moving to the next step.

Basketball Player's Fear Hierarchy for an Ankle Sprain★

1. You are going on the basketball court to practice.
2. You begin practice by running windsprints.
3. You are now in a "wave" drill and you practice your defensive step slide.
4. You are going to practice shooting with no defense.
5. You are running layups in practice.
6. You are in a scrimmage and you shoot over a defensive player.
7. You shoot over a defensive player and you are fouled.
8. You are in practice and will rebound a ball to start a fastbreak, and there is no defense.
9. You rebound a ball during a scrimmage and turn to give an outlet pass.
10. In a scrimmage, you jump high to rebound a basketball; when you come down you land on another player's foot, but you still turn and throw an outlet pass.

★ The athlete imagines doing each step successfully over and over while maintaining a relaxed state before moving to the next step.

Systematic Desensitization

Systematic desensitization may be used psychologically to rehabilitate the injured athlete. Desensitization helps the athlete handle anxiety[28] by combining relaxation training and visual imagery. It should be, when possible, supplemented by biofeedback training.

At the onset of rehabilitation, the sports psychologist should encourage the athlete to talk about anxieties over the injury and his return to competition. The athlete should then be introduced to relaxation training techniques and practice them by using a tape recording each day at home or in a private room next to the training room. When the athlete becomes skilled at relaxing on cue, he should then start desensitization procedures.

Systematic desensitization lasts for 20 to 30 minutes a day. It is timed so that psychological rehabilitation is completed when the athlete is physically ready to return to playing sports. A fear hierarchy should be established that applies specifically to the athlete's fears or to his anticipated fears. This hierarchy is a list of five to ten situations that elicit a progressive increase in his anxiety.

Desensitization starts with step one on the fear hierarchy. As the athlete imagines the first step, he tries to remain as relaxed as possible. Electromyography or thermal biofeedback may be used to measure muscle tension and relaxation. If this machinery is not available, the athlete should indicate his degree of relaxation on a scale of 1 through 10 (1 = very tense; 10 = very relaxed). The therapist calls off the numbers 1 through 10, and the athlete raises his index finger at the appropriate number. He may proceed to the next step after indicating deep relaxation and confidence while imagining the previous step on the fear hierarchy. The process is repeated until the athlete can relax on cue and stay relaxed while imagining each step on the fear hierarchy. After successfully completing the fear hierarchy, he should be ready mentally to return to athletics. In addition to mental desensitization, he should physically go through each step of the fear hierarchy before returning to competition.

The "Injury Prone" Athlete

Some athletes seem to be more prone to injury than are others, perhaps for physical reasons, such as limb malalignment, joints too loose or too tight, poor strength, or strength imbalance. Perhaps the athlete is not fully fit; his poor endurance leads to fatigue, a slower reaction time, and reduced coordination. In addition, he may not be warming up correctly.

Mentally, the athlete may be tense, depressed, or preoccupied with problems in school, with social problems, or with problems at home. The mental changes may be subtle, but the team physician, trainer, or sports psychologist can often tell that something is wrong. The athlete may uncharacteristically jump the gun, start fights, miss foul shots, or otherwise not be concentrating on his task. He may have trouble sleeping, show a changed behavior pattern, and have mood changes. Talking with the athlete will sometimes uncover the source of the problem, and the difficulty can then be resolved.

REFERENCES

1. AVERILL J: Personal control over aversive stimuli and its relationship to stress. Psychol Bull 80:286–303, 1973
2. BEAN KL: Desensitization, behavioral rehearsal, the reality: a preliminary report on a new procedure. Behav Ther 1:525–545, 1970
3. BECK A: Cognitive therapy: nature and relation to behavior therapy. Behav Ther 2:194–200, 1970
4. BLITZ B, DINNERSTEIN A: The role of attentional focus in pain perception: manipulation of response to noxious stimulation by instructions. J Abnorm Psychol 77:42–45, 1971
5. CHAVERS J, BARBER T: Cognitive strategies, experimental modeling and expectation in the attention of pain. J Abnorm Psychol 83:356–363, 1974
6. EVANS M, PAUL G: Effects of hypnotically suggested analgesia on physiological and subjective responses to cold stress. J Consult Clin Psychol 35:362–371, 1970
7. FOREYT JP, RATHJEN DP (eds): Cognitive Behavior Therapy. Research and Application. New York, Plenum Press, 1978
8. GREENE R, REYHER J: Pain tolerance in hypnotic analgesia and imagination states. J Abnorm Psychol 77:42–45, 1977
9. HAMBURG D, ADAMS JE: A perspective on coping behavior. Arch Gen Psychiatry 17:277–284, 1967
10. JACOBSON E: You Must Relax. New York, McGraw-Hill, 1934
11. JACOBSON E: Progressive Relaxation. Chicago, University of Chicago Press, 1938
12. JACOBSON E: Anxiety and Tension Control. Philadelphia, JB Lippincott, 1964
13. JANIS IL: Psychological Stress: Psychoanalytic and Behavioral Studies of Surgical Patients. New York, John Wiley & Sons, 1958
14. JOHNSON R: Suggestions for pain reduction and response to cold-induced pain. Psychol Rep 18:79–85, 1966
15. KAVANAUGH RE: Facing Death. Los Angeles, Nash Publishing, 1972
16. KÜBLER-ROSS E: On Death and Dying. New York, Macmillan, 1969
17. LAZARUS RS: Psychological stress and coping in adaptation and illness. Int J Psychiatry Med 5:321–333, 1974
18. LINDMANN B: Symptomatology and management of acute grief. Am J Psychiatry 101:1–11, September 1944
19. LIPOWSKI ZJ: Physical illness, the individual and the coping processes. Psychiatry Med 1:91–102, 1970
20. MAHONEY M: Cognitive and Behavior Modification. Cambridge, Massachusetts, Ballinger, 1974
21. MAHONEY MJ, THORESON CE: Self-Control: Power to the Person. Monterey, California, Brooks/Cole, 1974
22. MEICHENBAUM D: Cognitive Behavior Modification: An Integrative Approach. New York, Plenum Press, 1977
23. MEICHENBAUM D: Cognitive Behavior Modification. Morristown, New Jersey, General Learning Press, 1978
24. MELZACK R, CASEY K: Sensory motivational and central control determinants of pain. A new conceptual model. In Kenshalo D (ed): The Skin Senses. Springfield, Illinois, Charles C Thomas, 1968
25. MELZACK R, WALL P: Pain mechanisms: a new theory. Science 150:197, 1965
26. MOSS RH: The Crises of Physical Illness: An Overview in Coping with Physical Illness. New York, Plenum Medical Book Company, 1979
27. REEVES J: EMG-biofeedback reduction of tension headache: a cognitive skills training approach. Biofeedback Self Regul 1:217–225, 1976
28. ROTELLA RJ: Systematic desensitization. Psychological rehabilitation of injured athletes. In Bunker L, Rotella R (eds): Sport Psychology: From Theory to Practice. Charlottesville, Virginia, Deparment of Health and Physical Education, University of Virginia, 1978
29. SELYE H: The Stress of Life. New York, McGraw-Hill, 1956
30. STERNBACK R: Pain: Psychophysiological Analysis. New York, Academic Press, 1968

The Head

In some sports, the athlete must use his head as a prime impact area—for example, when heading a ball in soccer or landing on the forehead while carrying an opponent in Greco-Roman wrestling. In tackle football, the helmet and face-mask system is now so effective that some players illegally use the head as a battering ram and an offensive weapon. The risk of neck injury thus rises, especially if the player's neck is weak.

Although the number of fatal head injuries in tackle football has dropped over the last two decades, the number of paralyzing neck injuries has risen.[76] Moreover, although there are now fewer head injuries, such injuries are devastating. The doctor, trainer, coach, and athlete must try to prevent these injuries, recognize the danger signs of head injury, and be able to care for the head-injured athlete. Every effort should be made to protect the athlete's brain because brain injury may lead to epilepsy, dementia, or death.

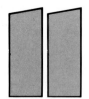

Athletic Injuries to the Head, Face, and Neck

Concussions

A *concussion,* derived from the Latin *concussus,* meaning "to shake violently," is a temporary disturbance of brain function that occurs without a structural change in the brain. About 50,000 concussions occur each year in tackle football as a result of blows to the head, and about one of eight collegiate football players sustains a concussion during his career. Although a concussion does not produce gross changes in the brain, it may produce neuronal, chemical, or neuroelectrical changes. This "scrambling of connections" takes time to reorganize.

Concussions may be graded as mild, moderate, or severe. The severity of a concussion seems to correlate best with the duration of unconsciousness.[66] A mild concussion produces a stunned, dazed athlete. The athlete is "out on his feet" but promptly regains awareness of the surroundings; no confusion, headache, dizziness, nausea, or visual disturbance results. The athlete feels well in 1 or 2 minutes and exhibits no unsteadiness or lack of coordination. It is easy for the athlete to hop on

225

one foot and tightrope-walk a straight line. Neurologic examination findings are normal.

The football player with a mild concussion should be kept out of action for a series of downs, a cautious approach that benefits both the athlete and the team. A dazed athlete is extremely vulnerable to further injury because his coordination is abnormal. Moreover, if the player returns to the game dazed, he may drop passes, miss handoffs and assignments, and fumble. The examiner should observe, examine, and question the athlete but should not return him to the lineup immediately. The player must be able to demonstrate that he can fully perform the techniques he must use in the game; when he does resume play, he should continue to be observed from the sideline.

A moderate concussion results in loss of consciousness, some mental confusion, and retrograde amnesia. Injured athletes sometimes have ringing in their ears, dizziness, and unsteadiness. Recovery may be fast, and after a few minutes the athlete may demonstrate good skill performance. But because he was knocked out and has amnesia for the plays and other events accompanying his injury, he should remain out of the game. He may return to the next practice if he is mentally clear, free of headache, and not confused, dizzy, or nauseated.

The severely concussed athlete will remain unconscious longer than the moderately concussed one. When he awakens, he will have a headache, dizziness, ringing in his ears, and be confused and unsteady. Memory is lost for the events associated with the injury, and he may have other recent memory loss. Of course, he may not return to play. If the athlete remains groggy or if his condition worsens, he should be hospitalized for observation. If he suffers a concussion and the examiner feels that he should be awakened at night for a check, the player had best be observed at the hospital.

Other players sometimes notify the trainer or physician that a teammate is acting strange in the huddle. The athlete may be able to walk normally but still have a concussion. If concussion is suspected, the player should be examined. He will usually be able to do simple mathematics, reverse spelling, and follow commands. The questions put to him, however, should involve recent memory. "What play was run when you were injured?" "Were you blocking or tackling?" "What happened at impact?" "What is the score?" The memory loss associated with concussion contrasts with the memory of the limb-injured athlete, who retains a lucid, explicit memory of the play and impact, as if the activity had occurred in slow motion.

The fixation of memories is an ongoing process that is damaged by the effects of a concussion. As information on the injury begins to be stored, the concussion disrupts the storage process. A player will recall the play signal or concussive impact when asked about it seconds after injury but lose this information permanently within minutes. It is thus important to sit the player out for a few minutes and to ask him again questions connected with recent memory.

In addition, the athlete should be asked if he has a headache, nausea, ringing in his ears, or dizziness. Inequality of the pupils, should be checked for, keeping in mind that some athletes have anisocoria (unequal pupils) normally. A baseline blood pressure and pulse rate should be recorded and the player then asked to close his eyes and to hold his arms out to his side with palms up. Downward drift of an arm is a sign of hemiparesis. More subtly, a forearm may pronate—the "pronator drift." The finger-to-nose test should be done, and as another test of control the athlete should be asked to reach out his foot to touch the examiner's hand.

If the athlete can easily hop on one foot, there probably is no corticospinal or corticocerebellar damage. He should be asked to tightrope-walk along a line and then stand with his eyes closed. If he wobbles, he should not be allowed to re-enter the game. Of course, waxing and waning of consciousness and continued grogginess are signs necessitating immediate hospitalization.

After a concussion, the athlete may be allowed to return to practice when he has no headache, has no trouble remembering, and is not irritable or tired.

Return to Contact Sports

The athlete must be thoroughly evaluated by a physician before being allowed to return to contact sports after a concussion. The dictum "three concussions and you're out" is too simple. One severe concussion may be sufficient for the team physician to recommend that the athlete avoid contact sports. Some doctors will not allow the athlete to play contact sports after he has had four moderate or two severe concussions. There is no simple rule, however, that applies to all athletes. Consciousness should be graded and a decision made based on severity of the concussions, their aftermath, and the risk to the athlete of serious, permanent brain damage.

"Knock-Out"

The most common knock-out blow is to the chin or "button." This twists and distorts the brain stem and overwhelms the reticular-activating mechanism (sleep-wake center), sending a sudden bombardment of impulses to the brain and rendering the boxer, for instance, unconscious. When a boxer is knocked down, striking the ring floor may cause more serious damage than the blow from his opponent. Ring floors are more safely constructed today than before, being made of canvas stretched over shock-absorbing Ensolite. The boxer may also be knocked out as his head strikes the cable ropes or ring posts or from a succession of hard blows. A blow to the eye or neck may produce severe pain, causing loss of consciousness, and a blow to the carotid sinus, heart, or solar plexus may block blood flow and cause the boxer to lose consciousness. Punches to the thin-walled temporal area may lead to loss of balance and dizziness.

Unfortunately, former fighters or steeple chase jockeys who have suffered many blows to the head may develop brainstem hemorrhages that result in diffuse neuronal destruction and the clinical appearance of dementia pugilistica ("punch drunk").[51] Such persons become irritable and depressed, with slurred and monotonous speech. They move slowly with an unsteady gait, have tremors, and must endure dull headaches and seizures.

Stroke

In young athletes with little or no atherosclerosis, brain stem stroke may result from vertebral artery trauma after neck rotation and extension. In this condition, the rotation or extension of the spine compromises vertebral artery blood flow.

The vertebral arteries ascend in transverse foramina up to the level of the axis. They then abandon their vertical course and are susceptible as they pass upward and outward to reach the transverse foramina of the atlas, from which point they enter the skull to form the basilar artery.

Most of the movement during neck extension and rotation occurs at the atlantoaxial and atlantooccipital joints, where the vertebral arteries lie unprotected. Excessive rotation may sublux the atlantoaxial joint, and the contralateral vertebral artery may be especially vulnerable to stretching and compression within the transverse foramen of the atlas, reducing blood flow to the brain.[35] Two thirds of all persons have significant discrepancies in the size of their vertebral arteries, with the left usually being larger than the right. Ischemia is more likely when the smaller vessel is compressed than when the dominant artery is compressed. Hyperextension causes the atlas to slide forward and stretch and compress the vertebral arteries within the transverse foramen of the atlas.

In one case, a wrestler who hyperextended and rotated his neck while bridging had several half-Nelsons applied to him shortly thereafter.[63] He then developed vertigo, ataxia, numbness of the left side of his face, and tingling in his body. Transient singultus prevented him from swallowing when he tried to drink water. Similar neck manipulations in yoga may also cause a stroke involving the brain stem.

Other Severe Injuries

One blow to the head, or the cumulative effect of many blows, may tear veins that pass from the brain to the dura, producing a subdural hematoma. Veins are usually torn on the side opposite the blow, a "contrecoup" injury. Veins may also be ripped when the brain strikes the sharp sphenoidal ridge, the bony prominence of the anterior fossa, or the free edge of the tentorium. The blood collects slowly over hours or weeks. The injured person notes a headache, intermittent drowsiness, lack of concentration, mild confusion, and slow deterioration of consciousness, and death may ensue. These persons should be examined serially, and the blood may require evacuation. A chronic subdural hematoma may be subtle, causing headache, nausea, blurred vision, irritability, and personality changes.

A skull fracture that extends across the groove of the middle menigeal artery may sever the artery, causing a rapid epidural accumulation of blood. Initially, in the so-called "lucid period," the athlete may seem well. Ten to 20 minutes later, however, danger signs of decreased consciousness and motor problems appear. X-rays may show a fracture line that is usually more lucent than are vascular markings because it extends through the entire thickness of the skull. The line also is usually sharply angled or straight, unlike the gentle arcs and branchings of vascular markings. Immediate surgery is imperative because an epidural hematoma is life-threatening.

A basilar skull fracture may cause periobital ecchymosis, or "raccoon eyes." Other signs of this fracture are subcutaneous ecchymosis in the mastoid area, or "Battle's sign," and blood that lies behind the tympanic membranes to produce a blue and bulging eardrum. The basilar fracture may be seen on a Towne's X-ray view that shows the vault of the skull without overlap from the facial bones. A petrous bone fracture may cause bleeding from the ear if the tympanic membrane has been ruptured. In these cases, a speculum should not be inserted into the ear canal, as it may cause contamination. Serious brain injury with herniation of the uncus produces a palsy of the third cranial nerve and anisocoria. Vertical nystagmus also connotes injury to the brain.

On-the-Field Evaluation of Head Injuries

If an athlete is lying on the field unconscious, a head and neck injury should be assumed until proven otherwise. The rescuer should grasp the athlete's jaw and pull it forward to protect him from swallowing his tongue. This should be done gently, as there may be a major neck injury. Ammonia ampules should not be placed under the athlete's nose because they may cause him to jerk his head away and damage his spinal cord.

The athlete is placed on a backboard with his head immobilized between sandbags or held fixed with a four-way strap. The face mask should be removed; the helmet usually is not removed because improper removal may cause undue neck motion. Some masks are hinged, or the rubber face mask mounting loops may be cut to allow the mask to swing away. If the face mask must be cut, heavy-duty bolt cutters will do the job efficiently. Bolt cutters should always be at hand, taped to the headboard. If the player's helmet must be removed, two persons must do the job:[43] One applies longitudinal traction while the second places his one hand behind the player's neck and grasps the player's jaw with his other hand. He maintains traction while the first rescuer spreads the helmet and removes it from the injured player's head.

Athletes who wear contact lenses should be identified so that the lenses may be removed if the athlete is knocked unconscious.

Footballer's Migraine

Blows to a player's head from a soccer ball, especially unexpected and accidental blows, may initiate migraine headaches by distorting the player's intracerebral vessels.[50] At the beginning of a match, the soccer ball will weigh 400 g, but old leather balls become much heavier on a wet pitch. The balls may travel at

50 km/h (30 miles/h); thus they may have a heavy impact. Migraine headaches have also been reported after blows to the side of the head in wrestling, a condition attributed to trauma-induced cerebral vasospasm. Tunnel vision, tingling in the hands, general headache, and vomiting may accompany a migraine headache. These cases demand a careful neurologic examination.

Helmets

Tackle Football

Tackle football helmets have changed dramatically since the 1890s, when the first unpadded leather headgear was worn. In the late 1930s, internal suspension systems were added, and in 1950, rigid outer shells with pneumatic and hydraulic inner suspension systems became available. The air-padded helmets are preferred by professional tackle football players today (Fig. 11-1).

Better energy-absorbing systems are being placed into helmets to protect against brain injury, and helmets have become so sophisticated and protective of the head that they now endanger the wearer's neck and his opponent's body.[59, 75] One study showed that helmets were responsible for 12% of the total injuries in high school football.[7] Similarly, almost 10% of professional tackle football injuries are produced by a blow from an opponent's helmet.

Minimum protective standards are now compiled by the National Operating Committee on Standards for Athletic Equipment (NOCSAE). Helmets are tested by dropping them from heights of 3, 4, and 5 feet to land on an Ensolite-covered steel block. The helmet is positioned to land on its top, front, rear, right and left front, and right and left rear sections under varied environmental conditions.[61] Football helmets must have rebound capabilities, unlike those used in motor sports racing which are designed to absorb a high impact only once. All National Collegiate Athletic Association institutions now require that helmets meet NOCSAE standards, and high schools must also meet these minimum standards.

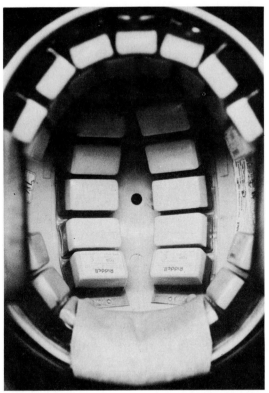

FIG. 11-1
The interior of this football helmet contains individual vinyl foam air cushions that conform to the shape of the player's head and absorb shock. Other helmets have inflatable air cells, liquid cells, and suspension systems.

A poorly fitted helmet is a dangerous piece of equipment, but when properly fitted it affords the athlete a remarkable degree of protection. Faulty technique and improper fit are the real villains in the rise of neck injuries. Most legal claims have been associated with such injuries, even though the helmet was not shown conclusively to be at fault. As a result of legal judgments against helmet manufacturers, about one half of the cost of a helmet is absorbed by liability premiums.[59]

Motorcycle

Although motocross competitors are required to wear crash helmets, motorcyclists are not required to wear a helmet on the highways in most states. Motorcycle crash helmets are designed to absorb a high impact only once, and they have poor rebound capability. The helmet also serves as a place to attach the facemask that prevents stones and bugs from striking the driver's eyes. The best protection against facial injury is a full-face helmet.

Laws requiring the use of crash helmets by motorcyclists have been repealed in many states, and deaths have doubled where such laws have been repealed.[37] Those who argue for repeal claim that a helmet decreases the driver's ability to hear, lowers his peripheral vision, and increases neck injuries and that the requirement is a violation of a person's rights.

These arguments are countered by studies showing that hearing is not reduced because there is no change in the signal-to-noise ratio.[37] Even wrap-around, full-face helmets allow 109° of peripheral vision on each side of the nose, an amount that satisfies Department of Transportation safety standards. There is no evidence of increased neck injuries. With respect to the rights issue, taxpayers must often underwrite lifelong medical bills and maintenance costs for head-injured cyclists, who frequently do not have insurance.

Bicycle

Many bicyclists forego helmets, even though they achieve high speeds on hard roads with potholes and traffic dangers. Among head protectors, the "leather hairnet" can prevent scrapes but provides only minimal shock-absorption. Vegetable bowl-shaped styrofoam helmets are better and can protect the cyclist's head in a fall from saddle height. They do not, however, cover the vital temporal region that can strike curbs. In addition to protecting the head, a white or fluorescent helmet helps to identify a cyclist.

Equestrian

Almost all serious head injuries in our equestrian study occurred to helmetless riders.[34] Fewer than 20% of all horseback riders wear a helmet, and even if they do, the helmet usually flies off when the rider falls, as most riders fail to attach the chin strap. Most helmets are little more than decorative shells anyway and afford little protection if they do stay on the rider's head.

Steeple-chase jockeys who suffer many falls may, like boxers, become "punch drunk" with traumatic encephalopathy and epilepsy.[46] The Jockeys Association in Great Britain and the British Standards Association have cooperated in the design of helmets for jockeys and for exercise boys and girls. These rigid shells contain energy-absorbing liners and floating cushions with temple protection and a secure cap retainer. Wearing this headgear has resulted in dramatically reduced numbers of severe, and sometimes fatal, head injuries.[34]

Baseball and Cricket

Little League baseball rules require protective helmets for batters, catchers, baserunners, first and third base coaches, and on-deck hitters. These helmets have saved many lives, as a pitched ball may travel 112 km/h (70 miles/h) and a batted ball more than 160 km/h (100 miles/h). For further protection, the on-deck circle should be in a safe location and all dugouts fenced in. Major leaguers usually wear a modified batting helmet while at bat, but the helmet only protects one side of the head, and if the batter ducks the wrong way he can be struck in the bare temple.

A cricket cap may soften a blow from the 154-g (5.5-oz) leather cricket ball. The bowler stands only 6.6 m (22 ft) from the batter, and the ball may bounce unpredictably at the batter from the turf or may glance off his bat. Peaked caps, such as baseball and kayak caps, block the sun's rays from striking the athlete's forehead and help to prevent headaches. The kayak cap may also be dunked in water and put on as a refreshing headpiece.

Hockey, Lacrosse, and Jai Alai

A hockey helmet should have a shock-resistant lining and padding in the temporal regions. The helmet not only protects a player's head but serves as an anchor for the facemask. A hockey helmet with a suspension system but without padding leaves the player's head susceptible to a depressed skull fracture from the hard puck. Lacrosse helmets, although only thin shells with a small visor, serve to anchor the face mask. Jai alai players also wear hard, plastic caps that are unfit to protect their heads from balls almost the size of baseballs and harder than golf balls that travel faster than 160 km/h (100 miles/h).

The Face

Face masks have helped significantly to reduce the number of facial injuries in tackle football, hockey, lacrosse, and motocross. In the 1950s most tackle football injuries were to the face, such as bloody noses, cut lips, and dental injuries. In 1955, face masks and mouth guards were recommended for high school football; by 1960 a face mask was required, and in 1962 the mouth guard was made mandatory. Players at first wore a single bar face mask, then a double bar. A vertical bar was added later, and more recently the birdcage face mask has become popular.

Quarterbacks, wide receivers, and running backs will often sacrifice protection for an unobstructed view. Face guards do restrict the visual field slightly at knee level and below, making it harder to see a low opponent.[67] Special face masks help to reduce injury; if a player must wear eyeglasses, for example, a specially designed face mask may be used. Mounting loops on a helmet allow the face mask to absorb blows.

The face mask must fit properly. If the bar style is fitted too low, it provides little protection for the facial area. If fitted too high, the bars obstruct vision and the mandible is exposed. By placing the face mask closer to the face, leverage is reduced if the face mask is grabbed by an opposing player. When a cage mask is fitted too close to the face, however, the angle of the mandible may be lacerated during violent contact as the cage is driven back and bent. Face masks should be checked each week for loosened screws and bolts. If no face masks were worn, the large number of severe neck injuries probably would be reduced, as a player wearing only a helmet and mouth guard would be less likely to head-tackle, butt-block, or spear.[66] Lost teeth or facial scarring would be a reasonable trade-off for serious head and neck injuries. Without a face mask, however, the player might tend to close his eyes and drop his head, and even more injuries could result.

Before introduction of the face mask, eye injuries were common in ice hockey.[58] Two thirds of those injuries were caused by the stick and the rest by the puck, but blindness resulted equally from both objects. Full face wire mesh and polycarbonate hockey masks reduce facial injuries by preventing the stick or puck from penetrating. Although goaltenders often wear an expensive, molded fiberglass mask, the puck can still get through to cause a hyphema or worse injury. Plastic shield face protectors are satisfactory if kept in good condition but may fog up and scratch.

When lacrosse face masks had only horizontal bars, the number of facial injuries was large, as the stick and balls could squeeze through (Fig. 11-2). The addition of a mandatory vertical bar has helped to reduce the number of facial injuries (Fig. 11-2).

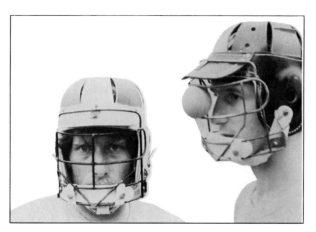

FIG. 11-2
A lacrosse ball could enter the old-style lacrosse mask to damage a player's eye (*right*). The recently mandated vertical bar should reduce the number of facial injuries (*left*).

Serious motocross competitors wear a face mask, and such masks and helmets should be worn by all motorcyclists. The motorcyclist's mask keeps flying objects, stones, and bugs from injuring his eyes and helps a driver avoid losing control of his vehicle. A full face helmet will give even better protection against severe facial injuries from motorcycle crashes.

Eye Injuries In Athletics

Because the opening to the eyeball is small, large objects, such as soccer balls and basketballs, may be deflected before their kinetic energy reaches the eye.[14] Almost any kind of ball, however, may become deformed and seriously contuse the globe, despite protection provided by the skull's bony rims. Moreover although the eyeball is surrounded by bony rims and is elastic and embedded in a resilient fat pad, minor trauma may cause eventual blindness, as when glaucoma develops after an injury,

Facial Cuts

The boxer's face may be cut by friction from laces rubbed over it, by pinching of the skin between the boxing glove and the orbital bone, and by head-butting. The cuts usually occur in the supraorbital region but may occur infraorbitally and in the lid. A supraorbital cut may trickle blood into the eye, interfering with the boxer's vision.

Cuts cannot be treated between rounds in the Olympic games, but a cut can be fixed in other amateur and professional bouts. The periorbital cut should be wiped clean, pushed shut, pressure applied, and then coated with an astringent. Pressure should not be used, however, if there is a chance that the globe has ruptured. A layer of flexible collodian is next applied and Vaseline smeared around the cut so that further blows will slide off. After the fight, the cut should be minimally debrided and closed in layers to keep it from scarring down to bone. If not so treated, the cut will open easily. Stitches should be placed about 2 mm apart, tied loosely, and a pressure dressing applied.

To minimize scarring, the stitches may be left in only 3 to 5 days, and the athlete should not box for 4 weeks.

The eyelid consists of two halves: The anterior half contains skin and orbicularis muscle; the posterior half contains the tarsus and conjunctiva. Vertical lid lacerations, and lacerations that include the canthal tendons and lacrimal drainage system, should be treated by a practitioner with experience in oculoplastic surgery. A thorough eye examination, including dilated fundus examination, should be done to exclude damage to the eyeball.

Boxers should wear headgear while sparring and during collegiate and service team bouts. The soft leather boxing headgear is padded with latex foam rubber or animal hair to protect the boxer's eyes, temples, and base of the skull; some models even protect the jaw.

Conjunctival Irritation

Dust and dirt from playing surfaces irritate an athlete's eyes, while sweat may be rubbed into his eyes by dirty fingers. If the conjunctiva becomes irritated, foreign bodies or corneal abrasions might be suspected. Antibiotic drops should be administered only by an ophthalmologist after a slit-lamp examination; they should never be given at the time of an initial corneal abrasion.

After a few hours in bright and reflected sun, a skier or yachtsman's cornea may suffer sunburn in which the eyes become irritated and the athlete is then unable to tolerate bright light. Dark glasses or goggles will prevent this type of sunburn.

Finger in the Eye

In basketball, fingers are sometimes poked in the eye while players scramble for the ball, and a fingernail may scrape the eyeball. During cross-country skiing, a skier's cornea may be abraded by a tree limb. Such minor accidents may result in serious injury to the eye, including hyphema (blood in the anterior chamber), dislocation of the lens, and a retinal detachment. These conditions should never be overlooked on examination. All fingernails should be inspected and trimmed before games and practices and players required to remove rings and other jewelry that may endanger opponents or their teammates. Cross-country skiers are advised to wear eyeglasses or goggles while skiing in the woods.

To assess eye problems and to protect an injured eye, the physician should carry a local anesthetic, fluorescein strips, a concentrated light source, a small, near-vision card, eye patches, hard protective shields, and tape.

Fluorescein drops demonstrate superficial eye scrapes as bright green marks where the epithelium is absent. The marks are especially easy to see when a cobalt blue light is used for the examination. Scratched eyes should be patched. In this procedure, a pad is folded into the hollow of the orbit and then topped with a second pad. The athlete should be instructed to keep both eyes shut while wearing a patch, since blinking only further irritates the eye. Corneal injuries should be checked by an ophthalmologist because the abrasion may be a laceration. The eye patch should be worn for 24 hours, then the eye rechecked and patched for another 24 hours, which is usually sufficient time for healing to take place.

Foreign Body in the Eye

If a foreign body enters the athlete's eye, it may lodge in the upper or lower fornix or on the conjunctival or corneal surfaces, producing the sensation of being under the upper lid. Oblique illumination from a concentrated light source may be needed to determine its precise location. A foreign body at the lower lid is easily removed by pulling the lower lid down and gently wiping it away with a cotton bud.

When a foreign body is under the upper lid, an attempt should be made to move it to the lower lid. The athlete should first be asked to look down, and the upper lid should then be gently pulled over the lower lid to produce tears that may flush the object to the lower part of the eye. If the foreign body remains under the upper lid, the lid should be pulled out before folding it upwards over a cotton bud to expose the tarsal conjunctival surface. Another cotton bud may be used to wipe away the object.

Tennis Eye

Eye injuries may occur unexpectedly if an athlete is off guard, as in tennis when a player's eye is struck during a warm-up when more than one ball is in play (Fig. 11-3). When volleying, players' eyes are vulnerable to hard-hit balls and to balls that skip off the net. Balls hit in anger or frustration after a player loses a point may strike an opponent who is not alert. Players with poor vision may have difficulty following the flight of the ball and be injured.

Squash balls and racquetballs are especially dangerous because they are small enough to fit into the orbit of the eye. The wild swings of inexperienced players send balls flying off at dangerous angles and velocities. In badminton, the 1.9-cm (0.75-in) diameter striking end of the shuttlecock similarly endangers the eyes.

In the excitement of a racket game, the player may underestimate the severity of a blow to his eye. The blow may cause temporary blurring with rapid recovery, but weeks or even years later the player may have serious vision loss from a detached retina that progressed from an asymptomatic peripheral break. For this reason, when a player's eye is struck by any small ball, an ophthalmologic checkup is desirable to rule out intraocular damage. An early fundoscopic examination, with the pupil fully dilated, may reveal hemorrhage and edema in the peripheral retina, indicating a small tear. Proper observation and treatment will prevent extension of the tear. Any player with subjective disturbance of vision, altered visual acuity, loss of visual field or diploplia, excessive edema, and chemosis or hemorrhage into the anterior chamber should consult with an ophthalmologist.

A player looking around at a partner who is serving should have his racquet up as a guard. Ordinary eyeglasses will not protect the eyes in tennis, as the lens may be pushed against the eye. To prevent this, tennis players should wear either an eyeguard or a sports frame with pop-

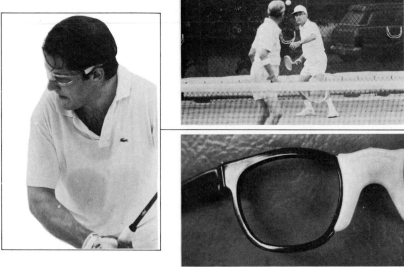

FIG. 11-3
Eyeguards help to protect the eyes in racquet sports (*left*). A tennis ball
may cause an eye injury as the player at the net glances around to see
what his partner is doing (*upper right*). Nylon frames with fly-away
temple pieces are the best type of frame (*lower left*), if "glasses" must
be worn.

out lenses and rotating earpieces (Fig. 11-3).
Closed eyeguards should be mandatory for
squash and racquetball players, and novice badminton players are especially well advised to
wear safety glasses because inexperienced players frequently suffer eye injuries.

"Black Eye"

Blows to a boxer's eye may rupture small
blood vessels in the subcutaneous tissue of the
eyelid. This skin is the thinnest in the body,
and the subcutaneous supporting structures are
equally tenuous. Hemorrhage here causes rapid
and extensive swelling, shutting the lid. The
eyeball should be checked for blood before it
swells shut and the orbital bones palpated. A
swollen eye should not be dismissed as a minor
contusion because a blow may dislocate the lens
or produce a hyphema, retinal edema, retinal
hemorrhage, vitreous hemorrhage, retinal tear,
or retinal detachment. The globe may have
ruptured, causing intraocular hemorrhage and
loss of vision. If the lids are swollen shut or if
the eye is clearly difficult to examine, it should

not be forced open, and an ophthalmologist
should be promptly consulted.

Swelling is usually self-limiting, and ice bags
may be applied during the first 24 hours. Instant cold packs should not be placed over the
eyes because they occasionally leak small
amounts of chemicals through tiny holes. Some
boxing handlers will cut a boxer's eyelid with
a razor blade to evacuate blood, an unacceptable
practice with little practical value, as the blood
has spread diffusely through the tissues and is
not loculated. The blood supply to the lids will
help to resorb such interstitial blood within a
few weeks.

Hyphema

A blow to the eye may damage small vessels
of the ciliary body, which hemorrhage into the
anterior chamber between the cornea and the
iris. The athlete reports blurred vision, photo-
phobia, and aching eye pain. The eye reddens
and blood appears, producing a fluid level in
the anterior chamber. Eyes with this condition
should be shielded immediately and the athlete

placed under the care of an ophthalmologist. Bedrest is obligatory, since further hemorrhage notoriously occurs in the first few days and the second hemorrhage may be worse than the first. The hyphema may prevent a clear view of the retina for several days, but most hyphemas are absorbed within a week. After absorption takes place, the ophthalmologist can dilate the pupil to check for retinal damage, and the patient should be followed for life to avert the development of secondary glaucoma.

Retinal Detachment

A blow to the eye may be followed by detachment of the retina, especially in athletes with a predisposing familial history. Detachment is most likely to occur in persons with retinal degenerative lesions, such as myopia. Constant agitation of the vitreous body may be accompanied by retinal traction sufficient to cause breaks in a retina that is thin or diseased. For this reason, some ophthalmologists caution myopic people, especially those who have had previous retinal detachment, against jogging. A retinal detachment may occur weeks or months after an injury. Retinal breaks, with or without detachment, require the expertise of an ophthalmologist for full assessment and appropriate treatment.

Blow-Out Fracture of the Orbit

If a fist, elbow, or ball strikes the orbit, blunt trauma may increase intraorbital hydrostatic pressure and break the inferomedial margin of the orbit. Because this weak bone may fracture even without an associated orbital rim fracture, the athlete should be sent to an ophthalmologist with the eye shielded after any blunt trauma.

An athlete with a blow-out fracture of the orbit will develop periorbital edema and hemorrhage; when this subsides, he may have double vision. The infraorbital rim may feel abnormal, and the inferior rectus muscle may become tethered to the fracture, interfering with ocular movements.

Water's x-ray view, Caldwell view, and a coned-down view of the orbital floor will reveal bone fragments that have been driven into the maxillary antrum from the orbital floor.

Tomography is the best means to evaluate the extent of the damage, and surgery is usually performed in 7 to 14 days.

Contact Lenses

Many athletes wear contact lenses to avoid the disadvantages of spectacles, which may have heavy frames, fog up, and require cages, masks, and elastic straps.[28] Spectacles can also be knocked off or a spectacle lens pushed into the orbit. Although hard contact lenses are particularly beneficial to athletes who have astigmatism, such lenses may slide off center, pop out, and be lost. Moreover, wind and dust particles may slide under them to cause serious eye abrasions. These sudden and often painful distractions may be dangerous in some sports, negating the advantages of such lenses. For the athlete who wears contact lenses, a cage or mask is still advisable because a broken contact lens may be more dangerous than a shatter-proof spectacle lens.

Soft contact lenses are generally more comfortable than hard contact lenses.[70] Vision is often not as crisp, however, and astigmatism not as well corrected with soft lenses. Swimmers usually can wear the soft lenses if goggles are used. These lenses require considerably more care than hard lenses and are more expensive. Proper care of soft lenses requires distilled water, saline solution, special lens cases, and a heating unit. The team physician and trainer should know which athletes are wearing contact lenses, and if a wearer is knocked unconscious the lenses should be removed immediately.

Eyeguards

Because a badminton bird, squash ball, or racquetball may cause eye injuries, some clubs require players to wear eye protectors. Such protection is important not only for myopic and novice players but also for skilled players. The skilled player is less likely to give up control of center court, thus increasing the risk of eye injury from the racquet or ball.

A myopic athlete's eyeglass lenses are concave, with the center section of the lens thinner than the outer edge, subjecting it to easy breakage. To give optimum protection, the lens center should be at least a 3-mm thick CR39 plastic or polycarbonate plastic.[17] Plastic lenses have a higher resistance to breakage than do glass lenses and are lighter, give less surface reflection, and are less likely to fog.

Although plastic lenses do not easily break, they can be broken and may pop through an ordinary frame. Such lenses should be mounted in a sports frame made of nylon with a steep posterior lip. When a lens in a sports frame is struck, it projects forward instead of being driven toward the eye. The athlete should wear a nylon frame with temples that rotate about 180°. Currently popular metal frames should be avoided because they can cut the face or damage the eye easily.

All open eyeguards do not provide equal protection, and direct shots from a racquetball or squash ball can strike and damage the eye through the space between the upper and lower rims of some guards. Closed eyeguards with either plain or prescription lenses will prevent such injuries. An open eyeguard is, however, better than none because it will prevent slashes from racquets and damage from off-center hits.[17] Sturdy goggles are recommended for skiers, as cheap plastic goggles can shatter into tiny pieces.★

Facial Bone Fracture

A blow to the angle of the jaw, the point of the chin, or the side of the chin may break an athlete's jaw and fracture the thin facial bones (Fig. 11-4).[24] Although the mandible is stronger than the maxilla, it is weak at the canine teeth, the third molars, and the condylar necks, the places where most mandibular fractures occur.

To diagnose a facial bone fracture, the physician should palpate the bone edges for a step-off or crepitus. He should then place traction on the chin to elicit condylar neck pain. To detect a midthird facial bone fracture, the examiner should press down on the vertex of the

★ For a copy of eye protection recommendations or other information on eye safety in sports, contact the National Society to Prevent Blindness, 79 Madison Avenue, New York, NY 10016.

athlete's head while pressing upward in the vault of his palate with the index finger. These maneuvers will produce pain and bony movement at the fracture. The upper incisors may be grasped with one hand and the nose with the other; the incisors are then wiggled. Facial bone fracture must be diagnosed early, as the excellent blood supply of the facial bones will otherwise allow them to heal rapidly in a poor position, resulting in an unacceptable malocclusion of the teeth.

Facial bone fractures may be wired and healing achieved in about 6 weeks. Most athletes may resume sport after 8 weeks, but a boxer must wait 3 months before returning to the ring. A special face mask will afford protection to an athlete after a facial bone fracture. In football, for example, an extra face bar may be added to the helmet to protect the player's injured jaw (Fig. 11-5).

Ear Injuries in Athletics

"Scrum Ear" and "Wrestler's Ear"

When an athlete's ear is repetitively rubbed or when it absorbs many blows or a single blow, blood may leak between the skin and the perichondrium. The ear then becomes throbbingly painful, tender, and swollen. After a few hours, a well-defined, smooth, rounded mass forms within the helix fossa. Blood and serum collects on both sides of the ear cartilage, isolating the cartilage from the soft tissue upon which its nutrition and vitality depend. The cartilage may then die and collapse. If the ear is not properly treated, the hematoma will organize and scar down within a few weeks, pulling the ear into a contorted, cauliflowerlike configuration—the gnarled ear of a boxer, the scrum ear of a rugby player, or wrestler's ear.

Hot spots from friction during wrestling practice may be prevented by smearing Vaseline on the ears. The lubricant is, however, prohibited during matches. Wrestlers should wear earguards, especially during wrestling practice, where the wrestler spends 95% of his time (Fig. 11-6). The headgear must be well

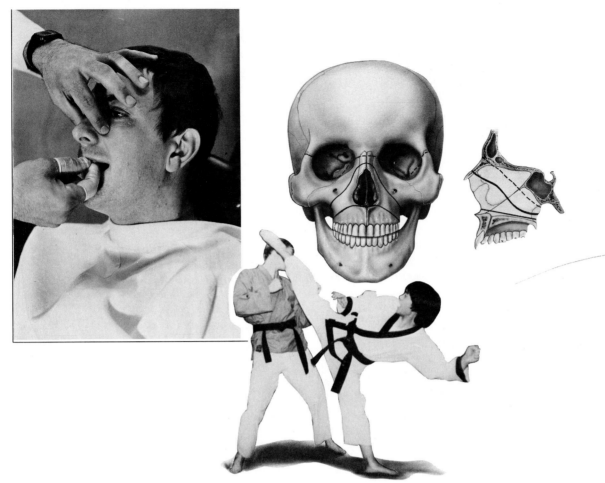

FIG. 11-4
A blow to the face (*lower right*) may produce a facial bone fracture
(lines on the skeleton). One diagnostic maneuver to diagnose a facial
bone fracture is for the examiner to grasp the upper incisors with one
hand and the nose with the other, and then wiggle the incisors to elicit
motion and pain at the fracture (*left*).

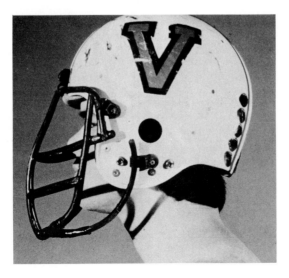

FIG. 11-5
An extension on the
face mask protects the
player's injured
mandible.

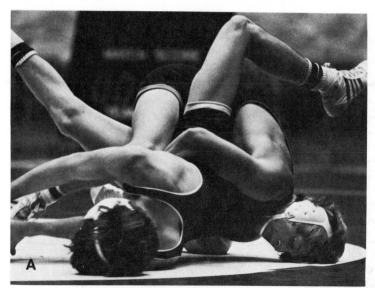

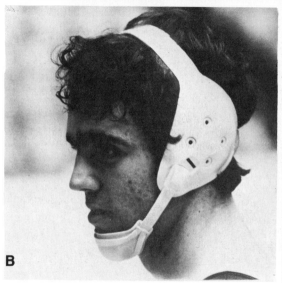

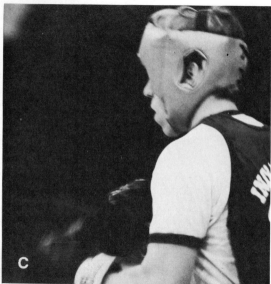

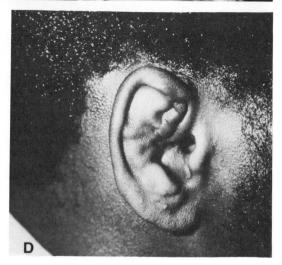

FIG. 11-6
Wrestlers (*A, B*) and boxers (*C*) wear ear protectors to protect against an auricular hematoma and a deformed ear (*D*).

fitted, as poor-fitting or loose headgear may rub and cause wrestler's ear.

If an ear has been rubbed and becomes hot, an ice pack should be applied promptly. Any hematoma should be aspirated sterilely because infection in this region may lead to chondritis, a long lasting problem. After the hematoma has been aspirated, the region may be compressed with a collodion pack, plaster of paris cast, mineral-oil-soaked cotton balls, or silicone mold. The collodion pack is a cast of cotton or strips of gauze soaked in flexible collodion.[12] The collodion applicator should be kept well saturated to place collodion on the ear before the layers of gauze are started. After 24 to 48 hours, the pack may be removed and the ear checked for any reaccumulation before being repacked. The new pack should be left in place as long as possible, and repeated if needed. Plaster of paris may also serve as a packing, but a Q-tip should be placed in the ear canal while the plaster sets. Another technique uses a cotton "stent" moistened with mineral oil and placed into all of the convolutions of the auricular folds and also postauricularly. A mastoid dressing holds the stent in position for 10 days. As an alternative to aspirating the hematoma, it may be evacuated by making multiple incisions through the skin and perichondrium.[19] Dental rolls are then sutured in place and a mastoid dressing applied.

These techniques are not without problems, as the collodion pack may easily dislodge and the collodion pack and plaster of paris cast usually lack a vent. The problems may be avoided by fashioning a silicone mold pressure dressing around the end of an applicator stick, providing a tunnel through the mold that equalizes pressure between the external auditory canal and the outside atmosphere.[33]

"Swimmer's Ear"

Swimmer's ear is an acute, diffuse external auditory canal infection usually caused by the bacterium *Pseudomonas aeruginosa* or, sometimes, by *Proteus, Escherichia coli,* or fungi.[18, 64] Humans lack the adaptations diving mammals have to prevent external ear problems. Porpoises, for example, have no external auditory canal opening, and a seal's ears are covered during dives by external skin flaps.

Swimmer's ear may develop even if pool water is sparkling clean,[73] as water washes away the ear's natural cerumen and the skin in the canal becomes irritated and itches. If the athlete then scratches in his ear, he may disrupt the continuity of the lining cells of the ear canal. These cells produce a protective acid mantle that retards bacterial growth, and individual variations in the mantle may explain why some athletes are more prone to develop swimmer's ear. An excessively curved, narrowed, or partly obstructed ear canal may trap water. Trapping also occurs when cysts, bone growths, ear wax,

ear plugs, allergies, or dermatitis blocks the canal. In some cases, the infection moves inward to cause a middle ear infection or to interfere with balance and hearing, or the infection may even advance to infect the brain.

Because the latency period for swimmer's ear is about 3 days, the association between swimming and swimmer's ear is sometimes overlooked. When the ear hurts and itches, the swimmer pulls the earlobe and rocks his jaw from side to side. On examination, the external ear canal is swollen and tender. Less often the infection is caused by a fungus; *Candida* produces yellow or white dots, and *Aspergillus nigra* forms a grayish-black membrane that coats the canal.

An infected ear canal should be reacidified with a solution of acetic or boric acid in alcohol.[18] Antibiotic and cortisone drop combinations may also be used, and alcohol and glycol drops will decrease the moisture. A cotton wick that has been soaked in Burrow's solution (aluminum acetate) should be inserted to limit further swelling. The ear debris is then carefully removed, and acid–alcohol drops are instilled. The wick should be kept moist with drops of Burrow's solution applied to it every 2 hours to bring the solution to the full length of the ear canal and keep the canal open.

The swimmer can remove trapped water and prevent swimmer's ear by vigorously shaking his head and jumping with his head tilted to one side. The ears should then be fanned or blown dry with a hair dryer. Three drops of 3% boric acid in alcohol may be put into the ear canals before and after each swim to dry the canals. For good aural hygiene, three drops of glycerin may be placed in each ear canal after a shower and the canal covered with a cotton pledget that is removed after 1 hour.

Vinegar dropped into an ear may macerate the ear canal. If cotton buds are stuck into the canal or if the concha or tragal areas are vigorously rubbed with a hand or a towel, the delicate skin surface may break. Cotton buds may also push wax against the tympanic membrane or remove too much of the protective wax. Ear plugs should not be used because they are not water tight and may trap water and cause pressure necrosis.

Osteomas and Exostoses

Some swimmers and surfers develop small, bony masses in front of the tympanic membrane.[15, 18, 23] Such growths are endemic in swimmers in cold California water but are not usually found in the ears of swimmers who swim in heated pools. Swimmers in cool ocean water should wear headgear to protect their ear canals.

A growth may be an attempt to protect against the cold water that bathes the tympanic membrane and may be an osteoma or an exostosis. An *osteoma* is a solitary unilateral bone growth attached to the tympanic squamous suture superficial or lateral to the canal isthmus. Exostoses are broad-based elevations of the bony canal that are usually multiple and bilaterally symmetrical. They lie deep or medial to the canal isthmus at the upper edge of the tympanic bone. These multilobed tumors of the external ear canal, unlike swimmer's ear, are painless but progressive. First, the inner bony part of the canal thickens with cobblestonelike swellings, and after further exposure to cold water the swellings become knucklelike. Eventually, they completely block the ear canal to produce a conductive hearing loss.

Osteomas and exostoses may be excised. If a defect remains that rings more than one third of the circumference of the ear canal, it may be closed with a skin graft.[15]

Barotrauma

Divers may experience serious problems such as cerebral arterial air embolism, joint pains (the "bends"), or venous gas pulmonary embolism (the "chokes").[78] Divers who have chronic obstructive pulmonary disease, bronchial asthma, or lung blebs sometimes trap air when they ascend from deep water, causing a pneumothorax.

More common problems affect the air-filled cavities of the sinuses and the middle ear spaces of divers.[73] These very susceptible air-filled structures have rigid walls and small openings, and the air within them must be equilibrated, continuously, with the external air pressure. Proper equilibration demands that eustachian tube and sinus ostia be patent.

The barometric pressure outside and inside the body at sea level is 14.7 lb/in², and for every 33 feet of descent in sea water the pressure increases by this amount. Barotrauma may occur even in relatively shallow dives because the greatest volume changes within tissue cavities per foot of descent occur near the surface.

"Ear squeeze" may develop during the descent phase of diving as pressure differentials cause vascular tissues to dilate and the epithelium of the sinuses and middle ear to swell. This swelling is an autoregulatory mechanism that functions to lower the pressure differential. The engorgement of the tissues decreases air volume in the cavity but may further occlude the ostia and prevent equalization of pressures. The pressure differential may then increase to produce transudation and, finally, blood vessel rupture, which reduces the pressure differential by adding blood to the cavity. With ear squeeze, the diver notices ear pain, decreased hearing, ringing in his ears, inability to clear his ears, and, sometimes, blood-tinged sputum.

When the external canal is blocked by cerumen, an osteoma, the diving hood, or an earplug, an artificial air-filled cavity external to the tympanic membrane is created. The middle ear becomes overpressurized in relation to the closed cavity between the plug and tympanic membrane, and the tympanic membrane distends outward to produce a "reverse ear squeeze."

Inexperienced divers may not be able to equalize pressure.[78] Infection, allergies, or vasomotor rhinitis may also swell the mucous membranes. Large adenoids, scarring from adenoidectomy, or congenital obstruction of the openings prevent pressure equalization.

The diver should keep the openings to his middle ear and sinuses clear by removing impacted cerumen. The ears should be checked for osteomas or exostoses, and pharangeal masses that block air passages should be removed. Divers are advised to practice equalizing pressure and are cautioned not to dive when suffering from sinusitis or during a seasonal flare-up of allergic rhinitis. Persons with disorders that might interfere with consciousness, such as seizure disorders or potential insulin reactions, should not dive.

A diver who takes a decongestant or antihistamine before diving should be aware that a "rebound" phenomenon may occur that produces swelling of the mucous membranes and barotrauma.

Tympanic Membrane Rupture

A blow to the ear in water polo, surfing, or water skiing may rupture the athlete's tympanic membrane. This injury used to be common in water polo, but players now wear caps with ear protectors, and thus the disorder is seen less often.

In competitive water skiing, the maximum boat speed is 58 km/h (36 miles/h), although the skier may go faster than the boat and a fall may rupture his tympanic membrane. The rupture occurs with a pop, and the athlete notices a decreased ability to hear. A ruptured membrane may admit cold water to produce a dangerous cold water caloric effect on the labyrinth, causing dizziness and nausea, which may panic the diver, water skier, or swimmer.

A ruptured tympanic membrane should be observed each day for signs of infection. If infection is present, antibiotic therapy should be administered; alternatively, antibiotic drops or systemic antibiotics may be given from the start to prevent infection. Steroid drops should be avoided because they retard healing. The membrane usually closes spontaneously within a week, although some otolaryngologists recommend early surgical closure of the rupture.[57]

Caloric Labyrinthitis

Stimulation of the labyrinth of the ear by cold water produces caloric labyrinthitis with vertigo, loss of balance, and nausea.

Pipkin reported on caloric labyrinthitis in an otolargyngologist who dove from a dock into a lake.[60] As cold water suddenly filled his external auditory canal, the doctor developed vertigo and lost his sense of balance. He understood, however, what was happening and, using his sense of touch, he crawled on the lake bottom to safety.

Ninety percent of all drowning victims drown within 9 m (10 yds) of shore; why so many strong swimmers drown is uncertain. Because caloric labyrinthitis may cause some of these drownings, no one should swim alone or in unfamiliar water and all boaters should wear life preservers.

Round Window Rupture

The round window membrane may rupture in skin divers, free underwater divers, snorkelers, scuba divers, and weight lifters.[18] The athlete's ear pops and a leakage of perilymph causes sudden deafness. This type of rupture demands prompt closure of the fistula, which may save some hearing. Unfortunately, the sudden hearing loss is often irreversible making prevention essential.

Divers should be advised to avoid wearing earplugs and to forego diving if they have an upper respiratory infection or allergic flare-up. Also, divers and weight lifters with already damaged ears should be advised that they risk more serious damage when they perform a Valsalva maneuver, which is increased pressure by forcible exhalation against a closed glottis.

Hearing Loss From Firearms

Repetitive impulse noise from the sudden explosive force of gunfire may produce hearing loss in marksmen and officials who must fire a starting gun at track meets. The "near ear" is subject to the greater acoustical trauma because it is closer and at a more direct angle to receive the assault.[56] The left ear is the near ear of a right-handed rifleman, whereas the right ear is the near ear of a right-handed pistol shooter.

The noise from most guns is loud enough to cause hearing loss.[55] The peak sound pressure level (PSPL) for the maximum endurable threshold of repeated impulses for ears of normal sensitivity is 150 dB. All shotguns and center-firing and rim-firing weapons have been found to exceed the damage risk level of 150 dB, except for the smaller 0.22 cartridges.

Less noise would preserve hearing and would allow marksmen to be more relaxed and to shoot more accurately.[74] The amount of powder in the cartridge and its characteristics could be reduced to decrease the PSPL, but this would alter ballistic findings.[55] Therefore, the most practical solution would be a modification of the gun barrel. In the absence of such a change, marksmen can help to reduce their hearing loss by firing on flat, open terrain and by wearing earmuffs that reduce noise by 20 to 45 dB.[56]

Nose Injuries in Athletics

Nose Bleed

The athlete with a nose bleed should sit or kneel in front of the physician and bend his head slightly forward. This position keeps him from swallowing blood, which may produce nausea and vomiting, and also lessens bleeding, since the head is above the heart. The physician places his thumb along the outside of the bleeding nostril and his index finger on the opposite side of the athlete's nose and applies steady pressure for several minutes.

When persistent, the nose should be packed, but cotton ball packings are unsafe because the athlete may inhale a piece of cotton. A regular-sized tampon will serve as packing and may be referred to as a "nose plug."[4] The tampon must be cut to fit inside the nose. Once in the nose, the material expands and conforms to the nostril. The athlete may return to the game, as the tampon is too large to be inhaled, and the nose plug can be removed later. Several tampons, with strings removed, may be carried in the trainer's kit.

Broken Nose

A nasal fracture may be determined by gently wiggling the athlete's nose at the cartilage line and above it on the bone to detect pain or grating. If displacement is noted, the nose should be splinted, and the fracture will need to be reduced. When swelling prevents a proper evaluation of external nasal deformity, ice should be applied and the nose re-evaluated in 3 days. If the diagnosis of a nasal fracture is delayed for 2 weeks, the fracture may no longer be reducible by closed means. Even though the nose contains very little bone, nasal defects may affect the eustachian tube, making clearing of the ears by inflating the middle ear difficult or impossible.

A hematoma in the nasal septum is an emergency and must be incised or aspirated and the nose packed to prevent cartilage destruction, necrosis, and development of a saddle nose deformity. A bulge may also cause nasal obstruction.

Mouth Injuries in Athletics

Mouthguards

Before face masks were added to football helmets, 50% of football injuries were in or about the mouth; after the addition of face masks, mouth injuries fell to 25% of the total. The face mask, however, offers little protection against blows under the chin from forearm blocking, from knees, or from kicks and does not block blows to the top of the head that snap the jaws shut.

Mouthguards were recommended for high school tackle football players in 1955 and made mandatory in 1962 but were not required for collegiate tackle football players until 1973.[40, 42] Today's combination of face mask and mouthguard has made mouth injuries very rare. Mouthguards have not only reduced injuries to the mouth, such as split lips and broken teeth, but also have helped decrease concussions by absorbing the energy from blows, thus damping the transmission of forces to the brain.[45, 71, 72]

Whether playing in recreational or competitive sport, every athlete should wear a mouthguard as a routine safety item,[41] whether in practices or in an actual game.

The major types of mouthguards include custom-made, mouth-formed, and stock. Custom-made mouthguards are heavy-duty ones, made of dental vinyl or plastic pulled by vacuum over a plaster mold of the athlete's teeth. A mouth-formed, thermal-set, boiled, pliable, plastic mouthguard (Fig. 11-7A) is satisfactory, but the stock rubber mouthguard is unacceptable because it may be a very poor fit. A well-

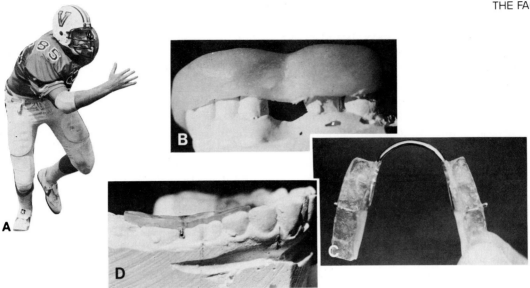

FIG. 11-7
A mouth-formed mouthguard attaches to the face mask (A). A latex mouthguard is custom-made and even fills in gaps (B). The MORA (C) is an acrylic device that corrects temporomandibular joint dysfunction; it rests on the lower teeth (D) to produce proper occlusion.

fitted mouthguard is comfortable and offers very little interference with the athlete's speech and breathing. The volume of air intake in an athlete pushed to exhaustion decreases only by about 5% with a custom-made mouthguard (Fig. 11-7B).[36]

In tackle football, the mouthguard is often attached to the player's face mask or chin piece to keep him from misplacing it. A safety strap feature allows the strap to be pulled free of the mouthguard under unusual pressure to avoid stress injury to the player's teeth. Mouthguards must be checked for wear, as many injuries occur when the guard has worn down.

Temporomandibular Joint

In addition to absorbing shocks, a mouthguard may also help to preserve an athlete's energy and to increase his strength by balancing the temporomandibular joints. When this joint is imbalanced, the nervous system picks up the fact of the malalignment when the athlete swallows and his teeth touch. As reflexes are activated, energy-sapping compensations for the malalignment occur in the athlete's back and limbs.

Some athletes have large mandibles with equally large mandibular condyles. If a large condyle is cradled in the base of an average size skull, there is less tolerance in the joint and a greater susceptibility to concussion. Athletes with deep overbite occlusion problems usually have small condyles and average-sized heads. These persons lack anterior muscle supports for their heads and necks, resulting in an overuse of the posterior cervical muscles and more strained necks and pinched nerves.[71, 72]

An orthodontist can place a resilient bite plate between the occlusal surfaces of the upper and lower teeth to suspend the condyle away from the fossa, providing the temperomandibular joint with more tolerance. The plate also gives posterior occlusal support needed to balance the head.

Richard Kaufman, a sports orthodontist, fit the American luge team with MORA (mandibular orthopedic repositioning appliance) mouthpieces to relax their tense head and neck muscles and reduce headaches and back pain.[80] The MORA mouthpiece (Fig. 11-7C) comprises two strips of acrylic that fit precisely over the lower molars and bicuspids (Fig. 11-7D). The mouthpiece is held painlessly in place by two small stainless steel clasps that latch between the first and second bicuspids. The orthodontist adjusts the appliances, repositioning the condyles and balancing them from left to right as needed. With the MORA mouthpiece in place, the athlete can speak and breathe normally. The temperomandibular joint is thus balanced, reflex activity at the joint is reduced, and the athlete has added strength and endurance.[80]

Tooth Problems

Tooth problems may be prevented by preseason checkups and early dental care. Equipment for dental emergencies should include a kit containing forceps, sterile cotton, sterile saline, oil of clove (Eugenol), calcium hydroxide (Dycal), and temporary filling material (Cavit).

If an athlete loses a filling, forceps and sterile cotton may be used to clean the area and oil of clove and calcium hydroxide placed in the hole before a temporary filling is added. When a toothache accompanies the lost filling, the area should be cleaned with sterile cotton and a small ball of oil-of-clove-wetted cotton placed into the cavity. The cotton is then covered with temporary filling material. The subject then bites down to compress the temporary filling. When a tooth is chipped and the nerve exposed, calcium hydroxide may be applied to the uncovered nerve area.

When knocked out, a tooth should be promptly washed with sterile saline but not rubbed. An ice pack may be applied to the face, with the athlete holding the tooth in its bed with his fingers or by keeping his mouth closed. He should then see a dentist, who may be able to align the tooth and keep it in place with arch bars or dental bands. If the periodontal membrane heals, the tooth will be reattached solidly.

A Panorex X-ray should be taken to rule out alveolar or mandibular fracture after all moderate or severe injuries to the mouth.

Swallowed Bubble Gum or Chewing Tobacco

If an athlete chews gum or tobacco, his temperomandibular joint becomes overworked, and the chewing induces fatigue by sapping strength and endurance. The chewing athlete also risks aspirating the gum or tobacco and strangling.

The Heimlich or abdominal-thrust maneuver may save a choking athlete.[38, 39] Using this technique, the rescuer wraps both of his arms around the victim, and the victim's head and torso are allowed to slump forward. The rescuer then clasps the back of his wrist with his other hand so that the fist is pressed against the victim's diaphragm just below the ribs with a quick, hard squeeze. The squeeze is repeated as needed until the foreign body pops out like a cork. The victim should *not* be slapped on the back to dislodge the foreign body because such a slap may cause further inhaling of the foreign body.

If an athlete is knocked out and has gum or tobacco lodged in his throat, an oral screw may be used to force the mouth open to remove the foreign body. For an athlete who has an uncorrectable upper airway obstruction to breathing, a cricothyreotomy may be lifesaving.

Laryngeal Injury

A laryngeal injury may threaten the athlete's life; for this reason, a boxer keeps his chin tucked in. Blows may otherwise cause swelling and spasm of the larynx, and the thyroid cartilage (Adam's apple) may be contused or fractured. Trail bike riders risk laryngeal injuries when they ride on trails where wires, ropes, or chains may be strung. The threat of such injury requires baseball catchers and hockey goaltenders to wear throat flaps to block the ball or puck (Fig. 11-8). An inexpensive flap can be made by attaching the spine pad from a football girdle to the catcher's mask by leather lacing.[52] The pad will also serve as a target for the pitcher. Full contact karate participants shun neck protection, risking fractures of the larynx from kicks or punches.

Laryngeal injury produces voice changes. Crepitus is felt and landmarks are lost. Stridor may be delayed, and a laryngeal hematoma may expand to obstruct the airway completely.

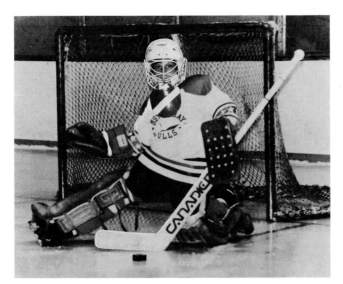

FIG. 11-8
The goaltender's protective gear includes a throat flap that attaches to his face mask and protects his larynx.

The Neck

The neck is subject to some of the most devastating injuries in athletics, and sports rank second only to automobile accidents as a leading cause of injury to this area. Three of four fatalities in organized tackle football are associated with head and neck injury, and one half of wrestling deaths follow a broken neck.

The National Athletic Trainer's Association (NATA) and the University of Pennsylvania Sports Medicine Center have established a National Head and Neck Injury Registry that solicits information on head and neck injuries in sports.[76] Injuries qualifying for the Registry include head and neck fractures or dislocations, injuries that require hospitalization for more than 72 hours or that require surgery, and injuries that produce permanent paralysis or death. The Registry provides information forms to record the diagnosis, treatment, disability, and current status of the athlete. The Registry also requests a record of the place of injury, the position the athlete played, and how the injury occurred—whether in a game, practice, or scrimmage, the mechanism of injury, and how it was verified. Other information requested includes the height, weight, and age of the player, whether he had a previous injury, the helmet manufacturer (if applicable), the type of field, and weather conditions at the time of injury.

Deadly head injuries in tackle football have declined during the last two decades, but neck injuries have risen during the same period.[7, 76] The helmet–face mask system effectively protects the player's head, but by so doing it allows the head to be used as a battering ram in tackling and blocking. Luckily, the helmet's slick outer plastic shell sometimes enables the head to slide off an opponent. At first glance, the proposal to place a soft outer lining on the football helmet may seem sound, but such a lining would produce increased friction, and the tackler's head would stick to his opponent and absorb more force.

Football helmets are not designed to protect a player's neck; thus most fatal or paralyzing injuries occur when the player's neck is hyperflexed as he spears, head tackles, or butt-blocks. In head tackling and butt-blocking, the top of one's head is used as the contact point, hitting the opponent "in the numbers." Knee blows to the head or grabbing of the face mask tilts the face mask violently and hyperextends the neck. Tacklers sustain more than 70% of all neck injuries; specifically, defensive backs, who must tackle bigger, running backs and ends, suffer the largest number of head and neck injuries.

Philo and Stine assert that the grave risk of quadriplegia in tackle football has been concealed from players and parents.[59] Feldick and Albright further state that "unless changes in technique are taught and rules are enforced, continued neck injuries and catastrophic paralysis will put football in severe jeopardy.[21] If the number of neck injuries does not decrease appreciably, litigation against equipment manufacturers could conceivably remove helmets from the market, and football could end by default."[21, 79] Such criticism has resulted in a change in the definition of spearing, tightening of the rules, and a reappraisal of blocking and tackling techniques. Spearing, for example, formerly referred to the impaling of a player who is out of action or the use of one's helmet after a blown whistle. It is now redefined as intentional use of the helmet to punish an opponent, and no player may now deliberately butt, ram, or strike an opponent with the top of his helmet. In "head tackling," the tackler drives in with his face to his opponent's numbers, propelling his helmet upward to the opponent's chin. Officials are now empowered to penalize players who use the head as a primary contact point. Instead of a 15-yard penalty for use of the head, the player should be banished from the game. Officials who neglect to call penalties for spearing and butting should be replaced, and coaches who teach spearing should be fired.

Running backs should run with their heads up, avoiding the dangerous, flexed position.[47] If the head nods slightly forward, the neck becomes a vulnerable straight column. In the correct "bulled" position, the player holds his head back some 10° and tucks his chin so that shocks are absorbed by the neck muscles and upper back muscles. Proper tackling is done head to side, with the tackler's head up, his eyes open, and initial contact made with the hands. The head slides up along the opponent's side, and chest-to-chest contact is made. Strong leg drive is needed. Players should work on their tackling form in preseason practice. Shoulder blocking and tackling with the neck extended and tucked in a "bulled" position must be taught, and players must be trained to fall for-

wards and backwards, rolling on their shoulders and quickly getting up.

Injuries will, however, continue to occur because the head is not easily controlled when the runner is moving and tackles must be made at high speed. Youths are accustomed to head contact, and because the helmet and face mask assembly are so effective, players become reckless, making head-first contact inadvertently.[66] If the face mask were removed from the helmet, damaged teeth and scarred faces might be traded for broken necks.[66] But without a face mask, the player might tend to close his eyes and drop his head, and even more neck injuries could result.

Types of Injuries

Diving

Immature, reckless young men with impaired judgment who lack training are the ones most likely to suffer a neck injury while diving, often ignoring warnings of shallow water. The water slows a diver's speed of fall, but only when a depth of 1.5 m (5 ft) has been reached. The force of the water spreads the unskilled diver's arms apart, and his head may strike bottom.[1] Many drownings may be due to tetraplegia, when the diver strikes his head on the bottom, resulting in wedge or burst fractures of C-5.[8]

Recreational divers rarely even lock their thumbs, but this precaution is insufficient to prevent their hands from pulling apart on entry. A stronger grasp may be achieved by holding the thumb with the opposite fist or by using the competitive diver's interlocking technique (Fig. 11-9).

Safety efforts are best directed toward the prevention of diving accidents, with widely publicized warnings about the hazards of diving into shallow water, including the fact that underwater rocks may not be clearly seen with changing light conditions later in the day.[1]

Equestrian

A fall from a horse may result in a cervical spine fracture and tetraplegia. Such injuries are

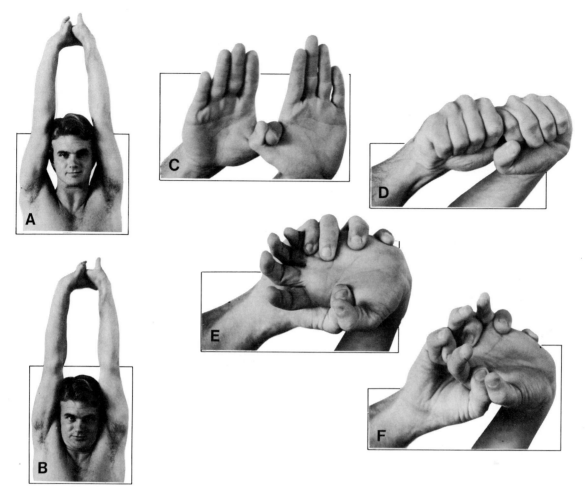

FIG. 11-9
Proper arm and hand positioning help to protect a diver's neck. In *A,* the shoulders do not cushion the neck as they do in *B,* the correct position. Locked thumbs (*C*) can be easily pulled apart, exposing the diver's head. A better grip is to grab a thumb (*D*). The best grips are with overlapping hands (*E*) or intertwining fingers (*F*).

a significant problem for steeplechase riders, who often tumble from their mounts.[46]

Equestrian athletes should practice dressage to bring the horse's hindquarters underneath the body and to achieve balance. As the horse's gymnastic skill increases, the horse should move more easily. Riders should stay on familiar terrain and check tack routinely. Learning how to fall and roll to protect the neck is advisable. A few steeplechase jockeys wear plastazote spinal protectors to prevent neck injury.

Young Tackle Football Players

Death rates do not accurately reflect the incidence of neck injuries in high school tackle football,[2] and juniors and seniors have especially high rates of injury. Many injuries in this age group go unrecognized; thus when the symptoms of neck injury, such as radiation of pain into an arm or numbness and tingling in a limb, are explained to high school players, they frequently reveal a history of such injury.

Of 108 college freshmen tackle football recruits in one study, 35 showed x-ray evidence of previous injury, such as old compression fractures, posterior element fractures, disc narrowing, and ligamentous instability.[21] Just over half of these athletes had been seen by a doctor, and x-rays had been taken only in 13 cases.

Youths complaining of neck pain should be examined. The examiner sometimes may find congenital instability in an immature neck. Lack of an odontoid, for example, puts the player at great risk for serious injury. Players should be informed about the symptoms of neck injury, and any player who misses a practice or game because of neck pain should have an x-ray taken. The player must have full, pain-free range of motion in his neck before returning to practice.

Fractures

The head weighs about 4.5 kg (10 lb) and is supported by the smallest, most delicate part of the spine. The first cervical vertebra, the atlas, comprises a ring with lateral masses and no central body. Its articulations are curved to provide flexion and extension between the overlying occiput and itself. The second cervical vertebra, the axis, has curved articulations that allow rotation between the atlas and the axis. Most of the rotation in the cervical spine occurs in this area.

The odontoid is the superior projection of the body of the axis. The transverse ligament holds the anterior tubercle of the atlas adjacent to the odontoid. Stability of the atlas and axis depends on the transverse ligament of the atlas and the odontoid process of the axis. The third through seventh vertebrae are similar to each other, providing some flexion, extension, tilt, and rotation. The vertebral arteries ascend in the vertebral foramen of each lateral mass from C–6 through C–1.

X-ray films of the cervical spine should include anteroposterior, lateral, and oblique views and an open-mouth view to show the odontoid and the lateral masses of the atlas. Sometimes the lower cervical spine is especially difficult to visualize after an injury because muscle spasms cause the shoulder shadow to obscure the region. In these instances, the athlete's head is stabilized, and his arms are gently pulled down to allow this area to be seen. If this technique is unsuccessful, a "swimmer's view" is obtained in which one arm is abducted 180° and the other arm is pulled down along the athlete's side (Fig. 11-10). To obtain a clear view of the lower cervical spine, the beam is then directed at a 60° angle to the neck.

Prevertebral soft tissue swelling of 5 mm or more at the anterior-inferior border of C–3 provides indirect evidence of a cervical spine injury. Although an x-ray may show normal alignment, momentary subluxation may have occurred at the time of injury, causing severe

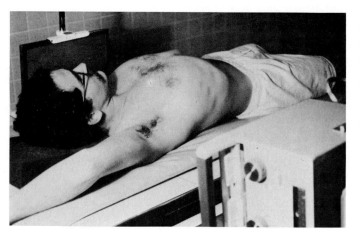

FIG. 11-10
Sometimes, lower cervical vertebrae are not seen on a standard lateral x-ray. The swimmer's view, with one arm raised, equalizes soft tissue densities and allows a clear view of these vertebrae.

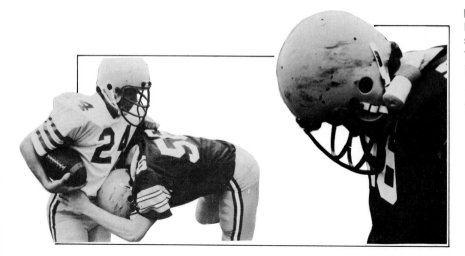

FIG. 11-11
Head tackling (*left*) can seriously damage the tackler's neck and even paralyze him. The "birdcage" mask (*right*) can help to block full flexion.

damage to the spinal cord. The mechanisms of cervical spine injury include neck compression, pure flexion, flexion and compression, flexion and rotation, hyperextension, and lateral flexion.

Compression Injuries

Compression injuries to the cervical spine occur in diving accidents and from head-on tackles.[5, 26] An axial load on the head causes the occiput to drive the atlas down onto the axis, producing a burst fracture of the ring of the atlas (Jefferson's fracture). The ring usually fractures posteriorly in two places weakened by grooves of the vertebral arteries. The atlas is a fragile ring, but fortunately its opening for the spinal cord is wide. This fracture is diagnosed on an open-mouth view by noting that the articular facets have slid laterally on the axis.

Vertical compression may also produce a comminuted, explosion fracture of a vertebral body and a posterior subluxation of the body. Even though the fracture itself is stable, serious neurologic damage may result. With the aid of tomograms or a computerized tomography scan, fragments may be found in the spinal canal. Such fragments may be pressing on the anterior spinal artery, producing cord ischemia. This ischemia leads to an anterior cervical cord syndrome consisting of complete motor paralysis and sensory anesthesia with dorsal column sparing so that proprioception and deep pressure sensation from the trunk and lower extremities are retained.

Flexion Injuries

In a pure flexion injury, the athlete's chin sometimes strikes his sternum before his neck breaks. A face mask, such as the bird-cage face mask used in tackle football, blocks further flexion (Fig. 11-11). Flexion of the neck may produce a stable wedge fracture of a vertebral body. A pure flexion injury, as from a fall on the back of the head, may also rupture the transverse ligament. The odontoid then is no longer restrained, and an atlantoaxial dislocation results. After such an injury, as the athlete leans his head forward, the atlas slides forward, and he becomes dizzy, developing a headache from pressure on the greater occipital nerve and a tingling in his feet. As he leans backwards, the dislocation reduces.

If the distance between the odontoid and the anterior arch of the atlas on a lateral x-ray exceeds 5 mm, the supporting structures probably have failed. A distance of more than 10 mm implies the loss of all ligamentous stability. A lateral x-ray with the neck flexed is most important, as overlooking this instability could result in an athlete's death. If he survives this dislocation, his neck is firmly immobilized, and an early occipitoaxial fusion or an atlantoaxial fusion with wire and an iliac bone graft is performed.

When an athlete falls on the back of his head, he may fracture his odontoid. Such fractures usually occur at the weakest part of the dens, its base. A slight tilt of the odontoid on the open-mouth view will serve as a clue to a fracture and is an indication for tomograms and flexion and extension films. When a fracture is suspected but no fracture line is seen, the lateral film should be checked for prevertebral soft tissue swelling as a clue to the presence of a fracture.

Flexion/Compression Fractures

A player's neck may buckle during head tackling (*see* Fig. 11-11). This happens most commonly in high school defensive backs who wear single or double bar face masks, the kinds least likely to block flexion. Major stress occurs at the C-5–C-6 level, where the mobile part of the cervical spine joins the less mobile part. Flexion and compression forces produce a wedge-shaped or a teardrop fracture, which is a chip broken off the anterior lip of C-5. The injured athlete's neck will be unstable if his posterior soft tissue elements are completely torn, but otherwise the compression fracture may be stable. The entire vertebral body may crumble, with the posterior part split off and displaced posterolaterally and the posteroinferior margin fracture pushed into the spinal canal. The disc between C-5 and C-6 may also be expelled back into the spinal canal. These fractures frequently produce a transverse lesion of the cord and tetraplegia.

Flexion and Rotation Injuries of the Cervical Spine

A combination of neck flexion and rotation may dislocate or fracture one or both facet joints. If a player is lying on the field with his head locked in one position, no attempt should be made to straighten it, since his facet joints may be locked. If the rotational component of the injury force is great, the pedicles may be fractured. With complete unilateral facet dislocation, x-rays show the vertebral body to be subluxed about 25% anteriorly. When both facets are locked, the body is displaced anteriorly about 50%. Traction may unlock the facet joints, but sometimes operative unlocking is needed.

Hyperextension Injuries

When a player's face mask is grabbed and levered backwards or an athlete's face is struck by a knee, his occiput may actually contact his thoracic spine, causing neck injury (Fig. 11-12). The force needed to hyperextend the neck is not too great, as the anterior muscles of the neck are far weaker than the posterior muscles. Such injuries may produce vertebral artery ischemia or thrombosis, with a momentary feeling of paralysis or tingling in the limbs. Compression and spasm of spinal arteries produce acute paralysis, numbness, and tingling in the lower limbs, then in the upper limbs, but the athlete may recover even before he is transported from the field.

Hyperextension is the most common mechanism of nerve root injury. Injury to the C-5 root affects the shoulder and deltoid muscle; the C-6 root controls the biceps and conveys sensation from the radial aspect of the arm and thumb; C-7 conducts sensation from the index and middle fingers; and C-8 controls the intrinsic muscles of the athlete's hand and innervates his ring and little fingers and his inner arm.

Hyperextension of an athlete's neck may fracture the laminas or pedicles of the axis, or a lamina may fracture along with an avulsion of an anterior-superior chip of a vertebral body. Tomograms and oblique x-rays may be needed to diagnose such a fracture. The athlete may have a complete cord injury, but an x-ray film may show only a widened interspace anteriorly. Hyperextension may also produce an odontoid fracture; the only external sign of the injury may be a bruise on the athlete's forehead or face.

Hyperextension may produce a central cord syndrome, the most common incomplete cord syndrome. This occurs mostly in middle-aged persons who have osteoarthritic spines. The spinal canal is narrow, and the cord is crushed between anterior osteophytes and an infolded ligamentum flavum posteriorly. Central spinal

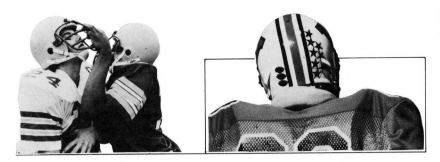

FIG. 11-12
A player's neck may be hyperextended by leverage on his face mask (*left*). A neck roll (*right*) can help to block hyperextension.

cord vessels are injured, venous circulation is impaired, and there is progressive hemorrhage and thrombosis of vessels with edema ensuing. Damage to the anterior horn cells in the central gray matter of the cord will produce a severe, flaccid, lower motor neuron paralysis of the upper extremities, whereas damage to the central part of the corticospinal and spinothalamic long tracts in the white matter produces upper motor neuron spastic paralysis of the trunk and lower extremities. The medial part of the lateral pyramidal tracts are affected, but there is sacral sparing. Motor and sensory function often return to the athlete's lower extremities and trunk, but recovery of hand function is poor.

Cervical collars will limit extension of the neck, but defensive backs and wide receivers object to collars, arguing that a collar restricts their movements.

Lateral Flexion Injuries

Lateral flexion of an athlete's neck may cause a fracture through the lateral mass of a pedicle, a vertebral foramen, or a facet joint. Such an injury may produce a Brown-Sequard syndrome, where damage is limited to the lateral half of the athlete's spinal cord, producing an ipsilateral corticospinal muscle palsy and contralateral hypesthesia to pain and temperature. Lateral flexion may also produce a nerve pinch.[10]

"Burners" and Nerve Pinch

An athlete may stretch his cervical plexus or his brachial plexus, damage a nerve root, or rupture a cervical disk that will press on a nerve root. These upper extremity nerve injuries are especially common in wrestling, hockey, and tackle football, as when a linebacker's neck is bent to the side when he tackles. Nerve injuries in motocross are quite severe and may include nerve root avulsions. Other athletes who may injure their upper extremity nerves are skiers whose poles catch on trees, diving soccer goalies, and mountaineers and hikers who carry heavy backpacks.

A "burner," also called a "stinger" or a "hotshot," is a stretch of the cervical plexus, the supraclavicular nerves, or the brachial plexus that occurs when the athlete's head is bent away from the side of his arm pain.[11] Supraclavicular nerves convey sensation from the top and front of the athlete's shoulder, and injury to them produces a sensory loss but no motor loss. An athlete's brachial plexus may be contused (neurotmesis) beneath his clavicle on the surface of the first rib. If a nerve root is avulsed (axonotmesis), the axon degenerates distally. A nerve root may be pinched when an athlete's head is abruptly flexed laterally, and pain then radiates down the arm on the side to which his head was bent.

When examining the athlete's arm for nerve damage, knowledge of neuroanatomy is essential. The first and second cervical nerve roots contribute to the spinal accessory nerve. This is the motor nerve to the trapezius, but it lacks a sensory part. The contour of the trapezius should be examined and compared to its counterpart. Trapezius strength may be tested by having the athlete shrug his shoulders against manual resistance. The rhomboid muscles are innervated by the nerve to the rhomboids from the C-5 nerve root; the examiner should observe for wasting of this muscle. The serratus anterior receives its nerve supply by way of the long thoracic nerve; the athlete should perform a wall push-up as a check of his serratus anterior's ability to protract the scapula. The suprascapular nerve supplies motor impulses to the supraspinatus and infraspinatus muscles; atrophy of these muscles should be looked for. For examination of the muscles supplied by the brachial plexus, the examiner should ask the athlete to abduct his shoulder, flex and extend his elbow, and pronate and supinate his forearm against resistance. The examiner should note any numbness or tingling in the arm and do a pinprick sensory examination.

If the athlete's neck is extended and tilted toward the involved side during an examination after a nerve pinch or cervical disc rupture, his symptoms are aggravated. After a brachial plexus injury, pain will increase when his neck is tilted away from the symptomatic side. An electromyogram may help in differentiating between a cervical disc protrusion and an injury to the brachial plexus. With cervical disc protrusion, the electromyogram will show fibrillation in the athlete's paraspinal muscles. When the injury is to the brachial plexus, the paraspinal muscles are normal.

If an athlete suffers a burner or a nerve pinch, his protective gear should be checked. His shoulder pads should be in good condition, fit correctly, be worn separately, and protect him from lateral flexion beyond safe limits. When he shows signs of clinical recovery, his neck, shoulders, and upper back should be restrengthened. He must recover full sensation and strength before being allowed to return to practice, and he may need protective straps or a neck roll. His blocking and tackling technique should also be re-evaluated.

If an athlete feels well after a burner and the clinical examination findings are normal, he may return to the game. He should, however, be checked after the game, the next day, and several days later, as there may be ischemia and delayed nerve damage. After neuropraxia, with damage only to the myelin sheath, the player may return to practice in 2 days to 2 weeks.

After the first injury, an athlete is more easily reinjured, possibly because of less space in the foramen owing to swelling and fibrosis. The nerve root remains trapped and vulnerable to movement that may stretch or compress it. An athlete may also have less range of lateral flexion toward the injured side and impaired facet joint function. Long after nerve pinches and burners, he may have neurologic changes and limited neck flexibility and note persistent weakness in his extensor-supinator or flexor-pronator groups of muscles, along with patches of radial or ulnar nerve numbness.

An athlete who suffers recurrent burners in a high-velocity collision sport may have an underlying cervical sagittal stenosis.[32] The stenosis is usually asymptomatic until spondylolysis develops or a hyperextension injury or vertebral subluxation occurs, whereupon the subject may become transiently or permanently quadriplegic. If sagittal stenosis is suspected, a lateral cervical spine film should be taken. The examiner measures the cervical canal width from the middle of the posterior surface of the vertebral body to the nearest point on the ventral surface of the spinous process. From C-3 through C-6, a sagittal diameter ranging from 14.5 mm to 20 mm is within normal limits.

On-the-Field Care of Neck Injuries

The team physician must be constantly alert for the mechanism of injuries. If a player is knocked out, it should be assumed that he has a neck injury.[47] Ammonia capsules should not be used because the injured player may jerk his head away and injure his spinal cord. If he is conscious, a rapid sensory and motor examination should be done to rule out spinal cord injury.

If an athlete has neck pain or a tender neck, he is assumed to have a fracture or a fracture-dislocation. His neck should be supported manually in a neutral position with his head and neck aligned with his spine. Forceful traction is unnecessary, and a pillow should *not* be placed under his head. If he holds his neck in a fixed position, he may have locked facets; no attempt should be made to straighten the neck out, maintaining it instead in the position in which he is holding it.

The player's helmet should remain on, with his face mask swung away or the bars cut with a high-quality, heavy-duty bolt cutter. If the helmet must be removed, two persons should do the job.[43] One rescuer applies inline traction by placing his hands on each side of the helmet with his fingers on the player's mandible, a position that prevents slippage if the chin strap is loose. The chin strap is unsnapped, and a second rescuer places one of his hands at the angle of the player's mandible, the thumb on one side, the long and index fingers on the other. With his other hand, he applies pressure from the occipital region. This maneuver transfers the inline traction responsibility to the second rescuer. The rescuer at the top then removes the helmet, which must be expanded laterally to clear the ears. Throughout the procedure, inline traction is maintained from below to prevent head tilt. After the helmet has been removed, the rescuer at the top replaces his hands on either side of the injured player's head with his palms over the player's ears. This traction is maintained from above until a backboard is in place.

A backboard, rather than a stretcher, should be used for transporting the neck-injured athlete, as it can be placed under him with minimal movement, is rigid, and has an outrigger and buckles that form a four-tailed chin strap. Five men carry the board while a leader at the head gives commands.

Neck Straps and Neck Rolls

To prevent excessive neck motion, a 3.8-cm (1.5-in)-wide semielastic strap may be snapped to the shoulder pad from the rear of the football helmet.[3] Potential liability exists, however, when a helmet is altered in this manner.

Neck collars are the most common shoulder-pad accessories and include standard types, inflatable types, and custom-made models that consist of a rolled towel in stockinette with a string through it. Some players wear an inexpensive collar made of pipe insulation with a shoestring running through it. Stockinette is placed around the pipe insulation and taped.

A cervical collar should circle the entire neck rather than leaving a "V" in the front. Interior linemen, linebackers, and especially those athletes who have had a neck injury should wear collars. A loose-fitting collar has little value, but a properly applied collar will prevent excessive neck motion.

The edges of poorly fitted shoulder pads may drive into the base of the wearer's neck in a pileup. If the pads are too low, they will allow excessive neck motion. On the other hand, a high cantilever pad may be struck by a player's neck and cause injury if he has increased his neck size through strengthening exercises. For this reason, the cantilever pads should be lowered when the player's neck size increases.

Many nerve pinches are associated with wearing professional-type shoulder pads.[10] These pads protect the shoulders adequately, but players of average build and flexibility are especially prone to lateral neck sprain while wearing them. The neck motion of bull-necked players is limited when they wear either high or low shoulder pads, whereas one half of those with average neck length get no protection for lateral flexion from professional shoulder pads. Long-necked, limber athletes receive more protection to lateral flexion than do athletes with average-size necks, since long-necked athletes have greater ranges of motion.

Neck Strengthening

All tackle football players must have strong and flexible necks. Thus, before the season begins, long-necked athletes should add at least 2.5 cm (1 in) of circumference to their necks. Weak-necked athletes should not play football. A strong neck will not prevent a neck fracture from occurring if great force is applied to the bone, but it will aid the athlete in keeping his head in a stable position.[47] This position prepares his neck musculature for contact: He holds his head in about 10° of extension with the occipital line about 10° above the horizontal and his shoulders elevated—the "bulled position." Players who tend to duck their heads need special coaching to lessen their chances of injury. Strong neck muscles also prevent fatigue resulting from wearing a heavy helmet.

The athlete may strengthen his neck by isometric, isotonic, isodynamic, intermedialis, or functional bridging methods. Isometrics may be performed either against the athlete's own hand resistance, the resistance of a hand-held towel, or the hands of a partner during buddy exercises. The contraction is held for 6 seconds and released for three sets of six repetitions.

Isotonic strengthening is achieved with weights attached to the athlete's head by a hal-

ter and strung over a wall pulley. The athlete flexes, extends, and obliquely and laterally flexes his neck. A 6-week isotonic wall pulley program can add 3 cm (1.25 in) of circumference to the neck, compared to a gain of only 1 cm (0.4 in) after an isometric program.[49] Because the shoulder is the base of support for the neck, the athlete should also do shoulder shrugs and high pulls with barbells.

A broad rubber tubing may be used isodynamically to resist neck motion. The athlete assumes the positions that may be encountered in his sport and strengthens his neck in these positions. Wrestlers may also perform intermedialis neck strengthening against the resistance of a knowledgeable partner, with the athlete stopping his neck motion for a brief isometric contraction, then resuming the mo-

FIG. 11-13
Young football players often lack good neck development (*A*). Neck exercises (*B*) play an important part in an athlete's preparation for tackle football. Bridging prepares and protects the athlete's neck but should not be done with a helmet on (*C*). Some face masks can swing away when rubber mounting loops (*arrow*) are cut (*D*).

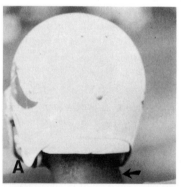
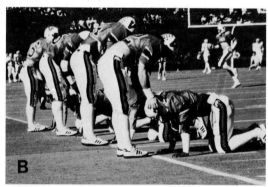
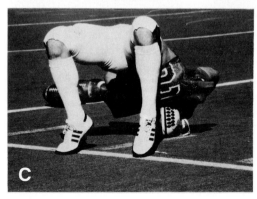
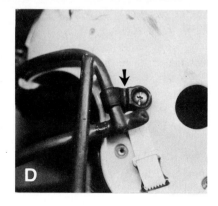

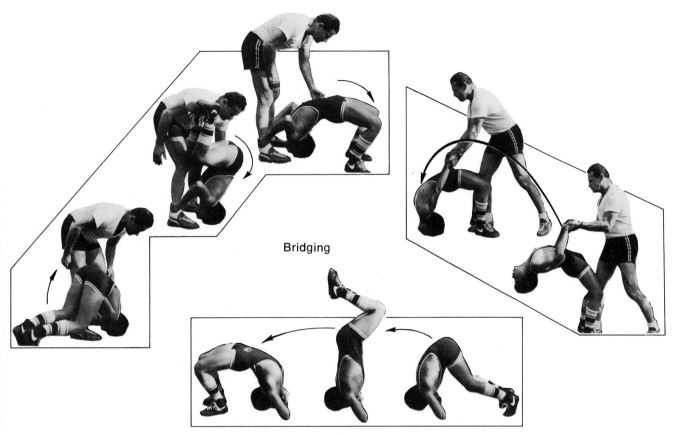

Bridging

FIG. 11-14
"Bridging" is taught stepwise by a skilled instructor.

tion against isokinetic resistance. This technique stimulates the common stops and starts at the different positions encountered in athletics.

Bridging is an athlete's best all-around neck strengthening and flexibility exercise because it tunes his neck to absorb shocks and develops proprioception. Bridging has been criticized unjustly as emphasizing excursion of the neck, causing ligamentous loosening, and "grinding up the neck." Equipment managers oppose bridging in tackle football because it damages helmet suspensions. Bridging on the top of the head in a football helmet produces shearing stress and damages the helmet and the player's neck (Fig. 11-13). A correct program will allow the athlete to bridge on his forehead and develop a strong, supple neck (Fig. 11-14).

REFERENCES

1. ALBRAND OW, CORKILL G: Broken necks from diving accidents: a summer epidemic in young men. Am J Sports Med 4:107–110, 1976
2. ALBRIGHT JP et al: Nonfatal cervical spine injuries in interscholastic football. JAMA 236:1243–1245, 1976
3. ANDRISH JT et al: A method for the management of cervical injuries in football. A preliminary report. Am J Sports Med 5:89–92, 1977
4. BAKER TE: A quick and easy method for controlling nosebleeds. First Aider, Cramer 48(5):14, January 1979
5. BAILEY RW: Fractures and dislocations of the C-spine. in Adams JP (ed): Current Practice in Orthopedic Surgery. Saint Louis, CV Mosby, 1969
6. BENNETT DR et al: Migraine precipitated by head trauma in athletes. Am J Sports Med 8:202–205, 1980
7. BLYTH C, MUELLER F: An Epidemiological Study of High School Football Injuries in North Carolina. Final Report of PHS Grant No. FDA00032-02, 1. Washington, D.C., U.S. Public Health Service

8. BURKE DC: Spinal cord injuries from water sports. Med J Aust 2:1190–1194, 1972

9. CARTER DR, FRANKEL VH: Biomechanics of hyperextension injuries to the cervical spine in football. Am J Sports Med 8:302–309, 1980

10. CHRISMAN OD, SNOOK G: Lateral flexion neck injuries in athletics. JAMA 192:613–615, 1965

11. CLANCY WG et al: Upper trunk brachial plexus injuries in contact sport. Am J Sports Med 5:209–216, 1977

12. COOPER DL, FAIR J: Treating "cauliflower ear." Phys Sportsmed 4(7):103, 1976

13. DANIELSON LG, WESTLIN NE: Riding accidents. Acta Orthop Scand 44:597–603, 1973

14. DEVOE AG: Injuries to the eye. Am J Surg 98:384–389, 1959

15. DIBARTOLOMEO JR: Exostotic ear tumors—sea water sport peril. Phys Sportsmed 4(7):60–63, 1976

16. DOVE A: Case report: rotary subluxation of the first cervical vertebra. Phys Sportsmed 7(9):115–119, 1979

17. EASTERBROOK M: Eye protection for squash and racquetball players. Phys Sportsmed 9(2):79–82, 1981

18. EICHEL BS: Otologic hazards in water sports. Phys Sportsmed 2(7):43–45, 1974

19. EICHEL BS, BRAY DA: Management of hematoma of the wrestler's ear. Phys Sportsmed 6(11):87–90, 1978

20. FARBER GA: Football acne—an acneiform eruption. Cutis 20:356–360, 1977

21. FELDICK HG, ALBRIGHT JP: Football survey reveals "missed" neck injuries. Phys Sportsmed 4(10):77–81, 1976

22. FOWLER BJ: Ocular injuries sustained playing squash. Am J Sports Med 8:126–128, 1980

23. FOWLER EP Jr, OSMUM PM: New bone growth due to cold water in the ears. Arch Otolaryngol 36:455, 1942

24. FRACKEL WH: Facial injuries in sports. Am J Surg 98:390–393, 1959

25. FUNK FJ, WELLS RE: Injuries of the cervical spine in football. Clin Orthop 109:50–58, 1975

26. GARBER JN: Fracture and fracture-dislocation of the cervical spine. In Hoyt WA Jr (ed): Symposium on the Spine. Saint Louis, CV Mosby, 1969

27. GARNER AI: Correct eye disorders to improve performance. First Aider, Cramer 46(8):2–3, 1977

28. GARNER AI: Athletes are endangered by unsafe eyewear. First Aider, Cramer 47(3):3, 1977

29. GARNER AI: Can your athletes really see? Athletic Training, 14:156–157, 1979

30. GIERUP JM et al: Incidence and nature of horse-riding injuries. Acta Chir Scand 142:57–61, 1976

31. GOOD RP, NICKEL VL: Cervical spine injuries resulting from water sports. Spine 5:502–506, 1980

32. GRANT TT, PUFFER J: Cervical stenosis: a development anomaly with quadriparesis during football. Am J Sports Med 4:219–221, 1976

33. GROSS CG: Treating "cauliflower ear" with silicone mold. Am J Sports Med 6:4, 1978

34. GROSSMAN JAI et al: Equestrian injuries: results of a prospective study. JAMA 240:1881–1882, 1978

35. HARDESTY WH et al: Study on vertebral artery blood flow in man. Surg Gynecol Obstet 116:662–664, 1963

36. HAYES D et al: Effects of intraoral mouth guards in ventilation. Phys Sportsmed 5(1):61–66, 1977

37. HEAD PROTECTION FOR THE CYCLIST: A Medical Inquiry. American Medical Association Meeting. Washington, D. C., 14 April, 1977

38. HEIMLICH HJ: The Heimlich Maneuver: where it stands today. Emergency Med 10:89, 1978

39. HEIMLICH HJ, UHLEY MJ: The Heimlich maneuver. Clin Symp 31(3):3–32, 1979

40. HEINTZ WD: Mouth protectors: a progress report. J Am Dent Assoc 77:632–636, 1968

41. HEINTZ WD: The case for mandatory mouth protectors. Sports Med 3:61–63, 1975

42. HEINTZ WD: Mouth protection in sports. Phys Sportsmed 7(2):45–46, 1979

43. HELMET REMOVAL FROM INJURED PATIENTS. American College of Surgeons Committee on Trauma. Q J Am Assoc Automotive Med 2(4):2, 1980

44. HERRICK RT: Clay-shoveler's fracture in powerlifting: a case report. Am J Sports Med 9:29–30, 1981

45. HICKEY JC et al: The relation of mouth protectors to cranial pressure and deformation. J Am Dent Assoc 74:735–740, 1967

46. LANDRO L: Riding injuries stir British medical concern. Phys Sportsmed 4(10):125–129, 1976

47. LEIDHOLT JB: Spinal injuries in athletes: be prepared. Orthop Clin North Am 4:691–707, 1973

48. MACFIE DD: ENT problems of diving. Med Serv J Can 20:845, 1964

49. MAROON JC et al: A system for preventing athletic neck injuries. Phys Sportsmed 5(10):77–79, 1977

50. MATTHEWS WB: Footballer's migraine. Br Med J 2:326–327, 1972

51. MAWDSLEY C, FERGUSON FR: Neurological disease in boxers. Lancet 2:799–801, 1963

52. MIDDLETON J: Football spine pad protection for baseball catchers: Athletic Training 15:82, 1980

53. NELSON WE et al: Syncope, bradychardia and hypotension after a lacrosse shot to the neck: management and prevention. Phys Sportsmed 9(8):94–97, 1981

54. ODESS JS: The hearing hazard of firearms. Phys Sportsmed 2(10):65–68, 1974

55. ODESS JS: Acoustic trauma of sportsman hunter due to gun firing. Laryngoscope 82:1971–1989, 1972

56. OGDEN FW: Effect of gunfire upon auditory acuity for pure tones and the efficacy of ear plugs as protectors. Laryngoscope 60:993–1012, 1950

57. OPPENHEIMER P et al: Repair of traumatic-myringorupture. Arch Otolaryngol 73:328–333, 1961

58. PASHBY TJ: Eye injuries in Canadian anateur hockey. Am J Sports Med 7:254–257, 1979

59. PHILO H, STINE G: The liability path to safer helmets. Trial Magazine 13:38–40, 1977

60. PIPKIN G: Caloric labyrinthitis: a cause of drowning. Case report of a swimmer who survived through self-rescue. Am J Sports Med 7:260–261, 1979

61. REID SE et al: Head protection in football. Phys Sportsmed 2(2):86–92, 1974

62. RICHARDS RN: Rescuing the spine-injured diver. Phys Sportsmed 1(9):63–65, 1973

63. ROGERS L, SWEENEY PJ: Stroke: a neurological complication of wrestling. A case of brainstem stroke in a 17-year-old athlete. Am J Sports Med 7:352–354, 1979

64. ROYDHOUSE N: Earaches and adolescent swimmers. In: Swimming Medicine IV. International Series on Sport Science, Vol 6, pp 79–85 (Eriksson B, Durberg B, eds). Baltimore, University Park Press, 1977

65. RYAN AJ (moderator): Round table discussion: eye protection for athletes. Phys Sportsmed 6(9):43–67, 1978

66. SCHNEIDER RC: Head and Neck Injuries in Football. Baltimore, Williams & Williams, 1973

67. SCHNEIDER RC, ANTINE BE: Visual fields impairment related to football headgear and face-guards. JAMA 192:616–618, 1965

68. SCHWARTZ R, NOVICH MM: The athlete's mouthpiece. Am J Sports Med 8:357–359, 1980

69. SEELENFREUND MH, FREILICH DB: Rushing the net and retinal detachment. JAMA 235:2723–2736, 1976

70. SMITH M: Contact lenses and athletes. Trainer's corner. Phys Sportsmed 6(4):124, 1978

71. STENGER JM et al: Mouthguards. J Am Dent Assoc 19:263, 1964

72. STENGER JM et al: Mouthguards. J Am Dent Assoc 69:273–281, 1964

73. STRAUSS MB et al: Swimmer's ear. Phys Sportsmed 7(6):101–105, 1979

74. TAYLOR GD, WILLIAMS E: Acoustic trauma in the sports hunter. Laryngoscope 76:863–879, 1966

75. TORG JS: Unusual fractures caused by football helmet impact. Phys Sportsmed 4(11):73–75, 1976

76. TORG J et al: The National Football Head and Neck Injury Registry: report and conclusions 1978. JAMA 241:1477–1479, 1979

77. TORG JS et al: Collision with spring-loaded football tackling and blocking dummies. Report of near fatal and fatal injuries. JAMA 236:1270–1271, 1976

78. TURCOTTE H: Scuba divers answer the challenge of the sea. Phys Sportsmed 5(8):67–68, 1977

79. UNDERWOOD J: The Death of an American Game: The Crisis in Football. Boston, Little, Brown, 1979

80. VERSCHOTH A: Weak? Sink your teeth into this. Sports Illustrated 54:36–42, 1980

81. VINGER PF: Sports-related eye injury. A preventable problem. Surv Opthalmol 25:47–51, 1980

82. VIRGIN HH: Cineradiographic study of football helmets and the cervical spine. Am J Sports Med 8:310–317, 1980

The shoulder comprises four joints: sternoclavicular, acromioclavicular, glenohumeral, and scapulothoracic. Although it serves as a base for the upper extremity, the shoulder is the most mobile of joints, with relatively little bony stability except that lent by the capsular and musculotendinous structures. Many shoulder injuries in athletics are to these soft structures.

The sternoclavicular joint is stabilized by ligaments and often contains a fibrocartilaginous meniscus. The acromioclavicular joint may also contain an intra-articular disc that degenerates with age. The joint capsule is weak but is strengthened by fibers of the deltoid and trapezius muscles. The coracoid process of the scapula is closely related to the acromioclavicular joint and extends forward like a crow's beak—hence the term "coracoid" from the Greek "korax," "the crow." Arising from the coracoid are the pectoralis minor, the conjoined tendon of the coracobrachialis and short head of the biceps, the coracohumeral ligament, the coracoacromial ligament, and the coracoclavicular ligaments. The coracoclavicular ligament comprises conoid and trapezoid portions that strengthen the nearby acromioclavicular joint and lend vertical stability to the clavicle. The coracoid and its attached muscles and ligaments stabilize the scapula while muscles flex the arm and forearm.

The glenohumeral joint is the major shoulder joint. The humeral head is three times larger than the glenoid socket, and the arcs of the joint surfaces differ. The socket is shallow but is deepened by the glenoid labrum, the fibrocartilaginous origin of the joint capsule. The tendon of the long head of the biceps starts at the supraglenoid rim of the scapula and extends extrasynovially, but intracapsularly, through the shoulder joint (Fig. 12-1). It then passes into the bicipital groove under the transverse humeral ligament. The bicipital groove angles medially about 30° from the course of the biceps tendon in the arm, and its medial wall may vary from steep to shallow. A supratubercular prominence on the humerus will sometimes irritate the biceps tendon above the point where the tendon passes into the groove.

The short rotators of the shoulder comprise the rotator cuff. They retain the humeral head in the glenoid and maintain the instant center of rotation in a fixed position while the deltoid abducts the shoulder. The supraspinatus does not initiate abduction of the shoulder but instead

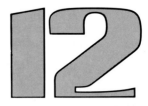

The Shoulder

259

has a quantitative action throughout abduction and forward flexion. This may be proved by paralyzing the supraspinatus muscle with local anesthesia around the supraspinous nerve.[58] The completeness of the paralysis is checked by electromyography. Even though the supraspinatus is paralyzed, the subject will be able to move his shoulder against gravity through a full range of motion. His abduction power and endurance, however, will decrease with his arm held in 90° of abduction and with weights in his hand. Since the same results hold for forward lifting, the supraspinatus thus has only a quantitative role in shoulder abduction and flexion. It functions to retract the joint capsule and to help hold the head in the glenoid while the deltoid abducts the arm.

The bony acromion and the coracoacromial ligament compose the coracoacromial arch. The ligament forms a soft roof for the rotator cuff, intra-articular portion of the biceps tendon, and humeral head. It may also be a stabilizer that counteracts the pull of the conjoined tendon during the skeletal development of the coracoid process. The underlying subacromial bursa and supraspinatus tendon may, however, impinge on this ligament and become irritated.

As the athlete abducts his shoulder, the humerus is depressed by the rotators so that the tuberosities may pass under the coracoacromial arch. If the arm is kept in internal rotation during abduction, the greater tuberosity impinges on the arch, and the arm can only abduct to about 60°. When the athlete externally rotates his arm, however, the greater tuberosity may pass under the arch.

Scapulohumeral motion should be smooth and coordinated. During the first 30° to 60° of abduction or forward flexion—the "setting phase"—the scapula seeks a stable position. The scapula then moves laterally with the humerus in a ratio of 1° of scapular movement for every 2° of humeral movement. Thus for every 30° that the arm is elevated, the humerus moves 20° and the scapula 10°. This scapular movement preserves the resting length of the deltoid.

FIG. 12-1
A shoulder seen from the anterior aspect (*left*), and then looking into the glenoid (*right*).

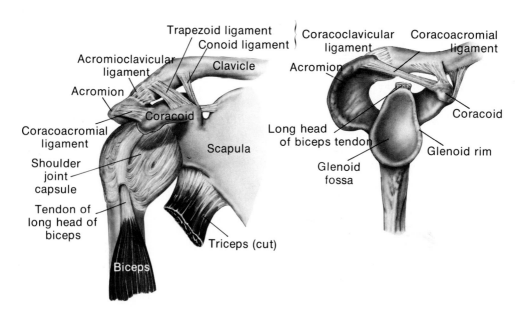

Examining the Shoulder

The athlete's shoulder should be examined systematically, with the examiner first observing for undue prominences, as from an acromioclavicular separation and for muscular hypertrophy or atrophy. Some athletes have normally hypertrophied muscles, as in the case of the latissimus dorsi of a baseball pitcher or of a veteran tennis player. Scapulohumeral rhythm is next assessed as the athlete abducts his shoulder to determine whether there are any hitches, hiking, or substitutions in this motion.

The athlete's neck should always be examined during a shoulder evaluation, since a neck disorder may be causing the shoulder pain. As the athlete rotates his neck, and with his neck turned to one side, the examiner presses on the vertex of the athlete's skull to see if he reports any discomfort or arm pain that may indicate a disc problem. Adson's maneuver is done by having the athlete turn his head away from the arm to be tested; the examiner then raises the arm to see if the radial pulse disappears, an indication of a possible thoracic outlet problem.

A systematic shoulder examination should start in front and work around the shoulder to the back. The sternoclavicular joint is first palpated. If the athlete has landed on his hand, forces may have been transmitted up to this joint; blows from the lateral side of the shoulder may also disrupt it. The examiner next walks his fingers along the entire clavicle, checking the area of insertion of the trapezius into the clavicle and the medialmost origin of the deltoid from the clavicle. The coracoclavicular ligament area and the acromioclavicular joint are palpated, and the clavicle is pressed at the acromioclavicular joint to see if it moves. The coracoid process is next felt; even a normal coracoid, however, may be somewhat tender to deep pressure.

The anterior capsule of the shoulder lies about one fingerbreadth lateral to the coracoid. While this area is being palpated, the athlete's arm should be rotated internally and then externally. If the tender spot does not move, the anterior capsule may be implicated.

The stability of the athlete's glenohumeral joint may be tested with the subject supine by pulling and pushing the humerus forward and back, trying to produce subluxation. In a more dynamic test for shoulder stability, the athlete externally rotates his arm and then presses forward against the examiner's manual resistance while the examiner pushes the humeral head forward. The examiner next feels over the bicipital groove for the long head of the biceps tendon, first with the shoulder rotated internally and then with it rotated externally. If the tender area moves with shoulder rotation, the biceps tendon is the probable structure involved. A test for a dislocating biceps tendon may also be made with the arm abducted to 90° and the examiner rotating it from internal to external rotation. If a slip is felt or a pop heard, the tendon of the long head of his biceps may be dislocating. The examiner next abducts the athlete's arm to 70° and palpates under the acromion for a tender supraspinatus tendon or subacromial bursa. At this level of abduction, the greater tuberosity is just passing under the coracoacromial arch where impingement may occur.

The rotator cuff may be tender, and sometimes the shoulder will pop when the arm is rotated. A roughened or torn anterior part of the cuff may be detected by rotating the arm and feeling under the deltoid. The arm is extended to palpate the anterior part of the cuff, and when the athlete grasps his opposite shoulder with his hand or lies prone with his arm hanging over the examining table, the posterior part of the cuff is uncovered and may be palpated. The examiner should ask the athlete to simulate the shoulder motion that hurts, and by offering resistance to this movement the examiner may be able to locate the trouble spot.

Throwers may develop latissimus dorsi tightness, and athletes who do heavy bench presses in the off-season may have pectoralis major tightness, resulting in an internal rotation contracture. This may be checked with the athlete supine: His chest is held down on the examining table and the shoulder rotated externally.

The scapula is examined with the subject prone and his arm hanging over the examining

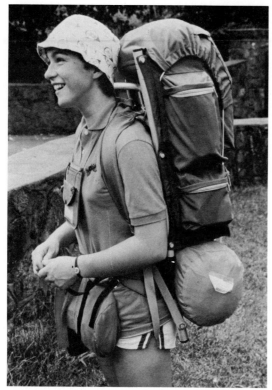

FIG. 12-2
A heavy backpack may cause "backpack
palsy."

table. The short rotators and the large muscles
that anchor the scapula to the thorax may then
be palpated from behind. The shoulder is
moved to uncover the region under the scapula,
and the chest wall may be palpated.

"Backpack Palsy"

Campers, hikers, and mountain climbers often
wear heavy backpacks, and the infantry type—
lightweight aluminum frame with heavy web
shoulder straps (Fig. 12-2)—may damage the
upper trunk of the backpacker's brachial
plexus, producing a severe and prolonged disability. There is a striking predilection for damage to the nondominant side, perhaps because
it is relatively weak. Such damage is similar to
Erb's paralysis from breech deliveries or from
lateral flexion injuries of the neck. An affected

backpacker may have significant radial and
musculocutaneous nerve dysfunction but usually only minimal median nerve deficit. The
ulna nerve is spared.

Early diagnosis allows a good recovery. The
suprascapular and axillary nerves are checked
by ascertaining the strength of the supraspinatus and deltoid muscles. Sensory changes are
checked over the lateral upper arm in the sensory region of the C-5 and C-6 nerve roots.

A backpacker with a nerve injury should refrain from wearing the backpack and should
strengthen his shoulder muscles, especially on
the nondominant side. When the hiker resumes
wearing the pack, he should limit the weight
he carries.

Thoracic Outlet Problems

Many anatomic abnormalities and some injuries may narrow the space through which an
athlete's arteries, veins, and nerves enter his
arm. These may include cervical ribs, a prominent transverse process of C-7, anomalies of
the first rib, excessive callus around a clavicle
fracture, or a malunited clavicular fracture in-
truding on this space. A shoulder drooped from
heavy use may also narrow this space. Moreover, during the abduction, extension, and extreme external humeral rotation phase of
throwing, the pectoralis minor stretches, transiently occluding the second portion of the axillary artery.

The symptoms of thoracic outlet compromise may be neurologic, venous, arterial, or a
combination of these.[54] Venous compromise
produces edema, limb stiffness, venous engorgement of the arm, and sometimes thrombophlebitis.[59] Arterial involvement may produce a cool, pale limb with claudication.[57] The
sympathetic nerves may also be irritated, causing a Raynaud's phenomenon, with worsening
after prolonged activity. Irritation of the brachial plexus produces numbness and tingling,
and the arm feels weak and heavy and tires
easily. The pain is usually around the elbow
but may also be in the chest, neck, shoulder,
forearm, or hand.

Arterial occlusion may occur in baseball

pitchers,[57] resulting in a painful, weak, and tired pitching arm. Arteriograms will show the occlusion, and thrombectomy and bypass vein graft, followed by rehabilitation, may enable the player to return to high-level pitching. In one case, a shortstop developed acute swelling and numbness in his throwing arm. Cinevenogram revealed acute occlusion of the subclavian vein from compression by his first rib. The compression was relieved by resection of the first rib.

Tennis players with a heavy, drooped, and internally rotated racquet arm shoulder may develop neck and arm pain owing to nerve compression.[47] This "tennis shoulder" may be helped by shrugging exercises that strengthen the shoulder elevators, elevating the shoulder to relieve the compression.

When examining athletes for thoracic outlet compromise, the examiner should ask them to mimic the activity that produces the discomfort. Local problems must first be ruled out before checking for referred causes. A cervical disc or compression in the quadrilateral space, for example, may be causing the shoulder or elbow pain. Tests such as a cervical myelogram, a Doppler examination of arterial and venous blood flow, cinevenography, arteriography, electomyography, or nerve conduction studies may be needed to ascertain the diagnosis.

Most compression problems may be initially managed nonoperatively with a sling, anti-inflammatory medicine, and exercises. The athlete's upper, middle, and lower trapezius muscle fibers are strengthened, along with the serratus anterior and erector spinae, to elevate the drooped shoulder.[7] Thrombectomy, bypass graft, or first rib resection may be needed.

The Sternoclavicular Joint

The sternoclavicular joint is at the base of the shoulder strut. Forces from landing on the hand may be transmitted to this area, and blows to the side of the shoulder may even dislocate this joint. In an anterior dislocation, the joint capsule is torn and may interpose to block reduction. This may be seen when a tangential view of the sternoclavicular joint is taken with the beam angled along the opposite clavicle. The dislocation may result in grating, clicking, and popping when the athlete moves his arm overhead or rotates his shoulder.

An anterior dislocation may be reduced by abducting the athlete's arm and pulling the shoulder girdle backwards with arm traction and then manipulating the clavicle. These reductions are often hard to hold with the usual figure-eight bandage; some surgeons, therefore, use a fascial sling between the clavicle and the first rib or perform a subclavius muscle tenodesis to hold the clavicle in place. Anterior dislocations usually do not require surgery.

Upon returning to athletic activity after anterior dislocation of the sternoclavicular joint, the athlete may note aching and swelling, grating, clicking or popping, and fatigue in that area. When these signs appear, a short portion of the inner end of the clavicle may be resected.

Retrosternal dislocation of the clavicle at the sternoclavicular joint may exert pressure on the trachea and great vessels, threatening the athlete's life.[1, 25] It may produce dysphagia, a snorting type of breathing, and even neurovascular trouble in the upper extremity. The dislocation should be reduced immediately. For this procedure, the athlete lies supine with a sandbag between his shoulders or with his shoulder extended over the table edge. Traction is then applied to his arm with his shoulder abducted and extended. His clavicle may have to be grasped through the skin with a towel clip and then maneuvered up and forward so that is snaps into place. After reduction, the athlete must wear a Velpeau bandage for 3 to 4 weeks and then begin motion exercises. Because of the contour of the joint and the ripped ligaments, these reductions are often unstable. Even so, pins should not be used to hold the reduction, as they may migrate.

The Clavicle

When an athlete falls, he may extend his arms to absorb the shock. The clavicle may snap, however, especially in jockeys, equestrians, or motocross racers who fall from a height or are thrown into the air. Rodeo cowboys who ride broncos and bulls, rope calves, and wrestle steers commonly fracture their clavicles. These men, however, usually know from experience how to fall, and they try not to land with their arms outstretched.

In youth ice hockey, broken clavicles are common, not so much from direct contact but from indirect transmitted force, when the skater falls on the ice or crashes into the boards.[40] Shoulder pads with a polyethylene cap protect the players from direct trauma but are not effective against forces transmitted up the arm.

An angled clavicle x-ray, with the athlete bowed backwards, will reveal any displacement. Clavicle fractures are usually treated with a figure-eight bandage and a sling with an ice-bag wrapped over the fracture. While wearing the figure-eight, the athlete must work to maintain the strength and endurance of his other limbs to avoid falling behind during the treatment phase.

Deltoid Strain, Bruised Shoulder, and "Shoulder Pointer"

Arm tackling may cause an anterior deltoid strain; these strained shoulders should be iced and taped before the athlete goes home and iced as needed later. Heat should *not* be applied. Shoulder bruises may follow firearm recoil in marksmen, but most marksmen wear a shoulder pad to prevent such bruising.

Shoulder injuries account for one third of all injuries in rugby union, and many of these impairments are bruises.[35] A "shoulder pointer" is a contusion to the trapezoid or to the deltoid muscle around the shoulder. Trapezius fibers may be avulsed where the trapezius inserts into the posterior edge of the clavicle close to, but not at, the point of the acromioclavicular joint. Cryotherapy is effective for shoulder pointers, and a local anesthetic and steroid may be injected, as in a hip pointer.

Modifications of rugby have led to tackle football. In rugby union, however, blocking is not permitted, and the object is to go after the ball rather than the runner. Some rugby players wear soft foam shoulder pads, and rugby forwards may have light felt pads sewn into the jerseys over the point of the shoulder. Rigid protective equipment probably would be counterproductive, since players would then increase their impact speed.

"Swimmer's Shoulder" and Subacromial Bursitis

A swimmer who trains by swimming up to 18,000 m a day may develop shoulder pain, as 80% of the power in swimming comes from arm action. If we assume 15 strokes for each 22.5 m, and if the swimmer trains at 9000 m a day, with 60% percent freestyle, butterfly, or backstroke, each arm goes through about 10,800 repetitive motions a week.[48, 49] The butterfly stroke is similar to the freestyle stroke, except for the body roll, and the backstroke is remarkably similar to the freestyle stroke. As the arm is near the swimmer's side or as the forward-flexed shoulder is rotated internally, the humeral head abuts against the acromion and the coracoacromial ligament. This impingement may irritate subjacent structures.

The microvascular pattern of the rotator cuff has been studied with micropaque injections.[34] The supraspinatus tendon is wrung out, especially when the swimmer adducts and then internally rotates his arm (Fig. 12-3A).[26] During internal rotation and forward flexion, the greater tuberosity abuts against the acromion. The supraspinatus tendon also has an avascular zone when the arm is abducted.[34] This has been found to be true even in cadavers of persons younger than 20 years old. The avascular zone is about 1 cm proximal to the point of insertion of the supraspinatus. The intracapsular part of the biceps becomes stretched over the humeral head and also has an avascular zone. These are vulnerable vascular patterns, in which chronic irritation leads to a death of cells and inflammation, subacromial bursitis, calcific tendinitis, and rotator cuff tears.

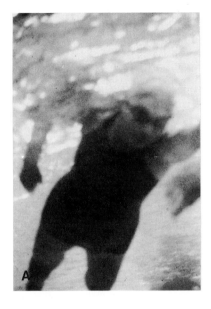

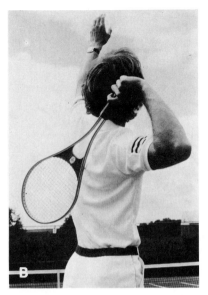

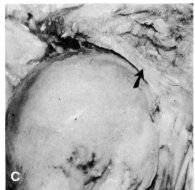

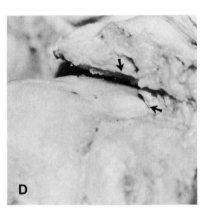

FIG. 12-3
The supraspinatus tendon is wrung out during the recovery phase of the freestyle stroke (*A*). Subacromial impingement may occur during overhead activities in tennis (*B*). The coracoacromial ligament (*C*) is responsible for many impingement problems. After the ligament has been resected (*D*), the supraspinatus moves much more freely.

The incidence of painful shoulders in swimmers ranges from 40% to 60%. It is slightly more common on the breathing side and most likely to occur in sprinters and middle-distance swimmers because of the "explosiveness" of each stroke. Women suffer from painful shoulders more often than do men, perhaps because of their higher stroke turnover rate. The condition is rare in swimmers younger than 10 years of age, probably because of shorter workouts. More than 50% of 13- to 18-year-old swimmers, however, complain of shoulder pain—mostly those not doing weight training or flexibility work.

The classification system that defines the severity of swimmer's shoulder is similar to that used to classify jumper's knee.[16] In phase I, the swimmer has pain only after activity; in phase II, he has pain both during and after activity but is still able to compete normally, and his condition is not disabling; in phase III, the swimmer is unable to compete at his normal level; and, in phase IV, he has pain even with everyday living.

Treatment should begin at phase I or II rather than at an advanced phase. During the early phases, a swimmer may be switched to sprints to decrease his training distance. In addition, a change to another stroke allows cardiovascular conditioning and avoids the aggravating movement. Thus the butterfly stroke may be free of pain though the freestyle stroke hurts. The swimmer should be on a full range-of-motion program during his training and should ice his shoulder immediately after a workout. A short course of phenylbutazone is sometimes used in diminishing doses to reduce the inflammation.

If the swimmer needs rest in phase III, he is put on dry-land exercises and a kickboard program. A steroid injection is sometimes given if a vital meet is upcoming. The swimmer may work on a high arm recovery technique because this technique seems to produce fewer shoulder problems. Bilateral breathing also helps; otherwise one arm catches deeper than the other.

Surgery is recommended in phase IV. The swimmer's coracoacromial ligament should be resected (*see* Fig. 12-3D), for if merely transected it will grow back. Older swimmers may need some bony decompression, achieved by shaving the undersurface of the acromion without disrupting the deltoid.[36]

There is a great reduction in swimmers' shoulder problems when swimmers stretch thoroughly before entering the water. The stretching increases the blood flow, lubricates, and gently stretches the rotator cuff.

Subacromial bursitis is a common problem for baseball pitchers and other athletes who use repetitive overhand motions and for some runners. If a runner hikes up his shoulders, his subacromial capacity is diminished, and the subacromial structures become inflamed. The pain is relieved when the runner relaxes his arms.

When an athlete abducts his arm, the subacromial space decreases. Wheelchair athletes, even those who race marathon distances, rarely have shoulder trouble. When the arm is used overhead, however, the supraspinatus tendon and the underlying intra-articular tendon of the long head of the biceps present a thickened anterior mass of tissue that must pass under the coracoacromial arch. The subacromial bursa becomes irritated and thickens to produce a snapping as the tendon passes under the coracoacromial arch. A throwing athlete with chronic rotator cuff impingement may have tenderness at the anterior aspect of his rotator cuff near the greater tuberosity. He may also report an audible "pop," or a popping sensation, when his arm travels through the acceleration phase of throwing.

The coracoacromial ligament may be resected before chronic changes occur. X-rays usually are normal, there is good shoulder strength and motion, and the cine studies and clinical examinations do not show instability. Arthrograms do not reveal any communication with the subacromial space, and subacromial bursagrams show the bursa to be normal or small. If these subjects do not significantly improve after a rest, including a minimum of 6 weeks free from the aggravating activity, they should undergo an operation. In this procedure, a strap incision is made under local anesthesia, extending from the acromioclavicular joint to the coracoid process. The deltoid is split and then detached for about 2 cm along the acromion. The athlete is asked to reproduce the pop, and the ligament is then cut and partly excised. He is then asked to reproduce the throw again and should volunteer that the impingement is no longer present. Postoperatively, he gradually regains motion, followed by strengthening and light throwing. Although the shoulder pain and popping are relieved after resection of the coracoacromial ligament, some athletes will feel a lack of constraint of the humeral head, as when spiking a volleyball.

Coracoid Injuries

A marksman's coracoid may be bruised from recoils in target or game shooting. A more severe reaction may occur during the acceleration phase of the tennis serve or when a young athlete pitches: Excessive traction on the tip may avulse the coracoid.

Because even a normal coracoid tip is usually tender to deep palpation, the one opposite the injury should be palpated for comparison. An axillary view will help to locate the avulsed fragment, but the examiner should be aware of secondary ossification centers to avoid misinterpreting the x-rays.

A fresh avulsion of the coracoid need not be fixed internally. If it later becomes symptomatic, however, the distal fragment may be excised and the conjoined tendon reattached.[3]

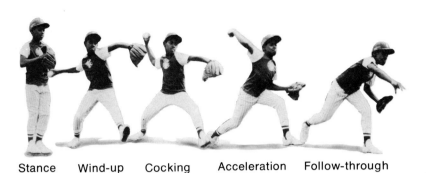

FIG. 12-4
Phases of throwing.

Stance   Wind-up   Cocking   Acceleration   Follow-through

Throwing

Throwing is an integral part of many sports, but different techniques are needed, depending on whether the object propelled is heavy or light and on the size and shape of the object.[18]

The baseball pitcher flings the baseball. The phases of pitching are stance, windup, cocking, acceleration, and follow-through (Fig. 12-4). During stance, the pitcher stands on the rubber and obtains signs from his catcher. In the windup phase, the pitcher steps back with his rear leg and extends his arms. During cocking, the shoulder is abducted in extension and marked external rotation. This prestretching phase prepares the muscles for the throw, and the anterior shoulder structures are also stretched. In the acceleration, or forward, phase, the arm is behind the body before being flung forward toward the catcher, and the ball is released at ear level. In the follow-through, the humeral head leaves the glenoid by more than 2.5 cm as the shoulder goes from external to internal rotation. The triceps decelerates the arm, and the thumb turns down as the forearm pronates. A unique aspect of baseball is the pitcher's need to master several pitches and different types of arm motions. The stress on the pitcher's shoulder is increased by having to throw from a pitcher's mound.

The tennis serve is a throwing motion, with a cocking, or backscratch, phase, acceleration, ball impact, and follow-through. The player essentially throws the racquet at the ball at high speed but then must decelerate from 300 miles/h within a very short distance.[38, 47] The large muscles that anchor the shoulder are stretched during the tennis serve.

The football pass is a pushing motion in which the cocking phase and follow-through are shorter than in a flinging motion. While the biceps tendon is tight, the quarterback is especially vulnerable to opponents' attacks on his throwing arm. Unlike a baseball pitcher, the football quarterback uses the same type of motion for each pass, with little variation.

Field event throws include the javelin, shot-put, discus, and hammer. Javelin throwers with good technique throw over the shoulder with elbow extension. "Round arm" throws are incorrect, and these throwers tend to develop shoulder and elbow problems similar to those of baseball pitchers. A shotputter's fingers support the heavy shot, and the large, scapular-anchoring muscles must slow the arm down after the shot has been released. Discus and hammer throws are centrifugal motions that do not produce as many shoulder problems as do overhead events.

Softball pitchers, hurlers, and ten-pin and duck-pin bowlers stress, and sometimes rupture, their biceps tendons during their underhand, flexion activities.

Diagnosis and Treatment of Injuries

When diagnosing a throwing injury, the examiner should obtain a detailed history to determine which phase of the throwing motion is involved.

During wind-up, the head of the humerus wears and roughens from leverage on the posterior glenoid and the tendon of the long head of the biceps stretches. In the cocking phase, the shoulder moves from internal to external rotation. Pitchers have increased external rotation of the shoulder and decreased internal rotation, but their total range of motion is usually normal. The cocking phase produces anterior shoulder pain sometimes associated with anterior cuff irritation, anterior "cuffitis," or subluxation of the long head of the biceps. Because both biceps and triceps are contracted, bicipital tendinitis and tricipital tendinitis may occur.

When his arm is abducted and rotated externally, the athlete who has had injury to the glenohumeral joint may have laxity of the anterior complex of the shoulder, consisting of the capsule and the subscapularis. A pitcher will note an unstable feeling as his humeral head begins to slip forward out of the socket and then pops back again. As the examiner pushes the humeral head forward, the athlete may wince in apprehension of the feeling of instability. This is the "apprehension shoulder" of anterior subluxation. Some pitchers normally sublux their shoulders and develop posterior shoulder pain first as their muscles go into spasm to prevent the humeral head from sliding forward. They later develop anterior shoulder pain.

At the start of acceleration, the pitcher's body is "opened up" and his arm is left behind. Strong internal rotation of the shoulder then

FIG. 12-5
During follow-through of a throw, the humeral head leaves the glenoid. The humerus pulls on the capsule, triceps, and teres minor, causing a bony outgrowth.

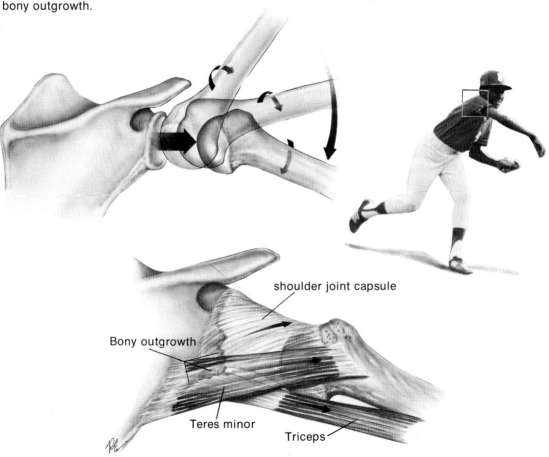

shoulder joint capsule

Bony outgrowth

Teres minor

Triceps

begins, a movement so forceful that a young pitcher may even avulse the coracoid tip. Apprehension shoulder may occur at the beginning of the acceleration phase, and anterior capsular pain may be reproduced when the examiner manually resists the acceleration motion.

Repetitive throwing too hard and too often may produce subacromial pain with subdeltoid and subacromial bursal adhesions. Frequently pitchers with these adhesions exhibit poor form, opening up too soon; that is, the pitcher leaves his arm behind his body after bringing his trunk around. As his arm drags behind, he tries to rush it forward to catch up by dropping his elbow, "short-arming" the ball.[41]

Subacromial symptoms subside with rest, but once mature adhesions form the pain returns whenever throwing is resumed. At surgery, the subdeltoid and subacromial bursa are often obscured by a thick adhesion that involves the whole bursal complex. The bursae are thick and show myxoid degeneration. Unfortunately, all modes of treatment for fully developed subdeltoid bursitis seem to fail.[41] For this reason, a pitcher should not be asked to pitch through a painful shoulder and to risk irreparable damage from formation of dense adhesions. The pitcher's motion should be analyzed by a pitching coach to identify and correct flaws in the delivery.

The force of strong internal rotation in the acceleration phase may rupture the pectoralis major or latissimus dorsi or fracture the pitcher's humerus. A pectoralis major rupture leaves a gap in the axillary fold.[60] Tears of this tendon should be repaired, but tears within the muscle will heal themselves.

A pitcher releases the baseball at ear level, and his arm then follows through toward the plate. The arm continues to rotate internally, soon catching up with the body. Now the arm must be decelerated by the long head of the triceps, which acts as a rein, putting traction on the area of origin of the triceps at the inferior lip of the glenoid. This traction may produce triceps origin microtrauma and the formation of new bone at this site (Fig. 12-5). A traction spur may later break off, move, and cause pain.

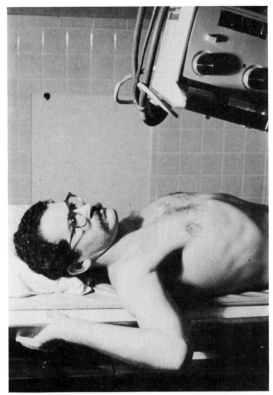

FIG. 12-6
Subglenoid bone growths are best seen on x-ray films taken with the pitcher's shoulder externally rotated and the tube angled upward.

To demonstrate this bone formation on x-ray, the pitcher lies supine and externally rotates and abducts his shoulder 90° (Fig. 12-6) as the x-ray beam is angled from his axilla to an x-ray plate placed above his shoulder.

Ossification at the posteroinferior part of the glenoid—"Bennett's lesion"—is often associated with tears of the glenoid labrum and posterior capsule. The ossification is, in part, an inflammatory response to microtrauma, and is also caused by posterior subluxation of the humeral head and posterior cuffitis in the region of the teres minor.

If a pitcher develops posterior shoulder pain and x-rays show bone at the posteroinferior glenoid, his arm should be rested, and oral anti-inflammatory therapy or a steroid injection may be given. A pitching coach should later evaluate his follow-through mechanics. Sometimes, the pitcher stays closed too long, not opening up to face the target, and his arm gets ahead of him. In addition, he should stop throwing sidearm. If the pain persists, the bony overgrowth may have to be excised. In this procedure, the surgeon makes an incision over the scapula spine with the pitcher prone. The deltoid is reflected from the spine, the posterior capsule and glenoid are then reached through the interval between the infraspinatis and teres minor. The capsule is opened longitudinally and the lesion noted and removed. After operation, the athlete must wear a sling for 1 week before beginning a strength and flexibility program. Light throwing resumes at about 8 weeks after the procedure.

If a pitcher is not fit, fatigue will decrease his coordination and change his pitching motion. If he is overweight, the excess fat serves as a brake on his contracting muscles. "A pitcher's legs go first": If his legs are not strong for push-off and balance, his pitching power will drop. This disrupts his delivery, and the change in his throwing motion may lead to injury.

Warming Up

A complete warm-up before pitching helps to prevent injury to a pitcher's throwing arm.[6] The trainer first applies moist heat to the pitcher's arm for about 20 minutes, followed by an ice rub or a cold, wet towel rub. The pitching shoulder may also be massaged with an analgesic rub. The pitcher then lies on his side, and the trainer moves the shoulder into abduction, rotation, and extension to stretch the shoulder capsule. These stretches are repeated with the pitcher on his back, and the trainer works on forearm and wrist motion, followed by a gentle shaking of the whole limb.[2]

After the massage and stretches, the pitcher suspends his full body weight from a bar by one arm and revolves slowly for 30 seconds. He may also hang from the roof of the dugout later to achieve the same stretching effect. Hanging stretches his shoulder and arm muscles and opens the joint to loosen the joint structures. He should not do chin-ups or pull-ups because they cause tightness. Once the shoulder is stretched and before he begins his warm-up throws, the pitcher performs a general warm-up, working up a sweat before stepping on the rubber.

The moist heat, massage, stretching, and general warm-up program enhances flexibility for optimal delivery, allowing the pitcher to get the most out of his arm. This program probably saves as many as 20 pitches from pre-game warm-up throws, giving the pitcher an extra boost late in the game.

When warming up, the pitcher should remove his jacket and throw in the direction he will be facing in the game.[6] He should begin at a distance shorter than the rubber to home plate, gradually moving to the full distance. The first pitches should be straight slow balls, with no curves thrown until the arm is fully warmed up. The pitcher should not throw hard until the umpire is on the scene.

A pitcher's normal 15 to 20 minute warm-up may start with 30 straight balls at medium velocity, then adding 10 curves, 10 sliders, and 10 fast balls of increasing speed. He finishes with sets of 5 pitches of various types, to total 80 pitches. The pitcher then rests for 5 minutes before game time but keeps his warm-up jacket on until he is ready to pitch, regardless of climatic conditions.

Arm Care After Pitching

After repetitive hard throwing in a game, edema and a fibrin exudate accumulate in the shoulder tissues. Some bleeding into the muscles may also occur that may result in scarring. After firing the last pitch, or after throwing a football or a javelin, the athlete can lessen this accumulation and assist in waste product removal by warming down, stretching the shoulder, and moving it through its range of motion.

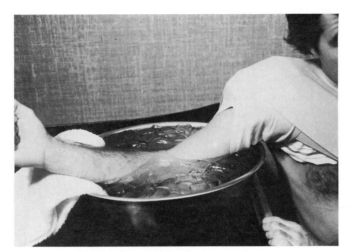

FIG. 12-7
After a game, the pitcher has an ice bag placed on his externally rotated shoulder and rests his elbow in ice water.

Pitchers who do not complete a game and relief pitchers who pitch only to a few batters need the same postgame arm care as pitchers who pitch complete games.

After the game, the arm should be iced down with a large ice pack held over the player's shoulder by an elastic wrap, and the elbow soaked in cold water (Fig. 12-7). The ice is analgesic, decreases swelling, and is antispasmodic. Cold reduces the metabolism of the tissues and lessens cellular damage and the inflammatory response. The ice should not, however, be left on for more than 15 to 20 minutes, or a strong reflex vasodilitation may occur.

Sore Arm

Because throwing too hard or too soon during the early season may lead to a sore arm, a good way to start the season is to throw without wearing a glove. If a sore arm occurs, the cause of the soreness should be carefully diagnosed. Pitchers must not be allowed to pitch through sore arms, as this may only worsen any condition.

The pitcher with a sore arm will experience a drop in strength with each day of rest. For this reason, a pitcher must exercise outside the soreness range to maintain strength and to keep his shoulder loose with a full range of motion. A sore shoulder exercise program will include sawing exercises, cross-overs, shrugs, and circumductions (Fig. 12-8). The circumductions are first done in a clockwise and then in a counterclockwise direction, making the largest possible circles. Each exercise should be repeated 50 times three times a day.

Anti-inflammatory medicines such as aspirin may be given 20 to 30 minutes before exercising. Some physicians give a decreasing dosage schedule of butazolidine, 200 mg four times daily for 2 days, then 200 mg three times daily for 2 days, and finally 100 mg three times daily for 3 days. Others use indomethacin (Indocin), ibuprofen (Motrin), tolmetin sodium (Tolectin), or naproxen (Naprosyn) for an anti-inflammatory effect.

The Fungo Routine

If a thrower is sidelined for a lengthy period and begins his return to throwing with short throws, neither a full range of motion nor a natural throwing motion will be achieved. A "fungo routine" of long easy throws is a better beginning. In this program, the fungo hitter bats balls to the player, who throws them back from the outfield in an easy manner, bringing his arm through a full range of motion. The

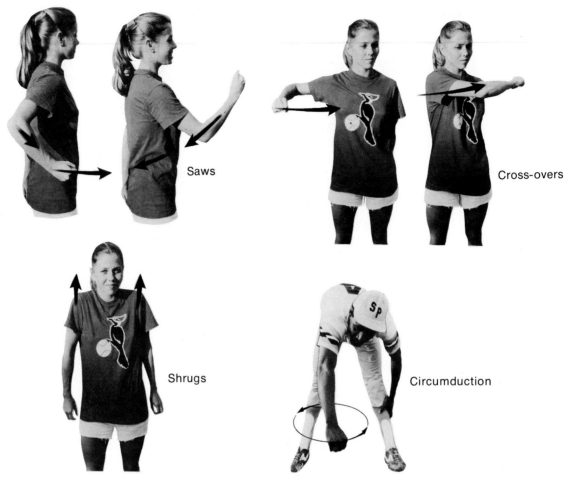

FIG. 12-8
Sore shoulder exercises include saws, cross-overs, shrugs, and circumduction. The athlete usually performs 50 repetitions of each exercise three times a day.

arm is thus stretched and strengthened without placing too much stress on the shoulder. The throws must be pain-free with normal form, and if the player substitutes movements or deviates from normal form, the workout should be halted.

The program starts with long easy throws from the deep outfield, and the ball should be allowed to roll into the plate, just reaching the fungo hitter. The sessions last 30 minutes for 2 days, then the player's arm is rested for 1 day. The player next moves to the middle of the outfield, making stronger throws into the fungo hitter on about five bounces. These sessions last for 30 minutes over 2 more days, followed by another day of rest. Next come stronger, crisp throws from the short outfield, with a straight trajectory, on one bounce to the fungo hitter. These sessions also last 30 minutes for 2 days, followed by 1 more day of rest. The pitcher should now be ready to return to the mound with a full wind-up, throwing at about half speed before increasing to three-quarter and then to full speed. The full program takes 3 to 4 weeks until the pitcher returns to the pitching rotation.

Shoulder Separations

The acromioclavicular joint is a satellite joint of the shoulder that moves throughout shoulder abduction, especially during the early and late stages of this motion. As it shifts and rotates, much of its stability is afforded by the deltoid and trapezius origins that surround it. With damage to the supporting ligaments of the acromioclavicular joint, the muscles may pull the distal clavicle into a dislocated position. If an athlete falls on the point of his shoulder or lands on the ground with an opponent on top, as in rugby, wrestling, or tackle football, the clavicle hits the first rib and is driven upward, and the acromioclavicular ligaments or the acromioclavicular and coracoclavicular ligaments may be disrupted, springing the joint.[35,46]

Acromioclavicular separations are graded I, II, and III (Fig. 12-9).[4] A grade I separation connotes damage to the acromioclavicular ligament fibers but no laxity. If an athlete comes to the sideline with shoulder pain, the examiner should feel under his shoulder pads for tenderness over the acromioclavicular joint. Before he is sent back into the game, his shoulder should be completely examined with the shoulder pads off. Otherwise, if the acromioclavicular joint has been damaged and the player is returned to the game, a second hit may transform a grade I separation into a grade II or grade III sprain. Ice and a sling are used in the initial symptomatic care of a grade I sprain,

FIG. 12-9
Acromioclavicular separations. A grade I acromioclavicular separation implies damage to the acromioclavicular ligament without displacement of the clavicle. A grade II separation means subluxation of the acromioclavicular joint and an increase in the coracoclavicular distance, owing to disruption of the acromioclavicular ligament and damage to the coracoclavicular ligaments. Both the acromioclavicular and the coracoclavicular ligaments are ruptured in a grade III separation, allowing the clavicle to ride high.

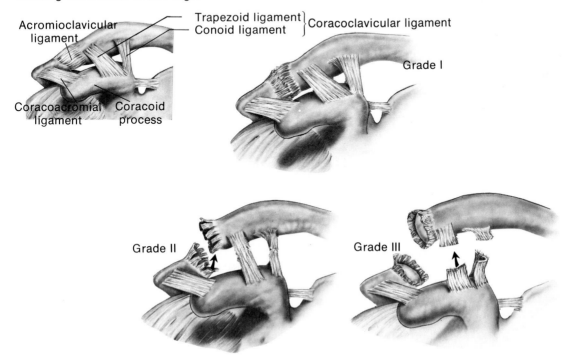

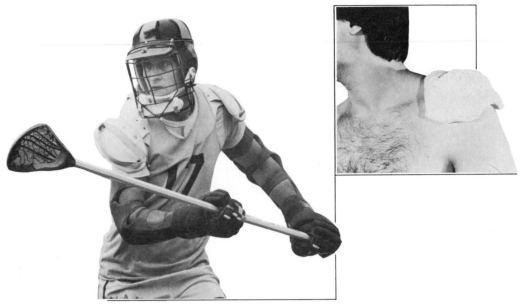

FIG. 12-10
Shoulder pads or a plastic and felt pad can protect an injured
acromioclavicular joint.

followed by cryotherapy and isodynamics or weightlifting out of the soreness range. The player may return to competition when soreness diminishes and he has regained full strength and flexibility. For added protection he may wear a foam donut pad or a plastic cap under his shoulder pads (Fig 12-10).

A tear of the athlete's acromioclavicular ligament, combined with a grade I sprain of the coracoclavicular ligament, ranks as a grade II shoulder separation. An x-ray film may show the distal clavicle to be elevated by about one half the width of the joint, and there is a slight increase in coracoclavicular distance. The resulting prominence at the acromioclavicular joint is sometimes obscured by swelling, but the distal clavicle is movable.

The risen clavicle may be best seen on x-ray when the tube is tilted up 15° and the exposure is decreased. Sometimes the athlete is asked to hold weights in his hands, or the weights may be strapped to his wrists to bring out the subluxation. These weights may, however, cause him to shrug his shoulder and reduce the subluxation. If weights are needed to demonstrate

the separation, the treatment is usually no different from that for a grade I separation.

A grade III, or major shoulder, separation connotes rupture of the athlete's acromioclavicular ligament and the conoid and trapezoid portions of the coracoclavicular ligament. The distal clavicle is movable, and because of swelling or spasm of the surrounding muscles, this type of separation may appear clinically to be a mildly elevated grade II separation. With the athlete in a supine position, the prominence may not be very apparent, but when he sits up the clavicle may be strikingly elevated. Some surgeons inject the injured area with xylocaine to see whether the athlete can abduct the shoulder completely or if there is abutment. If shoulder motion is blocked, the surgeon may decide to operate.

The treatments for grade II and grade III shoulder separations are subjects of controversy, varying from symptomatic programs and early motion and strength work, to special slings or tape jobs and operations to hold the clavicle down.

The nonoperative program emphasizes exercises. During the early sore period, while the athlete is lying down, he uses active-assistive overhead motion. About 5 days after injury, he may begin a trapezius and deltoid strengthening cryotherapy program that includes abduction against resistance and shoulder shrugs. Early strengthening of these muscles produces a strong shoulder, and there is usually not much functional difference between this early activity, nonoperative program and operative treatment. Allowing the distal clavicle to remain in a dislocated position may cause the athlete no trouble. Later, if the distal clavicle abuts in overhead activities, such as pitching a baseball, throwing a football, or grabbing rebounds in basketball, the distal clavicle may be resected.

The examiner may decide to inject a local anesthetic into the painful area, relocate the clavicle with the patient supine, and hold the re-duction with an acromioclavicular sling until the ligaments have healed. In practice, however, this technique is painful, prolonged, and only occasionally successful. Even if reduction is achieved and the coracoclavicular ligaments heal, the damaged acromioclavicular joint may become painfully arthritic.

The clavicle functions mainly as an attachment for the deltoid, trapezius, and sternocleidomastoid muscles. To maintain the effective length of these muscles, some surgeons pull the clavicle down and reconstruct the coracoclavicular ligaments. Occasionally, an athlete will not want a bump, preferring instead to trade the bump for a scar. There are many ways to stabilize the acromioclavicular joint (Fig. 12-11). Wires may be passed through the acromion into the clavicle, but they must be bent so that they will not migrate. Some surgeons place a

FIG. 12-11
Acromioclavicular repairs. A grade III acromioclavicular separation may be treated with a special sling or operatively with a screw, pins, or tape. In each operation, a short piece of the distal clavicle is also resected.

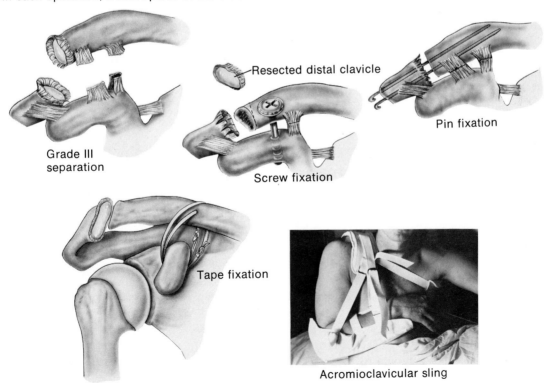

Resected distal clavicle

Pin fixation

Grade III separation

Screw fixation

Tape fixation

Acromioclavicular sling

lag screw through the clavicle into the coracoid, but the screw must be removed in 6 to 8 weeks or it may break owing to rotary motion between the coracoid and clavicle. To eliminate the need for removal of the fixation device, the clavicle may be lashed down to the coracoid with a 5-mm polyethylene fiber tape. Range-of-motion exercises and rehabilitation may start a few days after the operation. The tape does not stretch and need not be removed, and the athlete may return to sports as soon as the wound has healed. Before all operations that use the coracoid as a stabilizing post, the surgeon should take an x-ray film along the spine of the scapula to show the entire coracoid. If the coracoid has a fracture through its base, it could dislodge after the operation. Another operative approach entails attaching the short head of the biceps or the coracoid process itself as a "dynamic transfer" to the undersurface of the clavicle.

An important consideration in these operations is the disposition of the acromioclavicular joint when the clavicle has been reduced. The damaged acromioclavicular joint may become a trouble spot; thus an arthroplasty may be done in which 1 cm of the distal clavicle is resected (see section on Acromioclavicular Arthritis below). Some surgeons sever the acromial attachment of the coracoacromial ligament and use it to reinforce the shredded coracoclavicular ligament. However, unless the athlete is a swimmer, a throwing athlete, or a volleyball player who has been having subacromial trouble, the coracoacromial ligament is usually left in place to act as a soft cushion, preventing upward displacement of the humeral head.

Acromioclavicular Arthritis

Heavy use of the shoulder may cause the acromioclavicular joint to break down with arthritis, especially in athletes who use across-the-body motions, such as golfers, baseball players, and ice and field hockey players.[12] Osteoarthritic changes of narrowing and osteophyte for-

mation are apparent on x-ray film. The x-ray tube should be tilted up at an angle of about 15° and the exposure decreased to show the acromioclavicular joint, as the joint may be washed out in an ordinary shoulder x-ray.

With proper operative technique, a resection of the distal clavicle solves the problem of acromioclavicular joint arthritis. If too much of the distal clavicle and the posterior capsular ligament are removed, however, the distal clavicle will become hypermobile. No more than 1 cm of bone need be resected, and the resection should be angled wider posteriorly, with the posterior capsular ligament retained. The shoulder is then brought through a full range of motion to ensure that there will be no impingement during overhead activities. It is mobilized a few days after operation, and the athlete may return to contact sports in about 6 weeks.

Rotator Cuff Tears

The muscles of the shoulder maintain its instant center of rotation in a fixed position. While the rotator cuff muscles hold the humerus in the glenoid, the deltoid abducts the shoulder. With damage to the rotator cuff, the humerus skids in the glenoid, becoming unstable. The supraspinatus is the key muscle in the rotator cuff group, passing just below the coracoacromial ligament; it may be irritated by abutment against this structure.

Tears in an athlete's rotator cuff are usually short, longitudinal ones[39] occurring in the critical zone between the supraspinatus and the coracohumeral ligament (Fig. 12-12). This is an area of poor vascularity where degeneration of the tendon frequently occurs. Repeated microtrauma to the cuff may also provoke a significant tissue reaction with thickening, thus decreasing the already confined subacromial space (see "Swimmer's Shoulder" and Subacromial Bursitis above).

The most common rotator cuff lesion in throwers is a partial tear in which a few fibers are avulsed from the tuberosity in the deep

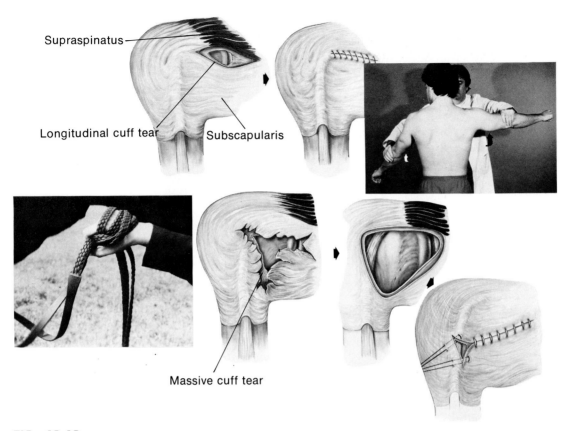

FIG. 12-12
Tears in the rotator cuff are usually longitudinal ones between the supraspinatus and subscapularis tendons that result in weakened abduction. A massive tear of the rotator cuff may occur if, for example, an equestrian's arm is yanked by her horse. The surgeon trims these rips and repairs them with a suture made from a fascial strip.

layers. The arthrogram may show this as an indentation, and the lesion may be seen during arthroscopy. Large tears of the cuff are less common. They are more likely to occur in a violent way, as when an equestrian's arm is jerked by a horse while the reins are wrapped around her hand.

If an athlete has a partial tear of his rotator cuff, he may feel pain during overhead motions. There may be crepitus or clicking and some weakness on abduction of the shoulder, although he will be able to abduct fully. Most of this weakness comes from deltoid atrophy from reduced use of the arm owing to pain. The examiner should look for atrophy of the supraspinatus in the suprascapular fossa and have the athlete abduct his shoulder through a full arc of motion to locate weakness. The examiner may place his palm over the painful shoulder to note grinding and compare this shoulder with the normal side. The rotator cuff may be felt by finding an interval between the deltoid fibers and by rotating the shoulder. The athlete may hesitate or grimace as his arm is raised. If a subacromial injection of xylocaine relieves the pain, an impingement syndrome is a likely diagnosis.

An arthrogram will reveal complete tears and deep surface tears but will not show partial tears within the substance of the rotator cuff

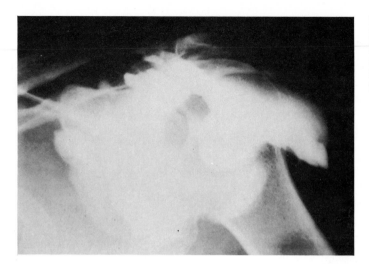

FIG. 12-13
In this arthrogram, a full-thickness rotator cuff tear allows injected dye to escape from the shoulder joint.

(Fig. 12-13).[55] Such interstitial tears do not occur in normal tendons, but as a person ages there is progressive tendon degeneration. Normal tendons separate in the muscle at the musculotendinous junction or at the insertion of the tendon into bone when loaded. Degeneration increases the potential for rupture.

If there is even a small full-thickness tear of the cuff, continued use will aggravate the lesion, and it can extend to become a major tear, much as a short tear of a knee meniscus can extend to become a bowstring tear.[2] A major tear of the rotator cuff will generate pain when the subject tries to abduct his shoulder. However, because the deltoid plays a large quantitative part in this action, he may be able to initiate abduction. Major tears should be repaired early to prevent retraction of the cuff.

Partial tears are repaired with synthetic sutures. Cat gut or silk is not used because it may cause a reaction. Larger tears can often be closed with synthetic suture, but if there is a gap that cannot be closed fully, a darning technique with fascia lata on a fascia needle will repair the defect. The biceps tendon can also be used as a free graft in large tears. The intra-articular part of the tendon may be spread out flat, and the remaining distal portion of the tendon may then be attached to the proximal humerus by the keyhole technique. In large retracted tears, an acromioplasty helps provide space in which to work on freeing the cuff to achieve closure. Acromionectomy is not recommended because it is difficult for the athlete to re-establish abduction when the point of origin of the deltoid has been removed.

Chronic tears of the rotator cuff usually produce pain at night. Such tears may require a fascia lata stitch or a free graft of the biceps tendon. A cantilever brace with a hinge that allows the arm to swing across the chest may be used postoperatively.

Bicipital Tendinitis

The tendon of the long head of the biceps arises at the supraglenoid tubercle and passes at an angle of 30° into the bicipital groove, where it lies deep to the transverse humeral ligament. During shoulder motion, the tendon does not glide but remains fixed as the humerus slides along the tendon. During the follow-through in throwing, the humerus actually leaves the socket by as much as 2.5 cm to 3.75 cm (1 in to 1.5 in). Rubbing of the tendon by the groove and ligament is worsened by a tight groove, especially if the channel has a steep medial wall (Fig. 12-14). In addition, many shoulders have a rough supratubercular area that irritates the tendon.[24]

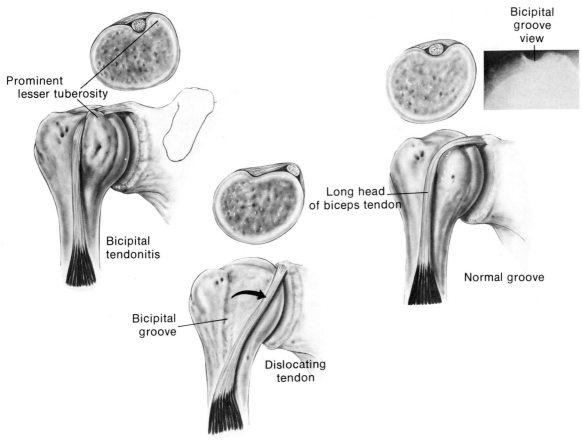

FIG. 12-14
The tendon of the long head of the biceps may be irritated in a bicipital groove that has a prominent lesser tuberosity. If the groove is too shallow, the tendon may dislocate.

The athlete with bicipital tendinitis usually reports a prodrome of shoulder pain. There is tenderness over the bicipital groove, and this area moves when the shoulder is shifted from internal to external rotation.[15] The examiner can press over the bicipital groove to locate the tender spot. The athlete's elbow is then flexed, with his arm at his side, and the shoulder is rotated. In bicipital tendinitis, the tenderness follows the movement of the bicipital groove. With the shoulder rotated internally, the tenderness is medial; at neutral position it remains medial. When the shoulder is externally rotated, however, the groove lies in front or even lateral to the midline, and this becomes the tender area. The examiner may also extend the athlete's elbow with the forearm pronated to fix the biceps at the bicipital tuberosity. The arm is then extended to produce pain.

Ice may be used in the early treatment of bicipital tendinitis and the athlete given a nonsteroidal, anti-inflammatory medicine. Painful maneuvers should be avoided, and if the pain persists the arm should be rested. A local steroid deposit around the tendon often relieves the pain, but if it is injected into the tendinous substance it may provoke rupture. The surgical procedure for recurring bicipital tendinitis is identical to that for ruptures of the tendon of the long head of the biceps.[11]

Dislocation of the Biceps Tendon

A checked swing in baseball, with a sudden forceful jerking back of the bat, or an attack on a quarterback's externally rotated passing arm, with the biceps tensed, may tear the transverse humeral ligament from its insertion on the lesser tuberosity. Where the transverse humeral ligament peels off, the long head of the biceps tendon can slide up and over the tuberosity, especially when the medial wall of the bicipital groove is shallow, with an inclination of 30° or less (*see* Fig. 12-14).[42]

The athlete with a dislocating biceps tendon has anterior shoulder pain with popping, cracking, and occasionally a locking sensation. The tendon slips and rolls over during throws, sometimes snapping back during internal rotation.

Shoulder pain may occur when the shoulder is abducted to 90° and then rotated externally and internally. The tendon dislocation can sometimes be brought out by manually resisting the throwing motion. Tenderness follows the movement of the bicipital groove. When the arm is internally rotated the tenderness is medial, and in neutral position the tenderness remains medial. When the arm is externally rotated, however, the groove lies in front of, or even lateral to, the midline, and the tenderness shifts to this position.

A tunnel x-ray view may be taken to evaluate the bicipital groove. The x-ray plate is placed at the top of the athlete's shoulder and the beam directed along the line of the groove. The picture provides information on the configuration of the groove and may reveal osteophytes at the edges of the groove.

For acute biceps tendon dislocation, the shoulder is iced and the arm rested in internal rotation. When dislocations recur, the repairs are the same as those for biceps tendon rupture.

Rupture of the Long Head of the Biceps Tendon

The biceps tendon becomes worn by persistent rubbing in a tight, steep-walled groove that has supratubercular rough spots. Further degeneration of the tendon occurs in swimmers as an avascular zone of the intracapsular part of the tendon is stretched over the humeral head. Rupture of the biceps tendon is not uncommon in the degenerated tendons of older athletes: It may follow an underhand delivery in softball or a snappy, underhand basketball pass (Fig. 12-15). However, even young athletes, especially gymnasts and weight lifters, may rupture the tendon of the long head of their biceps. This type of rupture produces a bulging biceps in the arm.

The biceps spans two joints, and repairs usually restore only the part near the elbow. If the tendon is left unrepaired, the athlete will lose about 20% of his elbow flexion power. Repair is usually not recommended for nonathletes, but repair may restore needed elbow flexion and supination to competitive athletes.[14]

In repairing this condition, the surgeon enters the shoulder joint through a small split in the rotator cuff. The intra-articular part of the tendon is then removed from the glenoid to prevent a buckling tendon remnant from interfering with shoulder action. Some surgeons roughen the floor of the bicipital groove and suture the tendon into the groove with mattress stitches.[24] Others use a staple, but the staple may loosen.[15] Still others choose a "trap door" technique in which the tendon is placed under an osteoperiosteal flap near the bicipital groove. After most of these operations, the shoulder must be rested. Because such long restriction of motion may freeze the shoulder, a keyhole technique that allows postoperative shoulder and elbow motion and rapid resumption of activities may be preferred (*see* Fig. 12-15).[17]

Acute Dislocation of the Shoulder

In an anterior dislocation of the shoulder, the shoulder abducts and rotates externally, and the acromion acts as a fulcrum on the humeral head, which breaks through the weak anterior capsule. The labrum rips from the glenoid, and the subscapularis and supraspinatis stretch. The

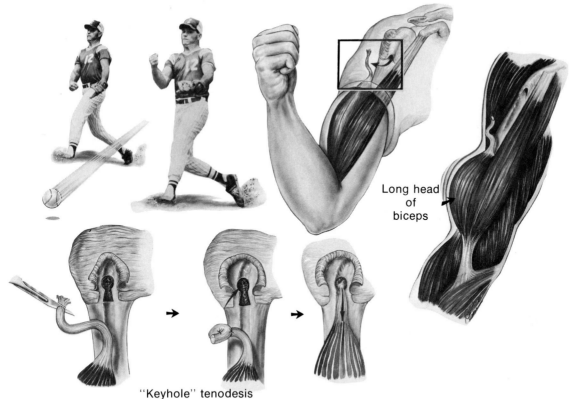

"Keyhole" tenodesis

FIG. 12-15
The tendon of the long head of the biceps may rupture in a softball pitcher, leaving him with a weakened arm. Some elbow power may be regained by reattaching the tendon in the bicipital groove.

humeral head then slides below the coracoid and sometimes pops back into place but more frequently stays dislocated (Fig. 12-16).

A player typically comes off the field supporting his arm and usually has a hollowed-out area at the shoulder. In a muscular athlete, this sign may be less apparent when the two shoulders are compared. However, an athlete with an anterior dislocation will usually not be able to touch his other shoulder.

Although the shoulder will sometimes pop back after gentle traction on the field or sidelines, in most cases the athlete must be taken from the playing field for reduction of the dislocation.

Early on, there is not much spasm. An icebag on the shoulder will provide analgesia and muscle relaxation. The athlete is then helped to a prone position on the training table, or on a car fender, with his arm hanging over the side. The physician gently pulls downward, with the athlete's elbow flexed to 90° and his forearm supinated to relax the biceps (*see* Fig. 12-16). An assistant then rotates the inferior angle of the scapula toward the spine so that the glenoid faces the humerus. The combination of traction and scapular rotation allows the humeral head to slide easily back into the socket. A dislocation will sometimes even reduce spontaneously when the athlete lies prone on the examining table with a pillow under his chest and his arm hanging over the edge of the table.

The "Hippocratic" is an alternative method of reduction. While an assistant applies countertraction around the chest, the athlete's arm is pulled at about 30° of abduction in line with

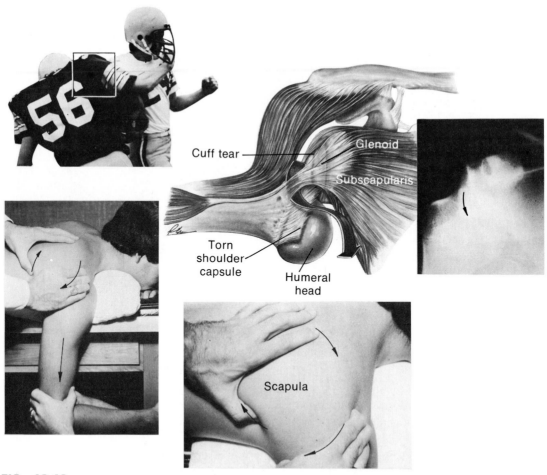

FIG. 12-16
Forces applied to the externally rotated and abducted arm during arm tackling may wrench the humeral head from the glenoid, ripping the capsule. A rotator cuff tear sometimes accompanies the dislocation. The dislocation, usually an anterior, subcoracoid one, is best reduced by traction and scapular rotation.

the trunk (Fig. 12-17). If the examiner's foot is placed against the athlete's chest for counter-traction, it may slip into the axilla to damage the brachial plexus. In a muscular athlete, a wrist-lock technique may be used with the athlete's elbow flexed to relax the biceps tendon and forestall fatigue during the traction phase. The dislocated shoulder will usually reduce, but in some muscular persons seen late and who have strong muscle spasm, a narcotic medicine and an intravenous relaxant, or even general anesthesia, may be needed to facilitate reduction.

Once the dislocation is reduced, a true anteroposterior x-ray of the shoulder should be taken. An axillary lateral or a transthoracic lateral view is also needed to be certain that the dislocation has been reduced. An icebag is placed on the shoulder over a towel, held with a figure-eight elastic wrap.

An athlete's first anterior dislocation should be immobilized for 3 to 4 weeks. Special immobilization devices or advanced exercise programs appear to have no effect on the recurrence rate.[50, 51] The arm is usually placed in a sling, with abduction and forward flexion resistive exercises starting as soon as the early pain subsides. Otherwise, the anterior deltoid will atrophy rapidly. The athlete should also perform shrugs but should avoid external rotation early in retraining.

A fracture of the humerus or of the scapula

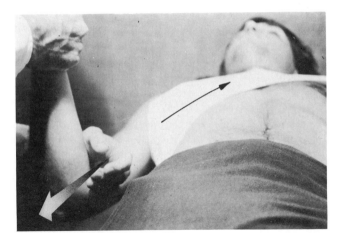

FIG. 12-17
An anteriorly dislocated shoulder may be reduced with sustained straight traction (*arrow*) against the countertraction of a sheet around the chest (*smaller arrow*).

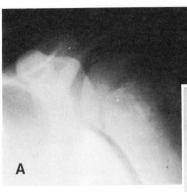

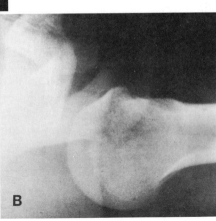

FIG. 12-18
Anteroposterior x-ray of posterior dislocation of the shoulder looks convincingly normal (*A*). The axillary view, however, shows the humeral head to be dislocated posteriorly (*B*).

sometimes accompanies a shoulder dislocation, and nerve damage may account for slow progress in regaining strength. In this situation, an arthrogram may be needed, as a rotator cuff tear may also be present, causing shoulder pain and a poor return of strength.

A blow to the front of the shoulder may drive the humeral head out of the socket posteriorly, or when a lineman comes up with shoulders abducted 90° and flexed forward, his humeral head may slip out posteriorly. This type of dislocation also occurs after falls on ski slopes. The athlete who has sustained a posterior dislocation will have his arm internally rotated and adducted at his side. The coracoid is

prominent and the anterior part of the shoulder flat. He will have limited ability to abduct and to rotate his shoulder externally, and the humeral head may often be felt posteriorly, below the acromion.

An anteroposterior x-ray film may look almost normal (Fig. 12-18A), but close inspection will show the medial margin of the humeral head to be overlapping the glenoid abnormally. Posterior dislocation should be suspected if there is a fracture of the lesser tuberosity. A lateral x-ray view along the spine of the scapula will reveal the humeral head to be dislocated posterior to the Y axis of the scapula (Fig. 12-18B).

Gentle traction is applied in line with the internally rotated, adducted humerus to reduce a posterior dislocation. Sometimes the internal rotation may have to be increased to disengage the head. Pressure is then applied to the humeral head from behind to push it forward. After the dislocation has been reduced, the humerus is most stable at midrotation and slight extension. If the arm is placed in a sling and rotated internally across the chest, the chance of redislocation increases to about 30%. Thus, a splint that will hold the shoulder in the internally rotated and slightly extended position for 3 weeks should be applied.[9] If an athlete should suffer recurrent posterior dislocations or subluxations, a posterior osteotomy and bone graft will change the angle of the glenoid, checking posterior dislocation.

Recurrent Anterior Dislocations of the Shoulder

The "essential lesion" and the humeral head wedge defect both promote recurrent dislocation of the shoulder. The "essential lesion" is a tear of the fibrocartilaginous glenoid labrum that occurs during the initial dislocation and does not heal back to the glenoid. As a result, the anteroinferior part of the shoulder joint capsule is not able to block redislocation of the shoulder, and the humeral head may slide out through the gap. The torn labrum is not visible on a plain x-ray film, but an arthrogram of the shoulder will show dye leaking from the shoulder joint through the defect into a bursa. The lesion may also be inspected arthroscopically.[37,55]

The wedge defect of the humeral head is visible on plain x-ray films taken with the shoulder rotated internally.[13] As the humeral head dislocates from the glenoid, it jams against the anterior glenoid rim. The firm cortical rim crushes the soft cancellous bone in the posterolateral part of the humeral head, producing a defect that appears on plain x-ray film as a posterolateral wedge of compressed bone.

Anterior dislocation of the should recurs frequently in contact sports that require abduction and external rotation of the arm. In ordinary activities, persons younger than 45 years of age have an 80% recurrence rate.[50, 51] The lower rate in older persons may be due to fibrosis at the glenoid rim and to less activity. These statistics, however, may not apply to older athletes.

Some football players who have had an anterior dislocation of the shoulder may compete while wearing a shoulder strap that prevents redislocation (Fig. 12-19). Gieck uses a 1.5-inch wide elastic belt,[19] riveting the buckle to the shoulder pad on the side opposite the dislocation. The remaining part of the belt is then looped around the affected arm while the arm is held adducted and flexed slightly forward. The belt has several notches to allow the athlete to adjust the tension. Because it tends to stretch, the belt must be adjusted every week or two.

The belt system is good for receivers, running backs, and defensive backs by allowing forward flexion of the shoulder for pass receiving and defending while limiting external rotation from a horizontal, extended, and abducted position. If the belt cannot be worn and dislocations recur, one of many surgical options may be recommended,[32] including capsulorrhaphies with sutures or a staple, transfer of the subscapularis, and transfer of the coracoid process.

A capsulorrhaphy is a replacement of the torn shoulder capsule to the glenoid rim from whence it came. Techniques for this procedure include the Bankhart, DuToit, and Putti-Platt operations.[43] In the Bankhart operation, the surgeon drills holes through the glenoid rim and reattaches the torn labrum to the rim by means of sutures. After the operation, the athlete wears a sling for 3 days before advancing to full range-of-motion exercises. Recurrences of dislocations are infrequent unless the athlete has a large defect in the humeral head (a Hill-Sachs lesion). The staple capsulorrhaphy (DuToit operation) requires a longitudinal incision through the subscapularis tendon (Fig. 12-20). The surgeon then peels the capsule off the subscapularis and staples the torn capsule to the glenoid. This corrects the essential lesion,

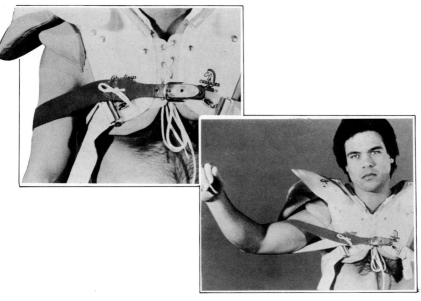

FIG. 12-19
An elastic strap attached to the shoulder pad (*left*) prevents full abduction and external rotation (*right*).

FIG. 12-20
The shoulder capsule may be repaired by reattaching it to the roughened glenoid rim with a staple.

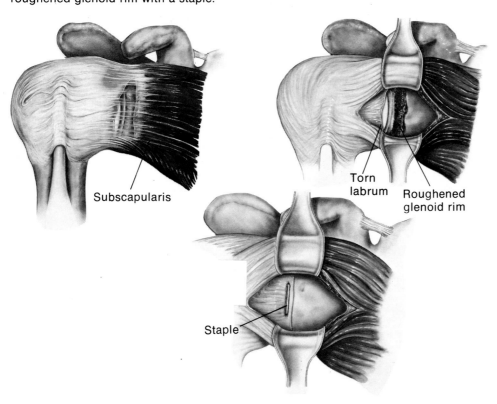

Subscapularis

Torn labrum

Roughened glenoid rim

Staple

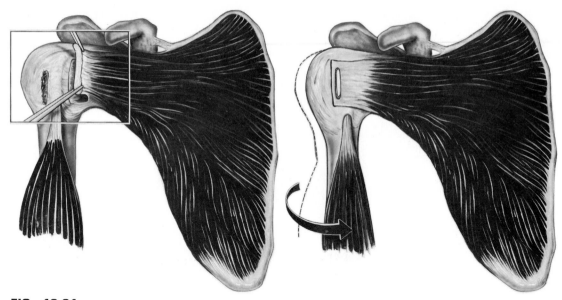

FIG. 12-21
The subscapularis tendon may be transferred from the lesser to the greater tuberosity, thereby limiting external rotation of the shoulder.

but the staple may loosen. In the Putti-Platt operation, the capsule and distal part of the subscapularis tendon are attached to the soft tissue around the glenoid rim. This operation limits external rotation of the shoulder.

The surgeon may elect to perform a subscapularis transfer (Magnuson and Stack operation), which entails transferring the subscapularis tendon from its insertion into the lesser tuberosity of the humerus, laterally across the bicipital groove to the greater tuberosity, about 1.5 cm distal to the original level of insertion (Fig. 12-21). The tendon may be placed into a trap door of bone, or the surgeon may use a serrated staple to secure the tendon. This operation also restricts external rotation, and the staple may loosen.

The Bristow operation is a coracoid transfer that protects against dislocation while allowing good external rotation (Fig. 12-22). In this procedure, the surgeon removes the tip of the coracoid process with the coracobrachialis and short head of the biceps still attached to it. He then roughens the bone at the junction of the middle third and lower third of the anterior glenoid rim and places the coracoid there. As the athlete abducts and rotates his shoulder externally after healing, the coracoid tip serves as

a bone block, and the conjoined tendon of the coracobrachialis and short head of the biceps work as a dynamic sling that prevents the humeral head from dislocating.

Some surgeons modify the coracoid transfer operation by using a screw to attach the coracoid tip to the glenoid, but the screw may loosen and even damage a blood vessel to produce an aneurysm. Although a coracoid transfer will sharply reduce dislocations, it limits external rotation to some extent. Because a throwing athlete needs the fullest external rotation of his throwing arm shoulder, only rarely is he able to return to the highest levels of performance and competition after repair of a recurrently dislocating shoulder.

Anterior Capsular Derangement

The humeral head may ride forward on the glenoid rim to produce pain, feeling as if it is slipping in and out of the socket. This instability is termed "apprehension shoulder" and occurs during the cocking and acceleration phases of throwing, in the backscratch position and acceleration phase of the tennis serve, and when

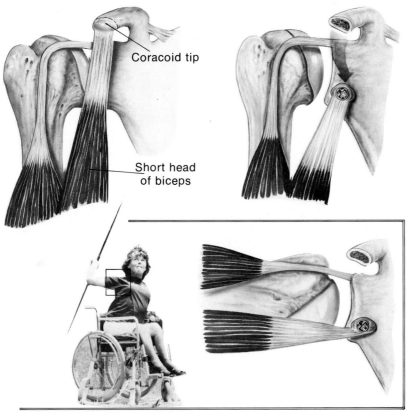

Coracoid tip

Short head
of biceps

FIG. 12-22
In a throwing athlete with a recurrently dislocating shoulder, the
coracoid tip and its conjoined tendon may be transferred to the glenoid
rim. When the arm is abducted, the tendon blocks dislocation of the
humeral head.

a backstroke swimmer goes into a turn (Fig. 12-23A). The slipping is felt in a position common to each of these activities when there is abduction and external rotation of the shoulder.

Anterior capsular derangement may be an aftereffect of an anterior dislocation that immediately popped back. An athlete may not even recollect having dislocated his shoulder, reporting that his shoulder "goes out" and hesitating to abduct and rotate it externally. The pain is in the anterior part of the shoulder, and the tenderness is about 2.5 cm lateral to the corocoid. As the examiner externally rotates the athlete's shoulder, the tender area does not move, thus differentiating it from bicipital tenderness. The examiner has the athlete flex his trunk and then rotates the shoulder passively while palpating anteriorly. Sometimes a

click is felt and the pain is duplicated as the humeral head slips over the glenoid rim and then back into the socket. With the athlete supine, the examiner may be able to pull the humeral head forward, but usually the scapula follows the humerus to invalidate this maneuver (Fig. 12-23B). To duplicate the subluxation dynamically, the athlete abducts and rotates his shoulder externally, and the examiner then resists the acceleration phase of a feigned throw and pushes the humeral head forward (Fig. 12-23C). This maneuver will often bring out the humeral head subluxation.

X-ray studies may help in diagnosing anterior capsular derangement. An internally rotated plain film may show a wedge defect in the posterolateral part of the humeral head, but most often findings will be normal. Arthrog-

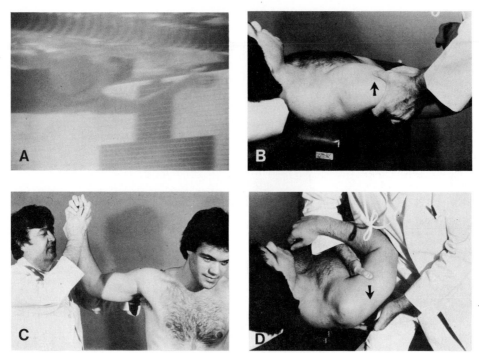

FIG. 12-23
The humeral head may slide partly out of the glenoid during a turn in the backstroke (A). The examiner tries to duplicate this subluxation by pulling the humeral head forward (B). In throwing athletes, the feeling of instability recurs when the athlete "throws" against resistance (C). The examiner may also test for posterior subluxation by pressing the humeral head posteriorly (D).

raphy may show dye extravasating into a large subscapular pouch that has resulted from avulsion of the glenohumeral ligaments from the glenoid.[30] The athlete should adduct and rotate his shoulder internally during the test because the subscapularis is tense in external rotation, and the underlying pouch would be obliterated radiologically.

If a backstroke swimmer has anterior capsular derangement, he may have to change his turning technique to a front flip turn in which he reaches across but remains on his back at the touch to avoid disqualification. If subluxation continues and interferes with the athlete's performance, the pouch may be obliterated by reattaching the capsule to the anterior glenoid through drill holes or with a staple. In this procedure, the capsule is opened to allow full exploration of the joint, and any capsular tears are sutured. In athletes who use their arms overhead, the coracoacromial ligament is resected to prevent future subacromial impingement. A baseball player should strengthen his anterior deltoid; if the anterior deltoid is weak, he will drop his shoulder when throwing and develop more problems.

The Humerus

Hypertrophy of the humerus is a normal response to prolonged heavy arm exercise,[22] and the cortical thickness of the humerus on the playing side of top-level male tennis players is thus 35% greater than on their nonplaying side. Top-level female players have a cortical thickness 28% greater on their playing side than on their control side.[47]

One half of a large group of college gymnasts showed an asymptomatic cortical irregularity of the proximal humerus that simulates the cortical desmoid often found at the distal medial femoral condyle. This benign reactive process is located at the insertion of the broad, strong pectoralis major on the anteromedial cortical border of the humerus. Most athletes with this irregularity are all-around gymnasts who regularly perform strength moves, especially on the rings—hence the term "ringman's shoulder."

The proximal humeral epiphysis of a young thrower may become disrupted, or a cyst in the proximal humerus may weaken the bone, making it more vulnerable to fracture. The normal humerus of a child may also fracture if it is subjected to excessive torque, and exostoses may develop from direct trauma to the arm.

"Little League Shoulder"

Injury to the proximal humeral growth plate in a young pitcher is called "Little League shoulder." This injury also occurs in catchers who throw as often as pitchers but use less windup. Rotary torques are applied to the humerus during the acceleration phase, and decelerating distraction forces are applied during the follow-through.[8]

If the proximal humeral growth plate is in-jured, the youngster's shoulder may swell and hurt. The examiner may reach into the player's axilla and feel for tenderness of the bone,[56] and an x-ray film may show "preslip" changes. These changes include a wide epiphyseal line, with demineralization and rarefaction on the metaphyseal side of the growth plate. A young pitcher's proximal humeral epiphysis may also slip off his humeral shaft (Fig. 12-24). The x-ray film will sometimes show a triangular chipped-off piece of metaphyseal bone that indicates a grade II epiphyseal fracture. New bone appears about 10 days after these fractures, which quickly heal with rest.

A fracture may also occur in youths through a thin-walled unicameral bone cyst just distal to the proximal humeral growth plate. This fracture produces a painful, swollen shoulder, and an x-ray film will show the cyst. The natural course of a cyst is to disappear in the diaphyseal region as the epiphysis grows away from it. The cyst may spontaneously fill in after a fracture as the callus forms. If fractures recur through a cyst, the surgeon may elect to curette out the cyst wall and insert a bone graft. The growth plate must first, however, be allowed to move away from the cyst before surgery is done to prevent damage at operation.

Fractures of the humeral shaft have been reported in throwing athletes and arm wrestlers.[20] During the acceleration phase of throwing, the latissimus dorsi and the pectoralis major strongly rotate the athlete's shoulder internally,

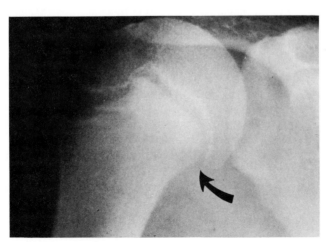

FIG. 12-24
"Little League shoulder" is a fracture at the proximal epiphysis of the humerus. Here, the humeral head has slipped partly off the shaft (*arrow*).

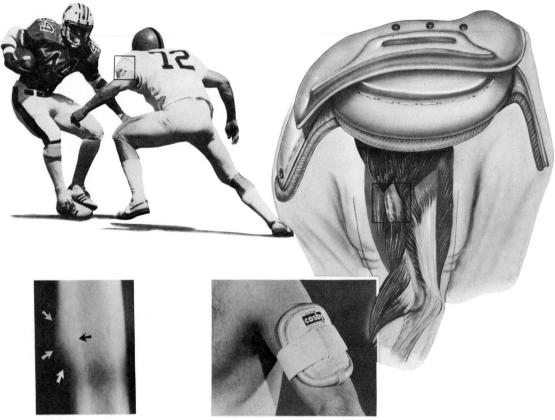

FIG. 12-25
Tackler's exostosis (*see* text for description). Blows that slide off a
shoulder pad may damage the humerus. An extra arm pad can protect
the area from these blows.

leaving his elbow behind. This torque may produce a spiral fracture of the humerus, especially
in the weak-armed but hard throwing teenage
pitchers with unrefined deliveries. When an
outfielder throws from next to a fence or wall,
he cannot use his body but must throw with
his arm only. The torque may be so great as to
fracture his humerus. Similarly, an arm wrestler may fracture his humerus during the losing
phase of a contest. In the losing position, his
elbow extends progressively, and there are
changes in the direction of applied force during
this eccentric muscle contraction. The humerus
fractures spirally in its middle third and lower
third with or without a butterfly fragment.
These fractures are treated with a hanging arm
cast.

Tackler's Exostosis

In tackle football, a linebacker's internally rotated and abducted arms receive direct blows
from the helmets of players he is tackling. The
linebacker also sustains blows as he holds his
arms internally rotated to ward off blockers,
and the arms are bruised from direct blows or
blows that slide off his shoulder pads.

The player may develop a painful bony
prominence at the subcutaneous part of the anterolateral humerus, just distal to the edge of
the shoulder pad (Fig. 12-25). This "tackler's
exostosis" results from damage at the insertion
of the deltoid or at the brachialis origin with
tearing of the periosteum. Bone forms in continuity with the cortex and grows by accretion.

The athlete's upper arm swells acutely, and within 4 weeks a hard mass can be felt. The elbow range of motion usually is full. Early x-ray films show swelling, and at 2 or 3 weeks the accretion of bone is confirmed as a "dotted veil" that later evolves into a mature exostosis. Because the exostosis may be disabling, early recognition and treatment are important.

When a blow to the arm brings tenderness and swelling, the area is iced and the arm rested. If a large hematoma develops, it is aspirated and a compression wrap is applied for 10 days. The contusion should not be massaged soon after injury, as this may cause further bleeding and irritation. If the arm is seen for the first time at 2 weeks after injury and bone is noted, the arm should be rested in a plaster splint. Sometimes, the bone will then spontaneously resorb. If mature bone forms, the area will be sore, despite extra padding. If the region continues to be painful, the mass may be removed surgically.

At surgery, a tackler's exostosis may be differentiated from myositis ossificans. A tackler's exostosis has no cleavage plane between it and the cortex of the humerus, and the anterior mass of the brachialis is not involved. The exostosis usually occurs in older players, whereas myositis ossificans occurs more frequently in high school players. The connective tissue associated with the bruised brachialis muscle becomes ossified in myositis ossificans.[23]

Tackler's exostosis can be prevented by requiring offensive linemen and linebackers to wear fiber doughnut pads attached to their epaulets or separate from the shoulder pads to cover the lateral humerus. A mature myositis ossificans lesion may be resected if it is large and painful, predisposes to further injury, has a pointed end that is easily reinjured, or restricts elbow motion to the point of being a functional handicap.

Tennis Shoulder

In the tennis serve, the racquet is thrown up at the ball and decelerated over a very short distance from a speed of about 480 km/h (300 miles/h).[38] The forces generated in this movement stretch the scapular-anchoring muscles, and the shoulder then droops, rotating forward from the pull of gravity on the increased mass of the arm (Fig. 12-26).

The player with a drooped shoulder may develop anterior rotator cuff symptoms. A relative abduction of the shoulder is produced as the scapula tilts downwards. There is less room for the rotator cuff, and it may be impacted, especially during serves and overhead returns. The player may also have pain on the backhand side when the arm ends high, especially with backhand volleys.

Signs and symptoms of compression at the thoracic outlet are thought by some to be associated with the drooped "tennis shoulder," causing neck and arm pain.[47] However, we have studied over a period of 5 years the players who compete in the United States Tennis Association National Clay Court Championships.[28] These players have an average of 50 years of playing experience. All have drooped racquet arm shoulders, but none have had symptoms of an outlet syndrome. We therefore conclude that the "tennis shoulder" of a veteran player is a normal response to exercise and generally will not produce shoulder difficulties. The younger and harder-hitting tennis professional may, however, develop outlet problems. If such a player is symptomatic, shrug exercises will help to elevate his shoulder, and if the symptoms persist, a thorough workup should be conducted.

Scapular Pain

The athlete's scapula is surrounded by muscles to stabilize his upper extremity. Several bursas between the scapula and the chest wall may become irritated.[52]

Periscapular pain is frequent in shotputters, tennis players, and weight lifters. In putting the shot, the scapula muscles anchor the arm and must restrain the scapula during the follow-through. Pain in the rhomboids and scapulocostal bursitis are treated with massage, ultrasound, and, occasionally, steroid injections.

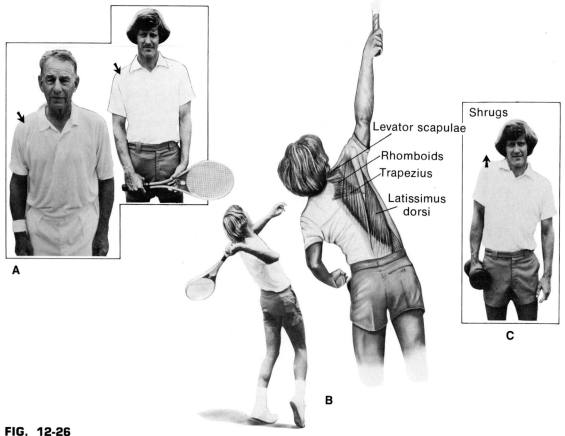

FIG. 12-26
The drooped but strong racquet-arm shoulder is characteristic of senior tennis players and young professionals (*A*). It follows a stretching-out of the scapular-anchoring muscles from repeated serves (*B*). These muscles may be strengthened with shrugging exercises (*C*).

During the backscratch position of the tennis serve, the inferior angle of the scapula may jam against the ribs to produce a bursitis, and the rhomboids may also be strained during the follow-through. Treatment is similar to that given for the shotputter's shoulder.

A weight lifter must strongly protract his shoulders. During this activity, the serratus anterior holds the scapula firmly to the lifter's chest wall. The muscle arises from his first eight ribs and inserts into the medial border of the scapula. A strong contraction of this muscle may fracture the first rib through the weak subclavian groove.

In weight training, standing pullovers may place traction on the long thoracic nerve, par-alyzing the serratus anterior. This injury may be diagnosed by having the athlete do a wall pushup to elicit scapular winging. An electromyogram will show serratus anterior denervation. This injury may be prevented if pullovers are done while the athlete is supine.[53]

A snapping scapula may be due to a prominent superomedial border of the scapula that passes over the underlying muscles and ribs. The examiner may move the scapula about and feel under it while the athlete lies prone with his arm hanging over the side of the examining table. If the snapping is painful and persists after a rest period, the superomedial angle may have to be resected.

When an athlete has intractible periscapular

pain, the examiner should look to the neck for diagnosis, as the pain about the scapula may have a radicular origin in the neck.[10] The athlete may report recurrent stiff necks but usually without neurologic or electromyographic changes. Pain in his trapezius or other shoulder muscles or at the occipital-cervical junction may be due to nervous tension or afternoon fatigue or may follow prolonged flexion and extension of the neck. In these cases, the athlete should strengthen his neck muscles and try neck traction for relief of the shoulder pain.

REFERENCES

1. ALLMAN F: Symposium on sports injuries to the shoulder. Contemp Surg 4:70–109, 1975
2. ANDREWS JR et al: Musculotendinous injuries of the shoulder and elbow in athletics. Athletic Training 11(2):68–70, 1976
3. BENTON J, NELSON C: Avulsion of the coracoid process in an athlete: report of a case. J Bone Joint Surg [Am] 53:356–358, 1971
4. BERGFELD JA et al: Evaluation of the acromioclavicular joint following first and second degree sprains. Am J Sports Med 6:153–159, 1978
5. BERSON BC: Surgical repair of pectoralis major rupture in an athlete—case report of an unusual injury in a wrestler. Am J Sports Med 7:348–351, 1979
6. BOYD R: Gradual warmup routine helps pitchers avoid arm injuries. First Aider, Cramer 47:6, February 1978
7. BRITT LP: Non-operative treatment of the thoracic outlet syndrome symptoms. Clin Orthop 51:45–48, 1967
8. CAHILL BR et al: Little League shoulder. Am J Sports Med 2:150–154, 1974
9. CAUTILLI RA et al: Posterior dislocations of the shoulder: a method of post-reduction management. Am J Sports Med 6:397–399, 1978
10. COVENTRY M: Recurring scapular pain. JAMA 241:942, 1979
11. CRENSHAW AH: Surgical treatment of bicipital tenosynovitis. J Bone Joint Surg [Am] 48:1498, 1966
12. COX JS: The fate of the acromioclavicular joint in athletic injuries. Am J Sports Med 9:50–53, 1981
13. DANZIG LA et al: The Hill-Sachs lesion—an experimental study. Am J Sports Med 8:328–332, 1980
14. DEL PIZZO W et al: Rupture of the biceps tendon in gymnastics: a case report. Am J Sports Med 6:283–286, 1978
15. DEPALMA AF, CALLERY GE: Bicipital tenosynovitis. Clin Orthop 3:69, 1954
16. FOWLER P: Swimmer problems. Am J Sports Med 7:141–142, 1979
17. FROIMSON AI, OH I: Keyhole tenodesis of biceps origin at the shoulder. Clin Orthop 112:245–249, 1975
18. GAINOR BJ: The throw: biomechanics and acute injury. Am J Sports Med 8:114–118, 1980
19. GIECK JH: Shoulder strap to prevent anterior glenohumeral dislocations. Athletic Training 11(1):18, 1976
20. GREGERSON HN: Fracture of the humerus from muscular violence. Acta Orthop Scand 42:506–512, 1971
21. HAWKINS RJ, KENNEDY JC: Impingement syndrome in athletes. Am J Sports Med 8:151–158, 1980
22. HUDDLESTON AL et al: Bone mass in lifetime tennis athletes. JAMA 244:1107–1109, 1980
23. HUSS CD, PUHL JJ: Myositis ossificans of the upper arm. Am J Sports Med 8:419–424, 1980
24. HITCHCOCK HH, BECHTOL CO: Painful shoulder. J Bone Joint Surg [Am] 30:263–267, 1948
25. KENNEDY JC: Retrosternal dislocation of the clavicle. J Bone Joint Surg [Br] 31:74, 1949
26. KENNEDY JC, HAWKINS RJ: Swimmer's shoulder. Phys Sportsmed 2(4):35–38, 1974
27. KENNEDY JC: Orthopedic manifestations of swimming. Am J Sports Med 6:309–322, 1978
28. KULUND DN et al: The long-term effects of playing tennis. Phys Sportsmed 7(4):87–94, 1979
29. KULUND DN et al: Tennis injuries: prevention and treatment. Am J Sports Med 7:249–253, 1979
30. KUMMEL BM: Arthrography in anterior capsular derangements of the shoulder. Clin Orthop 83:170–176, 1972
31. KUMMEL BM: When shoulder complaints limit athletic performance. Phys Sportsmed 2(8):46–51, 1974
32. LIPSCOMB AB: Treatment of recurrent anterior dislocation and subluxation of the glenohumeral joint in athletics. Clin Orthop 109:122–125, 1975
33. MARIANI PP: Isolated fracture of the coracoid process in an athlete. Am J Sports Med 8:129–130, 1980
34. MACNAB I, RATHBUN JB: The microvascular pattern of the rotator cuff. J Bone Joint Surg [Br] 52:524, 1970
35. MICHELI LJ, RISEBOROUGH EM: The incidence of injuries in rugby football. Am J Sports Med 2:93–98, 1974
36. NEER CS: Anterior acromioplasty for the chronic impingement syndrome in the shoulder. J Bone Joint Surg [Am] 54:41–50, 1972
37. NELSON CL: The use of arthrography in athletic injuries of the shoulder. Orthop Clin North Am 4:775–785, 1973
38. NIRSCHL RP: Throwing or swinging the shoulder pays. Phys Sportsmed 2(12):20–27, 1974
39. NIXON JE, DISTERANO V: Rupture of the rotator cuff. Orthop Clin North Am 6:423–447, 1975
40. NORFRAY JF et al: The clavicle in hockey. Am J Sports Med 5:275–280, 1977
41. NORWOOD LA et al: Anterior shoulder pain in baseball pitchers. Am J Sports Med 6:103–106, 1978
42. O'DONOGHUE DH: Subluxing biceps tendon in the athlete. Am J Sports Med 1:20–29, 1973
43. OSMOND-CLARKE H: Habitual dislocations of the

shoulder. The Putti-Platt operation. J Bone Joint Surg [Br] 30:19, 1948

44. PARK JP et al: Treatment of acromioclavicular separations. Am J Sports Med 8:251–256, 1980
45. PENNY JN, WELSH RP: Shoulder impingement syndromes in athletes and their surgical management. Am J Sports Med 9:11–15, 1981
46. PETTRONE FA, NIRSCHL RP: Acromioclavicular dislocation. Am J Sports Med 6:160–164, 1978
47. PRIEST JD, NAGEL DA: Tennis shoulder. Am J Sports Med 4:28–42, 1976
48. RICHARDSON AB: The shoulder in swimming. Swimming World 29:33–34, 1979
49. RICHARDSON AB: The shoulder in competitive swimming. Am J Sports Med 8:159–163, 1980
50. ROWE CR: Prognosis in dislocations of the shoulder. J Bone Joint Surg [Am] 38:957–977, 1956
51. ROWE CR, SAKELLARIDES HT: Factors related to recurrence of dislocations of the shoulder. Clin Orthop 20:40–48, 1961
52. RUSSEK AS: Scapulo-costal syndrome. JAMA 150:25–27, 1952

53. STANISH WD, LAMB J: Isolated paralysis of the serratus anterior muscle: a weight training injury. Case report. Am J Sports Med 6:385–386, 1978
54. STRUKEL RJ, GARRICK JG: Thoracic outlet compression in athletes: a report of four cases. Am J Sports Med 6:35–39, 1978
55. TIRMAN RM: Shoulder arthrography. Contemp Orthop 1(2):26–32, 1979
56. TORG JS et al: The effect of competitive pitching on the shoulders and elbows of pre-adolescent baseball players. Pediatrics 49:267–272, 1972
57. TULLOS HS et al: Unusual lesions of the pitching arm. Clin Orthop 88:169–182, 1972
58. VAN LINGE B, MULDER JD: Function of the supraspinatus muscle and its relations to the supraspinatus syndrome: an experimental study in man. J Bone Joint Surg [Br] 45:750–754, 1963
59. WRIGHT RS, LIPSCOMB AB: Acute occlusion of the subclavian vein in an athlete: diagnosis, etiology and surgical management. Am J Sports Med 2:343–348, 1974
60. ZEMAN SC et al: Tears of the pectoralis major muscle. Am J Sports Med 7:343–347, 1979

The Elbow

Anatomy

The elbow joint consists of three articulations: the humeral-ulnar, the capitellar-radial, and the radial-ulnar. The humeral-ulnar articulation determines the carrying angle of the elbow. When the elbow is flexed, the forearm is in line with the arm; as it extends, the trochlear course allows the forearm to move into valgus, producing the "carrying angle." Fractures at the elbow may alter this carrying angle. Pronation and supination take place about the capitellar-radial articulation, an area jammed during throwing. The radial-ulnar articulation is a small one that moves during pronation and supination.

The medial collateral ligament of the elbow has two parts: an anterior band and a posterior band. The thick anterior band is a major static stabilizer of the elbow, arising from the medial epicondyle to insert on the medial side of the coronoid process of the ulna. The thinner and weaker posterior band functions only when the elbow is flexed to more than 90°. The medial collateral ligament is stretched in baseball pitchers and round-arm-style javelin throwers, all of whom put extreme valgus stress on their elbows. Medial collateral ligament laxity may result from poorly reduced medial epicondyle fractures.

The flexor carpi radialis, palmaris longus, and parts of the flexor carpi ulnaris and flexor digitorum sublimis originate from the medial epicondyle. One head of the pronator teres arises from the metaphyseal flare just proximal to the epicondyle. The flexor muscle mass exerts a strong pull on the epicondyle and may be partly avulsed in the young thrower. Because it is not yet fused to bone, the epicondyle sometimes is jerked from its bed and pulled into the elbow joint. Older tennis players, especially professionals who use spin serves, develop a large medial epicondyle as a response to heavy use.

The extensor muscles of the wrist and fingers arise from the lateral condyle of the humerus. The origin of the extensor carpi radialis brevis is often the site of damage in tennis elbow. It inserts at the base of the third metacarpal, the center of the hand. A fracture through the lateral

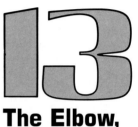

13

The Elbow, Wrist, and Hand

FRANK C. McCUE III

295

condyle into the elbow joint sometimes heals slowly, as the fracture site is bathed in synovial fluid containing fibrinolysin that prevents organization of the fracture hematoma.

The bony structures of the elbow joint are the capitellum, trochlea, and radial head. The capitellum lines up with the radial head on a lateral x-ray view of the elbow. If the radial head repeatedly jams against the capitellum, as in baseball pitching, capitellar avascular necrosis and osteochondritis dissecans may ensue. The trochlea sweep controls the carrying angle, and pieces from the medial edge of the trochlea may be chipped off during throwing.

Incongruity of the radial head after a fracture may result in osteoarthritis of the elbow with pain during pronation and supination. The orbicular or annular ligament arises from the humerus to surround the radial head. Adhesions between this ligament and the capsule of the elbow joint are responsible for some cases of tennis elbow.

When the elbow is fully extended, the olecranon fossa accepts the olecranon tip. The common supracondylar fracture in children extends through the very thin bone of this fossa and may lead to a bony buildup within the fossa that blocks full extension. Such a bony block affects throwing and also hinders a good follow-through in basketball shooting.

A posterior fat pad resides in the olecranon fossa just external to the elbow joint.[64] Intra-articular injury pushes this fat pad up so that it may be seen on a lateral x-ray film as evidence of intra-articular swelling. During throwing, the fat pad is normally pulled up by a slip of triceps, such as the articularis genu muscle of the knee, to prevent trapping and painful pinching of the fat pad between bone surfaces during rapid extension.

The biceps muscle is the main supinator of the forearm. Strong flexion of the elbow against resistance may avulse the biceps brachi from the bicipital tubercle of the radius. The brachialis muscle inserts into the coronoid process of the ulna. This muscle pulls chips from the coronoid in boxers, pitchers, and wrist wrestlers.

The major nerves near the elbow are the radial, median, and ulnar nerves. The deep and recurrent branches of the radial nerve may be trapped as they pass between the two parts of the supinator muscle. The median nerve may be impinged upon proximally in a tunnel under the ligament of Struthers, which sometimes runs from a supracondylar process of the humerus down to the medial condyle. Distally, the nerve may be trapped between the humeral and ulnar heads of the pronator teres as it seeks to lie on the substance of the flexor digitorum superficialis. The ulnar nerve courses behind the intermuscular septum and enters the forearm between the humeral and ulna heads of the flexor carpi ulnaris. It may be trapped and irritated by fascial thickenings in the ulna groove behind the medial epicondyle; in such a case, the ulna nerve may be decompressed or transplanted to the anterior compartment above the level of the medial epicondyle.

Fibers of the interosseous membrane descend medially from the radius to the ulna. If the athlete falls on his hand, the compression forces can be transmitted through this membrane from the strong lower radius to the strong upper ulna and humeral-ulnar joint. The triceps insertion fans out over the olecranon, and chips may be pulled off the olecranon tip in over-the-shoulder javelin throws or during missed jabs in boxing. The olecranon bursa lies at the elbow tip. It may become inflamed from repeated landings on the point of the elbow or after forceful elbow extensions. Sometimes loose bodies form within this bursa.

Fractures

Supracondylar

A fall from playground apparatus may fracture the thin bone in the supracondylar region of a child's humerus (Fig. 13-1). The fracture ends may then damage the intima of the brachial artery. Although the intima is torn, it may take days for it to block the circulation completely. If the brachial artery is blocked, Volkmann's ischemic contractures of the forearm may occur, wherein the muscles die and the

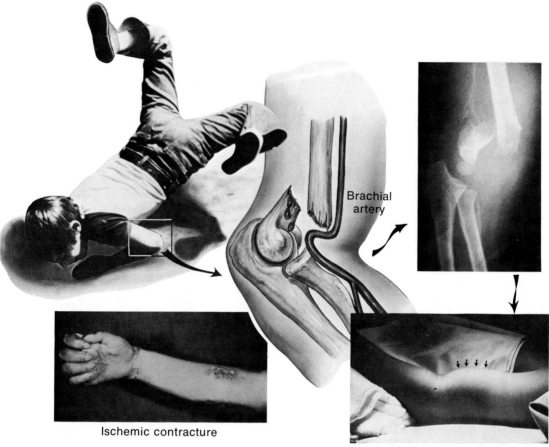

Brachial artery

Ischemic contracture

FIG. 13-1
A supracondylar fracture of the humerus may damage the brachial artery and lead to a severe ischemic contracture of the forearm and hand.

nerves fibrose, producing a useless limb. The vascular status and the nerve function of the limb should be evaluated both before and after reduction of the supracondylar fracture. The fracture is carefully reduced under axillary block or general anesthesia by applying traction and then flexing the elbow. The elbow should not be flexed initially without first applying traction, or else the brachial artery may be pinched.

A splint may be applied with the elbow in a flexed position for undisplaced or minimally displaced supracondylar fractures. If the elbow is flexed too much, however, the radial pulse may disappear. If this happens, it should be extended somewhat until the pulse returns. To treat a fully displaced fracture, a pin may be placed through the olecranon for overhead traction, and 10 days later a cast may be applied.

If there is no radial pulse and the youth has pain, pallor, paresthesia, and pain on passive extension of the fingers, overhead traction should be instituted. If pulse and feeling fail to return, then the brachial artery should be explored. Resection of a segment of the artery that contains the torn and folded intima may be needed to reduce the circulatory spasm. Prompt treatment of an elbow with danger signs may avoid the terrible complication of Volkmann's contracture.

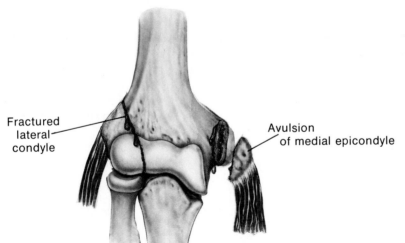

Fractured lateral condyle

Avulsion of medial epicondyle

FIG. 13-2
A lateral condyle fracture allows synovial fluid to flow in and hinder healing. The medial epicondyle may be avulsed and even rotate from its normal position and obstruct the joint.

Medial Epicondyle

The medial ligament of the elbow and flexor origin may be disrupted in a young thrower, gymnast, or wrestler who fractures the medial epicondyle (Fig. 13-2). Medial elbow stability depends on an intact medial collateral ligament and forearm flexors. Fibrous union of a displaced medial epicondyle fracture may cause chronic medial instability of the elbow and end a throwing career.

A routine elbow x-ray may not show much displacement of the medial epicondyle, compared to that which occurred at the time of injury. On x-ray, the epicondyle may appear to be reduced, but in fact it may be rotated 90°. This change in position of the medial epicondyle alters medial collateral ligament function and lessens the stability of the medial side of the elbow.

There are three types of medial epicondylar fractures.[85] Type I occurs in youths who have open epiphyses. Here, the entire apophysis is avulsed, along with the forearm flexors and the medial collateral ligament. In type II fractures, the young athlete's epiphyses have closed. If the fragment is large enough to include the proximal attachment of the anterior band, the medial collateral ligament will be intact. Marked displacement, however, may tear the ligament. Type III fracture occurs in older children and adults. Here, a small chip is avulsed

from the posterior aspect of the medial epicondyle with part of the musculature, and the midportion of the medial collateral ligament tears.

A gentle test, the gravity stress test, is available for diagnosing acute medial instability of the elbow. With the athlete supine, the shoulder is rotated externally. Then his elbow is flexed 20° to bring the olecranon clear of its fossa. The weight of the forearm and hand will usually exert enough valgus force to open the medial side. In larger, more muscular persons a 0.45 kg or 0.9 kg (1 lb or 2 lb) weight may be strapped around the wrist. If the elbow is unstable, gravity stress test x-rays will show that the joint has opened and that the medial epicondylar apophysis has become displaced distally.

Exploration of the medial side of the elbow is indicated if the medial epicondyle is displaced more than 1 cm, or if it lies in the elbow joint. Moreover, a throwing athlete's elbow is usually explored if it is unstable on the gravity stress test. Exploration is also indicated if an epicondylar fracture is associated with a posterior or posterolateral dislocation, since the epicondyle was probably very displaced and is now rotated.

Lateral Condyle

Fractures of the lateral condyle of the elbow are intra-articular ones that heal slowly and may become displaced (see Fig. 13-2). Synovial fluid seeps from the joint into the fracture site and contains fibrinolysin, which disrupts the fracture hematoma and may lead to a non-union.

A displaced fracture of the lateral epicondyle demands pin or screw fixation. Even if a lateral epicondylar fracture is undisplaced, however, the elbow should be x-rayed intermittently until it has healed, as an initially undisplaced fracture of the lateral condyle may become displaced. A malunited fracture alters the carrying angle of an athlete's elbow, and his range of elbow motion could also suffer.

Dislocation

Most elbow dislocations are posterior or posterolateral ones. Both of these types may have associated fractures of the medial epicondyle. Fortunately, even if the elbow is unstable medially, the forearm flexors are usually functionally intact and give satisfactory dynamic support for most elbow activities. In a thrower, however, a ligamentous repair is more likely to restore optimum function. Operative exploration is indicated in throwing athletes if the medial epicondyle has been fractured, since the epicondyle was probably very displaced and is now rotated.

The dislocation may be reduced on the field or in the locker room before muscle spasm sets in. It is best performed, however, with the athlete lying prone on an examining table with his elbow hanging off the side. First the lateral displacement is reduced, and then straight traction is applied. The elbow should not be directly flexed before reduction, as this flexion maneuver could damage the brachial artery.

The athlete's elbow is rehabilitated with active range-of-motion exercises. Passive stretch should be avoided because it may cause elbow stiffness or myositis ossificans. When the athlete is ready to return to practice, the elbow should be taped in slight flexion, or a custom-made padded elbow strap may be wrapped around the arm and forearm and connected to allow full flexion but prevent hyperextension (Fig. 13-3).[35]

The Elbow in Throwing

During the acceleration phase of throwing, the thrower's arm is pulled forward dramatically. The forearm lags behind, and thus a valgus stress is placed on the elbow (Fig. 13-4). The forearm flexors then flex the wrist and fingers to propel the baseball, which is released in a flinging motion at about ear level. During follow-through, the forearm pronates, and the olecranon jams into the olecranon fossa.[2]

Types of Elbow Injuries

"Little League Elbow"

Young baseball players may develop elbow problems from a heavy pitching schedule.[52] The Little Leaguer is allowed to pitch as many as six innings per week and averages 18 pitches per inning. A professional pitcher throws about 120 pitches in a nine-inning game, averaging 11 to 15 pitches per inning. Although a Little Leaguer throws fewer pitches than does a professional pitcher in a week of competition, he may throw hard on days between games. He may be a catcher for his team as well, and thus throw even more.

Adams studied the x-rays films of both elbows of 162 boys, aged 9 to 14 years, and compared pitchers to nonpitchers and to youngsters who were not playing organized baseball.[1] He found that changes at the medial epicondyle, the radius, and the capitellum were in direct proportion to the amount of throwing and whether the youngster threw curve balls. All of the 80 pitchers that he checked had some degree of bony hypertrophy and separation and fragmentation of the medial epicondylar apophysis. Only a small number of the x-ray films of nonpitchers and control subjects showed these changes.

In the "Houston study," 595 Little League pitchers were examined.[33] Seventeen percent had elbow symptoms, and 12% had a limitation of elbow extension. Many radiologic "anatomical variants" were noted at the elbow. The medial epicondylar lesions were thought to be stress fractures, and if the youngster rested his arm, these lesions were said to result in no functional deficits. The bony hypertrophy and enlarged medial epicondyles were considered to be normal anatomic variants.

In the "Eugene study," 120 pitchers, aged 11 and 12 years, were examined.[49] Twenty percent had elbow symptoms, and 23% had x-ray changes related to traction on the medial epicondyle. Ten percent of these pitchers had limitation of elbow extension. Five percent of these youths had more serious lateral compartment x-ray changes, but none of them had symptoms related to that area. The investigators concluded that the elbow symptoms of Little League pitchers did not correlate with the x-ray findings.

Studies that show negligible epiphyseal involvement in Little League baseball players may be misleading, since the youths present to physicians with symptoms when they are 13 or 14 years old and have already graduated from Little League baseball.[11] The elbow trouble has an insidious onset, symptoms being early but subtle.[5] These young athletes may fail to report elbow pain to the coach, and even if they do the coach may not have the soreness thoroughly investigated.

Most problems are at the medial side of the elbow, and Little League elbow has been defined as an avulsion of the ossification center of the medial epicondyle.[9,25,80] The valgus stress of throwing may cause fragmentation, irregularity, mild separation, enlargement, or breaking of the medial epicondyle. The worst, chronic problems, however, are found on the lateral side of the elbow where repeated jamming of the radial head against the capitellum may cause osteochondritis of the capitellum, avascular ne-

FIG. 13-3
Taping may prevent hyperextension of the elbow. Elastic tape serves as an anchor. Four strips of 3.8-cm (1.5-in) white tape are then stacked and folded longitudinally to form a strong band, which is held in place with more elastic tape. The ends of the band are folded over and secured with white tape.

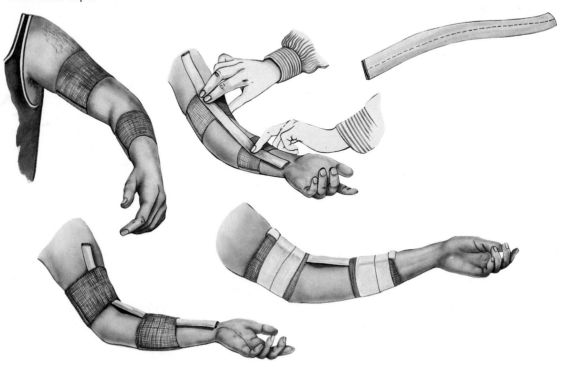

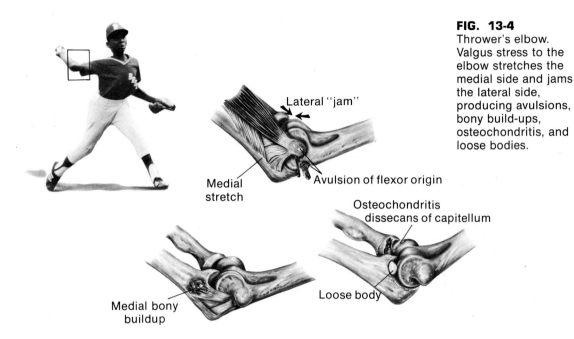

FIG. 13-4
Thrower's elbow. Valgus stress to the elbow stretches the medial side and jams the lateral side, producing avulsions, bony build-ups, osteochondritis, and loose bodies.

Lateral "jam"

Medial stretch

Avulsion of flexor origin

Osteochondritis dissecans of capitellum

Medial bony buildup

Loose body

crosis of the radial head, osteochondritic loose bodies, and osteoarthritis.[82] Eight percent of young pitchers have lateral changes, and it is not uncommon to see loose bodies in the olecranon fossa of teenagers who began pitching at a young age.

The most serious of the elbow findings in young pitchers is osteochondritis dissecans of the capitellum. Valgus elbow stress during the acceleration phase stretches the medial collateral ligament of the elbow, and ultimately the radial head impinges against the capitellum. Osteochondritis dissecans occurs mostly in pitchers but does occur in some catchers. The average age of onset is 12.5 years, with the youths having played organized baseball for an average of 3.5 years.[11]

X-ray films show ill-defined, patchy decalcification or cystic areas on the capitellum, radial head irregularity and hypertrophy and early partial closure of the proximal radius growth plate. In contrast to normal closure, however, the fusion of the radial head growth plate begins on the lateral aspect and proceeds medially. These conditions are not benign but mark the end of hard, painless throwing for the teenage athlete. The prognosis is poor despite treatment, and these side problems may well reduce the athlete's ability to participate in throwing or racquet sports later in life.[79]

When elbow symptoms are marked and rest measures fail, the most consistent results follow curettage of the fragmented capitulum down to bleeding bone and removal of all fragments that are either loose or attached to bone. In a study of young throwers with osteochondritis of the capitellum 13 of 15 operated on had loose bodies.[30] Surgery will not produce a normal elbow, but the pain does lessen and the youngster usually regains more elbow extension.

To prevent elbow problems in young pitchers, good throwing mechanics must be taught, and youngsters should especially avoid just "throwing with the arm." Proper pregame warm-up is important, and the pitcher should ice his shoulder and elbow after the game. Young pitchers should be encouraged to report elbow soreness. In youth baseball, sore arms are often treated like the sore arms of professional players with ice, reducing the pitching or missing a rotation. Soreness in youngsters, however, is more likely due to epiphysitis, and thus x-ray films are needed. If x-ray findings are abnormal, the youngster should refrain from pitching during that season.

Little League pitchers are at a disadvantage

compared to their Big League counterparts. Foremost, the Little Leaguer's elbow is always immature. Professional pitchers have skilled pitching coaches who emphasize good body mechanics, using the large muscle groups, body turn, and proper push-off and follow-through. The professional pitcher has conditioning programs for muscle strength, endurance, and flexibility, postgame icing, and expert medical care. The Little Leaguer usually lacks these advantages. Coaching is not expected to improve because there is no requirement that these well-meaning coaches be trained and certified to instruct their young players.

"Baseball Elbow"

When pitchers throw hard for years, their elbow joints wear out. Veteran pitchers develop an elbow flexion contracture, medial collateral ligament traction spurs or medial collateral ligament rupture, tardy ulnar nerve palsy, articular cartilage degeneration, posterior compartment lesions, and loose bodies.[75]

The flexion contracture results from traction on the anterior capsule, biceps, and brachialis, microtears of the wrist and finger flexors, and pronator tears with resulting fibrosis.[5, 36, 40] Bone may build up on the coronoid process and chip off to cause acute elbow pain.[19]

Reactive bone spurs form in the distal part of the medial collateral ligament owing to valgus overload. Sometimes a spur breaks off to entrap and irritate the ulnar nerve. Spurs can be removed before they break off. The ulnar nerve may sublux during pitching to produce tingling pain in the fourth and fifth fingers with each pitch. When chronic neuritis develops, the nerve may be decompressed at the elbow. If the ulnar nerve is subluxing, it may have to be translocated anteriorly. With the nerve in this new anterior position, the pitcher can usually continue a high level of throwing.

Sometimes, the stress is so great on the medial collateral ligament that it ruptures. An attenuated ligament may be replaced by a tendon, such as the palmaris longus, through drill holes. During rehabilitation, the tendon will assume ligamentous properties and become stronger.

Articular cartilage degeneration at the radiohumeral joint may disable a player. Moreover, in the acceleration phase, as valgus stress is applied to the elbow and it rapidly extends, an osteocartilaginous piece may be chipped from the trochlea, and the athlete will feel an acute, severe pain.

Posterior compartment lesions may be equally disabling. The olecranon process jams into the fossa, especially in pitchers with a poor follow-through who snap the elbow into extension. This jamming produces "olecranon fossitis" and new bone formation. The overgrowth of bone from the olecranon tip may fracture, causing severe elbow pain and leaving loose bodies at the tip of the olecranon.

Surgery on a pitcher's elbow usually comprises a combination of medial soft tissue surgery with removal of spurs and posterior intra-articular surgery. A posterolateral incision is generally chosen so that after the olecranon is observed and the loose bodies removed, the radial head and capitellar articular surfaces can be evaluated. The operation may well be effective if only one loose body is found and removed. The prognosis for a pitcher, however, is generally not good when many loose bodies are found because of coexisting traumatic arthritis. The surgeon's observations of the radiohumeral joint allow a prognosis as to when the pitcher may return to competition and a realistic appraisal of his future in baseball.[36]

"Javelin Thrower's Elbow"

A javelin thrower may develop elbow trouble with either the correct arm action or an incorrect, round-arm method.[62] The types of injuries suffered with each of these throwing styles are, however, different.

The correct arm action for throwing a javelin is an over-the-shoulder throw with a bent-arm carry. The elbow is flexed and held well above and in front of the shoulder and close to the head. The elbow is then brought forward early and forcibly extended to launch the javelin. This violent extension may fracture the olecranon tip.[84]

When the javelin is thrown with an incorrect

round-arm method, the elbow comes around at the level of the shoulder, and internal rotation of the shoulder transmits force to the javelin. These throwers, like baseball pitchers, sprain the medial collateral ligament of the elbow and spurs form. The athlete may be able to develop the correct arm action by changing to a middle-finger hold, with the index finger extended under the javelin and the middle finger placed behind the binding. This change twists the hand inward to reduce the stress on the medial collateral ligament.

"Tennis Elbow"

"Tennis elbow" most often refers to pain at or near a player's lateral epicondyle[72] and is generally caused by faulty backhand stroke mechanics.[34, 70] The player with a faulty backhand often uses an Eastern forehand grip or a fistlike grip with the thumb extended behind the handle for more power (Fig. 13-5). His stroke usually starts high with a hurried backswing. His body weight is on the back leg and power is generated at the wrist and elbow.

FIG. 13-5
A good backhand will have a relaxed backswing, low starting position, weight transfer, "L position" of the wrist at contact, and a full follow-through (*A, B*). The novice who has poor technique starts high with a leading elbow and a hammer grip and hooks his wrist (*C*). A two-handed backhand may improve the mechanics of the stroke (*D*).

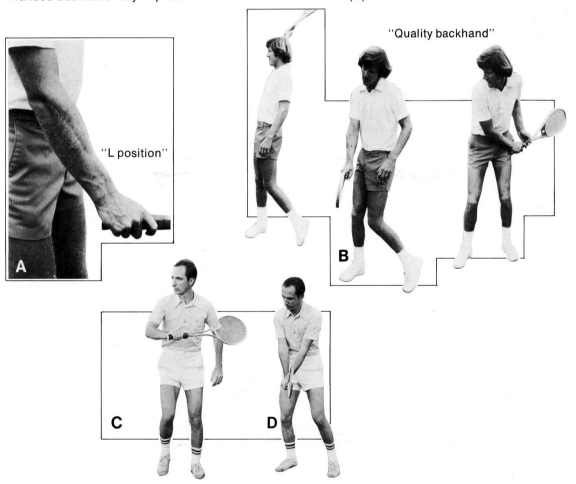

As the elbow extends, the wrist strongly hooks into ulnar deviation, which is a strong, commonly used motion for opening doors, chopping wood, and swinging a baseball bat. The beginner, however, may incorporate this motion, which comes so easily, into his stroke as a bad habit. His follow-through usually will be short and low and end with a jerk.

Combined elbow extension and ulnar hooking of the wrist cause the extensor mass, especially the deeply located extensor carpi radialis brevis, to rub and to roll over the lateral epicondyle and the radial head. Along with this irritation from rubbing over bony prominences are tugs on the extensor origin resulting in microtears. Rubbing, rolling, and microtears result in a painful elbow.

In an attempt to heal the damage, nerve-laden granulation tissue forms. This tissue is ill-suited to withstand constant use because it swells, stretches, and becomes painful. Adhesions also form between the annular ligament and the joint capsule. The pain worsens from the constant strain of the faulty backhand and the transmission of vibrations to the elbow from a too tightly strung racket with too small a handle or from heavy, wet balls and off-center hits.

Players with tennis elbow have pain in the region of the common extensor origin, especially when they try to extend their middle finger against resistance with the elbow extended. The extensor carpi radialis brevis inserts into the base of the third metacarpal, and extension of the middle finger tightens the fascial origin of the muscle. The lateral epicondyle is tender, and the player notes pain when he grips the racket and extends his wrist.

For a quality backhand, either an Eastern backhand or a Continental grip is used. The arm and racquet form an "L."[77] The racquet is unhurriedly taken back low, and the stroke starts low. The player's other hand can help support the racquet during the backswing. He then shifts his body weight and swings from the shoulder to achieve pace. At impact, his weight has been transferred to his front foot. His wrist is firm and locked in a cocked position, a position that corrects the hooked wrist, which in turn cures the leading elbow. The ball is met in front, and the follow-through is long and high.

The player with a faulty backhand should be taught proper form and master the wrist-cocked "L" position (see Fig. 13-5). If this cannot be learned, then he should work on a two-handed backhand, as tennis elbow only rarely affects players who use a two-handed backhand. A right-handed player hits a two-handed backhand like a one-handed left-handed forehand, with the right elbow slightly bent at contact. The player's left hand prevents the right wrist from hooking and also absorbs most of the impact and vibration. The player follows through by driving with the left arm.

A proper grip size prevents torque. A player determines his grip size by measuring from the proximal palmar crease to the tip of the ring finger, along the radial side of the ring finger (Fig. 13-6A). More simply, he can grip his racquet and then place the free index finger between the ring finger and the base of the thumb. If the index finger just fits, then the grip size is usually correct (Fig. 13-6B).

A player with "tennis elbow" should avoid a rigid racquet.[32] A racquet with a large sweet spot, or a fiberglass or graphite racquet, helps to reduce vibration. Some metal racquets vibrate like a tuning fork. A racquet should not be strung too tightly, usually between 50 and 55 pounds of tension is best.

Stretching and strengthening the wrist extensors are effective and major parts of the treatment for tennis elbow.[6, 45] Soreness is a guide for all stretching, isometric, and weight work. If the elbow becomes sore, the player has done too much exercise. The player's elbow is first immersed in a 40 °C (104 °F) whirlpool before he begins his exercises. He then performs isometric radial deviation-extension wrist cocking, holding each contraction for 6 seconds. When he is able to do these at full force without pain, he advances to cocking a tennis racquet. Next, a 0.67-kg (1.5-lb) weight is added to the neck of the racquet. More weight is added slowly until the player is lifting 2.25 kg (5 lb). He may have been lifting 6.75 to 9 kg (15 to 20 lb) before this episode of tennis elbow; thus it

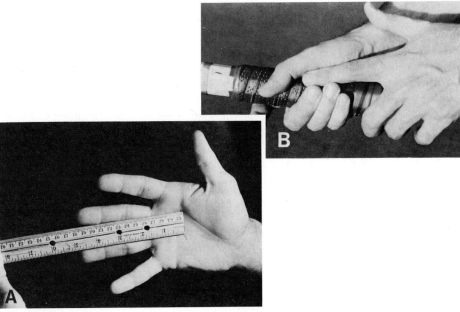

FIG. 13-6
Proper grip size may be determined by measuring along the radial side
of the ring finger, from the proximal palmar crease to the finger tip (A).
Another way to determine grip size is to hold the racquet and see if a
finger fits in the gap between the thumb and fingers (B).

must be explained to him that he should start off with lighter weights.

The tennis player may also wind up a weight attached to a broomstick by a rope. He starts with 20 repetitions of 0.56 kg (1.25 lb) and then gradually increases to 2.25 kg (5 lb), or he can twist a towel. After the acute period, deep friction massage is an excellent way to break up adhesions at the elbow, to increase circulation, and to eliminate wastes.

After doing well in flexibility, isometrics, and weight programs, the player may hit against a wall for 5 minutes and then build up to 7.5 minutes, 10 minutes, and 15 minutes a day. It is important that he use an Eastern backhand or Continental grip, hold his wrist cocked, and that his arm and racquet form an "L." Theoretically, however, hitting against a wall invokes a longer grip time than hitting with a partner, and therefore places a prolonged stress on the extensor origin. The grip pressure of better players is of short duration and peaks just before ball impact and then immediately relaxes. In average players the grip lasts longer. If there is no soreness after hitting against a wall for 15 minutes a day, the player may begin rallying. His elbow should be iced for 15 minutes after the stroke work.

Tennis players should keep their elbows warm, especially on cool or windy days. Some tennis players cut the toe section out of a wool sock, place the sock around their elbows and secure it with a light strip of adhesive tape to prevent it from sliding down. Neoprene elbow sleeves perform the same function. While the player sleeps, he should wear a splint that cocks his wrist up, as he may otherwise be flexing his wrist at night and stressing his extensors.

The symptoms of tennis elbow may resolve with rest, but they are sure to recur unless the player starts a strengthening and flexibility program and hits with a cocked wrist. If his arm were put in a cast, his muscles would atrophy, his proprioception would decrease, and recovery would take longer.

The "counterforce brace," a nonelastic, curved strap that the player fastens around his upper forearm,[26] is supposed to remove stress from the extensor origin. When his extensor muscles contract during the stroke, the brace serves essentially as a new origin for the muscles. It may reduce the sliding of the extensors over the lateral condyle. The brace also acts as a flag, reminding the player to concentrate on his backhand stroke mechanics.

A short, tapering course of phenylbutazone will usually alleviate the symptoms of acute tennis elbow. The chance that the drug may cause aplastic anemia or other serious problems is, however, too great for routine use. A white, chalky residue may accrue if a long-acting steroid is injected, and Steroid injections may cause some of the tissue necrosis seen at operation for tennis elbow.

If tennis elbow does not resolve after the above changes have been made and the player has followed a complete flexibility and strengthening program and improved the mechanics of his stroke, an exploration of his lateral epicondyle region and an extensor slide operation may be proposed.[45, 73] The extensor origin is explored and the extensor carpi radialis brevis exposed. This muscle lies under the extensor carpi radialis longus. Damaged tissue is removed from its undersurface. The elbow joint is then entered and checked for adhesions and synovial pannus. Any adhesions that bind the capsule to the orbicular ligament are lysed, and a partial synovectomy is performed. The extensor origin is then allowed to slide distally and left in this position. After operation, the player resumes the same exercise program recommended for the treatment of acute tennis elbow. Less successful operations include removal of the "radiohumeral meniscus"—a pannus of synovium growing between the radial head and the capitulum—which may be pinched, excision of the orbicular ligament to relieve tension in the elbow joint, and a procedure to elongate the extensor carpi radialis brevis.

A medial tennis elbow most commonly affects veteran tennis players and professionals who hit hard with good stroke mechanics.[66] Their strong wrist flexion in the tennis service and forehand ground strokes leads to medial epicondylar hypertrophy, avulsion of chips of bone from the medial epicondyle, and tears at the flexor origin. In the acute phase, rest and anti-inflammatory drug therapy may be beneficial. A player's warm-up procedures should be checked, especially his shoulder warm-up. The elbow must be iced after practice and after matches. Massage to the sore area rids it of waste products and breaks up scar.

"Boxer's Elbow"

When a boxer misses a jab, pieces of bone may chip from the tip of his olecranon process as it jams into his olecranon fossa.[31] These chips may then become loose bodies in his elbow joint. Direct impacts of the olecranon against the trochlea may shear off pieces of the trochlea, and traction on the coronoid process may avulse bone. Elbow pain is usually not related to one specific blow and is most painful when a jab is missed.

These elbows are operated on arthroscopically if the loose bodies cause locking or catching. The joint is irrigated, loose bodies are removed, and any pieces of articular cartilage that are partly attached, but appear ready to break free, are removed.

Olecranon Bursitis

Direct blows to the point of an athlete's elbow, or repetitive rubbing there, may irritate the olecranon bursa to produce synovial fluid that swells the bursa.[24] Olecranon bursitis is common in football receivers who land on hard artificial turf and has also been noted in recreational dart throwers trying to throw the darts *through* the board.[50] If the bursa is often irritated, the bursal wall will thicken. Fibrinous or cartilaginous loose bodies may form within the bursa and feel like bone chips.

An acutely swollen olecranon bursa should have an ice pack. The bursa is then sterilely aspirated of fluid and an elastic wrap snugly applied over a cotton roll for 24 to 48 hours. If the wall of the bursa has been thickened from recurrent bursitis or if it contains cartilage chips, the bursa may have to be removed. The incision should not be placed over the point of the elbow, as such placement may produce an adherent, painful, and easily bumped scar. Olecranon bursitis may be prevented by wearing well-fitting elbow pads.[69]

The Wrist and the Hand

Injuries of the hand are common in athletics, probably because the hand is characteristically in front of the athlete in most sports and frequently absorbs the initial contact.[61] Further, the hand is used in almost every sport in one way or another. There is a tendency to minimize the severity and importance of these injuries because the hand does not bear weight and injuries to the hand usually do not totally disable the athlete. This is particularly true of young, poorly supervised athletes who may return to vigorous activity and unprotected use of the extremity long before adequate healing.

The key to proper care of hand injuries is early, accurate diagnosis and precise and proper treatment, which must be followed by an appropriate rehabilitation program.[13] Conservative treatment measures are preferable for most injuries of the hand, and most athletes can be rapidly returned to their normal activities.[23] Primary surgical repair is indicated, however, in a small number of cases, and secondary reconstructive surgery may be needed in injuries that have been neglected or improperly treated.

Types of Injuries

Scaphoid Fractures

The scaphoid spans the proximal and distal carpal rows. The proximal part of this bone is intracapsular, and the distal portion has many soft-tissue attachments. The vulnerable waist of the scaphoid is adjacent to the styloid tip of the radius, and most of the scaphoid fractures occur here. A fall on the outstretched hand or direct impact on the hand may fracture the scaphoid by forcing it against this styloid process. The athlete notes pain on power grip and is tender over the "anatomic snuffbox."

Scaphoid fractures often are diagnosed inaccurately as sprains, and inadequate treatment may result in nonunion. If an athlete has the above symptoms but x-ray findings are negative, a cast is applied, which incorporates the proximal phalanx of the thumb. Then, in about 2 weeks, the wrist is re-examined and another x-ray film taken. If a fracture is noted, another cast is applied that extends from three fourths up the forearm down to the interphalangeal joint of the thumb and is carefully molded about the base of the thumb.

Most scaphoid fractures are through the waist, some are through the proximal pole, and the least frequent are of the distal pole. Fractures of the distal pole heal fast because of good blood supply. Fractures at the waist or proximal pole may require prolonged immobilization, and nonunion, avascular necrosis, and collapse may occur.

Those scaphoid fractures that are unstable and displaced need primary open reduction and fixation and sometimes primary grafting. Delayed unions require prolonged casting; a decision should then be made as to whether the fracture should be grafted. If the decision is made to treat the fracture with a bone graft, I favor a volar approach and use the volar aspect of the distal radius as a donor site. Postoperatively, patients with these fractures are treated with the standard scaphoid cast, and postoperative healing still takes about 3 to 4 months. While the fracture is healing, the athlete may sometimes return to athletics wearing a silicone rubber splint.

Protective Splint of Silicone Rubber Under the rules of collegiate tackle football, sole leather or other hard or unyielding substances are prohibited on the hand, wrist, or forearm no matter how well they are covered or padded. Mindful of this rule, a protective silicone rubber splint has been developed.[4] The splint allows the safe return to competition of athletes who have had wrist sprains or fractures, such as a healing scaphoid fracture.

The silicone rubber protective splint (Fig. 13-7) is constructed with gauze impregnated with silicone rubber-RTV 11. The splint is easy to apply, conforms to the injured part, and is du-

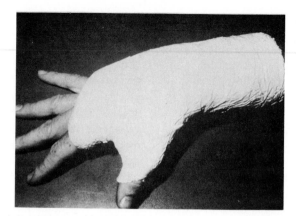

FIG. 13-7
A silicone cast may allow an earlier return to practice and competition.

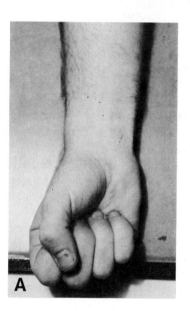

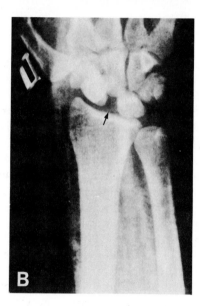

FIG. 13-8
A supinated x-ray view with the athlete's fist clenched may show the gap between the scaphoid and lunate (*arrow*).

rable. First, a thin coat of lubricant cream is applied to the skin, and the gauze is wrapped smoothly on the body part. A catalyst is mixed with the silicone, and a generous first coat of silicone is applied. Usually three or four thicknesses of gauze are used, and the silicone is worked into each layer of the gauze with a spatula. The silicone takes about 3 hours to cure at room temperature. For removal, the splint is cut along the ulnar side. It can be secured again with adhesive tape. Since the silicone splint does not breathe, it is not used as a permanent cast but may be worn during practice and competition. A bivalved hard cast is worn at other times.[4]

Rotary Subluxation of the Scaphoid

The scaphoid links the proximal and distal rows of the carpal bones. In rotary subluxation of the scaphoid, the strong ligamentous attachment between the scaphoid and the lunate is disrupted. This may occur after reduction of a perilunate dislocation. If the subluxation is overlooked, pain, clicking, and wrist weakness develop.

A closed-fist x-ray view in supination should be taken along with the standard views of the wrist to diagnose this rotary subluxation (Fig. 13-8). An enlarged gap between the scaphoid and the lunate may be seen in this view. The normal gap between the scaphoid and lunate is 1 to 2 mm, and a 3-mm gap is abnormal. The rotated scaphoid also appears foreshortened on the anteroposterior view. Lateral x-ray films show increased volar rotation of the distal pole of the scaphoid.

The acute subluxation may be reduced and held in radial deviation, but usually open repair is needed to give the best results. A combined volar and dorsal approach should be used to repair the ligaments on both sides. In chronic cases with disability, reconstruction is carried out, but the results are not as good as after a primary repair.

Lunate Dislocations

Lunate dislocations are seen more often than perilunate dislocations, but the lunate dislocation probably follows a perilunate dislocation that has spontaneously reduced. The lunate rotates and is pushed volarly, where it may compress the medial nerve. The volar radiolunate ligament remains intact, preserving the blood supply to the lunate. The diagnosis of a lunate dislocation is made on a lateral x-ray film of the wrist.

The lunate is reduced by applying longitudinal traction, extending the wrist, and then pressing the lunate dorsally. Sometimes the perilunate dislocation must be recreated to reduce the lunate, and then the perilunate dislocation itself is reduced. Wrist dislocations are protected in a cast for 4 weeks with the wrist in slight flexion. Asymptomatic athletes are then allowed to resume competition, protected for 4 more weeks in a silicone splint.

If a lunate dislocation has gone unrecognized and is seen late, open reduction is usually necessary. The most common complication of a lunate dislocation is a late rotary instability of the scaphoid. Other complications are median nerve palsy, flexor tendon constriction, and avascular necrosis of the lunate.

Avascular Necrosis of the Lunate

Avascular necrosis of the lunate (Kienböck's disease) is an infrequent complication of lunate dislocation, because the blood supply to the lunate is usually preserved. Avascular necrosis,

however, may follow an unrecognized fracture of the lunate. The athlete notes wrist weakness, stiffness, and pain with motion. X-ray films show the increased density of avascular necrosis.

If the athlete has avascular necrosis of the lunate but no change in the shape of the bone, a cast is applied. If the lunate has already collapsed and fragmented, however, then it should be excised early and replaced with a silicone prosthesis. Proximal row carpectomy or wrist fusion are salvage procedures.

Perilunate Dislocation and Trans-scaphoid Perilunate Dislocation

A direct blow to the hand may produce extensive ligamentous damage and dislocate the distal carpal bones dorsal to the lunate. In a perilunate dislocation, the entire scaphoid dislocates with the rest of the carpus. Frequently, however, the scaphoid is fractured through its waist and the distal part of the scaphoid dislocates dorsally, while the proximal part stays attached to the lunate. This is a trans-scaphoid, perilunate dislocation.

Straight longitudinal traction is applied to reduce these dislocations, and the lunate is pressed dorsally, while the rest of the carpus is pressed volarly. Sometimes the ligamentous tears render the reduction unstable. Rotary subluxation of the scaphoid may be present after reduction and should be repaired. The wrist anatomy should be restored to as near normal as possible. If the scaphoid fragments are displaced, an open reduction is performed with pin fixation.

Hamate Hook Fractures

The hook of the hamate projects toward the palmar surface of the hand as a long, thin process of bone. The transverse carpal ligament and the pisohamate ligament both attach to the hook, and the flexor digiti minimi brevis and opponens digiti both arise from it. The tendon of the flexor digitorum profundus to the little finger lies on its radial side, and the motor branch of the medial nerve on its ulnar side.

The hook of the hamate may be fractured in a fall, but it breaks more commonly during a

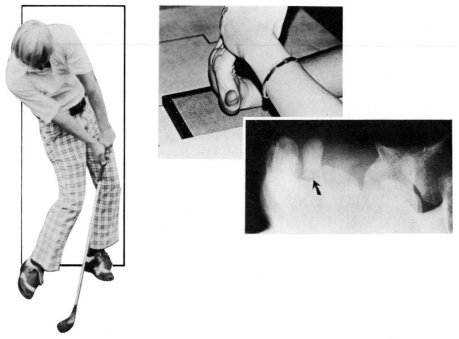

FIG. 13-9
The hook of the golfer's hamate may be fractured during a swing. The fracture line may be seen on a carpal tunnel view. The fracture sometimes fails to unite and irritates the nearby motor branch of the ulnar nerve; it may also cause a rupture of the flexor profundus to the little finger.

tennis, baseball, or golf swing (Fig. 13-9).[81] The butt of the handle may strike the hook and fracture it, or a violent contraction of the flexor carpi ulnaris can pull through the pisohamate ligament and jerk the hook.

An athlete with a hook of the hamate fracture will have wrist pain, a poor power grip, and a tender hook of the hamate. Routine x-ray films often do not show the fracture, so a carpal tunnel view should be included with the wrist in maximum dorsiflexion. If the wrist is too painful for this view to be obtained, a maximum radial deviation view, with the wrist partly supinated, may show the fracture.

A short gauntlet cast, with an extension to the little finger, is applied for acute undisplaced fractures of the hook of the hamate (*see* Fig. 13-9). The nonunion rate for this fracture is high, owing to the intermittent pull of the muscular attachments. For a badly displaced fracture or a symptomatic nonunion, the displaced hook is removed.

The ulnar nerve or the flexor digitorum profundus to the little finger may become irritated at the fracture site and give symptoms of ulnar nerve neuritis or flexor tendinitis. To prevent a later tendon rupture, some surgeons remove the hook of the hamate even in painless nonunions. So that the ulnar nerve is not damaged during this procedure, it is exposed in the canal of Guyon and carefully followed.

Nerve Compression

An athlete's median nerve may be compressed in a tight carpal tunnel, or the ulnar nerve may be compressed in the canal of Guyon. In the young, healthy athlete, rest and an anti-inflammatory medication will usually relieve median nerve compression, but sometimes surgical decompression is needed.

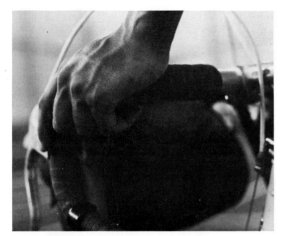

FIG. 13-10
A cyclist's ulnar nerve may be compressed at the wrist from pressure on the handlebars.

Touring cyclists, especially on bumpy, gravel roads, often develop numbness of the little finger and the ulnar half of the ring finger, with associated ulnar intrinsic muscle weakness.[20, 43] The numbness and weakness are caused by pressure from the handlebars on the ulnar nerve (Fig. 13-10), and may be relieved by wearing cycling gloves and thickly padding the handlebars. The ulnar nerve may also be compressed after a fracture of the pisiform or the hamate bone, and blunt trauma to the heel of the palm may also result in scarring within the canal of Guyon. This acute trauma may even produce a false aneurysm of the ulnar artery that may compress the ulnar nerve. Treatment consists of release of the ligament overlying the canal of Guyon and appropriate measures for the underlying lesion.

"Bowler's Thumb"

The hard edge of the thumb hole in a bowling ball may press against the base of a bowler's thumb during delivery and cause perineural fibrosis of the relatively subcutaneous ulnar digital nerve of the thumb.[20, 21, 42, 53, 54, 74] If fibrosis develops, the bowler will note pain, paresthesia when pressure is applied to this region, numbness of the ulnar-volar aspect of the thumb, and a fusiform mass.

If "bowler's thumb" is detected early, the bowler should modify his grip and use a larger, padded thumbhole. If the condition is noted later, after a mass has formed, the thumb is operated on. The thick, perineural sheath is incised and meticulously dissected free from the nerve fascicles. After neurolysis, the nerve may be transposed to a more dorsal-ulnar aspect of the thumb. Awareness of the entity of bowler's thumb neuroma prevents unnecessary removal of the digital nerve. The symptoms may be relieved without excising the neuroma, and the critical sensation is maintained along the medial border of the thumb.

Thumb Metacarpal Fractures

Axial compression may injure a hockey player's thumb metacarpal when he takes off his gloves to throw a punch. The thumb may be driven down to shear off the base of the thumb metacarpal. A small medial fragment remains hooked to the strong volar ligament, as the abductor pollicis longus pulls the main portion of the metacarpal proximally. This Bennett's fracture-dislocation may be treated by closed reduction and percutaneous pin fixation. In some cases, however, open reduction is needed to accurately approximate the articular surfaces. A Rolando's fracture is a proximal, intra-articular, T-shaped fracture of the first metacarpal. Here the flexor and extensor muscles pull the fracture fragments apart over the trapezium.

Although fractures of the metacarpal shaft are often angulated by muscle pull, a well-molded gauntlet cast can usually hold the reduction. Fractures of the proximal phalanx of the thumb may follow a twisting injury, such as when an equestrian's thumb becomes caught in a halter as the horse rears. These fractures are usually treated by a closed reduction and a gauntlet cast. Internal fixation may be required if the fracture slips.

Thumb Metacarpophalangeal Joint Dislocation

When the metacarpophalangeal joint of the thumb is forcefully hyperextended and dislocates, the membranous part of the volar plate

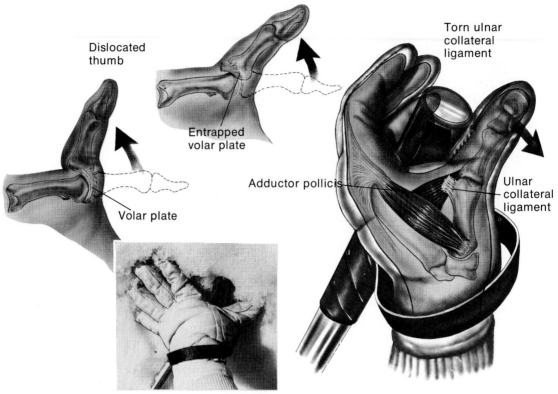

FIG. 13-11
Landing on a ski pole may dislocate the metacarpophalangeal joint of the thumb, and the volar plate may become trapped in the joint. In other instances, the ulnar collateral ligament of the thumb may tear from its insertion into the proximal phalanx, and the tendon of the adductor pollicis may interpose to prevent healing.

may tear (Fig. 13-11). In a simple dislocation, the proximal phalanx lies dorsal to the metacarpal head and is standing straight up. Longitudinal traction should be avoided because the volar plate may slip between the metacarpal and the proximal phalanx, converting the simple dislocation into a complex one. Instead, the physician should push against the dorsal surface of the proximal phalanx and push the metacarpal dorsally.

When the volar plate is caught between the metacarpal and the proximal phalanx, the dislocation may be irreducible. X-ray films show a sesamoid bone within the widened joint space, and there is a dimple in the palmar skin. To reduce such a dislocation, the thumb metacarpal is first adducted and the thumb flexed to

relax the intrinsics. Then the proximal phalanx is hyperextended, and the physician pushes against the dorsal surface of the proximal phalanx and pushes the metacarpal up. If closed reduction fails, open reduction may be performed through a volar or dorsal approach.

After reduction, the thumb is immobilized in a plaster splint for about 2 weeks. The athlete often is allowed to resume competition while wearing a silicone splint. When the joint is completely stable and has a full range of motion, the immobilization may be discontinued.

Ulnar Collateral Ligament Injury of the Thumb

Ulnar collateral ligament injuries of the thumb are often overlooked in young, poorly

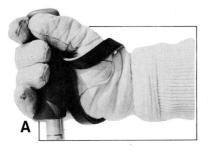
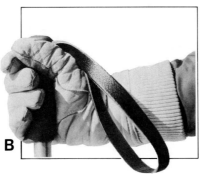

FIG. 13-12
If a skier wraps the pole strap around his wrist (*A*), he may injure his thumb in a fall. If he does not use the pole strap (*B*), however, another skier may be injured by the lost pole.

supervised athletes.[59, 60] There is a tendency to minimize the injury, but it may lead to a weakness of pinch and instability when the thumb is stressed in abduction. The injury occurs mostly in tackle football, from forced abduction of the thumb, but also in hockey players, who take off their gloves to fight, and in soccer goalkeepers, skiers, wrestlers and baseball players.[10, 15, 16, 27, 28, 71] The skier's pole strap allows him to plant the pole harder by pulling down on the strap, and thus the pole need not be gripped as tightly. When the strap is wrapped around the wrist discarding the pole is difficult, and the skier may land on it in trying to break the fall (Fig. 13-12A). A better method of holding the pole is with only the hand put through the loop.

The ulnar collateral ligament is usually torn from its attachment to the proximal phalanx. Sometimes a displaced and rotated chip from the proximal phalanx may be seen on x-ray films. Most of the tears are partial and can be treated by closed means, but acute, complete tears are treated with open repair and reconstruction. In more than half of these complete tears the intrinsic aponeurosis is found to be lying between the ends of the ulnar collateral ligament and would block healing.[59] The avulsed ulnar collateral ligament is reattached by a pull-out wire technique. If the ligament has been torn in its midportion, sutures are placed in it with the metacarpophalangeal joint flexed to 15° to 20°, and the athlete must wear a splint or a thumb spica for 5 weeks.

Taping of the thumb allows an athlete to continue playing without jeopardizing a mild or moderate sprain and to play after surgery (Fig. 13-13). First the metacarpophalangeal joint is stabilized with the tape, and then the athlete's index finger is taped to his thumb, holding the thumb adducted and preventing abduction at the metacarpophalangeal joint. Alternatively, elastic tape may be used to hold the thumb adducted (Fig. 13-14).

An athlete with an old ulnar collateral ligament injury may have a long history of pinch weakness, pain, and instability at the metacarpophalangeal joint of the thumb. When the ulnar collateral ligament is thin or missing, it can be replaced by a slip of the abductor pollicis longus, or a slip of the adductor pollicis may be advanced to the proximal phalanx as a dynamic repair.

Soft Tissue Injuries at the Metacarpophalangeal Joint of the Fingers

What may at first appear to be a dorsal dislocation of the proximal phalanx of a metacarpophalangeal joint is actually a volar dislocation of the metacarpal head (Fig. 13-15A). The head breaks through a buttonhole rent in the volar plate and is caught in this rent and between the lumbrical tendon and long flexors. This dislocation is usually referred to as an "irreducible dislocation," as closed reduction often fails. Although the index finger is most often affected, the little finger metacarpal or other metacarpals may also be dislocated. The af-

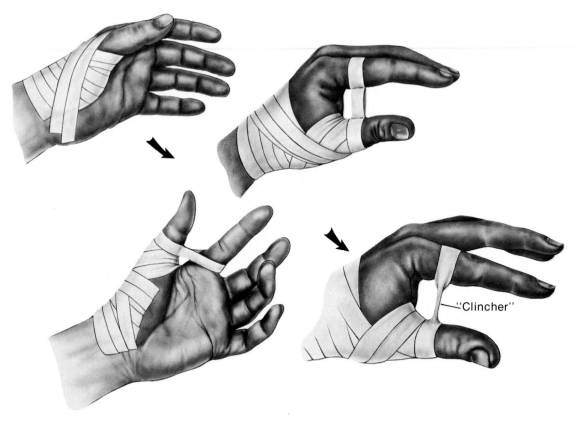

FIG. 13-13
A thumb taping with a "clincher" strap restricts thumb movement.

fected finger is generally angled toward the ulnar, overlapping the adjacent finger, and a dimple appears in the skin at the midpalmar crease. Longitudinal traction actually prevents reduction, as the surrounding structures form a nooselike constriction around the metacarpal neck. An acute dislocation may sometimes be reduced by increasing the deformity and attempting to return the proximal phalanx through the tear in the volar plate. Once swelling has occurred, however, an open reduction is usually needed.

The dislocation may be reduced surgically through a volar approach (*see* Fig. 13-15B). Great care must be taken to avoid damaging the very prominent palmar structures, especially the digital nerve and artery. Once reduced, the joint is surprisingly stable. The metacarpophalangeal joint is kept flexed about 30° for 7 to 10 days, and then active flexion is begun from this position. An extension-block splint is worn, and extension and hyperextension are not permitted until 5 weeks after surgery. Nearly full flexion is usually accomplished by the time the splint is removed.

A collateral ligament injury of a metacarpophalangeal joint is not nearly as common or as disabling as one involving a proximal interphalangeal joint. However, a piece of the proximal phalanx may be avulsed by the collateral ligament into the joint. Swelling, thickening, and the possible inclusion of the collateral ligament in the joint are the most disabling findings. Lateral instability is usually not a functional problem, as radial or ulnar control is maintained by the intrinsics.

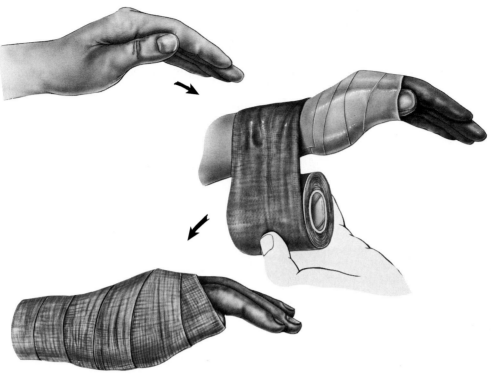

FIG. 13-14
A "pancake" thumb taping may protect a damaged ulnar collateral ligament of the thumb.

FIG. 13-15
A volar dislocation of the index finger metacarpal head presents as a bulge and a dimple in the palm (*A*). At operation (*B*), the metacarpal head (*arrow*) is reduced.

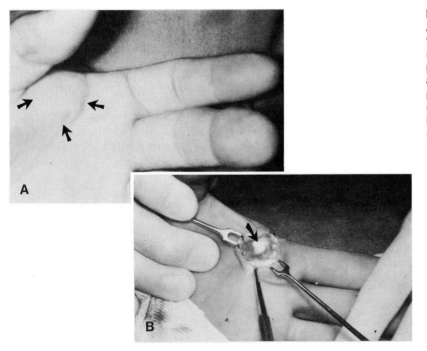

Another soft tissue injury at the metacarpophalangeal joint is rupture of the extensor hood of the extensor digitorum communis. The extensor tendon can then slip into the valley between the metacarpal heads and produce a disabling snapping. A large mass of granulation tissue may form from hypertrophic synovium in the tear, preventing an athlete from gripping. The mass should be removed and the extensor hood repaired.

Hand Injuries in Karate

Karate means "empty hand" in Japanese. The fighting technique began in India more than 1500 years ago for self-defense against bandits, was later taught to Chinese monks and developed further in Okinawa. In 1920, the martial art was exported to Japan and, after World War II, to the United States.[17, 29]

Karate enthusiasts scarify their limbs, converting them into weapons to strike the sensitive areas of their opponents. This toughening may be achieved by striking a straw-covered, pliable post over a number of years, or the hands and feet may be driven into sacks of sand, gravel, grain, or leather scraps.[47] Scar tissue slowly increases, but if rigid adherence to this program is replaced by a desire for quick results, the hands may be damaged.[78]

Hypertrophic infiltrative tenosynovitis may develop about an extensor tendon that is greatly enlarged proximal to where it is trapped by a mass of scar tissue at the metacarpophalangeal joint.[29] The scar tissue may be removed, but the incision should be placed so that it does not interfere with striking.[29]

A correctly executed thrust and hand strike uses the index and middle finger metacarpal heads. Axial compression forces are transmitted from these metacarpals to the distal carpal row, which is dynamically splinted by the taut wrist extensors and flexors. These forces may produce intra-articular fractures.[46] In contrast to correct technique, inaccurate thrusts, roundhouse blows, and the blocking of kicks will transmit angular torsional forces to produce oblique diaphysial fractures of the metacarpals.[39]

To lessen the chance of hand injury, a fist must be made properly (Fig. 13-16). A loose fist leaves the second and third metacarpals unsupported, and only their thick cortex and shaft may save them from breaking. To make a proper fist for karate, the interphalangeal joints are first maximally flexed. Then the metacarpophalangeal joints are flexed so that the thenar eminence gives support. The thumb is tucked out of the way. Striking is done only with the index and middle finger knuckles, and with a maximally tightened fist. At impact the wrist is pronated, reminding the striker to maximally tighten the fist and also tearing an attacker's skin.

Metacarpal Fractures

Fractures of the finger metacarpals include proximal fracture-dislocations at the base of the fifth metacarpal that may be similar to a fracture-dislocation of the first metacarpal; metacarpal shaft fractures; fractures through a metacarpal neck, the "fighter's fracture"; and intra-articular fractures at the metacarpophalangeal joint.

A proximal fracture-dislocation of the fifth metacarpal may behave like an unstable Bennett's fracture-dislocation of the first metacarpal. Such a fracture is reduced and fixed with pins. Fracture-dislocations of the second, third, or fourth metacarpal are extremely rare, and the treatment must be individualized. Fractures of the proximal shaft of the metacarpals are controlled by metacarpal ligaments and are generally stable. They are protected in a short arm cast.

A fracture of a metacarpal shaft is usually only minimally displaced and may be controlled in a well-molded short-arm cast that is worn for 4 to 6 weeks. Occasionally percutaneous pins or an open reduction is necessary. Long, spiral fractures are more likely to require internal fixation to avoid compounding, rotatory deformity, and shortening of the metacarpal. When these fractures are treated closed, care must be taken to control the rotation of the digit, and it is often taped to an adjacent finger. Open reduction of a metacarpal shaft fracture may produce complications such as compromise of the bone's blood supply, fibrosis of the interosseous muscles, adherence of the extensor tendons, and local infection.

A "fighter's fracture," or "punch fracture," through the neck of the fifth metacarpal may follow a roundhouse punch. A boxer, with proper punching technique and taped hands, will more often fracture his second or third metacarpal than his fifth metacarpal. The boxer has the advantage of good technique, bandaged hands, and boxing gloves. His hands are bandaged with his fingers spread (Fig. 13-16). When he flexes his fingers, the metacarpals are held strongly together. A boxing "glove" is really a mitten, with a firm leather band in the palm of the glove that supports all four finger metacarpals.

The fourth and fifth metacarpals are structurally weak, the fourth being the slenderest, while the fifth is shorter and has a paper-thin cortex. The thenar eminence supports only the second and third metacarpals, leaving the lateral two metacarpals without support in a bare-knuckled fist. The volar articular ridge of the metacarpal heads acts as a reinforcement and explains the obliquity of the fracture lines.

A fighter's fracture is common and often overtreated. Any rotation can usually be corrected by closed reduction with the metacarpophalangeal joint flexed so that the fragment is controlled by a tightening of the collateral ligament. Volar and dorsal felt pads are placed after the reduction. Then a molded plaster cast is applied, with an outrigger or with the little finger buddy-taped to the ring finger. Up to 40° of angulation is acceptable in the more mobile fourth and fifth metacarpals. Holding the metacarpophalangeal and proximal interphalangeal joints in flexion with pressure

FIG. 13-16
In a properly made fist, the thumb supports the second and third metacarpals, but the lateral two metacarpals remain unsupported, allowing a fracture to occur. The taping supports the boxer's metacarpals.

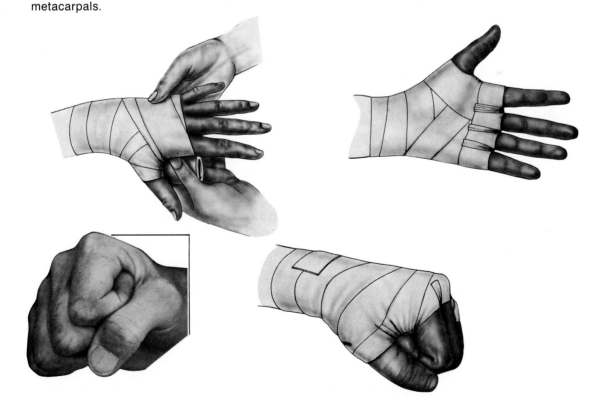

over the dorsum of the proximal phalanx is unnecessary. Serious secondary stiffness and skin problems frequently follow such treatment. A fracture that is very unstable may require percutaneous pinning and, occasionally, open reduction with internal fixation.

If an appreciable part of the articular surface is involved in a fracture, the fracture must be anatomically reduced, usually by open reduction. An arthroplasty with a silastic prosthesis may be needed in a joint that has been left grossly deformed by an old injury.

The complications of metacarpal fractures include rotatory deformity, localized Volkmann's ischemic contracture, limitation of flexion and extension at the metacarpophalangeal, proximal interphalangeal, or distal interphalangeal joints, and nonunion of the bone. In these cases, reconstructive procedures may be needed to improve function.

Fractures of the Proximal Phalanx

The periosteum of the proximal phalanx is in contact with the extrinsic extensor and flexor tendons and the lateral bands. Because of this close association, these tendons readily adhere to fractures of the proximal phalanx, especially if they have been imperfectly reduced. Tethering of the tendons limits active and passive motion at the proximal interphalangeal and distal interphalangeal joints. Moreover, a fracture of the proximal phalanx may affect the metacarpophalangeal or the proximal interphalangeal joint. Restricted motion in either of these joints is disabling, but restriction of motion in both joints is disastrous.

The intrinsic and extrinsic muscles exert deforming forces on the fracture fragments. The proximal fragment is flexed by the intrinsics, and the distal fragment is controlled by the extrinsic flexors and extensors that span it. The collateral ligaments of the metacarpophalangeal joints aid closed reduction, controlling the metacarpophalangeal joint when it is flexed and maintaining control of the proximal fragment. A flexed position also lessens the deforming force of the intrinsic muscles, and flexion of the proximal interphalangeal joint relaxes the extrinsic flexors, reducing their deforming force.

An epiphyseal fracture of a young athlete's proximal phalanx may be angulated. Closed reduction is usually successful. The tough periosteum is often intact and aids in obtaining and maintaining the reduction. After reduction the finger is splinted, and when the reaction has died down the injured finger is taped to an adjacent finger.

Inherently stable fractures of the shaft of the proximal phalanx and those that are stable after reduction may be controlled by splinting. After a thin felt pad is placed between the fingers, the injured finger is taped to an adjacent finger. For less stable fractures, a forearm split is applied with an outrigger that holds the finger in the position of greatest stability. Remember that all the fingers should point toward the proximal tubercle of the scaphoid. Malrotation will occur if this relationship is not maintained. Early motion is particularly important after a fracture of the proximal phalanx, to regain optimal finger motion.

Some proximal phalanx fractures present special problems. The spike of an oblique fracture may encroach upon the proximal interphalangeal joint just proximal to the articular surface and severely disrupt joint function. A spiral fracture can easily rotate and shorten to produce a deformity if it is not held well reduced. These are usually fixed percutaneously with pins, but when a closed reduction is not possible open reduction and pin fixation are done. A fracture involving the articular surface must be reduced anatomically and held with pins. When a proximal phalanx fracture is treated by open reduction and internal fixation, incisions must be placed properly and the tissue handled gently; otherwise, functional loss may be even greater than that after closed treatment. Prompt, appropriate treatment for proximal phalanx fractures is imperative. Secondary reconstructions for nonunions or for other bony or soft tissue abnormalities may not produce a fully functional finger.

Injuries to the Proximal Interphalangeal Joint

The anatomy of the proximal interphalangeal joint is complex for such a small articulation and must be understood for correct diagnosis and effective treatment of injuries to this joint. A hinged joint, it has a range of motion of from 0° to 120° in the plane perpendicular to the palm. The lateral ligaments and volar plate are thick and strong. They are supplemented dorsally by the central slip of the extensor tendon and by the flexor tendons, less closely on the volar surface. The lateral bands and their extensions, the oblique and transverse retinacular ligaments, and Cleland's ligament radiating dorsal to the neurovascular bundle add some stability and must move and glide freely to allow proper motion. The volar cul-de-sac must be free of scar to allow full flexion of the finger, during which the base of the middle phalanx glides into the sac.

The proximal interphalangeal joint has limited lateral mobility and is particularly vulnerable because of its relatively long proximal and distal lever arms that transmit lateral stress and torque.[57] Any fixed deformity of the proximal interphalangeal joint, either in flexion or extension, is extremely disabling. Because it is a small, non-weight-bearing joint, there is a tendency to minimize the severity of injuries to it. Poorly supervised athletes often return to unprotected use of the digit long before adequate healing has taken place.[58]

Injuries to the proximal interphalangeal joint include articular fractures, fracture-dislocations, dislocations, collateral ligament injuries, buttonhole deformities, and volar plate injuries such as hyperextension and pseudobuttonhole deformities.

Articular Fractures at the Proximal Interphalangeal Joint

Commonly seen articular fractures at the proximal interphalangeal joint include those that pass through one condyle of the head of the proximal phalanx, long and short oblique fractures, T fractures that split the condyles, fractures of the base of the middle phalanx, avulsion fractures of the articular surface, and comminuted fractures.

Stable fractures with little or no ligamentous instability, such as small chip fractures and avulsion fractures, should be splinted for 3 weeks with the proximal interphalangeal joint flexed to about 30°. In most cases, the athlete may return to competition, wearing the splint for protection. Early protected flexion begins

as soon as the acute reaction abates. Either a dorsal or volar splint should be worn during sports and other strenuous activities for an addition 4 to 6 weeks or until a full range of motion has been regained.

The indications for open reduction and internal fixation include displaced articular fractures that comprise more than one fourth of the articular surface, displaced volar lip fractures that invite subsequent dorsal subluxation, comminuted or displaced fractures, and dorsal avulsion fractures that include the insertion of the central slip of the extensor tendon into the base of the middle phalanx. Accurate restoration of the articular surface in this little, tight-fitting joint is important for a maximum return of function. Secondary reconstructive procedures, including silastic implant arthroplasty, give less predictable results. Arthrodesis is a treatment of last resort and is rarely indicated.

Fracture-Dislocations of the Proximal Interphalangeal Joint

The most common fracture-dislocation of the proximal interphalangeal joint is one through the volar lip of the proximal phalanx (Fig. 13-17A). Here the buttressing effect of the volar lip is lost, and, if untreated, the finger becomes stiff and painful and its function greatly impaired. The volar fragment may vary in size and comminution. If the joint is stable, the digit may be splinted in flexion with a splint that blocks extension; if unstable, operative reduction and pinning are needed (Fig. 13-17B). Early flexion exercises should begin in 3 weeks, and the finger should be protected during athletics for an additional 4 to 6 weeks.

An avulsion of the central slip of the extensor mechanism, with or without a bony fragment, and volar subluxation of the middle phalanx are rare injuries. They often demand an open reduction because the head of the proximal phalanx may be entrapped by the lateral bands to block a closed reduction.

Dislocations of the Proximal Interphalangeal Joint

If the proximal interphalangeal joint is hyperextended, the volar plate may rupture at its distal attachment, with or without an avulsion

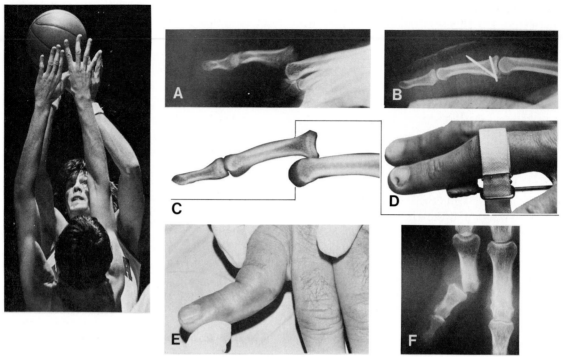

FIG. 13-17
A fracture of the volar lip of the middle phalanx may allow dislocation
(*A*). Pins are used to fix this fracture (*B*). A dislocated proximal
interphalangeal joint (*C*) may yield a buttonhole deformity that can
sometimes be corrected with a safety-pin splint (*D*). In a collateral
ligament tear (*E, F*), the proximal end of the ligament catches within the
joint and may need to be operatively removed.

fracture from the base of the middle phalanx,
and the middle phalanx will dislocate dorsal to
the proximal phalanx (Fig. 13-17C). Reduction
is usually easy and the joint generally stable
because the collateral ligament system has usually remained intact. Once reduced, the joint is
immobilized in 20° to 30° of flexion for 3
weeks, whereupon the splint is removed and
the athlete begins an active exercise program.
The finger should be taped to an adjacent normal digit during athletics for at least 2 more
weeks until it is asymptomatic. With proper
care and protection, full recovery should be
expected, with an asymptomatic finger and a
full range of motion.

For a lateral dislocation of the proximal interphalangeal joint to occur, a collateral ligament and the volar plate must tear. The method

of treatment for these dislocations depends on
what instabilities exist after reduction. Some
dislocations have a rotatory component, and
the head of the proximal phalanx may become
buttonholed between the central slip and the
lateral band. These dislocations usually require
open reduction. Open dislocations are meticulously cleaned, and then the torn tissues may
be repaired. The athlete may begin active protected motion as soon as his skin heals.

"Buttonhole Deformity"

A disruption of the central slip of the extensor digitorum communis tendon over the proximal interphalangeal joint produces a classic
buttonhole (boutonniere) deformity (Fig. 13-
17D) that consists of hyperextension at the distal interphalangeal joint.[56] A central slip rupture

is difficult to diagnose acutely. Unopposed pull of the flexor digitorum sublimis and pain and swelling at the proximal interphalangeal joint keep the joint flexed. The athlete's inability to extend his proximal interphalangeal joint is often attributed to the pain and swelling from the injury. The finger is splinted in the usual semiflexed position. When the extensor tendon is disrupted, however, this position favors a continued separation of the central slip and prevents healing. Later, as the athlete attempts to extend the finger, the tension on the lateral bands increases, causing them to drop volarly. These bands then become flexors, aggravate the deformity, and produce hyperextension at the distal interphalangeal joint.

To avoid developing a buttonhole deformity, a person with any injury associated with a lag of more than 30° in proximal interphalangeal extension and tenderness dorsally directly over the base of the middle phalanx should be treated for an acute extensor rupture. The digit should be splinted with the proximal interphalangeal joint in full extension, and this splint should be worn for 6 to 8 weeks. Protective splinting should be continued during competition for another 6 to 8 weeks or until full flexion and maximum extension of the finger have returned. The metacarpophalangeal and distal interphalangeal joints may be left free to move. If there is residual restricted passive extension at the proximal interphalangeal joint, correction with a safety-pin splint is needed (Fig. 13-17D). In many of these cases, however, surgical reconstruction will be required. Many surgical procedures have been designed to correct chronic deformities, but owing to a variety of findings, the results of these procedures are not predictable.

Volar Plate Injuries

The volar plate of the proximal interphalangeal joint has a proximal membranous portion attached to the proximal phalanx and a thick, cartilaginous distal portion attached strongly to the base of the middle phalanx. An acute volar plate injury requires splinting for at least 5 weeks. The athlete may begin early protected

motion at 3 weeks, wearing an extension-block splint to prevent extension of the digit.

An injury to the volar plate may result in either a hyperextension deformity or a flexion deformity at the proximal interphalangeal joint. Distal disruption of the plate may produce a "swan-neck" deformity. Surgical reconstruction is indicated only if the proximal interphalangeal joint locks in extension and interferes with normal function of the hand.

Damage to the proximal, membranous part of the plate may produce a "pseudoboutonniere" deformity. This resembles the classic boutonniere deformity, but the central extensor slip is intact. With a pseudoboutonniere deformity, there is usually a history of a hyperextension or a twisting injury to the proximal interphalangeal joint. The signs of a pseudoboutonniere deformity include a flexion contracture of the proximal interphalangeal joint, which is more resistant to correction by passive extension than is the typical boutonniere, slight hyperextension of the distal interphalangeal joint, and radiologic evidence of calcification under the distal end of the proximal phalanx.

Static safety-pin splinting is used in subacute, less-fixed pseudoboutonniere deformities. After correction, these fingers must still be followed closely because the deformity may recur. Chronic pseudoboutonniere deformities are much more resistant to extension with a safety-pin splint. If the deformity is disabling—usually past 40° of flexion—or if it progresses or is a problem to the athlete, surgery is indicated.

Collateral Ligament Injuries

Collateral ligament injuries to the proximal interphalangeal joint are most common on the radial side of the digit (Fig. 13-17E, F). The proximal attachment of the collateral ligament is avulsed, and the volar plate may be partly or completely ruptured, depending on the magnitude of the injury force. If part of the collateral ligament is intact, as evidenced by some stability, the joint may be splinted in 30° of flexion. The finger is splinted protectively for at least 3 weeks, but active motion exercises may begin at 10 to 14 days after injury. The splint is worn for another 4 to 6 weeks during athletics or until the joint is asymptomatic.

The treatment of choice for complete collateral ligament tears at the proximal interphalangeal joint is controversial. Some surgeons maintain that nonoperative treatment is satisfactory; however, the proximal end of the ligament frequently folds into the joint at the time of injury and remains stuck there. Thus, closed treatment often leaves the athlete with a swollen, tender, and unstable joint susceptible to further injury and prone to develop degenerative changes. Surgery allows inspection of the joint and repair of the torn ligament. The surgeon must, of course, be well versed in surgery of the hand, or further damage may result from the operation. Reconstructive surgery may be needed in chronic cases, but the results are less satisfactory and less predictable than after a primary repair.

Fractures of the Middle Phalanx

Fractures of the middle phalanx are usually slow healing, oblique, or transverse fractures through the hard cortical bone in the narrow waist of the shaft. The central slip of the extensor tendon inserts dorsally into the base of the middle phalanx, whereas the two slips of the flexor digitorum sublimis insert further distally into the volar surface of the shaft. This anatomy accounts for the characteristic deformities seen in the fractures.

The most common fracture site is distal to both insertions. In these, the stronger flexor sublimis tendon flexes the proximal fragment. Longitudinal traction and flexion of the distal fragment aligns the fracture, especially if there is an intact periosteal bridge. When a fracture occurs more proximally in the shaft, between the central slip of the extensor tendon and the insertion of the flexor digitorum sublimis, the proximal fragment will be extended and the distal fragment flexed. These fractures are reduced with longitudinal traction without flexion.

Fractures of the middle phalanx are held in a splint for about 3 weeks, whereupon exercises are begun. When the athlete is engaged in athletic competition, however, the splint must be worn for 6 to 8 more weeks or until the fracture is healed completely. Unstable fractures are fixed with percutaneous K wires and protected similarly. Occasionally, when satisfactory alignment cannot be obtained by closed means, open reduction and internal fixation are needed.

Avulsion of the Flexor Digitorum Profundus

Avulsion of the flexor digitorum profundus, "football finger," is more common than was earlier thought.[8, 14, 51, 68] The injury was misdiagnosed often or missed entirely, but increased suspicion and thorough examinations have led to an appreciation of its true incidence. The injury may occur in any digit but is most common in the ring finger. When a football player grabs an opponent's jersey, his little finger may slip, leaving only his ring finger holding on, the finger least able to be extended independently. The pull of the jersey forcibly extends the distal phalanx while the finger is being flexed actively. As a result, the flexor digitorum profundus is pulled from its insertion on the distal phalanx.

Even though the flexor digitorum is avulsed, it does not produce a diagnostic deformity. The examiner may decide wrongly that the athlete's inability to flex the tip of his finger is due to the marked soft tissue swelling and pain. The athlete's grip is weak and his proximal interphalangeal joint motion limited. The examiner should feel for a tender mass where the avulsed tendon has retracted into the proximal part of the finger or into the palm. X-ray films may show a small, avulsed fragment of bone.

The three common levels of retraction of the profundus tendon depend on the force of the avulsion. The least retraction occurs with an avulsion fracture of the volar lip of the distal phalanx as the volar plate remains attached to the fracture fragment. The plate tethers the flexor tendon near the distal interphalangeal joint to prevent further retraction. Greater force produces an avulsion of the tendon itself, which retracts to the level of the hiatus of the flexor digitorum sublimis and is held there by the vinculum longum. Intense force will completely avulse the tendon, and it will retract up into the palm.

The surgeon who treats these injuries must be familiar with the principles of hand surgery and well versed in the techniques of flexor tendon repair. Treatment must be individualized and adapted to each situation. In injuries that cause a large fracture through the volar lip of the distal phalanx with the volar plate attached, the fracture fragment is replaced. This re-establishes the continuity of the flexor digitorum profundus tendon. Postoperatively the finger is splinted in flexion for 3 weeks. The athlete then begins protected range-of-motion exercises, and the finger is splinted for another 2 weeks.

If the tendon has retracted to the hiatus, it still may be reattached for up to 3 weeks after the initial injury, and in some cases up to 6 weeks. If the injury is missed or neglected for a longer time, however, contractures will necessitate a secondary reconstructive procedure. When the tendon has retracted all the way into the palm, it may be reattached if the athlete is seen within 7 to 10 days after injury. However, the complete retraction of a sublimis tendon may disrupt its blood supply through the vinculum longum, and the tendon may die. By 10 days after these injuries, contractures develop, and a secondary repair is then indicated. The surgeon uses a free tendon graft because a primary repair at this time would result in a permanent flexion contracture of the digit. In reconstructing the tendon, any method that entails acute flexion of the finger must be avoided, as this would produce a flexion contracture. For some surgeons, a fusion of the distal joint may be the treatment of choice. A solidly fused, pain-free distal interphalangeal joint at the end of a proximal interphalangeal joint that has a normal range of motion is far better than a stiff finger.

Distal Interphalangeal Joint Dislocation

In the usual dislocation of the distal interphalangeal joint, the distal phalanx dislocates dorsally. The injured athlete himself or a teammate usually reduces the dislocation by traction and manipulation before the trainer or doctor sees it. After the reduction, the distal interphalangeal joint is generally stable; however, collateral ligament damage or interposition of the volar plate must be carefully checked for. After the dislocation has been reduced, a splint is worn during athletics for at least 3 more weeks or until tenderness is gone and a good range of motion is regained.

Volar dislocations of the distal phalanx are much less common than dorsal ones. They are associated with damage to the extensor tendon mechanism or fracture of the dorsal lip of the distal phalanx. Open wounds are not uncommon with distal interphalangeal joint dislocations; they are cleaned and closed whenever possible and treated appropriately to prevent infection.

Injuries to the Extensor Mechanism of the Distal Interphalangeal Joint

Extensor mechanism injuries at the distal interphalangeal joint are common in athletics, especially in football receivers, baseball catchers or fielders, and basketball players (Fig. 13-18).[56] Compared to flexor tendon injuries, however, these extensor mechanism injuries are often inappropriately minimized. Two types of forces may cause extensor mechanism injuries: An extrinsic force can flex the distal interphalangeal joint against the active contraction of the extensor mechanism and rupture the extensor mechanism; and an extrinsic hyperextension can compress the athlete's distal phalanx against his middle phalanx. The middle phalanx then acts like an anvil to break off a large fragment of the articular surface, disrupting the extensor mechanism. In any type of drop finger deformity, the proximal interphalangeal joint must be examined clinically and roentgenographically. An injury to this joint frequently accompanies a drop finger injury and may result in serious residual disability if unrecognized and untreated.

The extensor tendon most commonly ruptures at the insertion of its conjoint tendon into the base of the distal phalanx to produce a "mallet" or "drop" finger deformity. The flexion deformity of the distal interphalangeal joint is, in many cases, associated with a hyperextension deformity of the proximal interphalangeal joint.[1] The proximal interphalangeal

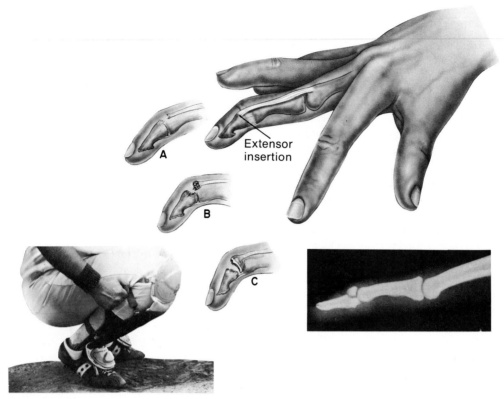

FIG. 13-18
"Baseball finger." The extensor mechanism may be disrupted at the distal phalanx by being stretched or torn (*A*). A bony fragment may be avulsed (*B*), or, in a youngster, a fracture may occur at the growth plate (*C*). Flexible catcher's mitts reduce the incidence of baseball finger by allowing the catcher to keep his throwing hand protected.

joint deformity develops after the central slip of the extensor mechanism is disrupted distally. As the athlete repeatedly attempts to extend his distal interphalangeal joint, he has increased extension at the middle joint, with resultant dorsal subluxation of the lateral bands and a stretching of the volar plate. The intrinsic muscles thus gain a mechanical advantage, and the deformity increases. The flexor digitorum profundus, now lacking an antagonist at the distal joint, is placed under increased tension owing to the hyperextension of the middle joint. This gain in the mechanical advantage of the profundus produces an even greater flexion force across the distal joint.

There are several distinct anatomic types of

distal interphalangeal joint extensor mechanism injuries, and the treatment needed depends on the type of injury. In some instances, the fibers of the extensor mechanism have been stretched and attenuated without being divided completely. In other cases, the tendon itself may rupture, or it may be avulsed from the base of the distal phalanx without any bony involvement (Fig. 13-18A). The tendon may also be avulsed with a small fragment of bone attached to it. This bony fragment appears on the x-ray film and may be used to localize the distal end of the retracted tendon.

A fracture may involve the articular surface of the distal phalanx (Fig. 13-18B). The fragment is usually large enough to affect the collateral ligaments of the distal interphalangeal joint and allow volar subluxation of the distal fragment in addition to the dropped finger deformity. Children may sustain a fracture-dislocation through the growth plate, which often involves the nail bed (Fig. 13-18C). The nail bed must be replaced to prevent later deformity and to facilitate healing.

A mallet finger, particularly in a young athlete, is usually treated by splinting alone if a large fragment of bone has not been avulsed. Stretching injuries often correct with time, but reinjury with complete rupture is a danger; thus they are treated like true ruptures. The distal joint is splinted in full extension or very slight hyperextension. If the distal joint were placed in extreme hyperextension, the blood supply to the skin might be impaired, resulting in a skin slough over the distal joint. Immobilization of the distal joint alone is satisfactory, allowing increased use of the hand and preventing proximal interphalangeal joint stiffness that follows use of a longer splint (Fig. 13-19A). I have used this method successfully to treat mallet fingers that were first seen up to 12 weeks after the injury had taken place.

An athlete may continue to participate in sports with the finger splinted. The splint is worn continuously for 6 to 8 weeks and then for an additional 6 to 8 weeks just during athletics. The splint may be placed either volarly or dorsally. A dorsal splint allows more fingertip sensitivity, which is particularly important for football receivers and basketball players (Fig. 13-19B). The splint must be kept dry to prevent skin maceration and should be checked at regular intervals. When the splint is changed, however, the finger must not be allowed to drop down into any flexion.

When the articular surface of the distal joint is involved significantly, an open anatomic reduction with internal fixation is needed to correct the deformity, forestall volar subluxation, and prevent later traumatic arthritis. If there is any question about being able to maintain the splint properly, a thin wire is passed across the distal joint as an adjunct to the splint. The pin is removed after 4 weeks, but the finger must be splinted for an additional 3 to 4 weeks during athletics.

If an untreated drop finger is disabling to the athlete, a secondary surgical reconstruction may be indicated. Although these procedures are not technically difficult, the results are not

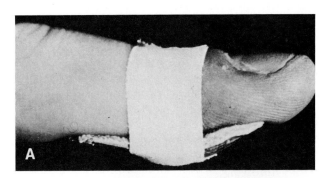

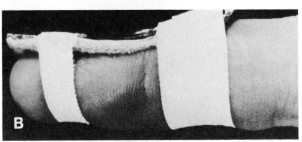

FIG. 13-19
A short splint (*A*) is used for "baseball fingers." The splint is worn dorsally (*B*) by ball handlers.

entirely predictable. A good alternative for the symptomatic athlete is a fusion of his distal interphalangeal joint.

Fractures of the Distal Phalanx

Fractures of the distal phalanx mostly are direct crush injuries and usually are not displaced. If the fragments are displaced, the displacement is due to the initial traumatic force, as no deforming tendons span the fracture site. The distal phalanx is covered dorsally by the nail bed, which rests directly on the periosteum, and volarly, by the fingertip pulp.

Undisplaced fractures of the distal phalanx are treated with a compressive dressing and splint. A painful subungual hematoma can be drained aseptically by piercing the nail with a heated paper clip. If the fracture of the distal phalanx is a displaced one, the nail and matrix may be disrupted. The matrix may lodge between the fracture fragments, block healing, and even cause a nonunion. A disrupted nail matrix must be replaced and repaired anatomically to allow proper healing and to prevent a nail deformity. The edges of the nail bed are approximated and repaired with fine absorbable sutures.

A nondisplaced nail may be used as a splint but should be removed unhesitatingly if the nail bed needs to be repaired. In addition, a nail may act as a foreign body or as a sequestrum. Although a nonunion is unusual in this area, it may occur, and reconstruction may be needed.

Hand Blisters and Calluses

Friction of the palm may cause blisters, which are collections of fluid between separated layers of epidermis, or produce calluses, which are protective build-ups of epidermis at friction areas.

During the season, calluses build up on a gymnast's hands.[7] They should be kept trimmed or else will catch on the equipment and rip. They may be shaved down with a safety razor or reduced with sandpaper or a callus file. Ideally, calluses should be trimmed to the level of the surrounding skin. If they are completely removed, the underlying skin will be left tender and may tear.

Gymnasts follow a daily routine of cleansing and moisturizing their hands and controlling calluses. To keep rips to a minimum, a gymnast changes apparatus if his hands begin to feel hot from friction. If his hands begin to feel hot while he is working on parallel bars, for example, he may switch to floor exercises to rest his hands. After a workout, he washes his hands to removed the gym chalk, which would otherwise dry his skin and increase its susceptibility to blisters and rips. He also applies a hand cream or a glycerin-based massge lotion a few times daily.

A gymnast's hands need protection, but to perform well he must have a feel between his hands and the bar. A leather hand protector may be worn, or one may be fashioned out of tape. Holes are cut through the elastic tape for the index and middle fingers, and the tape is placed over his benzoin-coated palm. The elastic tape is anchored at the wrist with adhesive tape and can be chalked with magnesium carbonate.

If the skin rips, it should be cleaned and an antiseptic applied. The skin should then be kept clean and should be moistened with massage lotion to decrease the chance of the underlying skin's cracking.

Weight lifters suffer blisters, especially when they use a bar that has deep knurling. Blisters may also trouble baseball pitchers.[83] A curve ball may cause a blister to form on a pitcher's thumb, and a fast ball may cause blistering on his fingertips. Although blisters on his fingertips indicate that the pitcher is releasing the ball correctly, they can certainly interfere with his throwing.

To prevent finger blisters, ballplayers can apply benzoin to their fingers, especially during the preseason but also during layoffs from pitching. All players are advised to report blisters early because an ice cube applied to a hot spot or to a blister may reduce the formation of fluid. A blister may also be aspirated sterilely. If a blister tears, it is cleaned, and the shreds are removed. The main covering is then replaced and attached with benzoin adherent.[67]

Gloves for Athletes

Gloves protect an athlete's hands. Lacrosse gloves have a flexible thumb and extra padding over the scaphoid. The palm is open so that the lacrosse player has a feel for his stick. To gain an even better feel for the stick, some players cut out the fingers of their gloves up to their fingertips, but a finger may then slip out and be injured.

The baseball catcher's mitt is now flexible so that the catcher may catch one-handed, thus protecting his ungloved hand from damage. The catcher may wear a pad inside his mitt to absorb shocks and to help prevent thromboses or aneurysms of the radial and ulnar arteries. An aneurysm occurs most commonly at the hook of the hamate where the vessels are least protected.

The boxer's glove is actually a mitten, since the thumb is separated from the other fingers. An extra pad guards the thumb, and a firm leather pad in the palm of the glove supports all four finger metacarpals.

Long ski gloves protect a skier's wrists from cuts from a ski edge.[55] Skiers should *not* wear short gloves. A young skier's gloves should be checked to be sure that he has not outgrown them, leaving his wrists susceptible to a sharp ski edge.

Platform tennis enthusiasts, who play in cold weather, may wear a mitten or a wool sock that has a hole cut in it to receive the handle of the paddle. While wearing this ingenious glove, the player's hand stays warm, yet he retains a feel for the paddle.

Still other athletes use gloves. Cyclists may use cycling gloves or, alternatively, pad their handlebars to avoid pressure on the ulnar nerve as it passes through the canal of Guyon. Fencers use a gauntlet to protect their wrists from blows. Wheelchair racers wear gloves to prevent possible damage to hands that have impaired sensations. Tennis or racquetball players may wear light, cotton gloves inside outer gloves to prevent skin irritation when the player sweats. They should carry a number of these as replacements when one pair becomes wet.

REFERENCES

1. ADAMS JE: Injury to the throwing arm: a study of traumatic changes in the elbow joints of boy baseball players. Calif Med 102:127–132, 1965
2. ALBRIGHT JA: Clinical study of baseball pitchers: correlation of injury to the throwing arm with method of delivery. Am J Sports Med 6:15–21, 1978
3. BARNES D, TULLOS H: An analysis of 100 symptomatic baseball players. Am J Sports Med 6:62–67, 1978
4. BASSETT FH et al: A protective splint of silicone rubber. Am J Sports Med 7:358–360, 1979
5. BENNETT GE: Shoulder and elbow lesions of the professional baseball pitcher. JAMA 117:510–514, 1941
6. BERG K: Prevention of tennis elbow through conditioning. Phys Sportsmed 5(2):110, 1977
7. BLACK SA: Blistered and torn hands disrupt gymnast's training. First Aider, Cramer 48(6):10–11, 1979
8. BLAZINA ME, LANE C: Rupture of the insertion of the flexor digitorum profundus tendon in student athletes. J Am Coll Health Assoc 14:248–249, 1966
9. BROGDON BG, CROW NE: Little leaguers elbow. Am J Roentgenol 83:671–675, 1960
10. BROWNE EZ JR et al: Ski pole thumb injury. Plast Reconst Surg 58:17–23, 1976
11. BROWN R et al: Osteochondritis of the capitellum. Am J Sports Med 2:27–46, 1974
12. BUCKHOUT BC, WARNER MA: Digital perfusion of handball players: Effects of repeated ball impact on structures of the hand. Am J Sports Med 8:206–207, 1980
13. BURTON RI, EATON RG: Common hand injuries in the athlete. Orthop Clin North Am 4:809–838, 1973
14. CARROLL RE, MATCH RM: Avulsion of the flexor profundus tendon insertion. J Trauma 10:1109–1118, 1970
15. COMMANDRE F, VIANI JL: The football keeper's thumb. J Sports Med Phys Fitness 16:121–122, 1976
16. CURTIN J, KAY NR: Hand injuries due to soccer. Hand 8:93–95, 1976
17. DANEK E: Martial arts: the sound of one hand chopping. Phys Sportsmed 7(3):140–141, 1979
18. DANGLES CJ, BILOS ZJ: Ulnar nerve neuritis in a world champion weightlifter. A case report. Am J Sports Med 8:443–445, 1980
19. DeHAVEN KE, EVARTS CM: Throwing injuries of the elbow in athletes. Orthop Clin North Am 4:801–808, 1973
20. DOBYNS JH et al: Bowler's thumb: diagnosis and treatment: a review of seventeen cases. J Bone Joint Surg [Am] 54:751–755, 1972
21. DUNHAM W et al: Bowler's thumb. Clin Orthop 83:99–101, 1972
22. ECKMAN PB et al: Ulnar neuropathy in bicycle riders. Arch Neurol 32:130–132, 1975
23. ELLSASSER JC, STEIN AH: Management of hand injuries in a professional football team. Am J Sports Med 7:178–182, 1979

24. FARNUM S: Traumatic bursitis. Phys Sportsmed 6(5):147, 1978

25. FRANCIS R et al: Little League elbow: a decade later. Phys Sportsmed 6(4):88–94, 1978

26. FROIMSON AI: Treatment of tennis elbow with forearm support band. J Bone Joint Surg [Am] 53:183–184, 1971

27. Gamekeeper's thumb on the ski slopes (editorial). Br Med J 1:213–214, 1974

28. GANEL A et al: Gamekeeper's thumb: injuries of the ulnar collateral ligament of the metacarpophalangeal joint. Br J Sports Med 14(2–3):92–96, 1980

29. GARDNER RC: Hypertrophic infiltrative tendinitis (HIT syndrome) of the long extensor. The abused karate hand. JAMA 211:1009–1010, 1970

30. GRANA WA, RASHKIN A: Pitcher's elbow in adolescents. Am J Sports Med 8:333–336, 1980

31. GRENIER R, ROULEAU C: Boxer's elbow: an extension and hyperextension injury. Am J Sports Med 3:282–287, 1976

32. GRUCHOW HW, PELLETIER D: An epidemiologic study of tennis elbow: incidence, recurrence and effectiveness of prevention strategies. Am J Sports Med 7:234–238, 1979

33. GUGENHEIM JJ et al: Little League survey: the Houston study. Am J Sports Med 4:189–200, 1976

34. GUNN CC, MILBRANDT WE: Tennis elbow and the cervical spine. Can Med Assoc J 114:803–809, 1976

35. HARRIS G: Elbow flexion strap for dislocated elbows. Athletic Training, 13(1):12, 1978

36. INDELICATO PA et al: Correctable elbow lesions in professional baseball players: a review of 25 cases. Am J Sports Med 7:72–75, 1979

37. KALENAK A et al: Athletic injuries of the hand. Am Fam Physician 14:136–142, 1976

38. KAPLAN EB, ZEIDE MS: Aneurysm of the ulnar artery: a case report. Bull Hosp Joint Dis 33:197–199, 1972

39. KELLY DW et al: Index metacarpal fractures in karate. Phys Sportsmed 8(3):103–106, 1980

40. KING JW et al: Analysis of the pitching arm of the professional baseball pitcher. Clin Orthop 67:116–123, 1969

41. KIRK AA: Dunk lacerations—unusual injuries to the hands of basketball players (letter). JAMA 242:415, 1979

42. KISNER WH: Thumb neuroma: a hazard of ten pin bowling. Br J Plast Surg 29:225–226, 1976

43. KULUND DN, BRUBAKER CE: Injuries in the Bikecentennial Tour. Phys Sportsmed 6(6):74–78, 1978

44. KULUND DN et al: The long term effects of playing tennis. Phys Sportsmed 7(4):87–94, 1979

45. KULUND DN et al: Tennis injuries: prevention and treatment. Am J Sports Med 7:749–753, 1979

46. LAROSE JH, SIK KD: Knuckle fracture: a mechanism of injury. JAMA 296:893–894, 1968

47. LAROSE JH, SIK KD: Karate hand-conditioning. Med Sci Sports 1(2):95–98, 1969

48. LARSON RL, MCMAHAN RO: The epiphyses and the childhood athlete. JAMA 196:607–612, 1966

49. LARSON RL et al: Little League survey: the Eugene study. Am J Sports Med 4:201–209, 1976

50. LEACH RE, WASILEWSKI S: Olecranon bursitis (dart thrower's elbow): a case report illustrating overuse/abuse in the sport of darts. Am J Sports Med 7:299, 1979

51. LEDDY JP, PACKER JW: Avulsion of the profundus tendon insertion in athletes. J Hand Surg 2:66–69, 1977

52. LIPSCOMB AB: Baseball pitching injuries in growing athletes. Am J Sports Med 3:25–34, 1975

53. MARMOR L: Bowler's thumb. J Trauma 6:282–284, 1966

54. MARMOR LL: Bowler's thumb. J Bone Joint Surg [Am] 52:379–381, 1970

55. MATCH RM: Laceration of the median nerve from skiing. Am J Sports Med 6:22–25, 1978

56. MCCUE FC III, ABBOTT JL: The treatment of mallet finger and boutonniere deformities. Va Med Monthly 94:623, 1967

57. MCCUE FC III et al: Athletic injuries of the proximal interphalangeal joint requiring surgical treatment. J Bone Joint Surg [Am] 52:937–956, 1970

58. MCCUE FC III et al: The coach's finger. Am J Sports Med 2:270–275, 1974

59. MCCUE FC III et al: Ulnar collateral ligament of the thumb in athletes. Am J Sportsmed 2:270, 1974

60. MCCUE FC III et al: Ulnar collateral ligament of the thumb in athletics. Am J Sports Med 2:70–80, 1975

61. MCCUE FC III et al: Hand injuries in athletics. Am J Sports Med 7:275–286, 1979

62. MILLER JE: Javelin thrower's elbow. J Bone Joint Surg [Br] 42:788–792, 1960

63. MINKOW FV, BASSETT FH III: Bowler's thumb. Clin Orthop 83:115–117, 1972

64. NORELL HG: Roentgenologic visualization of the extracapsular fat: its importance in the diagnosis of traumatic injuries to the elbow. Acta Radiol 42:205–210, 1954

65. NORWOOD LA et al: Acute medial elbow ruptures. Am J Sports Med 9:16–19, 1981

66. PRIEST JD et al: Elbow injuries in highly skilled tennis players. Am J Sports Med 2:137–149, 1974

67. RAYMOND P: Care of the hands. Oarsman 9(2):40–41, 1977

68. REEF TC: Avulsion of the flexor digitorum profundus: an athletic injury. Am J Sports Med 5:281–285, 1977

69. REICHELDERFER TE et al: Skateboard policy statement. Pediatrics 63:924–925, 1979

70. ROLES NC, MARIDSLEY RH: Radial tunnel syndrome: resistant tennis elbow as a nerve entrapment. J Bone Joint Surg [Br] 54:499–508, 1972

71. ROVERE GD et al: Treatment of "gamekeeper's thumb" in hockey players. Am J Sports Med 3:147–151, 1975

72. RYAN AJ (moderator): Round table: prevention and treatment of tennis elbow: Phys Sportsmed 5(2):33–54, 1977

73. SAVASTANO AA et al: Treatment of resistant tennis elbow by a combined surgical procedure. Int Surg 57:470–474, 1972

74. SIEGEL IM: Bowling thumb neuroma. JAMA 192:163, 1965

75. SLAGER RF: From Little League to big league, the weak spot is the arm. Am J Sports Med 5:37–48, 1977

76. SPINNER M: The arcade of Froshe and its relationship to posterior interosseous nerve paralysis. J Bone Joint Surg [Br] 50:809, 1968

77. STOLLE F: How to put topspin on your backhand. World Tennis 27:85–88, 1980

78. STREETONG JA: Traumatic hemoglobinurina caused by karate exercises. Lancet 2:191, 1967

79. TIVNON MC et al: Surgical management of osterochondritis dissecans of the capitellum. Am J Sports Med 4:121–128, 1976

80. TORG JS et al: The effect of competitive pitching on the shoulders and elbows of preadolescent baseball players. Pediatrics 49:267–272, 1972

81. TORISU T: Fracture of the hook of the hamate by a golfswing. Clin Orthop 83:91–94, 1972

82. TULLOS HS: Unusual lesions of the pitching arm. Clin Orthop 88:169–182, 1972

83. VERE–HODGE N: Injuries in cricket. In Armstrong JR, Tuckers WE (eds): Injury in Sport, pp 168–171. Springfield, Illinois, Charles C Thomas, 1964

84. WARIS W: Elbow injuries of javelin throwers. Acta Chir Scand 93:563–575, 1946

85. WOODS W, TULLOS HS: Elbow instability and medial epicondyle fractures. Am J Sports Med 5:23–30, 1977

Chest Injuries

Runner's Nipple

Friction from a runner's shirt may cause nipple irritation, pain, and bleeding in both women and men.[44, 45] For protection, a Band-Aid or a piece of tape may be placed over the nipples. Alternatively, the nipples may be coated with petrolatum or talcum powder and a silk shirt or a shirt made of synthetic material worn in place of a T-shirt.

Breast Pain from Jogging

A woman's breasts bounce when she runs, contusing the breast tissue and causing soreness. When a brassiere is not worn, the breasts may slap against the chest wall with as much as 70 foot-pounds of force. Bouncing and bruising are problems especially for large-breasted women, just before menstrual periods, during pregnancy, in women with fibrocystic breasts, and for those who run braless or who wear a nonsupportive brassiere.

A sports brassiere may help to prevent premature ptosis of the breasts by reducing the stress on Cooper's ligaments, which hold the breasts to the chest wall (Fig. 14-1).[28, 29] The supportive brassiere should prevent motion of the breasts relative to the body and should contain at least 55% cotton for absorbency. The brassiere's elasticity should be minimal, although some elastic is needed to allow easy breathing. Wide, nonelastic straps will stay on the shoulders but should not be the entire support of the brassiere, as the brassiere should be designed to provide some lift from below. All hooks should be well covered to prevent scratches; if the cups have seams, the seams should not pass over the nipples or should be reversed to avoid nipple irritation. The female athlete should wear a sports brassiere and wrap a 10-cm (4-in) elastic wrap binding over the brassiere for the best control of breast motion. The binding will provide additional support for the breasts, reducing motion by almost 50%.[28]

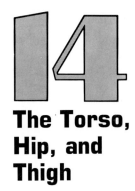

14

The Torso, Hip, and Thigh

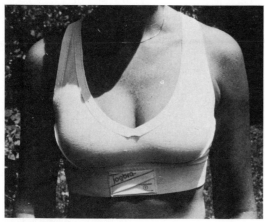

FIG. 14-1
A sports bra should have wide straps and no seams against the skin. In addition, an elastic wrap may help to hold the breasts against the chest wall.

Rupture of the Pectoralis Major

The powerful pectoralis major muscle arises from the medial part of the clavicle, the sternum, the first six ribs, and the aponeurosis of the external oblique. The strong tendon of this muscle has a twisting insertion into the humerus, and the clavicular and upper sternal part attach distally on the humerus while the lower sternal and abdominal portion cross over the upper part to insert higher up on the humerus. The pectoralis major adducts, flexes, and rotates the shoulder internally.

Rupture of the pectoralis major results from excess tension on the muscle. It may occur in a power lifter, wrestler, or an athlete doing bench presses with a heavy barbell, and it is not unusual for a champion power lifter to have had many of these muscle tears. The tear may be within the muscle itself, at the musculo tendinous junction, or an avulsion of the tendon from bone. The symptoms of a tendinous injury are a "snap" or a "pop," sudden sharp pain in the upper arm or chest, ecchymosis, and swelling. Adduction, flexion, and internal rotation of the arm are weakened, and the pectoralis muscle belly bulges on the chest with resisted adduction. With tendon avulsion, a de-fect can usually be felt in the anterior axillary fold. With a tear at the musculo tendinous junction, however, continuity may seem intact when the fascial covering remains intact. A chest film will usually show an absent pectoralis major shadow.

An injured person can do normal activities after a pectoralis major tendon rupture but has much less strength for strenuous activities. Surgery is advised for professional athletes or young athletes in strenuous sports to restore full strength and function.[68] In this procedure, a deltopectoral incision is made, the large hematoma evacuated, and the tendon reattached with sutures through bone. The athlete then wears a shoulder harness for 3 weeks, gradually increases his range of motion and does progressive resistance exercises. A power lifter must be restricted from heavy training for 3 to 6 months after surgery.

Rib Fractures

Because the athlete's first ribs are protected by the muscles and bones of the shoulder girdle, direct trauma usually will not produce a fracture. Nonetheless, first rib fractures do occur, generally from indirect forces. The scalene muscles and the upper slip of the serratus anterior muscle insert on the first rib, exerting opposing traction forces at the subclavian sulcus. When the athlete throws a ball or serves in tennis, a sudden strong scalenus anterior muscle contraction, combined with traction on the arm, may crack the first rib. As a weight lifter presses the barbell overhead, strong protraction of the scapulas fixes them against the thorax to form a solid base for the arms. The first rib may snap from overpull of the serratus anterior during this maneuver (Fig. 14-2).

As the rib fractures, the athlete usually feels an acute, knifelike pain, although some first rib fractures are stress fractures, which produce relatively little pain. An x-ray will show a crack through the weak subclavian groove. A fracture through the groove is rarely a surgical emergency unless the subclavian artery is torn.

More commonly, first rib fractures are treated with a sling followed by a graduated exercise program.

In contrast to first rib fractures, fractures of other ribs usually result from direct blows to the chest by balls or implements. The fast-pitched, 154-g (5.5-oz) cricket ball may fracture a wicket keeper's ribs, and jabs from the upper end of a hockey stick or blows from the head of a lacrosse stick may cause a similar fracture. Indirect forces may also cause rib fractures, as when a novice golfer fractures the posterior part of an upper rib during his golf swing.

Diagnosis of a rib fracture is most often clinical with tenderness or crepitus over the involved rib. Such fractures are mostly of the crack type and may not be seen on initial films. Focal, spot films may be needed, and a chest x-ray should also be taken to check for underlying lung damage or a pneumothorax.

Protective equipment such as the rubber chest protector of the lacrosse goalie (Fig. 14-3) or the tackle football blocking vest serves to cushion blows to the chest. When a rib is fractured, the area is usually taped to reduce motion and to support the segment. The older athlete with obstructive lung disease should not be taped, however, as taping restricts tidal air and encourages the retention of secretions. Intercostal nerve blocks will help to control pain. Protective padding or a "flak vest"—a rubber air bladder covered with a plastic shield—may

FIG. 14-2
A weight lifter may sustain a fracture through the weak subclavian groove of his first rib as he protracts his scapula.

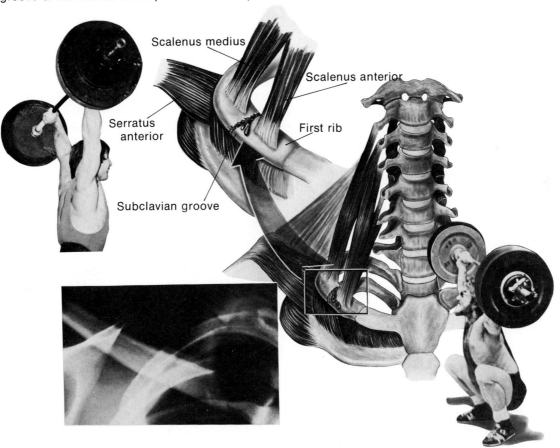

Scalenus medius

Scalenus anterior

Serratus anterior

First rib

Subclavian groove

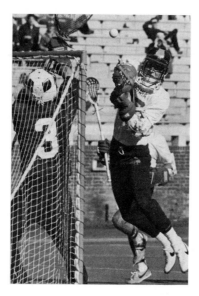

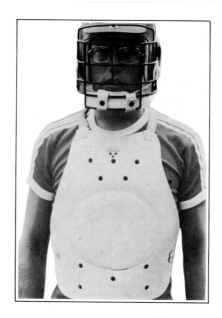

FIG. 14-3
A lacrosse goalie's chest is protected from hard shots by a rubber chest-protector.

FIG. 14-4
A rib may be fractured from a blow from an implement. The sore area may be protected by a "flak vest," an inflatable bladder with a plastic shield.

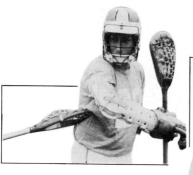

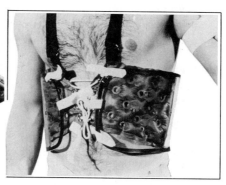

be worn to block blows to the injured chest (Fig. 14-4).

If an athlete's sternum is fractured, the heart may also be contused, the aorta may tear at the left subclavian, or a hemopericardium may follow. A baseline electrocardiogram should be obtained for comparison with changes that may later occur. Aortography is needed if the athlete is in shock or if a chest film shows mediastinal widening.

Costochondral Separation

A deforming force to the chest may cause a rib to separate from the costocartilage that attaches it to the sternum. A blow to the anterolateral part of the chest and a twisting injury in wrestling or in a rugby scrum all may lead to this type of separation.

With separation, the costochondral region is very tender, and trunk motion causes sharp pain. The athlete may feel a "slipping-out" and snapping sensation or a popping with crepitation.

The acute injury may be so painful that a local anesthetic must be used to dull the pain. An elastic rib belt is applied to support the chest, and the player is kept out of contact activities until he is almost totally asymptomatic, a period of 3 to 4 weeks for wrestlers, although the pain sometimes lasts more than 6 weeks.

Rib separation may also occur at a transverse process. The paravertebral area will be locally tender. Rarely, if the pain persists, the junctional area is resected.

Pneumothorax

A pneumothorax may occur during strenuous activity or even at rest without a direct blow to the chest.[52] If a lung bleb breaks, air is released into the pleural cavity.

The onset of symptoms may be insidious, with shortness of breath and vague chest discomfort, or the subject may have acute and dramatic shortness of breath. Diagnosis is made by percussing the chest and listening to the breath sounds. In a small pneumothorax, the chest film has an arc of lucency peripheral to the lung margin, while the lung may be partially collapsed in a larger one, and there may be a mediastinal shift.

The athlete with a small pneumothorax should avoid unnecessary physical activity and should be followed with serial chest films. The lung re-expands as free air is absorbed. If the lung has collapsed more than 30%, the athlete should be admitted for the placement of an intercostal catheter, which allows re-expansion, and the leak usually seals spontaneously after 24 hours. After discharge from the hospital, the athlete should be restricted from sports for 2 or 3 weeks to allow healing, and he should be warned that recurrence on the same or opposite side is quite possible. A third episode usually calls for operative intervention, at which time the nest of blebs in the apex is selectively re-sected and the parietal pleura is abraded to promote adherence.

Hyperventilation

The injured and upset athlete may breathe too fast, and hyperventilate. Carbon dioxide is lost and the blood becomes more acidic. Dizziness develops, and the athlete's fingers, toes, and lips tingle. These symptoms lead to greater apprehension, faster breathing, and panic. The athlete should be reassured that there is no cause for alarm and advised to breathe slowly and to hold his breath intermittently. He should then breathe in and out of a paper bag placed over his mouth and nose to effect rebreathing of exhaled carbon dioxide. The bag may be removed when the athlete is calm and breathing properly.

Abdominal Injuries in Athletics

The athlete's abdomen is usually not covered by protective gear and therefore is susceptible to injury in most sports. Fortunately, the lower ribs and strong abdominal and back muscles help to protect abdominal organs from blows. Although an alert athlete will tense the abdominal muscles to guard the underlying viscera, internal damage may occur as a player reaches over his head for a pass or is otherwise not on guard for a blow.[64]

In the case of a blow to an athlete's abdomen, the physician should suspect an injury to the spleen, liver, or small bowel. Apparent rapid recovery in a healthy young athlete after an abdominal blow does not exclude internal injuries. Even a small laceration within the abdominal cavity may lead to considerable intraperitoneal bleeding, as resistance to blood flow in the abdominal cavity is very low. Solid organs and hollow viscera may both be injured, but the former are more often injured than the latter.

A high index of suspicion, coupled with careful repeated examinations, will assure early diagnosis and avoid the overlooking of serious injury. At examination, the athlete should lie on his back and bend his knees to relax the abdominal muscles. The abdomen may then be checked for tenderness, guarding, absent bowel sounds, rigidity, and rectal bleeding.

Peritoneal lavage may help in the diagnosis of intra-abdominal injury when the athlete has associated injuries that preclude serial physical examinations, or when the neurologic status of the injured athlete makes abdominal findings difficult to evaluate. In this procedure, a liter of fluid is instilled into the abdomen, and the fluid that is siphoned back is placed in a glass test tube. When the examiner is unable to read newsprint through the fluid-filled tube, a positive tap is indicated. This degree of haziness of the fluid is considered significant, indicating that there are at least 20,000 to 30,000 cells/ml of fluid. Isotope scans and computerized axial tomography scans have also been used as aids in the diagnosis of internal injuries but have limited value in acute cases. Repeated physical examinations are the best means of diagnosing intra-abdominal injury.

Abdominal Wall Contusion and Muscle Tears

An abrupt twist, as in fast bowling at cricket, may rupture the rectus abdominus muscle. A hematoma then forms, and the pain that accompanies any motion restricts all activities.

For early treatment, ice should be applied, along with a compressing elastic wrap. The region is taped to appose the torn muscle ends. Infrequently, the athlete's inferior epigastric artery may also tear, and the hematoma will rapidly expand. In this case, the artery should be ligated. Isometrics will help to restrengthen the athlete's abdominal muscles, and with soreness as a guide, the athlete may progress to sit-ups, abdominal hangs, and leatherball raisers.

Blows to the Solar Plexus

When an athlete is not on guard, a blow to his upper abdomen by an opponent or from an implement or ball may "knock his wind out." He may be unable to catch his breath and feel as if he is in danger of death. In such cases, the physician or trainer should hurry to make certain that the athlete's airway is not being blocked by his mouthpiece, his tongue, or some turf. His belt should be loosened and his knees bent. A cold towel or "magic sponge" should be applied to his forehead, and he must be quietly reassured that he will recover in a short time.

Even when recovery from a solar plexus blow is rapid, a high index of suspicion should be maintained, along with repeated examinations for intra-abdominal injuries, such as a hematoma of the mesentary, pancreatic damage, or an injury to a solid or hollow organ.[64] A laparotomy is probably indicated if recovery is slow and the athlete has persistent local pain, tenderness, or shock.

Ruptured Spleen

The spleen is usually protected by the left lower ribs. It may, however, be injured as a player extends his arms overhead to receive a pass, when the muscles are relaxed and not guarding the abdomen, or when it is enlarged from mononucleosis and extends beyond the protective ribs.[22, 54]

In mononucleosis, the spleen is made large and weak from white pulp hyperplasia and extensive lymphocytic infiltration into the trabeculi and into the cores of the red pulp. The capsular and trabecular changes take 14 to 28 days to advance; thus the soft spleen probably will not rupture during the first 2 weeks of the disease. After 2 weeks, however, it may rupture from even the lightest blow, or from a Valsalva maneuver that suddenly compresses it by diaphragmatic and abdominal wall contraction. Thus, when mononucleosis is diagnosed, the athlete should be restricted from contact activities to protect the spleen from injury.

Infectious mononucleosis mostly affects athletes of high school and college age. The cardinal signs are lymphadenopathy, sore throat, fever, and fatigue. A positive mono spot test clinches the diagnosis. The examiner should gently palpate for an enlarged spleen. Care must be taken because repeated examinations, especially forceful ones, may rupture a large, soft spleen.

Mononucleosis should not be overtreated. The subject should rest while he has a fever, but when the fever abates he should resume ordinary activities. Before he returns to sport, however, he should feel well, have normal strength, normal spleen and liver size, a normal serum glutamic-oxalacetic transaminase, serum glutamic-pyruvic transaminase, bilirubin, complete blood count, erythrocyte sedimentation rate, and urinalysis.[61] Return to noncontact sports is usually possible in 3 to 4 months, but the athlete may have to be barred from contact sports for about 6 months, since delayed rupture of the spleen is a persisting danger. A ruptured spleen is, in fact, the most frequent cause of death in abdominal injuries. In one study, 17 of 22 splenic ruptures occurred in football, and in 8 of these cases, mononucleosis had been diagnosed *before* the rupture occurred.[23] The physician therefore must be alert to *delayed rupture* of a weak, large spleen of an athlete with mononucleosis. Such a rupture may occur even after all clinical, hematologic, and serologic criteria appear to be normal. Obviously, the athlete with mononucleosis should be instructed to seek immediate medical consultation if he develops any abdominal pain.

When an athlete receives a blow to the left upper quadrant of the abdomen, the spleen may rupture without a rib being fractured.[30] Initially, the left side will have a dull pain, but sometimes the symptoms quickly disappear and the player can return to the game. Thirty minutes later he may develop left shoulder pain, called "Kehr's sign," as free intraperitoneal blood irritates the diaphragm and excites the phrenic nerve reflexly. Less often, the blood will irritate the athlete's right diaphragm and pain will be referred to the right shoulder, or the spleen may be injured in the absence of any shoulder pain.

A delayed rupture of the spleen may follow an injury that produces a subcapsular hematoma. Such a spleen is highly susceptible to blows or strains, and the athlete may suddenly bleed to death days or weeks after the injury. The diagnosis of a subcapsular hematoma depends on a high index of suspicion and repeated abdominal examinations.[22] Radionuclide scans and computerized tomography scans help in the diagnosis by showing a definite separation of the capsule from the spleen.[12, 58] If the spleen is removed, the abdominal muscles require about 3 months to heal. Reconditioning is achieved by a graduated program, from isometrics to weighted abdominal hangs. The athlete should refrain from contact sports for about 6 months after splenectomy.

Ruptured Hollow Viscus

Rupture of a hollow abdominal organ, although uncommon in sports, is so dangerous that the medical team should have a high index of suspicion for such damage after a blow to the abdomen. A blow to a soccer player's unguarded abdomen may rupture a segment of bowel fixed across the spine. The abdomen is also a target in karate, where kicks may rupture a viscus. During hip circles on the uneven parallel bars, a gymnast's iliac bones normally bear the brunt of the force (Fig. 14-5), but intraabdominal injury may occur if the bar strikes

FIG. 14-5
A gymnast may injure her abdomen on the uneven bars.

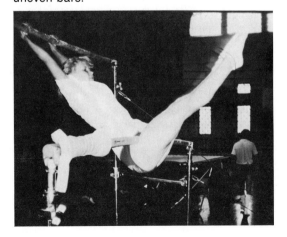

the abdomen above the iliac crests.[21] Visceral injuries also occur in equestrian accidents; thus a rider should be carefully checked for internal injuries after a fall from a horse.

A ruptured viscus usually produces pain, guarding, tenderness, loss of bowel sounds, abdominal rigidity, clammy, sweaty skin, and shock.[7] In addition, blood may irritate the diaphragm and cause shoulder pain from reflex stimulation of the phrenic nerve. A symptom-free interval after the injury may occur, however, as in the case of retroperitoneal injury, where it may take hours, or even days, for pain, guarding, and shock to develop.

If a ruptured viscus is suspected, an upright or right-side-up decubitus abdominal X-ray film should be taken and examined for free air under the diaphragm.[65] For the X-ray film to have maximum value, the athlete should remain in the upright or decubitus position for at least 3 minutes before the film is shot. The athlete's stool should also be checked for blood, as a submucosal bowel hemorrhage may leak into the stool.[21]

Solid abdominal organs, especially the soft and vulnerable spleen in mononucleosis, are more frequently injured than hollow organs.[54] Hemorrhage from a solid organ is more life-threatening than peritoneal contamination or bleeding from an injury to a hollow viscus. The liver may be torn or "fractured," especially when enlarged by hepatitis. Most liver lacerations will respond to simple tamponade, but if the liver is severely damaged, part of it may have to be resected. Also, an athlete's pancreas may rupture if it is stretched over the spine. This type of injury will reveal all the usual signs of intra-abdominal injury, but these signs sometimes appear late. Serial determinations of serum amylase may be helpful in diagnosing pancreatic injury.

The duodenum is vulnerable where it crosses the spine. If an athlete sustains severe, blunt trauma to the abdomen, the examiner should suspect a retroperitoneal rupture of the duodenum. The signs of intra-abdominal disorder or shock may take days to appear, and a late diagnosis may have a fatal outcome. Even during an abdominal exploration, there may be no intraperitoneal signs of duodenal damage; for this reason the surgeon should take care to examine the retroperitoneal portion of the duodenum. Suspicion of intra-abdominal injury is the key to its diagnosis, and methodical re-examination is the best way to uncover these serious injuries.

"Stitch in the Side"

A "stitch in the side" refers to sharp pains in an untrained runner's right side, behind his lower ribs. Possible causes of a stitch include gas in the large bowel, local anoxia of the diaphragm, diaphragmatic spasm, and liver congestion with stretching of the liver capsule. A runner may be able to "run through" the pain by breathing out forcefully through pursed lips or by breathing deeply and regularly. If the pain persists, the runner should lie on his back with his arms raised above his head, or a stitch can sometimes be relieved by the opposite movement of flexing the chest toward the thighs. When the pain leaves, the runner is usually able to resume his workout without a recurrence during the training session, and as fitness improves, stitches become less common.

Genitourinary Injuries

The athlete's kidneys, bladder, and genitals are relatively well protected from injury. The upper third of the right kidney and the upper half of the left kidney lie above the 12th rib, and there are three layers of abdominal muscle anterior to the kidneys. When these muscles are tensed, they help to protect the kidneys. Splenic and hepatic flexures of the colon lying between the kidneys and the abdominal wall also cushion the kidneys. The kidneys rest closer to the posterior abdominal wall than to the anterior wall, and the psoas muscles cushion them from the vertebrae. These organs are covered posterolaterally by the lower ribs and the paravertebral and flank muscles and rest in shock-absorbing pericapsular fat. They are fixed only by their vascular attachments to the aorta and the vena cava, affording an ability to move that reduces the impact of external blows.

An athlete's bladder is rarely injured in its protected location. When there is an urge to urinate, the bladder still lies below the pubis, protected by the pubic bones. Urinating before going out to the field empties the bladder, leaving the thickness of the bladder wall in its maximum and most protective state. The penis and testes are protected from injury by the athletic supporter, which holds them close to the body.

Renal Injury

A blow to the flank may damage a kidney, but abdominal blows, as when a player is tackled as he reaches up to catch a pass, are more often responsible for such injuries.[56] Injury to a kidney produces pain and tenderness, sometimes ecchymosis, and often hematuria, but the examiner may be fooled unless he is aware that normal urinalysis findings do not rule out renal injury, as the damage may not have interfered with the collecting system. Although kidney injury will usually produce hematuria, correlation between the degree of hematuria and the degree of kidney injury is weak. An indication of bleeding is loss of the kidney outline and obliteration of the margin of the psoas muscle on a plain x-ray film of the abdomen. If an athlete's urinalysis findings are normal and kidney injury is doubtful, however, there is no need for special studies.[66]

If an athlete has flank pain but the urine is normal, successive urine studies should be done to ensure that the urine remains clear. If kidney injury is strongly suspected, however, an intravenous urogram should be performed. Such a study certainly is needed if an athlete complains of flank pain and develops hematuria after a blow to the flank or abdomen.

Most kidney injuries are intracapsular and usually heal without complications or sequelae, but an athlete should be placed at complete bedrest until the urine is clear. Half of the athletes with extracapsular injuries respond well to bedrest and close follow-up. The other half may continue to bleed or leak urine. If the

intravenous urogram shows a nonfunctioning kidney or a major injury with extracapsular extravasation, a renal angiogram should be done. The angiogram can pinpoint and elucidate the lesion, resulting in more surgical repairs of kidney lacerations and fewer losses to nephrectomy.

The athlete's lumbar and flank muscles guard the kidneys, and protection is gained by strengthening these muscles.[47] Hip pads do not extend high enough to protect the kidneys, but the kidneys may be protected by kidney pads hung by straps from the shoulders. The flak vest is an excellent kidney protector.

Hematuria

Hematuria commonly accompanies or follows vigorous athletic activity. During intensive exercise, blood is shunted to active muscles, and renal blood flow decreases by about 50%, leading to relative renal ischemia and hematuria.[4] Other possible causes of exercise hematuria include direct kidney damage, renal vein kinking, damage to the kidney tubules, and bladder contusion.[3, 10, 41]

Erythrocytes, albumin, and erythrocyte casts have been found in the urine specimens of 80% of lacrosse players, swimmers, and runners and in 55% of tackle football players and oarsmen.[6] Distance swimmers and long distance runners show greater abnormality than do other athletes, but the urine usually clears within 48 hours.[25, 57] After a heavy football scrimmage or game, the player's urine sediment resembles that of a person with acute glomerulonephritis, containing erythrocyte casts, epithelial casts, and leukocyte casts.[11] Such findings have been termed "athletic pseudonephritis."[27] The frequency of abnormal urines parallels the severity of exertion, and the abnormalities disappear with reduction of the athlete's daily exercise load.

Although a boxer's urinalysis must be normal before he is permitted to enter the ring, after a fight most boxers have hematuria and abuminuria and their urine sediment may contain granular or hyalin casts.[4] These findings are related to exertion, the boxer's crouched position, his "grunt reflex," and direct damage from body blows. The more rounds boxed, the more chance that the boxer will have blood in his urine. The boxer assumes a crouched position for better balance, but this position increases intra-abdominal pressure and compresses his renal vessels. Boxers emit a loud grunt during attacks—the grunt reflex—that is timed with the delivery of a punch, causing the diaphragm and abdominal muscles to contract. The diaphragm may partially displace the kidneys and perhaps cause ptosis.

Effective body blows are infrequent in boxing. About 85% of all blows are directed to the head and face, and many body punches are blocked or slipped. Loin blows usually land near the left kidney, but they are indirect, and their force is thus attenuated. Blows to the right upper quadrant of the abdomen, however, are transmitted to the right kidney, making renal damage to this area more common.

Punches to the kidneys may produce recurring capillary damage that leads to scarred distortions. The term "athlete's kidney" refers to an impaired contour of the upper calyx, mostly of the right kidney, resulting from such scarring.[41] Many boxers with hematuria also have congenital anomalies, particularly hydronephrosis. Incompressibility of contained urine makes the hydronephrotic kidney more susceptible to injury than a normal kidney. A study of retired boxers might elucidate whether residual renal changes follow a boxing career.

Bladder trauma is another cause of hematuria in athletes, especially distance runners. The long distance runner with hematuria—"10,000 meters hematuria"—may pass small clots and have dull suprapubic discomfort and mild dysuria. What causes this bladder trauma in a runner? The pelvic floor muscles contract and intra-abdominal pressure simultaneously increases with exertion, forcing the flaccid, mobile posterior wall of the bladder against the bladder base. The base is a thicker, more rigid structure than the bladder wall and is relatively fixed by the ureters and lateral ligaments and continuous with the prostate. In an empty or near-empty bladder, the bladder surfaces are in contact, and minor impacts can summate to produce contusions, loss of the urothelium, and formation of a fibrinous exudate.

Blacklock performed cystoscopy on distance runners within the first few days after the onset of hematuria.[10] The bladder sites affected included the posterior rim of the internal meatus, the interureteric bar, and the area overlying the intramural ureter on each side. A mirror image of these lesions was found on the lower half of the posterior wall of the bladder. These findings suggest that there was contact of the posterior wall with the prominences of the interureteric bar and intramural ureter on each side and with the raised rim of the internal meatus. The rim of the internal meatus is rigid, prominent, and fixed because of the immediately underlying prostate. In some cases, the midline lesion on the posterior bladder wall featured a ring of contusion with a central area of normal urethelium. This pattern suggested contact of the posterior wall with the firm rim of the internal meatus, the island of normal urethelium being accommodated in the central depression of the meatus. Cystoscopy 1 week later showed only mild hyperemia at the affected sites.

Even when bladder knocking is presumed to be the reason for an athlete's hematuria, other potentially progressive abnormalities must be searched for, such as tumor, polycystic kidney, or renal cyst.

Investigating Hematuria

A fresh urinary sediment should be checked for erythrocytes, as hematuria may be the first sign of serious urinary tract disease. A count greater than one to two erythrocytes per high-power field is considered microscopic hematuria. The supernatant should also be checked with a dip stick for hemoglobin and for proteinuria. The sediment is then examined for bacteria, since infection may cause hematuria, erythrocyte casts, and leukocyte casts. Black athletes with hematuria should have a sickle cell preparation because hematuria may accompany each variety of sickle cell disease.

A complete history affords clues to the source of the hematuria. The athlete may have injured his flank or pelvis or may have engaged in heavy exercise. Does the hematuria appear at the beginning of urination? If so, "initial hematuria" indicates a urethral source. If the blood is noted chiefly at the end of urination, "terminal hematuria" connotes a source near the bladder neck or in the posterior urethra. Uniformly bloody urine, "total hematuria," indicates a source in the bladder, ureters, or kidneys.

An examination of the urine with the naked eye may produce a clue to the source of the bleeding. The longer the blood has been in contact with urine, the more it changes from bright red to a rusty or smokey brown, owing to the formation of acid hematin.[66] Upper tract bleeding produces dark brown urine and, sometimes, wormlike clots molded by the ureter. Lower urinary tract bleeding produces a pink-red or salmon-pink urine and irregularly shaped clots.

If a person has asymptomatic gross hematuria, the probability of a tumor is about 20%, whereas with microscopic hematuria the possibility is less than 2%. An exercise history, however, lowers the probability for tumor because hematuria is so common in athletes. A person's exercise program may have to be revised or even stopped briefly to eliminate the possibility of exercise-induced hematuria.

The athlete with hematuria should also be checked for high blood pressure, and the flank and pelvis should be examined for a mass or tenderness. In addition, skin abnormalities should be noted, including signs of injury and evidence of renal disease, such as purpura, edema, hemangiomas, or telangiectasia. The athlete with hematuria may need an intravenous urogram to determine the cause of the disorder.

Exercise After Kidney Transplantation and for Persons with End-Stage Renal Disease

A person with a new kidney should refrain from engaging in contact sports because the transplanted kidney is much more vulnerable to damage in its new pelvic location than is a kidney in the normal retroperitoneal position. Transplant recipients should, however, be encouraged to pursue endurance activities. Maximal comfortable exercise is appropriate to improve the appetite and retard muscle wasting in subjects on dialysis and in those with end-stage renal disease.

Hemoglobinuria

Runners sometimes pass a dark red urine that contains hemoglobin pigment. The source of this hemoglobin pigment has been elucidated by placing narrow, soft, compressible polyvinyl chloride tubes in the insoles of three runners.[57] Each runner had a tube of his own blood placed under one foot and a tube filled with another runner's blood placed under his other foot. As a control, another sample of his own blood was attached to one of his legs. Hemoglobinemia constantly appeared in the tubes underfoot if these runners ran on hard surfaces. When they switched to soft grass surfaces, the hemoglobinemia ceased. The test indicated that hemoglobinuria is probably due to mechanical damage to the erythrocytes in the soles of the runner's feet. The condition can be eliminated by running on softer surfaces and using a light foot fall with a sliding style and cushioning shoes.

Traumatic hemoglobinuria may also follow ill-designed karate exercises, where the enthusiast pounds his hand for a long time against a firm object. When a foam cushion is interposed, the hemoglobinuria ceases.

Myoglobinuria ("Squat-Jump Syndrome")

Myoglobin may appear in the urine of an athlete who performs squat-jumps. In this exercise, the athlete starts from a squatting position and jumps into the air. Myoglobin, hemoglobin, albumin, erythrocytes, and erythrocyte casts are found in the urines of military recruits who perform squat-jumps. The hemoglobinuria may come from hemolysis of extravasated erythrocytes in the swollen muscles. The squat-jump syndrome is distinguished from acute glomerulonephritis in that the dark urine follows excessive exertion, the muscles are sore and swollen, and there is myoglobinuria and a normal anti-streptolysin O titer.

Acute tubular necrosis may follow rhabdomyolysis, the breakdown of muscle. Acute tubular necrosis has been noted in a young wrestler, with elevated serum glutamic-oxalacetic transaminase, creatinine phosphokinase, lactic dehydrogenase, and aldolase enzymes after vigorous exertion. He had severe myalgia, muscle tenderness, dark brown urine, and clear blood plasma. The diagnosis of myoglobinuria may be missed, however, if the examiner always expects to see gross pigmenturia.

Torsion of the Spermatic Cord

The scrotal ligament normally prevents mobility of the testis by attaching the lower end of the spermatic cord and epididymis to the scrotum. If the tunica vaginalis is loosely attached to the scrotal lining, however, *extravaginal torsion* may occur as the spermatic cord rotates above the testis. With *intravaginal torsion,* the tunica vaginalis attaches unusually high on the spermatic cord, allowing freer motion of the testis below—the "bell clapper" deformity. Forceful contraction of the athlete's cremasteric muscle may draw his testis up over the pubis and twist the cord. Torsion is unlikely, however, if the athlete wears an athletic supporter.

Wyker and Gillenwater cite the primary physician's failure to suspect torsion of the spermatic cord as the most frequent cause for delayed treatment of testicular torsion.[66] This diagnosis must be kept in mind whenever an athlete has scrotal pain or swelling. Testicular torsion usually occurs in a young athlete who develops slowly increasing abdominal or groin pain. The athlete will sometimes, however, suffer abrupt, excruciating testicular pain, vomiting, and collapse. He also may convey a history of a mobile testis. The examiner should check for local tenderness, edema, and hyper-emia of the scrotal skin with the scrotal contents adherent to the skin. Also, the vas deferens will be inseparable from the swollen, twisted cord. In epididymitis, elevation of the scrotum usually relieves the pain. In contrast, when a twisted testis is manually elevated, the pain increases.

If testicular torsion can be reduced by external manipulation, an orchipexy should be performed later. If the torsion is irreducible, early operative exploration is necessary to save the testis, since infarction of the testis can occur within hours of the onset of torsion. At surgery, the testis is fixed to the scrotum with sutures. Because the anatomic defect is most often bilateral, an orchipexy should be done on both sides.

Hematocele

A kick in the groin or a straddle injury on a motorcycle, or on a bike with a long, thin saddle, may trap a testis against the thigh or bony pubis. Blood can collect in the tunica vaginalis, and a testis may be ruptured. Hematoceles do not transilluminate. A tense hematocele is treated at bedrest with scrotal elevation and an ice pack. If a hematoma is rapidly developing, a bleeding vessel may have to be ligated.

Gynecologic Injuries in Water Skiers

Although the female athlete's sex organs are well protected behind the pubis, the vagina, uterus, and fallopian tubes may be injured in water skiing. Inexperienced water skiers have difficulty standing up, and as the skier squats, water may damage the vulva and enter the vagina or the rectum. Such injuries may also cause incomplete abortions and salpingitis. Salpingitis, with right upper quadrant and iliac fossa pain, may begin about 3 days after a forced vaginal douche from squatting in the water, and the skier may be unaware of the association between water skiing and the disorder.

To avoid injection injuries to the vagina or

rectum, water skiers should wear rubber pants while skiing. In the case of vulvar hematoma, ice packs should be applied.

Penile and Urethral Injuries

The athlete's penis is only rarely injured because his athletic supporter holds it firmly against his body. Traumatic irritation of the pudendal nerve in bicycle racers or touring cyclists may, however, cause priapism or ischemic neuropathy of the penis. Priapism and the numbness from ischemic neuropathy resolve when the race or tour is over. Cyclists should be advised to use a furrowed saddle (Fig. 14-6) and not to squeeze the saddle on uphills, which can cause irritation from the saddle and numbness.

A fall astride a fixed object may rupture an athlete's urethra partially or completely, resulting in immediate pain, swelling, and perineal ecchymosis. Straddle injuries on motorcycles may produce a pelvic diastasis, rupture of the driver's bulbous urethra, and extravasation of the urine into the scrotum, perineum, and lower abdominal wall.

The early passage of a catheter into the bladder may obscure a complete rupture of the urethra after a urethral injury and may convert a partial urethral rupture into a complete one. A diagnostic retrograde urethrogram should

therefore be done before a urethral catheter is passed. A catheter may be inserted if a minor injury is diagnosed. The completely ruptured urethra should be operatively repaired and a suprapubic cystotomy added for urinary diversion.

Lower Back Injuries

Lower Back Pain

An athlete's lower back pain usually results from a strain or sprain with muscle spasm. If the pain persists, however, the examiner must look for a more serious condition.[60]

Runners may develop lower back pain. On downhill runs, the lumbar spine is hyperextended and the pelvis tipped posteriorly, occasionally generating pain, especially in the runner with lordosis. There is excessive forward flexion of the lumbar spine during uphill runs, as the runner "leans into the hill." The pelvis tips anteriorly, limiting forward hip flexion and putting greater stress on the lower back muscles. In the midstance phase of running, the unsupported side of the pelvis tilts downward, bringing a shearing force to the sacroiliac joint.

The runner with one leg shorter than the other may develop lower back pain with shearing at the sacroiliac joint. One leg may be functionally shorter than the other because one foot pronates excessively. The feet should be put into a neutral, balanced position. If one leg is still shorter after balancing with an orthosis, a heel lift should be prescribed. Limb shortness of one-quarter inch may not be a problem while walking but should be treated with a lift in a runner.

Adolescents may have a functional hyperlordosis while standing that may cause lower back pain.[49] The combination of a tight lumbodorsal fascia and tight hamstrings posteriorly with weak abdominal muscles anteriorly may be corrected by proper stretching of the lower back and the hamstrings, strengthening the abdominals, and attention to proper posture. Moreover, an athlete's iliopsoas muscles may

FIG. 14-6
This padded bicycle seat has a longitudinal furrow (*arrow*).

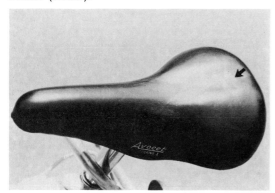

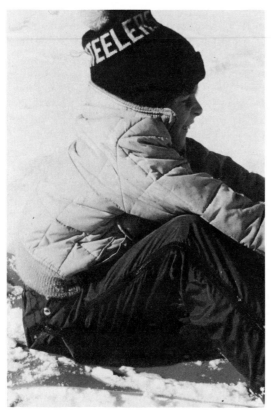

FIG. 14-7
In sledding or tobogganing, the preflexed
spine is susceptible to compression fractures.

be tight if he has been doing sit-ups with his
legs straight, and these muscles should be
stretched.

Almost half of all young athletes with lumbar
pain for more than 3 months are found to have
spondylolysis.[35, 37, 38] A few have spondylolisthesis with segmental instability, and some
have a symptomatic disc rupture. End-plate
fractures, growth plate injuries, altered disc
spaces at many levels, and even neoplasms are
also found. In some cases, however, a specific
diagnosis is never confirmed.

The differential diagnosis of back pain in an
adolescent athlete may include spondylolysis,
spondylolisthesis, Scheuermann's epiphysitis,
a mild vertebral body fracture, ruptured disc,
disc space infection, ankylosing spondylitis,
gynecologic problems, and aneurysmal bone

cysts or tumors, such as osteoid osteoma or
chondroblastoma. In older athletes, rectal tumors and myeloma sometimes occur.

Epiphysitis of vertebral end plates in the thoracic region is known as Scheuermann's disease
and mostly affects young men from 10 to 25
years of age. X-ray films show irregularities in
the superoanterior part of the epiphyses that
result in vertebral wedging. Subjects with this
disorder report back pain during sitting and
lying and after sports, but the pain often decreases during sports activities. With kyphosis,
long-term back pain develops, along with increasing thoracic spine deformity. Subjects' activity should be limited, especially avoiding the
butterfly stroke during swimming and activities
such as bench presses and dumbbell flies that
strengthen the pectoral muscles but accentuate
the kyphosis. Sometimes these youngsters require a kyphosis brace to halt progression of
the deformity.[50]

Mild vertebral body fractures may go unrecognized since x-ray films of the back are not
often taken; these fractures may cause lower
back pain later in life. Preflexion of the spine
on a toboggan (Fig. 14-7) reduces the force
needed to produce a fracture at the vulnerable
T-12 and L-1 level. If the toboggan hits a bump
or a rough area, the rider may be thrown into
the air and strike down with compressive loading on his preflexed spine. This force bursts the
vertebra, driving bone and disc material into
the spinal canal, perhaps paralyzing the athlete
or leaving him with long-term back pain.

A ruptured disc usually occurs in an athlete
who has had repeatedly injured discs and disc
degeneration, but a disc rupture may hamper
a young athlete for whom spontaneous recovery has been the rule. The ruptured disc is usually first diagnosed as a back sprain or strain;
however, intermittent lower back pain and
stiffness develop, usually without sciatica, although true sciatica may develop years later.
Pain extending to the knee but not beyond is
usually due to hamstring spasm. The straight-
leg-raising test that produces pain only to the
knee indicates hamstring tightness. The pain of
true sciatica goes all the way to the foot. Water-

soluble agents are now used for diagnostic myelograms, and epidural cortisone may hasten recovery in young athletes with chronic radicular symptoms.

The examiner should look for ankylosing spondylitis in older adolescents and young adults who have lower back pain as well as dorsal spine and sacroiliac area pain, with or without sciatica. Both hips are forcibly abducted to stress the sacroiliac joints for sacroiliitis. Oblique x-ray films of the sacroiliac joints are then taken and a sedimentation rate and histocompatibility antigen (HLA) typing obtained.

Because a gynecologic problem may also present as lower back pain, the female athlete should be examined for an ovarian cyst or gynecologic tumor.

An older athlete's lower back pain may be caused by facet overload with disc degeneration or may result from myeloma.[60] A rectal examination to check for a rectal tumor or a tumor of the prostate is also appropriate for older athletes with lower back pain.

Distant problems may be responsible for lower back pain.[33] The latissimus dorsi muscle, for example, which arises from the pelvis and spine and extends to the arm, may become strained because of poor use of the throwing arm. In such cases, good coaching in throwing technique helps to reduce back trouble. When an athlete sits on the bench, his hip flexors, hamstrings, and calf muscles are shortened, causing him to become more susceptible to a muscle pull or back strain if he enters the game without proper warm-up. Coaches can help to prevent injuries by advising athletes well in advance that they may be entering the game to allow time for adequate warm-up.

Lower Back Strain and Treatment

If an athlete strains his lower back, an ice pack is wrapped in a towel and applied to the back for 30 minutes, or ice massage is given to trigger points for 10 minutes. These cryotechniques surpass systemic muscle relaxants in their ability to provide relaxation and to prevent spasm and swelling. The athlete may be given sedatives to keep him drowsy and resting in bed. Butazolidin reduces acute inflammation: Some physicians start with a dose of 200 mg every 8 hours with meals, and after 48 hours drop the dose to 100 mg every 8 hours with meals in a rapidly tapering program. Back strapping will lend external support and allow the athlete some mobility (Fig. 14-8). A crisscross or chairback taping method may be used. An elastic wrap applied snugly around the injured athlete's abdomen will give added support.

During the acute phase of lower back pain, the athlete sets his extremity muscles but does not work his abdominal muscles (Fig. 14-9). As the pain and spasm lessen, he starts gluteal sets (tightening the buttocks) and abdominal sets. He performs pelvic tilts with his knees bent by pulling his abdominal muscles in and up to flatten his back to the floor. Near the end of the first week, during the subacute phase, ultrasound treatments should be started, and lateral stretches to stretch the lumbodorsal fascia should be begun. Anterior hip stretches in the lunge position stretch the rectus femoris, the fascia lata, and the iliofemoral ligament. To stretch his lower back further, the athlete may sit on a stool and flex his trunk while trying to touch his folded elbows to the floor. Next, while lying on his back, he brings his knees to his chest and holds this position.

The athlete with a lower back injury follows the stretches with single leg lifts, flexing one knee onto his chest and holding it there. He then lifts his opposite leg ten times for three sets. The leg lifts are followed by head and shoulder curls. First he raises his head and follows it with his shoulders while keeping the small of his back flat on the ground. This position is held for three counts. When the injured athlete is able to perform this series of exercises painlessly, he advances to side sit-ups, abdominal hangs, weighted hangs with a leather ball, and back extensions. After resuming his full warm-up program and functional exercises, he may return to practice.

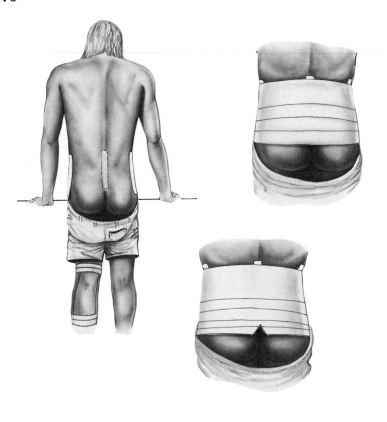

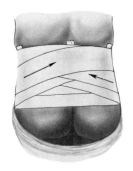

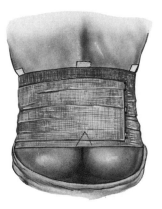

FIG. 14-8
An athlete whose back is to be taped bends slightly and supports himself on the trainer's table. A felt strip is placed over his spine to prevent irritation. Lateral anchor strips extend to just above his trochanters. Horizontal bands of 7.5-cm (3-in) tape are then stretched from anchor strip to anchor strip, followed by criss-crossed strips covered by more horizontal strips. Finally, the athlete is asked to tighten his abdominal muscles, and an elastic wrap is pulled snugly around his abdomen.

All athletes must understand the need for a full warm-up before practice or competition to prevent back strains. A qualified coach should check the athlete's form and his training routine. Rotational weight work may be added to the strength program to strengthen the rotator muscles of the spine. The athlete should be taught to lift with his knees bent and to hold the lifted object close to his body. Athletes should also avoid sitting in backache-producing swivel chairs.

Spondylolysis

Spondylolysis is a break in the narrow bony neck (the pars interarticularis) between the articular processes of the vertebrae. It commonly occurs in the lower lumbar region where high shearing forces tend to generate stress fractures resulting from repeated hyperextension of the athlete's lumbar spine. Hyperflexion may also cause stress fractures by placing great leverage on the neural arches, with the vertebral bodies

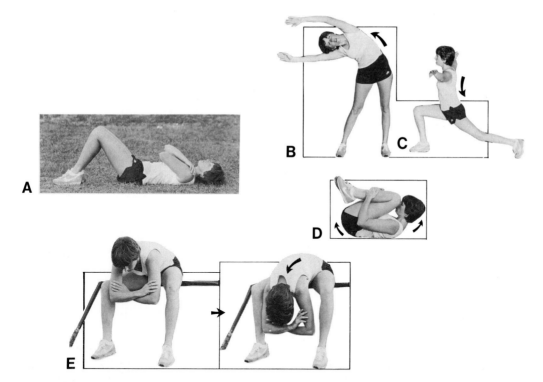

FIG. 14-9
Back exercises start with extremity setting, gluteal and abdominal setting, pelvic tilts (*A*), lateral stretches (*B*), anterior hip stretches (*C*), and the athlete bringing her knees to her chest (*D*) and flexing her trunk (*E*). As her back improves, she progresses to single-leg lifts (*F*), shoulder curls (*G*), side raises (*H*), abdominal hangs (*I*), and back extensions (*J*).

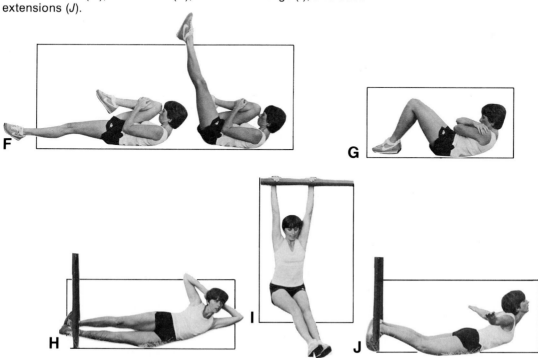

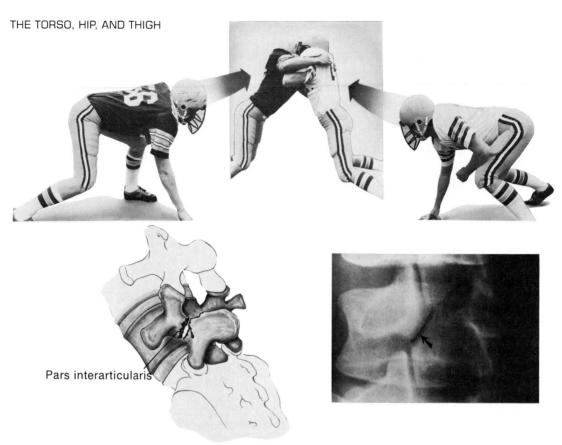

Pars interarticularis

FIG. 14-10
Spondylolysis, a break in the continuity of the pars interarticularis,
follows repeated hyperextension of the spine, as in football linemen.

serving as fulcra. A dysplasia in the cartilage model of the arch probably combines with these overbendings to render the pars susceptible to the physical forces.

Spondylolysis had been thought to result from a congenital defect in the pars, a dual ossification zone. Now that we know that there is only one ossification center, a congenital cause seems less likely, but there does appear to be a hereditary predisposition to this defect. Persons with a family history of spondylolysis need only the trauma of normal living to produce a defect. A defect is sometimes noted on x-ray films, although no pain is reported by the subject. Stressful athletic competition may, however, produce pain in such cases.

Spondylolysis most often affects athletes who must hyperextend their spines (Fig. 14-10). Young female gymnasts performing front and back walkovers, vaults, flips, and dis-

mounts have a high incidence of the condition. Defects in the pars interarticularis occur in 2.3% of the general white female population, but 11 of 100 young female gymnasts were found to have these defects.[35, 37, 38] Football linemen, butterfly-stroke swimmers, and weight lifters hyperextend their spines.[24] Hyperextension also accompanies the hiking in sailing, the tennis serve, the volleyball spike, hurdling, pole vaulting, and high jumping. Even divers who hyperextend on entry into the water, or jerkily distort their lumbar spines on entering the water after an imperfectly executed dive, show spondylolysis.

The athlete with spondylolysis has aching lower back pain that is usually unilateral or has started on one side. The pain is worsened by twisting and hyperextension, and there may be hamstring spasm and limited extension of the spine. Oblique x-ray films may show a lucent line in the pars interarticularis, but a cephalad-angled oblique view or a tomogram may be needed to demonstrate the defect. The first films may be normal. If pain persists after a rest period, the films should be repeated 6 weeks later. These serial films may show a developing defect. In contrast to these subtle defects, a defect may sometimes be so prominent as to be easily visible on a lateral film of the lower lumbar spine. Some athletes have a unilateral pars fracture with hypertrophy of the opposite pars.

If successive oblique x-ray films do not show a defect but lower back pain persists, an oblique technetium bone scan may be done that will show the developing defect as a "hot spot." A positive scan is usually associated with the athlete's being disabled for 3 months or more.[37] Resolution of this pain closely corresponds with resolution of the bone scan activity, although the athlete usually returns to competition before the bone scan activity returns to normal.

Lower back pain and muscle spasm in young athletes should always be heeded. Restricting vigorous activity may allow a stress fracture or fatigue fracture to heal, thus preventing a subroentgenographic reaction from becoming an x-ray detectable defect. Some defects heal without restriction of activities, whereas others require bedrest. If restriction or bedrest is required, the athlete should perform hamstring stretching and antilordotic abdominal strengthening exercises. A polypropylene antilordotic brace may allow a hyperlordotic youth to participate in sports.[50]

Spondylolisthesis

Spondylolisthesis (Fig. 14-11) is a slippage of one vertebra on another, and the disorder may occur in senior athletes with facet joint degeneration. It is more often seen, however, in youngsters between the ages of 9 and 14 years, and it is usually L-5 that slips forward on S-1. High-grade slips are more common in females, although pars defects are more likely in young male athletes.[37]

When the lumbosacral joints are loaded, a bilateral spondylolysis may convert to a spondylolisthesis. X-ray films should be taken while the athlete is weight bearing.[6] A first-degree slip means that a vertebra has slipped 25% over the body of the vertebra underlying it. A second-degree slip denotes that the vertebra has slipped 25% to 50%. About 5% of the general population have some degree of spondylolisthesis, but few have significant disability at a young age. If a slip reaches 50%, the athlete's sacrum becomes vertical. His flexibility lessens and his hamstrings become tight, making him incapable of high-level gymnastic performance. Pars defects in older athletes have rounded edges. Flexion and extension views should be taken or cineradiography used to see if motion is occurring at the defect.

With "spondylolisthesis crisis," an acute slippage of one vertebra over another, there are pain, tight hamstrings, and a peculiar gait, as the hips do not fully extend owing to the vertical sacrum. Nerve root tension may produce a sciatic scoliosis.

A high-grade slip produces a typical spondylolisthesis build with a short torso and heart-shaped buttocks.[37] The rib cage looks low, the iliac crests are high, and because of the vertical sacrum the buttocks are flat. If a preadolescent or adolescent athlete has slippage and lower back pain, he is restricted from vigorous activity until pain and muscle spasm abate. He may then resume all sports, but if the pain and spasm recur he must stop activity. X-ray films are repeated at 4- to 6-month intervals to rule out any further slip. A spine fusion may be needed when there is a spondylolisthetic crisis or nerve root irritation, a significant slip, or progression of the slip. The surgeon uses a paraspinal approach rather than a midline approach, so that the athlete may be up immediately after the operation. Heavy contact sports, skiing, or gymnastics are not allowed after the fusion.

The college athlete with spondylolisthetic lower back pain may engage in contact sports provided that he has no nerve root irritation. Younger athletes with grade II or greater slips are, however, usually barred from skiing or contact sports.[49]

Although pars defects alone do not seem to

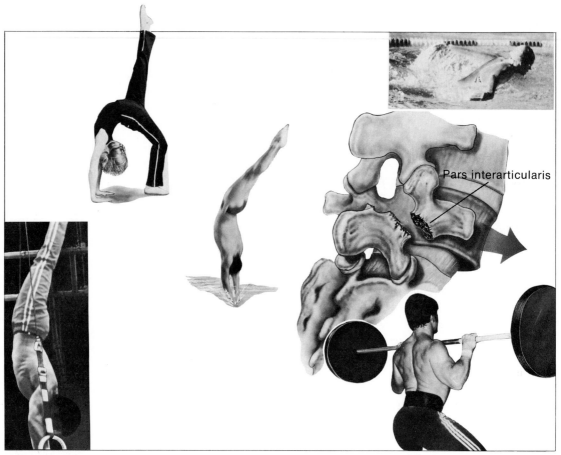

FIG. 14-11
Repeated hyperextension of the spine may produce a defect in the pars interarticularis. Further damage may cause spondylolisthesis, a sliding forward of one vertebra on the subjacent one.

predispose an athlete to later significant degenerative disc disease, those who have defects with slipping have more chronic pain and future disability.

Pelvic and Hip Injuries

The powerful hip and buttock muscles are the body's "seat of power." From here power radiates outward like a pebble dropped in a pond, with muscle groups generally growing weaker with greater distance from the center of the body.

The pelvic muscles are links to the limbs.

The latissimus dorsi, for example, arises on the iliac crest and spine, inserting into the humerus to rotate the arm internally. The hip abductors arise on the ilium and insert on the greater trochanter of the femur. The hip adductors arise on the pubis and insert on the femur. The gluteus maximus, a strong hip extensor, arises on the ilium to insert on the femur, and is also extended to the tibia by way of the iliotibial band. The iliopsoas arises from the lumbar spine and ilium and inserts at the lesser trochanter to flex the hip.

The strong rectus femoris part of the quadriceps arises from the anterior superior and the anterior inferior iliac spines to insert on the tibia, flexing the athlete's hip and extending his knee. The hamstrings arise from the ischium to insert on the tibia and fibula to extend the hip and flex the knee. Thus, muscles arising from the pelvis have distant action, and damage to these powerful muscles greatly limits athletic activity.

"Hip Pointer"

A direct blow to the iliac crest, as when a football helmet mashes muscle against bone, may painfully contuse the rim of the iliac crest. Such "hip pointers" may also result from a separation of muscle fibers pulled from the crest.

When an athlete is warmed up and involved in a match, a bruised iliac crest may not cause him immediate concern. Without first aid, however, slow internal bleeding overnight will result in swelling and pain the next morning. For this reason these injuries should be noted and treated early. An x-ray film is taken to rule out an iliac crest fracture, especially in high school athletes who may avulse the iliac crest apophysis.[14] A fluctuant hematoma should be aspirated, an ice pack applied, and the area compressed with an elastic wrap over a felt pad.

As soreness, swelling, and ecchymosis subside, contrast treatments are begun with ice massage for 10 minutes, moist heat for 10 minutes, ultrasound for 10 minutes, and ice massage once more. The area is then covered with a wide elastic wrap; the player should also change from girdle pads to old style hip pads.

Hip pads are now mandatory in college tackle football and are usually constructed of hard polyethylene sandwiched between layers of Ensolite. The pads protect a player's iliac crests, his greater trochanters, and coccyx. Three types of hip pads include snap-in, girdle, and wrap-around pads. Snap-in pads fit on the belt in the player's pants and are most effective if the pants are pulled up to keep the pads in place. The girdle pad is the most difficult to keep in place, and players should be advised to keep these pads from sliding down over their iliac crests, or they will lose protection. A pop-

ular trend today is to imitate professional players by removing the coccyx pad and using only a light foam padding over the iliac crest. This, however, means a loss of needed protection.

Iliac Apophysitis

The ossification center of the iliac crest first appears anterolaterally, and as the athlete matures it advances posteriorly until it reaches the posterior iliac crest. The average age of closure of this ossification center is 16 years for boys but may range up to 20 years. The age of closure for girls is 14 years but may range to 18 years.

High school runners now train harder than ever. Where they formerly ran 3 miles a day, they now run from 6 to 8 miles, and some youths are running more than 80 miles a week. Repetitive contractions by the oblique abdominal muscles, gluteus medius, and tensor fascia lata on the iliac apophysis as the pelvis swings and tips may cause an inflammatory response, iliac apophysitis, or a subclinical stress fracture at the iliac apophysis.[16] This occurs especially in runners with cross-over arm swings, and the athlete is usually unable to relate the onset of pain to a specific injury.

Iliac apophysitis presents as local pain over the anterior iliac crest while the athlete runs. To diagnose the condition, the examiner checks for tenderness at the origin of the tensor fascia lata, the gluteus medius, and the abdominal obliques. When the athlete abducts his hips against the examiner's resistance, the pain worsens. X-ray films may, however, be normal

A young runner may also develop a posterior iliac crest apophysitis. He will have pain when he tries to abduct his hip against manual resistance as he lies on his sound side with his affected upper hip flexed. A fracture should always be suspected and an x-ray film taken to rule it out.[14, 16] Both types of iliac apophysitis, anterior and posterior, resolve with 4 to 6 weeks of rest. Running resumes with less mileage, fewer hills, and care to avoid arm swings across the body.

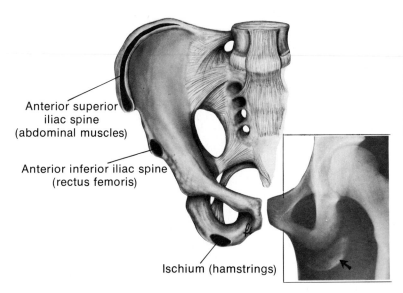

Anterior superior iliac spine (abdominal muscles)

Anterior inferior iliac spine (rectus femoris)

Ischium (hamstrings)

FIG. 14-12
Strong muscles may avulse bony fragments from the sites of their origin or insertion on the pelvis. In this case, the ischial apophysis has been avulsed (*arrow*).

Avulsion Fractures of the Pelvis

The sartorius muscle originates from the anterior-superior iliac spine, the rectus femoris from the anterior-inferior iliac spine, and the hamstrings from the ischial tuberosity. If a place kicker's cleats catch in the turf, his rectus femoris may be pulled from his pelvis to produce a defect in his upper thigh. A strong hamstring muscle contraction may similarly avulse a large bony fragment from the ischium (Fig. 14-12). If the fragment is separated far from its source, operative replacement may be needed.

Osteitis Pubis

Although muscle attachments cover the pubic symphysis externally, a large area on its internal aspect is covered only by periosteum and parietal fascia. The pubic symphysis has a poor blood supply, and this region is not well equipped to withstand irritation or infection.[1]

While an athlete runs, jumps, and kicks, the symphysis moves up and down, forward and backward, and rotates. Shear forces are transmitted to the symphysis, especially in soccer players and race walkers.[34] In the midstance of running, the unsupported side of the pelvis tilts downward, producing a shearing force at the pubic symphysis. Tension from the rectus abdominus or adductors, or direct trauma, may produce periosteal or subperiosteal damage to this weak bone, causing a subacute periostitis.[17, 31] Thromboembolic occlusion of the end vessels may allow a subsequent transient bacteremia to cause an infection there and accelerate bone absorption.

Osteitis pubis is common in soccer players and race walkers[43] and is also seen in runners who abruptly increase their mileage or add interval training with speed work. The onset is usually gradual, with local pain and tenderness at the symphysis. Sudden tension may, however, produce intense pain at the symphysis and groin pain. The athlete may think that he has strained a muscle and do stretching exercises that only aggravate the problem.

The pain of osteitis pubis may also be confused with an inguinal hernia, prostatitis, orchitis, urolithiasis, or a groin pull. Although a digital examination of the prostate may be painful, the pain may be due to pressure on the athlete's underlying pubic symphysis. Ankylosing spondylitis may also produce a periostitis of the pubic symphysis; thus an HLA-B27 antigen study should be gotten before affixing a trauma diagnosis to the osteitis.[31] A pulled groin muscle will be tender.

X-ray changes at the symphysis sometimes lag about a month behind the onset of pain. The lower half to lower two thirds of the symphysis should be checked for widening, loss of definition of the bones with demineralization, sclerosis, and periosteal reaction. The examiner should keep in mind, however, that marked osteoporosis with rarefaction is a normal x-ray picture in a 20-year-old whose pubis is ordinarily weak at this time.[62] A technetium pyrophosphate bone scan may allow early detection of inflammation around the symphysis.

After infection is ruled out, the athlete rests and uses an anti-inflammatory agent, such as aspirin or phenylbutazone (Butazolidin), then begins an adductor stretching program and returns, in a graded fashion, to running.

A soccer player may develop an unstable symphysis pubis in which the symphysis becomes tender, and he may also have lower abdominal pain. "Flamingo views" may show a shift of his symphysis. X-ray views should include an anteroposterior taken with the subject standing on one leg and another anteroposterior view taken with the subject standing on his other leg.

Groin Strain

An athlete may strain his groin if the thigh is violently rotated externally while his leg is widely abducted. This injury is commonly seen during early workouts in tackle football when players are not raising their legs and in slips on muddy fields. Groin strains are common in ice hockey players who forcefully adduct the thigh in the pushoff and rapidly shift their weight to the opposite leg to initiate the glide stroke.[48] Middle-aged bowlers may also strain their adductor muscles if they slip or stop suddenly. Bowlers at cricket suffer groin strains, especially at the beginning of the season when the ground is quite firm.[63]

An adductor strain is especially painful when the athlete adducts his thigh against the examiner's manual resistance. A psoas muscle strain produces deep groin tenderness and pain that radiates to the lower abdomen, and external rotation of the hip in extension worsens the pain. A very severe psoas strain may avulse the lesser trochanter.

All athletes should stretch their adductors diligently to prevent groin strain. This is best done with a partner stretching program. A gymnasium floor should be swept with a damp towel before each practice and game to clear it of dust that may cause players to slip.

If an athlete strains his groin, any fluctuant hematoma is aspirated and ice applied. Four days later, the strained region should be treated with heat and low-intensity ultrasound. The groin may be stretched with ice on it. For practices and games, a felt pad should be placed over the region and snugly wrapped on with a spica wrap. An extra long elastic wrap is best. The athlete's adductors, iliopsoas, and rectus femoris may be strengthened by squeezing and lifting a medicine ball with his legs. Hip flexion may be strengthened by lifting weights with the hip muscles on a knee table.

Dislocated Hip

Major trauma or a high-velocity collision in a sport such as tackle football will dislocate an adult athlete's hip, but a youth's hip may dislocate with much less force. Because the hip usually dislocates posteriorly, the subject lies with his hip in a flexed and adducted position. Oblique x-ray films are taken to see if any fragments of bone have been knocked from the posterior lip of the acetabulum. The dislocation may sometimes be immediately reduced by holding the athlete's pelvis down, flexing his hip to 90°, and then pulling up. However, because of the strong muscles in spasm around his hip, anesthesia is often needed. When the hip has been relocated, it may be tested for stability by trying to press it back out of the socket, and if stability has been restored, skin traction is applied to the leg to decrease muscle spasm around the hip.

The main danger of his dislocation is the possibility of damage to the blood supply to the femoral head, which may cause part or all of the head to die. Long-term crutch walking is therefore prescribed, with only a gradual return to athletic activity.

Avascular Necrosis of the Femoral Head

Hip pain in a young athlete between 5 and 12 years of age may be due to synovitis, an irritation of the hip joint with inflammation. As the hip joint fills with reactive synovial fluid, pressure from the fluid may occlude the blood supply to the femoral head, and part or all of the femoral head may die.[39]

The youngster with a complaint of pain in the hip must be evaluated fully. X-ray films should be taken and examined for rarefaction of the head characteristic of Legg-Calvé-Perthes avascular necrosis. Avascular changes usually involve the superior and anterolateral weight-bearing part of the head, and in later stages this area becomes irregular, collapsed, and sclerotic.

Because synovitis of the hip may be a cause of avascular necrosis, subjects should be put at bedrest. Skin traction will relax muscle spasm around the hip. These problems should be dealt with early to prevent the development of an incongruent hip, which leads to later osteoarthritis. Depending on the age of the subject, the stage of the process, and its severity, a special brace may have to be worn, or an operation may be needed to realign the joint.

If a youth develops severe hip pain with a marked limitation of hip motion, he may have a pyarthrosis. Hip aspiration will prove the diagnosis.

Slipped Capital Femoral Epiphysis

A young athlete's capital femoral epiphysis may slip even after a minor injury. The disorder occurs mostly in lanky or heavy youngsters between the ages of 9 and 15 years who are entering a growth spurt or who have an endocrine imbalance. There is often a prodrome or "preslip" phase, with vague aching around the hip or knee for weeks and a limp. X-ray films at this stage show widening of the growth plate and rarefaction at the metaphysis just below the physis.

The youngster with hip or knee pain should be checked to rule out a preslip phase or slippage of the femoral head. Although he reports knee pain, examination of the knee may be normal, with pain originating in the hip and referred to the knee by way of the obturator nerve. Youngsters with hip pain and x-ray evidence of preslip should be put at bedrest to prevent a slip. In some cases, prophylactic pinning may be needed.

Minor slips of the capital femoral epiphysis in childhood have been found to cause idiopathic osteoarthritis of the hip in adulthood.[51] Adults who were quite active in sports as children often show evidence of old slips, whereas such slips are infrequent in less active, age-matched control subjects. Many former athletes have old slipped capital femoral epiphysis that reduce joint congruence and presage osteoarthritis. A measurement technique and index to check for earlier slips will show the femoral head to be in a slightly drooped position. Care should be taken to catch these slips in the preslip phase by attending to hip or knee pain in youngsters, with the aim of preventing slippage and later arthritis.

A major slip of the capital femoral epiphysis may occur on the playing field, followed by hip or knee pain (Fig. 14-13). When the hip is flexed, it swings into external rotation instead of flexing (Fig. 14-13A). The player should be transported carefully from the field to have a hip x-ray, as he may have a major slip that movement could convert into a disastrous full slip.

The slipped capital femoral epiphysis may be seen best on a frog-leg lateral view. The slipped femoral head is tilted or in a drooped position, the "tilt deformity," and is eccentrically placed on the femoral neck (Fig. 14-13B). The head slips posteromedially on the neck, or as some describe it, the neck slips anterolaterally from the head.

Major slips deserve a short course of traction that may gently reduce the slip, and the head then may be stabilized with pins. If traction is unsuccessful, the head should be pinned *in situ*

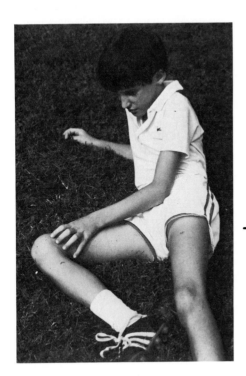

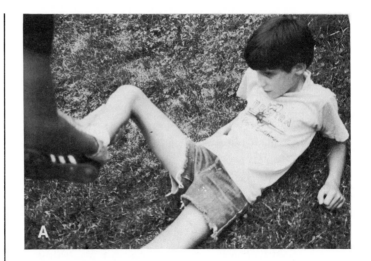

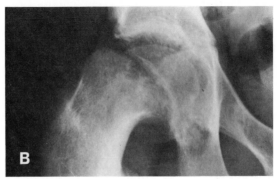

FIG. 14-13
A youth who complains of knee pain should have his hip examined. The hip should flex normally. External rotation of the thigh during hip flexion (*A*) may connote a major slip of the capital femoral epiphysis (*B*).

to prevent further slippage. A later osteotomy will restore good hip mechanics. Attempts to manipulate the head back onto the femoral neck may, however, cause the head to die.

Hip Cysts

Unicameral bone cysts are sometimes noted in the femoral neck of youngsters and in older athletes. A fracture through this weakened area may jeopardize the femoral head. Steroid injections have been recommended as a means of obliterating the cysts, but the cysts often remain after such injections. Filling the cyst with

a bone graft is the surest way to reduce the risk of a fracture.

Greater Trochanteric Bursitis

Inflammation of the bursa overlying the greater trochanter commonly occurs in female runners who have a broad pelvis and increased Q angle. The condition also occurs in runners who have a leg length discrepancy, which causes the pelvis to tilt abnormally. It is not uncommon in novice runners whose feet cross over in the midline, thus increasing the adduction angle. More experienced runners may develop a greater trochanteric bursitis when they train or compete on banked surfaces. Treatment includes rest, ice, and sometimes a steroid injection to reduce the inflammation. Leg length discrepancy and faulty running technique should also be corrected.

Thigh Injuries

Quadriceps Contusion ("Charley Horse")

A blow to the front of an athlete's thigh may produce a contusion with bleeding into the quadriceps.[55] The more relaxed the quadriceps at the moment of contact, the more severe the injury. Such blows are most often anterior or anterolateral, since the medial part of the thigh usually is protected by the athlete's other leg. If the thigh is struck dead-center on a thigh pad, it is safe, but if the periphery of the pad is struck the pad edge is driven against the thigh.

The severity of a quadricips contusion is nearly always underestimated. There may be little pain or discomfort while the athlete is warm and competing, but stiffness and pain develop within hours of the injury.

If a player receives a sharp blow to his thigh in football, treatment should be started at half time. If he is limping, immediate attention is needed to prevent worsening. The player should not try to run out the quadriceps contusion. These injuries deserve respect because they may be followed by myositis ossificans, a bony growth within the muscle.

Initial hemorrhage and muscle spasm may be reduced by stretching the quadriceps. The athlete's knee should be flexed and held in flexion with an elastic wrap until the next day and an ice bag placed over the wrap.[20] Early heat, massage, and whirlpool treatments should not be used, as these will bring in more blood and produce further swelling. The athlete may, however, take a shower as long as he keeps ice bags in place over the area.[40]

A mild quadriceps contusion produces little pain and swelling and some tightness but leaves a normal range of knee motion.[20] The athlete is able to flex the knee to 90° or more. For treatment, ice is applied for 10 minutes, followed by a transcutaneous electrical nerve stimulator for 20 minutes, and the quadriceps is stretched by slow, full knee flexion until the tightness is gone. A foam pad is then secured over the area with an elastic wrap.

A moderate quadriceps contusion produces more severe pain and swelling and limits the range of knee motion. The muscles are in spasm, and the athlete will not be able to flex his knee to 90°. Treatment comprises cold towels applied for 72 hours with the leg up and resting, and the athlete then uses crutches.[40] The athlete may return to practice when his thigh is pain-free and he has normal range of knee motion and normal muscle power and can fully perform functional exercises such as jumps and cuts.

A hematoma and muscle herniation exist in severe quadriceps contusions. If swelling has occurred very rapidly or is extreme, a bleeding diathesis or a significant vascular injury must be suspected. Clotting studies should be performed when there is a markedly swollen thigh. Minor clotting deficiencies are probably more common than is realized, and partial deficiencies of varying degrees may be noted in all types of hemophilias. If there is fluctuance, some physicians try to aspirate or remove the hematoma surgically, since the removal of a large blood clot may minimize subsequent fibrosis. Even when the thigh is quite swollen, blood often resists aspiration, since it is contained in the muscle, much as if it were in a sponge. Local anesthetics, enzymes, and steroids are sometimes given to aid in the absorption of the hematoma, but these injections always pose danger of infection.

The athlete with a severe quadriceps contusion should remain at bedrest with his thigh wrapped and iced. The circumference of the thigh should be checked serially. The athlete may do quadriceps sets for 5 minutes each hour but should avoid flexing the knee until the soreness diminishes. A plaster splint will keep the knee from bending while the athlete is up; otherwise, traction on the quadriceps will in-

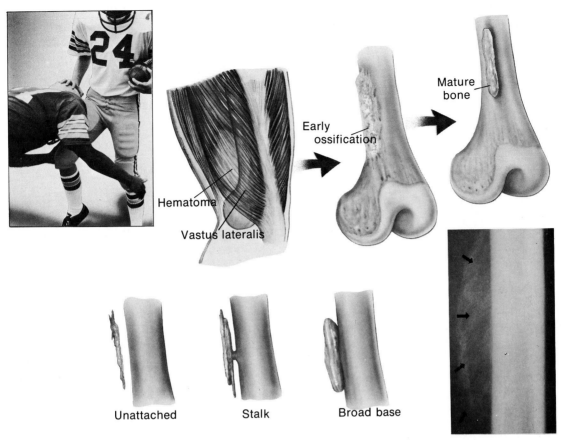

FIG. 14-14
A blow to the thigh may produce a hematoma that ossifies. It may take many forms as it matures and may need to be excised (*see* text for description).

crease the inflammation. A pair of cutout sweatpants will allow the plaster slab to fit comfortably.

An elastic thigh support will provide constant circumferential pressure and support during recovery. A foam rubber pad or an air pad covered with a football thigh pad will give added protection, and the player's pants should be tight enough to keep this pad from slipping.

Myositis Ossificans Traumatica

A blow from a helmet to another player's thigh or a knee to the thigh, or even a quadriceps muscle strain, may cause bleeding into the quadriceps. Heterotopic bone may later form adjacent or attached to the femur (Fig. 14-14).[36]

Although the swelling usually stabilizes in about 24 hours, the hemorrhage may be followed closely by acute inflammation. The thigh will be tender, firm, and hot the next day, and the athlete's body temperature may even be elevated. Fibroblasts from the endomysium or primitive mesenchyme from the injured fascia and connective tissue may then form osteoid and chondroid tissue. The reaction is similar to callus formation, and experiments show that the periosteum plays a role. Trauma to rabbit periosteum produces periosteal bone proliferation, but myositis ossificans does not occur without injury to the periosteum.[67]

In developing myositis ossificans, initial x-ray films will show a soft tissue mass. After 2 to 4 weeks, flocculations will be noted, and these evolve into one of three types of bone formation:[36] The stalk type is connected to the adjacent bone; the broad-based, periosteal type is more broadly connected, and the third type has no direct connection to the bone.

Bony myositis ossificans masses have been mistaken for a malignant bone tumor, the juxtacortical osteogenic sarcoma. The tumor differs in many ways, however, from myositis ossificans. Fifty percent of the sarcomas occur in people older than 30 years of age, and there is often pain with activity and at night. The tumor usually is located in the distal and posterior one third of the femur, the alkaline phosphatase level in the blood is raised, and the tumor expands in size. Histologically, the juxtacortical osteogenic sarcoma has wild bone at its periphery, in contrast to the mature peripheral bone of myositis ossificans.

Myositis ossificans usually follows significant trauma by 2 to 4 weeks, often occurring in a young athlete who has active bone turnover. After the acute phase, the mass is usually painless and is typically anterior to the midshaft of the femur. The alkaline phosphatase level is usually normal, and the mass decreases in size, becoming more compact and rounding off at the edges. Histologically, the ominous fields at the interior proceed to a more innocent osseous tissue at the periphery in a centrifugal pattern of maturation.

After 3 to 6 months, the myositic bone mass usually stabilizes, remaining unchanged, or it may shrink. If the mass is in a muscle belly, it sometimes is almost fully resorbed. When it is near a muscle origin or insertion, it is less likely to be resorbed and more likely to cause functional impairment. If the mass is tender or inhibits motion after 1 year, it may be removed.[36, 46] Earlier removal may provoke unwanted bone to recur in even greater amounts. Clotting studies should be performed if an athlete has recurring myositis ossificans because the athlete may have a clotting deficiency.

Hamstring Strain

The hamstring muscles decelerate hip flexion, extend the thigh, and flex the leg when the foot is not weightbearing. The hamstrings antagonize the quadriceps during most of leg extension in running and assume an extensor action with footstrike. The sudden change from a stabilizing flexor to an active extensor may cause a hamstring strain.

Quick starts with sudden, violent hamstring contraction or stretching may tear an athlete's hamstring. A strain may occur as a sprinter leaves the starting blocks, in the lead leg of a hurdler, or in a jumper's takeoff leg. It may also occur when a football lineman charges, especially late in a game if the player has failed to warm up properly before the beginning of the second half.

The short-head of the biceps femoris is of little help in the running pattern and is the most frequently strained hamstring.[13] It arises from the linea aspera, the upper part of the supracondylar line, and the lateral intermuscular septum and has two motor points, one innervated by the tibial part of the sciatic nerve, the other by the peroneal division of this nerve. This dual innervation of the biceps femoris causes problems, as the short head of the biceps may contract at the same time as the quadriceps, resulting in a hamstring pull.

Hamstring strains are associated with poor flexibility, inadequate warm-up, fatigue, deficiency in the reciprocal actions of opposing muscle groups, and imbalance between quadriceps and hamstring strength. With conventional isotonic testing, an athlete's hamstrings should have 60% to 70% of the strength of his quadriceps. Cyclists are an exception because their hamstring strength is roughly equal to their quadriceps strength. Strength ratios change with isokinetic testing at higher speeds, where the quadriceps and hamstrings of most athlete's balance out.

In a mild hamstring strain, there is no tear, only spasm of the hamstrings. The thigh usually does not hurt until the athlete cools down. In moderate pulls the athlete feels a "pop" or a snap, and there is immediate pain and loss of function. The examiner should palpate the hamstrings to see if there is a gap resulting from torn fibers. There may also be a lump or a hematoma. Severe pulls generally occur at the origin or at the insertion of the hamstring into bone.

Athletes should not try to "run out" a hamstring strain.[19] Instead, an elastic wrap and an ice bag should be applied. Crushed ice will conform to the shape of the thigh. A felt or foam rubber pad may be cut out and wrapped over the injured area with an elastic wrap to provide compression overnight. With varying effects, some physicians have the athlete ingest trypsin-chymotrypsin enzyme tablets or inject enzymes locally to help decrease the hematoma. Once further swelling is controlled, cryotherapy and contrast treatments of ice massage and ultrasound may begin. The athlete may work through an active range of motion in chest-deep water. When the soreness is gone, he may begin knee curls, knee extensions, and high-speed cycling. Later, light massage will break up intramuscular adhesions that exercise and heat cannot handle.

Mild pulls heal in a few days to a week, and moderate pulls heal in 1 to 3 weeks. Avulsion fractures at the ischial tuberosity or at the head of the fibula, however, take a month or more to heal.

On returning to practice, the athlete should wear an elastic support around his thigh. The support has a seamless circular knit and a rubber-elastic construction, is sized to fit tapered circumferences, and will help to keep the area warm and lessen swelling. Adhesive tape is too restricting, and elastic wraps may work loose.

REFERENCES

1. ADAMS RJ, CHANDLER FA: Osteitis pubis of traumatic etiology. J Bone Joint Surg [Am] 35:685–696, 1953
2. ALLMAN FL: Problems in treatment of athletic injuries. J Med Assoc Ga 53:381–383, 1964
3. ALYEA EP, PARISH HH Jr: Renal response to exercise—urinary findings. JAMA 167:807–813, 1958
4. AMELAR RD, SOLOMAN C: Acute renal trauma in boxers. J Urol 72:145–148, 1954
5. BAILEY RR et al: What the urine contains following athletic competition. NZ Med J 83:809–813, 1976
6. BAILEY W: Observations on the etiology and frequency of spondylolisthesis and its precursors. Radiology 48:107–112, 1947
7. BAKER B: Jejunal perforation occurring in contact sports. Am J Sports Med 6:403–404, 1978
8. BENSON DR et al: Can the Milwaukee brace patient participate in competitive athletics? Am J Sports Med 5:7–12, 1977
9. BERSON B: Surgical repair of pectoralis major rupture in an athlete. Am J Sports Med 7:348–351, 1979
10. BLACKLOCK NJ: Bladder trauma in the long-distance runner. Am J Sports Med 7:239–241, 1979
11. BOONE AW et al: Football hematuria. JAMA 158:516–517, 1955
12. BROGDON BG, CROW NE: Observations on the "normal" spleen. Radiology 72:412–413, 1959
13. BURKETT LN: Investigation into hamstring strains: the case of the hybrid muscle. Am J Sports Med 3:5, 1975
14. BUTLER JE, EGGERT AW: Fracture of the iliac crest apophysis: an unusual hip pointer. Am J Sports Med 3:192–193, 1975
15. CASTENJORS J: Renal clearance and urinary sodium and potassium excretion during supine exercise in normal subjects. Acta Physiol Scand 70:204–214, 1967
16. CLANCY WG, FOLTZ AS: Iliac apophysitis and stress fractures in adolescent runners. Am J Sports Med 4:214–218, 1976
17. COCHRANE GM: Osteitis pubis in athletes. Br J Sports Med 5:233–235, 1971
18. COLLIER W: Functional albuminuria in athletes. Br Med J 1:4–6, 1907
19. COOPER DL, FAIR J: Trainer's corner. Hamstring strains. Phys Sportsmed 6(8):104, 1978
20. COOPER DL, FAIR J: Trainer's corner. Treating the charleyhorse. Phys Sportsmed 7(6):157, 1979
21. DAUNEKER DT et al: Case report: intra-abdominal injury in a gymnast. Phys Sportsmed 7(6):119–120, 1979
22. deSHAZO WF III: Case report: ruptured spleen in a college football player. Phys Sportsmed 7(10):109–111, 1979
23. deSHAZO WF III: Returning to athletic activity after infectious mononucleosis. Phys Sportsmed 8(12):71–72, 1980
24. FERGUSON RJ et al: Low back pain in college football linemen. Am J Sports Med 2:63–80, 1974
25. FRED HL, NATELSON EA: Grossly bloody urine of runners. South Med J 70:1394–1396, 1977
26. FUNK FJ Jr: Injuries to the extensor mechanism of the knee. Athletic Training 10:141–145, 1975
27. GARDNER KD Jr: "Athletic pseudonephritis"—alteration of urine sediment by athletic competition. JAMA 161:1613–1617, 1956

28. GEHLSEN G, ALBOHM M: Evaluation of sports bras. Phys Sportsmed 8(10):89–98, 1980

29. GEHLSEN G, ALBOHM M: Evaluating sports bras. First Aider, Cramer 50(4):4–5, 1980

30. HAHN DB: The ruptured spleen: implications for the athletic trainer. Athletic Training 13(4):190–191, Winter 1978

31. HANSON PG et al: Osteitis pubis in sports activities. Phys Sportsmed 7(10):111–114, 1978

32. HEYMSFIELD SB et al: Accurate measurements of liver, kidney and spleen volume and mass by computerized axial tomography. Ann Intern Med 90:185–187, 1979

33. HORNER DB: Lumbar back pain arising from stress fractures of the lower ribs—report of four cases. J Bone Joint Surg [Am] 46:1553–1556, 1964

34. HOWSE JJG: Osteitis pubis in an Olympic road walker. Proc R Soc Med 57:88–90, 1964

35. JACKSON DW, WILTSE LL: Low back pain in young athletes. Phys Sportsmed 2(11):53–60, 1974

36. JACKSON DW: Managing myositis ossificans in the young athlete. Phys Sportsmed 3(10):56–61, 1975

37. JACKSON DW et al: Spondylolysis in the female gymnast. Clin Orthop 117:68–73, 1976

38. JACKSON DW: Low back pain in young athletes: evaluation of stress reaction and discogenic problems. Am J Sports Med 7:361–369, 1979

39. JACOBS B: Legg-Calvé-Perthes disease, the "obscure affection." Contemp Surg 10:62, 67, 1977

40. KALENAK A et al: Treating thigh contusions with ice. Phys Sportsmed 3(3):65–67, 1975

41. KLEIMAN AH: Athlete's kidney. J Urol 83:321–329, 1960

42. KNOCHEL JP et al: The renal, cardiovascular hematological and serum electrolyte abnormalities of heat stroke. Am J Med 30:299–309, 1961

43. KOCH RA, JACKSON DW: Pubic symphysitis in runners—report of two cases. Am J Sports Med 9:62–63, 1981

44. LEVIT F: Nipple sensitivity. Med Aspects Hum Sex 12:135, 1973

45. LEVIT F: Jogger's nipples. JAMA 297:1127, 1977

46. LIPSCOMB AB et al: Treatment of myositis ossificans traumatica in athletes. Am J Sports Med 4:111–120, 1976

47. MELVIN M: Trainer's corner. Protecting the kidney. Phys Sportsmed 7(3):161, 1979

48. MERRIFIELD HH, COWAN RF: Ice hockey groin pulls. Am J Sports Med 1:41–42, 1973

49. MICHELI LJ: Low back pain in the adolescent: differential diagnosis in low back pain in athletes. Am J Sports Med 7:361–369, 1979

50. MICHELI LJ et al: Use of modified Boston brace for back injuries in athletes. Am J Sports Med 8:351–356, 1980

51. MURRAY RO, DUNCAN C: Athletic activity in adolescence as an etiologic factor in degenerative disk disease. J Bone Joint Surg [Br] 53:406–419, 1971

52. PFEIFFER RP, YOUNG TR: Case report. Spontaneous pneumothorax in a jogger. Phys Sportsmed 8(12):65–67, 1980

53. PRIEST JD, NAGEL DA: Tennis shoulder. Am J Sports Med 4:28–42, 1976

54. RUTKOW IM: Rupture of the spleen in infectious mononucleosis. Arch Surg 113:718–720, 1978

55. RYAN AJ: Quadriceps strain, rupture and charleyhorse. Med Sci Sports 1:106–111, 1969

56. RYAN AJ (moderator) Round table: diagnosing kidney injuries in athletes. Phys Sportsmed 3(1):48–49, 1975

57. SIEGEL AJ et al: Exercise-related hematuria. Findings in a group of marathon runners. JAMA 241:391–392, 1979

58. SIGEL RM et al: Evaluation of spleen size during routine liver imaging with 99mTc and the scintillation camera. J Nucl Med 11:689–692, 1970

59. SMODLAKA VN: Groin pain in soccer players. Phys Sportsmed 8(8):57–61, 1980

60. STANISH W: Low back pain in middle-aged athletes. Am J Sports Med 7:361–369, 1979

61. TAYLOR KJ, MILAN J: Differential diagnosis of chronic splenomegaly by gray-scale ultrasonography: clinical observations and digital A-scan analysis. Br J Radiol 49:519–525, 1976

62. TODD RW: Age changes in the pubic symphysis. Roentgenographic differentiation. Am J Anthropol 14:255–271, 1933

63. VERE–HODGE N: Injuries in cricket. In Armstrong JR, Tucker WE (eds): Injuries in Sport, pp 168–171. Springfield, Illinois, Charles C Thomas, 1964

64. WILLIAMS RD, SARGENT FT: The mechanism of intestinal injury in trauma. J Trauma 31:288–294, 1968

65. WYMAN AC: Traumatic rupture of the spleen. Am J Roentgenol 72:51–63, 1954

66. WYKER AW Jr, GILLENWATER JY: Method of Urology. Baltimore, Williams and Wilkins, 1975

67. ZACCALINI PS, URIST MR: Traumatic periosteal proliferations in rabbits. J Trauma 4:344–357, 1964

68. ZEMAN SC et al: Tears of the pectoralis major muscle. Am J Sports Med 7:343–347, 1979

Anatomy

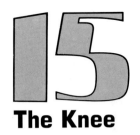

15
The Knee

The knee joint is a large and complex one in which the medial femoral condyle extends more distally than the lateral femoral condyle and prominence of the lateral femoral condyle serves to block the patella from sliding laterally out of the femoral groove. The lateral plateau of the tibia is convex, and the medial plateau is concave.

The quadriceps muscle group comprises the rectus femoris, vastus lateralis, vastus intermedius, and the vastus medialis and serves to extend the knee. These muscles join to form the quadriceps tendon, which is central to a fascialike retinaculum that is lateral and medial to the patella (*see* Fig. 15-1). The articularis genu is a small part of the quadriceps that extricates the suprapatella pouch to prevent its being pinched during knee motion. The oblique part of the vastus medialis usually inserts about one half of the way down the medial side of the patella. Because this part rapidly atrophies after a knee operation or immobilization, and terminal extension of the knee weakens, it had been thought that this part of the quadriceps was solely responsible for the last 15° of knee extension. It has since been shown that such limited extension is related to total quadriceps strength and is not an indication of selective weakness of the vastus medialis obliquus.[78]

Thus, the vastus medialis obliquus serves a patella-centering function.[77] In amputated limbs, a solitary vastus medialis obliquus will not extend the knee, whereas all of the long components of the quadriceps—the vastus lateralis, vastus intermedius, vastus medialis longus, and rectus femoris—effect full extension. Normally the last 15° of knee extension require 60% more force than is needed for extension up to the 15° position. When a weight is attached to the vastus medialis obliquus to keep the patella centered in the femoral groove, however, the force needed for the vastus lateralis to extend the knee decreases by 13%.

The patella usually has two major facets: a large lateral facet and a smaller medial one. The smallest facet is a medialmost "odd facet" of the patella, where osteoarthritis begins. The articular cartilage at the apex of the patella, the junction between the medial and lateral facets, is the thickest patellar cartilage. The earliest softening and chondromalacia appear here because it is so thick that diffusion of nutrients to its

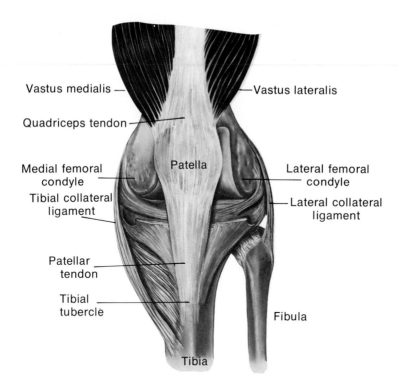

Vastus medialis

Vastus lateralis

Quadriceps tendon

Patella

Medial femoral condyle

Lateral femoral condyle

Tibial collateral ligament

Lateral collateral ligament

Patellar tendon

Tibial tubercle

Fibula

Tibia

FIG. 15-1
This anterior aspect of the knee shows the extensor mechanism (*see* text for description).

depths is difficult. Patellar-femoral, patellar-meniscal, and patellar-tibial ligaments arise from the patella. These ligaments sometimes hold the patella laterally and may be sectioned to relieve patella subluxation and to allow it to glide better in the femoral groove.

The patellar tendon passes from the distal pole of the patella to the tibial tubercle, where it has a sinuous insertion. The usually prominent tibial tubercle is the tongue portion of the tibial epiphysis, which eventually fuses to the rest of the tibia. There are two bursae in this region, one lying between the patella tendon and the tibia just before the tendon inserts into the tibial tubercle, and a second resting subcutaneously just anterior to the patella tendon.

Ligaments

The knee is encased in a fibrous capsular sleeve, weak in its anterior half and strong in its posterior part. Ligaments, menisci, and bone of the knee joint are responsible for the static stability of the knee, whereas muscles and tendons

provide dynamic stability. The ligaments work as an integrated network of bundles and fans with complex functions. In full knee extension, the cruciates and collateral ligaments are taut and the knee cannot rotate, but when the knee is flexed the tibia may rotate as the lateral ligaments relax. Although the ligaments work as a unit, they may be divided into a medial complex, a lateral quadruple complex, and the cruciates.

The Medial Side of the Knee

The medial capsular ligament comprises three parts: an anterior capsule, the medial capsular ligament, and the posterior oblique ligament. It joins with the medial meniscus by way of the coronary ligament and has a strong meniscal-femoral and a weaker meniscal-tibial part (*see* Fig. 15-2).

The tibial collateral ligament is phylogenetically a remnant of the adductor magnus tendon, arising high on the medial femoral condyle, separated from the medial capsular ligament over the joint line. It inserts into the medial face of the tibia beneath the pes anserinus and is the strongest medial structure and the primary stabilizer of the medial side of the knee (*see* Fig. 15-2). Its tension is maintained during the entire range of knee motion by a reciprocal tightening and loosening of its fibers (Fig. 15-3). This ligament stabilizes the knee against excessive external rotation as well as valgus forces and resists rotational forces better than the more centrally located cruciates. If the deep ligament and posterior capsule are resected to the midline of the popliteal space but the long tibial collateral ligament is left intact, the knee is still stable to valgus and rotatory stress.[84]

The posterior oblique ligament is strong, forming a sling around the medial femoral condyle.[48] It might better be termed the postero-

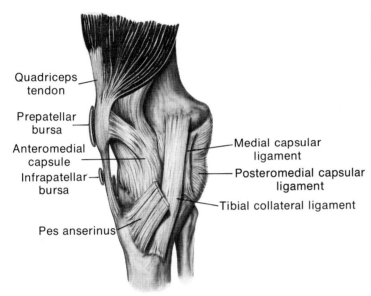

FIG. 15-2
The medial side of the knee contains static and dynamic structures (*see* text for description).

Quadriceps tendon
Prepatellar bursa
Anteromedial capsule
Infrapatellar bursa
Pes anserinus
Medial capsular ligament
Posteromedial capsular ligament
Tibial collateral ligament

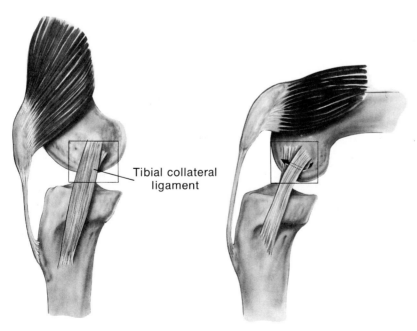

FIG. 15-3
Some part of the tibial collateral ligament is always taut as its fiber bundles shift with flexion and extension.

Tibial collateral ligament

medial capsular ligament to avoid confusion with the oblique popliteal ligament, a part of the insertion of the semimembranosus into the posterior capsule. The semimembranosus, through its capsular arm, tightens the posteromedial capsular ligament and retracts the posterior horn of the medial meniscus during knee flexion. The semimembranosus also has a direct head that inserts into the tibia and one to the oblique popliteal ligament that tenses the posterior capsule.

The Lateral Quadruple Complex

The lateral quadruple complex consists of the iliotibial band, lateral collateral ligament, popliteus tendon, and the biceps femoris.

The iliotibial band has a dynamic proximal origin as the fascial extension of the tensor fascia lata and the gluteus maximus. It attaches to the intermuscular septum at the level of the lateral femoral condyle and proceeds to insert into the lateral epicondyle of the femur and the lateral tibial tubercle of Gerdy. The iliotibial band is a static lateral stabilizer of the knee but, owing to its tensor fascia lata origin, has some dynamic function as well. It is tense as it moves forward in extension and back in flexion.

The lateral collateral ligament, shaped like a pencil, arises at the lateral femoral epicondyle and inserts on the fibular head. It is tight in extension but relaxes as the knee flexes. The popliteus muscle is peculiar, arising from the lateral femoral condyle as a tendon that passes deep to the lateral collateral ligament, and also from the posterior horn of the lateral meniscus and the posterior aspect of the fibula and inserting on the tibia (Fig. 15-4). This muscle stabilizes the knee in flexion and helps govern movement of the lateral meniscus. A popliteus bursa lies between the popliteus tendon and the lateral collateral ligament.

The biceps femoris, an important lateral stabilizer, inserts at the fibular head, the posterolateral tibia, the joint capsule, and the iliotibial tract. The lateral capsule, with its strong mid-third capsular ligament, completes the lateral structures. In flexion, the iliotibial band, popliteus tendon, and lateral collateral ligament cross each other to enhance lateral stability.

The Anterior Cruciate Ligament

The anterior cruciate ligament is intracapsular but extrasynovial. It has a crescentic origin from the lateral femoral condyle behind the intercondylar shelf, extending forward and medially into the medial plateau of the tibia in

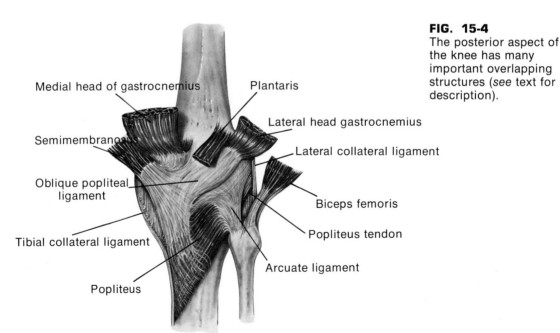

FIG. 15-4
The posterior aspect of the knee has many important overlapping structures (*see* text for description).

Medial head of gastrocnemius

Plantaris

Semimembranosus

Lateral head gastrocnemius

Lateral collateral ligament

Oblique popliteal ligament

Biceps femoris

Tibial collateral ligament

Popliteus tendon

Arcuate ligament

Popliteus

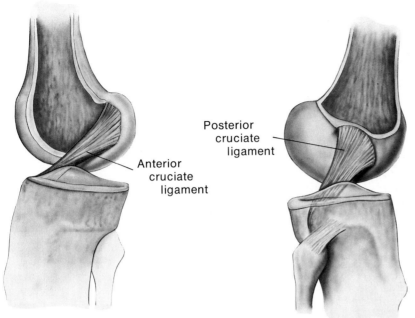

FIG. 15-5
The anterior and posterior cruciate ligaments form axes for knee rotation (*see* text for description).

Posterior cruciate ligament

Anterior cruciate ligament

front of the intercondylar eminence (Fig. 15-5). The blood vessels course up into the ligament from the infrapatellar fat pad and the synovium, and the nerves in the ligament probably relay position sense.

The anterior cruciate contains three coiled bundles: anteromedial, intermediate, and posterolateral. In extension, the anterior bundle is tight against the intercondylar shelf of the femur; in flexion, the anterior bundle relaxes while the posterolateral becomes tight.[106] Most of the anterior cruciate fibers are longitudinally oriented, but they also spiral from one insertion to the other; for this reason, the geometry of the ligament would be difficult to duplicate with an artificial ligament.

The anterior cruciate is tightest at the extremes of motion, full extension, and full flexion. In midflexion, it is tight when the tibia is internally rotated, but it is otherwise lax. Tightness in various parts of the anterior cruciate at all degrees of flexion acts reciprocally with the posterior cruciate, so that some cruciate fibers are tight at all times.

The anterior cruciate ligament prevents the athlete's femur from sliding backwards during weight bearing while also preventing abnormal internal rotation of the tibia by tightening up

and twisting on the posterior cruciate. In addition, this ligament exerts control over abnormal external rotation of the tibia. During external rotation of the tibia on the femur, as in a side-step cut, the cruciates unwind. With continued external rotation, the anterior cruciate wraps around the medial side of the lateral femoral condyle to limit further external rotation.

The Posterior Cruciate Ligament

Like the anterior cruciate, the posterior cruciate ligament is intra-articular but extrasynovial, with a crescentic insertion into the medial femoral condyle and a complex architecture (*see* Fig. 15-5). Its thin posterior part fans out on the tibia, and its bulk fans out on the femur. It is twice as strong as the anterior cruciate, working reciprocally with the anterior cruciate.[43]

This ligament is a basic knee stabilizer that is tightest in the midranges of motion. Because of its fan-shaped insertion, some part of it is tight during each degree of knee motion, and it becomes tighter with internal rotation of the tibia, resisting anterior slide of the femur when the athlete is bearing weight. The posterior cruciate also resists hyperextension and contributes to medial stability of the knee.

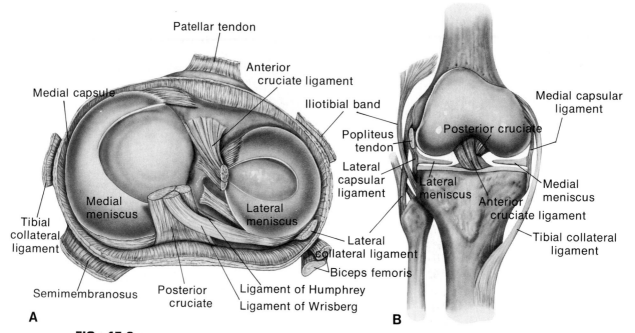

FIG. 15-6
The many structures in and around the knee joint are each important in athletic injuries. (*A*) Coronal view of the tibial plateaus. (*B*) Frontal view of the knee joint.

Posterior Capsule

The posterior capsule helps to stabilize the knee in extension. It is reinforced by the oblique popliteal ligament, an expansion from the semimembranosus tendon. The capsule is governed by a complex system of dynamic motors that include the popliteus, biceps, gastrocnemius, and medial hamstring muscles.

Menisci

The menisci of the knee arise from wedge-shaped condensations of mesenchyme between the developing femur and tibia,[87] whereas the remaining mesenchyme forms the cruciate ligaments. The menisci are mobile buffers with a circumferential arrangement of collagen fibers that suits them to their weight-bearing, shock-absorbing function. They also help to guide and to synchronize knee motion and are important for knee stability. The outer third of each meniscus has a blood supply that accounts for the healing of some peripheral tears and the regeneration of a tough, fibrous meniscus after some meniscectomies. The nonvascularized part of the meniscus receives its nutrition through the diffusion of synovial fluid.

The medial meniscus is C shaped, covering 30% of the surface of the medial tibial plateau (*see* Fig. 15-6). It is firmly attached anteriorly and posteriorly to the tibia and securely attached peripherally to the joint capsule by the coronary ligament.

The three types of medial menisci[19] include type I menisci with anterior and posterior horns of equal size; type II with large posterior horns; and type III with a very large posterior horn. The posterior horn is thick, making diffusion of nutrients into the depths of this horn difficult, hence degeneration is likely to occur here.

The blind side of the medial meniscus is an area that is not easy to see from an anterior operative approach to the knee joint.[41] It includes the posterior horn and its capsular and synovial attachments and the meniscal attachment to bone. The meniscus dives into a deep, wide hole behind the intercondylar eminence to attach posteriorly. This strong attachment is best seen through an arthroscope. When the meniscus is completely freed from the joint capsule, it pops straight up, owing to its vertical deep hole attachment.

The lateral meniscus is O shaped, covering 50% of the lateral tibial plateau (Fig. 15-6). Its anterior and posterior horns attach to the tibia, whereas the meniscus is only loosely attached to the capsule.[73] The popliteus tendon arises partly from the posterior part of the lateral meniscus and is probably important in coordinating meniscal motion with knee joint motion.[46]

Pes Anserinus

From above downwards, the pes anserinus is the combined insertion of the sartorius, gracilis, and semitendinosis on the anteriomedial face of the tibia. Although the tendons insert individually, they are connected by an aponeurosis, the combined structure resembling a pes anserinus, or "goose's foot." The pes works mainly as a flexor of the knee but also rotates the leg internally. The pes anserinus bursa sits between the pes, near its insertion, and the overlying tibial collateral ligament.

Examining an Athlete's Injured Knee

When examining an athlete's knee, the physician should first ask if he has had previous injury to the knee and what sort of treatment he has received. Then, how was the knee hurt this time, and what was the mechanism of injury? What did the injury feel like? Did the knee pop or give way? Was the athlete able to stand up immediately after the injury? Did the knee swell, and, if so, when did it swell—immediately or overnight? Swelling is estimated by a comparison to the sound knee. Is the athlete bowlegged or knock-kneed, or does he

have recurvatum or external tibial torsion? The quadriceps must be checked for wasting and the thigh circumferences measured.

The sound knee should be examined first to establish baselines for strength and stability and to observe whether the athlete is tight jointed or loose jointed. This procedure tends to increase the athlete's confidence in the examiner. The dynamic Q angle—the angle that the patella tendon makes with the long axis of the thigh with the knee flexed 30° and the tibia rotated externally—is also measured.

The examiner should feel along the distal femoral growth plate of the young athlete, searching for a fracture. He should also palpate the adductor tubercle for an osteochondroma or bone spikes and bursae. With the athlete sitting, hip flexion strength should be manually tested, furnishing a good guide as to whether the athlete has been favoring the knee. The tone of the quadriceps is felt, the quadriceps is palpated, and the knee is extended against the examiner's manual resistance. The examiner next feels around and under the patella and over the femoral condyles for defects or tender areas.

The athlete is then asked to flex and extend his knee. While the knee is being flexed and extended, the examiner may cover the patella with his palm and feel for crepitus. At less than 30° of flexion, the patella is mobile and all of its facets may be felt, including the most medial portion, or odd facet, where osteoarthritis commonly begins. Next, with the knee extended and the examiner's thumbs placed laterally, the patella should be pressed medially at the same time as the fingers press it into the groove. This maneuver may bring out the pain of chondromalacia. The examiner then palpates the athlete's patella tendon from its patellar origin to its insertion at the tibial tubercle. With the knee flexed to 45°, the examiner should try to sublux the patella by pressing it laterally. An athlete whose patella has previously been dislocated may reach down in fear that his patella is sliding out laterally, a positive apprehension sign. The lateral capsule is considered tight if the examiner, is unable to push the patella more than 1 cm medially with the knee flexed to 30°.

With the knee flexed over the table, the examiner next feels along the medial and lateral joint lines for tender areas or bulges that may mean meniscal cysts. Such cysts usually are posteromedial or posterolateral, bulging through a weak area in the capsule. The examiner then feels the pes insertion on the medial face of the tibia for a swollen and tender pes anserinus bursa. The athlete is asked to assume a figure-four position with his knee bent to 90° and his ankle placed on his other knee. In this position, the examiner may feel the prominent lateral collateral ligament and the popliteus tendon that passes deep to it. Examination of the iliotibial band, which may be snapping over the lateral femoral epicondyle, is made at this juncture. The athlete then lies prone with his feet hanging over the examining table as he is checked for a popliteal cyst, and his hamstrings are palpated as they course toward their insertions.

The athlete should be asked to do a deep squat, and if there is pain as he goes down or comes up, patellar femoral problems are indicated. Pain at the deepest part of the squat, usually posteromedial, is characteristic of a posterior horn tear of the medial meniscus. To bring out the symptoms, the athlete may be asked to duck-walk and do squat jumps. The click test is next performed. The athlete's hip is first flexed and then his knee fully flexed. The examiner rotates the leg with one hand, and with the other feels over the joint line for any clicks or pops. Any knee can be made to click, but a painful click is evidence for a meniscal tear. A similar analysis, the compression grind test (Apley), may be made with the athlete prone. This is done with the examiner holding the athlete's thigh in place with one hand while his other hand flexes the knee and rotates the leg. If the grinding phase hurts, the leg is pulled up and the same maneuver performed. The grinding may disappear when the leg is lifted, signaling that the pain and crunching on the grind test was probably due to a meniscal tear. The athlete may also sit in a yoga position with soles together while the examiner presses his knee downwards, a maneuver that sometimes causes the meniscus to be caught, eliciting pain.

With the athlete supine and relaxed, his injured leg is gently lowered over the side of the examining table to relax his muscles for valgus and varus stress tests. With the knee fully extended, it should have good stability unless there is major ligamentous damage. The knee is then flexed to 30°, and the same valgus and varus stress tests are performed to measure any damage to the medial and lateral sides.

Testing for anterior cruciate integrity was formerly done by flexing the knee to 90°, sitting on the foot, and checking that the hamstrings were relaxed before pulling the leg forward. Now, a more accurate way to test for anterior subluxation of the tibial plateau is a drawer test, with the knee flexed to just 15° (the Lachman test). The examiner holds the thigh steady with one hand while pulling the tibia forward with the other. This test is more accurate than the drawer test because it is not hindered by hamstring contraction and the concavity of the posterior horns of the menisci that lend stability and act as secondary restraints to the drawer. To test for posterior cruciate integrity, the examiner flexes the knee to 90° and firmly presses the tibia backwards. At this time he should also observe whether the tibia sags backwards compared to the sound side.

Because some muscles cross both the hip and the knee and the knee and the ankle, it is important during a knee examination to examine the hip flexors, extensors, abductors, and adductors and to perform a thorough examination of the foot and a check of heel-cord flexibility.

To study the knee with plain x-ray films, anteroposterior, lateral, tunnel, sunrise, oblique, and "skin pin" views may be taken. The anteroposterior and lateral views are taken with the athlete bearing weight. The tunnel view is taken with the knee flexed 45° to show the intercondylar notch, which may house the lesion of osteochondritis dissecans, most often noted on the lateral side of the medial femoral condyle. "Sunrise" views, taken with the knee flexed to 30°, 60°, and 90°, reveal the position of the patella in the femoral groove, the slope of the femoral groove, the form of the lateral condylar buttress, the patellar shape, and whether the patella is tilted. Oblique views may be needed to show avulsion fractures. If a tender spot is noted, a pin is taped to the skin at the site and a "skin pin" x-ray film taken.

Running

A runner's knee problem may be caused by an abnormality of the leg or foot, such as a tight heel cord, a pronated foot, or a cavus, high-arched foot. Shocks are normally absorbed at the knee by knee lexion, at the ankle by dorsiflexion, and in the foot by pronation. A tight heel cord puts a burden on the knee to flex further to absorb shock. As a result, even when the runner is on a flat surface the knees are flexed, putting extra strain on the quadriceps, which presses the patella painfully against the articular surface of the femur. A pronated foot leads to valgus forces at the knee, putting stress on the medial knee capsule. In this condition, the foot stays on the ground longer, and the patella may thus translate, or slide side-to-side, to produce shearing stress. Lateral capsular knee sprains are caused by jamming of the inflexible cavus foot. Tight hamstrings may also produce knee problems because the quadriceps must work harder against these tight hamstrings, and the kneecap is thus further compressed against the femur. To prevent or to treat these problems, the athlete should stretch his heel cords, use orthotic devices for pronated feet, wear padding for cavus feet, and stretch his hamstrings.

The surface on which the athlete runs may

affect his knees. Subchondral bone trabeculae absorb shock at the knee, amounting to a force of about three times that of body weight during running. These trabeculae may fracture and cause knee pain, although the fractures are too fine to be seen on x-ray films. Healed microfractures cause increased density in the subchondral region and decrease its shock-absorbing capacity. The articular cartilage must then absorb the shocks, a job for which it was not designed and which causes the cartilage to break down, resulting in incongruities and arthritis.

A 59-kg (130 lb) person puts about 390 pounds of force on his tibial plateaus with each walking step. If an average day of walking consists of about 8000 steps, the knees must accept more than 3 million pounds of force a day.[97] If the person weighs 200 pounds, almost 5 million pounds of force reach the plateaus of the knees each day. These forces are much greater in running than in walking because, while walking, one supportive foot is always on the ground, whereas running is a series of jumps. These figures underline the value of weight loss in the heavy person to avoid arthritis of the knee.[74]

The terrain on which the athlete runs may affect his knees. On crowned roads or banked tracks, the uphill leg pronates to cause medial knee pain, and the downhill leg jams to produce latereal knee pain (*see* Fig. 15-7). During downhill runs, quadriceps contractions decelerate the runner's femur, pressing the kneecap against the articular cartilage of the femur and possibly causing retropatellar pain. The popliteus also

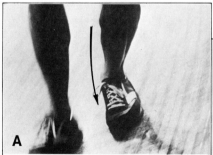

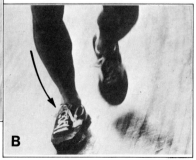

FIG. 15-7
The uphill leg on a banked track (*A*) pronates (*arrow*) and places stress on the medial side of the knee. The downhill foot (*B*) jams and supinates (*arrow*), stressing the lateral side of the knee.

aids in holding the femur back during downhill runs, and popliteus tenosynovitis may arise. A temporary change to flat terrain will often correct some of these problems, and stretching, orthoses, or shoe changes may effect a cure.

Unusual running styles sometimes promote knee problems. Some inexperienced runners run with their knees turned in, externally rotating their legs to clear the ground. This style may result from femoral anteversion and tibial torsion, but it can be improved by lifting the knees to clear the ground. Strange running styles may be quite effective, however, for some athletes.

Cutting

Cutting is the term used to describe an athlete altering his running gait and changing direction by a few degrees or as much as 90° or more.

Cuts involve three phases.[3] The first is preliminary deceleration. There is no foot descent phase. Instead, the heel jams into the ground, and the foot flattens. The quadriceps and hamstrings provide the power for deceleration, which is achieved by knee flexion instead of the normal dorsiflexion of the foot. After deceleration, the plant and cut involves a twist toward the new direction. In the final phase, takeoff, the athlete pushes off and moves in the direction of the cut.

There are two major cuts: the sidestep and the crossover (*see* Fig. 15-8). In the side-step cut, the foot opposite the direction of the cut is planted, and the other foot then takes the first step in the new direction. In the crossover cut, the athlete plants the foot that is on the same side as the new direction. The opposite leg then crosses in front of the planted one to move in this new direction.

Because these are such strong forces on the knee, many athletic injuries occur during cutting. The sidestep cut stresses the medial knee ligaments of the planted leg. Also, the twisting motion of the planted leg in this cut and quad-

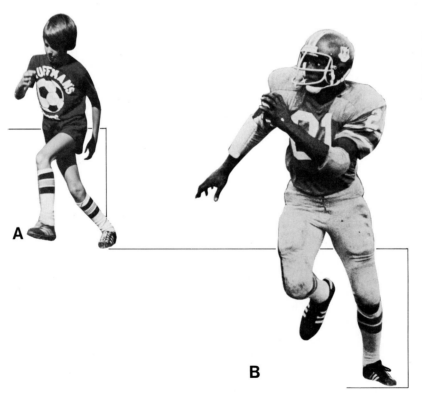

A

B

FIG. 15-8
A cross-over cut (*A*) and side-step cut (*B*) affect the pivoting knee differently.

riceps contraction at pushoff may snap the patella laterally into a dislocated position. In a crossover cut, the lateral knee ligaments of the planted leg are stressed.

During cuts, the athlete's knee is placed in a vulnerable, partly flexed position in which its inherent stability drops and a blow from an opponent may damage the knee. The ligaments are further loaded if shoe cleats catch in the turf. Cutting drills come last in knee rehabilitation programs because they are the most stressful moves. Thus, one of the prime determinants as to when the athlete may return to practice or games is how well he performs cuts.

Kicking

The energy contained in an athlete's leg just before a kick is equivalent to the energy of a fall of almost 1 m by a 90-kg person.[33] During a kick, 15% of the leg's kinetic energy is transferred to the ball to accelerate it. Most of the remaining 800 pounds of force is dissipated by knee flexion and a pulling back of the leg by the hamstrings. Hamstring strains are common in kicking, as the forces on these structures are very strong and there is not much time in follow-through to dissipate the energy.

Flexibility and good technique are important in preventing injuries in kicking sports. In the martial arts, many American enthusiasts suffer knee injuries, whereas these are only minor problems in Asiatic competitors.[65] Some have attributed this injury distribution to racial differences in knee anatomy,[65] but the variations more likely are related to the athlete's technique and flexibility, since Caucasian European competitors also have a low knee injury rate.

The athlete may injure an opponent or himself while kicking and may develop quadriceps tendinitis or pes anserinus bursitis. If a placekicker's foot catches in the turf or strikes an opponent, he may strain a muscle or avulse a piece of bone. For this reason, soccer cleats are stubby at the toe to avoid catching. Medial hamstring strain is commonly seen in older persons new to soccer football, resulting from attempts to kick with the medial side of the foot.

Bicycling

Bicycling is safe and beneficial for the knees. It develops the thigh muscles, improves muscular endurance and flexibility, enhances the nutrition of knee cartilage, and possibly postpones arthritis. The hamstrings of a cyclist often are equal in strength to his quadriceps because toe clips allow him to pull, and when the crank is just 15° past the horizontal, the vastus muscle group is turned off, but the hamstrings continue to act. Cycling also enhances muscular endurance by stimulating mitochondrial enzyme systems.[29] In addition, the cyclist nourishes the knee by gently pumping in nutrients, rather than jamming the knee, as in running.

Knee safety in cycling depends on proper saddle height, avoidance of pushing too hard in high gears, proper cleat placement, and keeping the knees warm. In a study of persons of all ages who participated in the Bikecentennial 80-day tour from Reedsport, Oregon, to Yorktown, Virginia,[68] it was found that each cyclist used about 2 million pedal strokes to pedal the 7200 km (4500 miles) over varying terrain. Knee pain was rare, however, and was easily relieved by altering the saddle height. Older cyclists with osteoarthritis reported that their knees vastly improved during the tour.

Proper saddle height is determined by placing the heels on the pedals and pedaling backwards while the bicycle is supported. The cyclist's knee should be slightly bent when the pedal is at its lowest point. If the pelvis rocks, the seat is too high, causing the rider to reach for the pedals. To be sure that the saddle is not too low, it should be run up until the pelvis starts to rock and then should be slightly lowered.[140]

Another method often used to measure saddle height is the crotch-to-heel measurement.[36] One-hundred-nine percent of the cyclist's inside leg measurement is transposed along the tube from the pedal surface to the top of the saddle. The 109% value serves as a starting point. The saddle is then lowered a bit, and the cyclist keeps it at this height for about 150 km (100 miles). A mark is placed on the post, and the saddle height is changed again. Eventually, the most comfortable position will be found, and the saddle height is set at this point. This method may, however, result in the saddle's being placed too high.

Knee pain frequently occurs from pushing too hard in high gears. Many cyclists have their saddles too high and are unable to pedal fast enough because they cannot reach the pedals. Instead of spinning, they end up pushing gears that are too high. Ideally, cyclists maintain the same revolutions per minute in different gears. Bicycle tour riders may strive to maintain an 80-per-minute cadence.

A cyclist's knee pain may often be relieved by a slight change in the saddle height, thus altering the contact points on the patella. Even a 2.5 cm (1 in) change of saddle height, up or down, alters the action of almost every muscle in the lower extremities involved in pedalling. For this reason, the saddle must be adjusted carefully to avoid knee soreness.

Proper adjustment of the saddle on a stationary exercise bicycle is as important as it is on a touring bicycle. This is evident during bicycle ergometer graded exercise testing of noncycling subjects, when quadriceps muscle soreness sometimes prematurely ends the test. A proper saddle height adjustment before the test begins will avoid the problem.

Faulty placement of the feet on the pedals or incorrect cleat placement may stress the knee. The cyclist's toes should point slightly medially. Medial knee pain may result when the foot is turned out, and lateral pain occurs if the foot is pointed in too far.[36]

Proper cleat placement may be determined by having the cyclist ride a good distance in his new shoes so that an impression of the pedal forms on the bottom of the shoe. The cleat is then aligned to this impression to orient the shoe properly. Although the cyclist's tibia rotates in when the knee is flexed and rotates out when the knee extends, the cleats do not hinder this movement, since flexibility at the ankle and foot adapts to these movements.

Cyclists tend to think like runners. Just as runners often wear shorts at air temperature of 10°C (50°F), so do some cyclists, overlooking the wind-chill factor. Shorts should not be worn until the temperature reaches about 18°C

to 21°C (65°F to 70°F). When the temperature drops to −7°C to −1°C (20°F to 30°F), the wind-chill factor on a bicycle is 0° to 10°, making long underwear obligatory. When a cyclist pedals home on cool evenings, he should wear a cut-off wool sock around each knee to keep them warm. Cyclists should stretch before cycling, just as runners stretch before running.

Knock-knees, bowlegs, and foot pronation cause knee stress in cyclists, and these problems must be balanced with shims or orthotic devices in the shoes or with shims affixed to the pedals. A bowlegged cyclist's lateral knee pains may be eliminated by building up the lateral side of the pedals, and medial ligament pains may be relieved by building up the medial side of the pedals or by adding arch supports to the shoes.

The Knee Extensor Mechanism

Quadriceps Tendon Rupture

Quadriceps tendon rupture is most likely to occur in an older athlete with a degenerated tendon.[32] Soreness often precedes the quadriceps tendon rupture, and in this phase the athlete's activity level should be reduced and a gentle quadriceps cryotherapy stretching program begun. If the athlete is taking inflammatory drugs, he must not be allowed to use the affected part in training or competition during the course of treatment, as the drugs mask pain. Steroids should not be injected into or about this major weight-bearing tendon[59] because they will mask pain and may cause collagen necrosis, which can weaken the tendon.

The quadriceps tendon usually ruptures when the knee is flexed to about 90° and is subjected to abnormal stress, as when an older athlete slips on sand or leaves on an unswept tennis court or the Olympic-style weight lifter does a split in the clean-and-jerk.

Although it is a major injury, quadriceps tendon rupture is sometimes overlooked. Initial x-ray films may fail to show a fracture; an athlete's knee may then be wrapped, only to give out a day later. Careful examination will pre-

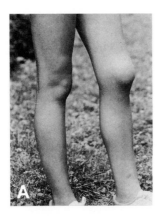
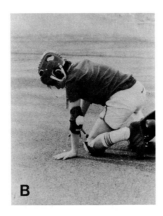
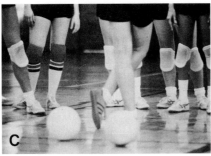
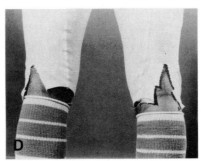

FIG. 15-9
Prepatellar swelling may be quite marked (*A*). Knee pads (*B, C*) may prevent such damage. If, however, a player's football pants are too tight and he cuts them (*D*), the knee pads will slide up and lose their protecting value.

vent such delays in diagnosis. The examiner should feel for a gap above the patella and test for knee extension. X-ray films may show a low patella, and occasionally a fragment of bone is seen to have avulsed from the superior pole of the patella.

If a quadriceps tendon rupture occurs, the tendon is reattached to the patella through drill holes, or the avulsed fragment of bone is replaced on the patella and the rest of the tendon attached through drill holes. In recurrent or old quadriceps tendon ruptures, some of the proximal tendon is reflected distally and incorporated into the repair.

Postoperatively, a major goal is to restore the fullest flexion to the knees without damaging the repair. Full flexion is especially important to collegiate and free-style wrestlers, rodeo cowboys, and hockey defensemen, who must drop their knees into acute flexion. A

bicycle is used in rehabilitation, and the contract-relax stretching method usually obtains further flexion. In this technique, the athlete first contracts his quadriceps isometrically against resistance, then relaxes as the trainer passively flexes the knee.

Prepatellar Bursitis

Inflammation and swelling of the prepatellar bursa may follow a single blow to the kneecap from a lacrosse stick, or when the athlete lands on synthetic grass that rests on asphalt (*see* Fig. 15-9A). Repetitive rubbing of the knee in collegiate or free-style wrestling sometimes inflames the bursa. The prepatellar region becomes puffy, and flexion of the knee decreases as the skin becomes tense over the tender, swollen bursa.

The prepatellar bursa may also become infected from a "turf burn," as "green dust" is ground into the abrasion.[71] An acutely or chronically inflamed prepatellar bursa may occasionally be contaminated from an overlying infected artificial turf burn. In such cases, the red, inflamed, and contaminated bursa may be hard to differentiate from an abrasion with cellulitis.

An inflamed prepatellar bursa usually is aspirated and an elastic wrap applied. If the needle is placed into the bursa through cellulitis, however, the bursa may become infected. Thus, if cellulitis is suspected, warm, moist packs should be placed around the knee, the knee immobilized, and antibiotics started. The knee must then be systematically reappraised to arrive at a precise diagnosis.

To prevent prepatellar problems, an athlete may smear petroleum jelly on his legs to ease a slide on artificial turf. Knee pads should be worn when repetitive knee contact is anticipated on hard surfaces or in tackle football, where forces on the prepatellar area are increased by the weight of other players piling on.

The most widely used knee pad is flat and fits in the front knee pocket of the pants. Basketball players use an elastic sleeve with a flat insert. The pads should be large enough to cover the knee region, and athletes should not be allowed to cut them down for any reason.

The athlete's pants must be long and tight enough to prevent the knee pads from sliding. Newer stretch materials allow players to select pants as tight as may be comfortable, but sometimes pants are too short, and the patellar area is exposed as the knee pads ride up. This causes the pants to become too tight in the popliteal region, and when the player cuts the back of the pants the knee pads flop around.

Subluxation of the Patella

During the pushoff phase of a side-step cut, extension and valgus forces act on the knee of the planted leg. The kneecap may then slide out laterally, especially in a female athlete who has a weak vastus medialis obliquus or a high insertion of this muscle. Many female athletes have a wide pelvis and anteverted hips, a shallow femoral groove and a flat lateral femoral condyle, a high-riding and flat patella, and ligamentous laxity with recurvatum and externally rotated tibias, all favoring subluxation. However, the male athlete may also sublux his patella with hard cuts. In the past, this condition was often overlooked in male athletes, resulting in unnecessary meniscectomies.[47] In younger athletes, the sliding often disappears as the sulcus deepens and the shape of the patella changes as the bones mature.

The athlete with subluxation of the kneecap reports "catching," "giving way," and medial knee pain, a symptom complex that resembles that of a medial meniscus tear. The laterally sliding patella causes pain by tugging on and tearing the medial capsular structures. On examination of the seated athlete, the kneecaps sometimes point laterally like "grasshopper eyes," often with more mobility than is normal and occasionally more proximal than normal. To ascertain whether the kneecap is abnormally high (patella alta), the athlete should sit with his knee flexed to 90° over the edge of the table. If his kneecap faces upwards, it is high, if it faces straight ahead, it is at a normal level. The Q angle, the angle that the patella tendon makes in reference to the long axis of the thigh, is usually more than 15°; however, a large Q angle is not diagnostic of subluxation, as even Q angles of more than 20° may not be associated with subluxation. The dynamic Q angle is found by flexing the knee to 30° and rotating the tibia externally. It is more significant than the static Q angle because it shows what happens when the athlete cuts.

The sunrise x-ray view of the knee is very helpful because it yields a tangential view of the flexed knee that shows the intercondylar sulcus, the shape of the lateral condyle, how the patella sits in the sulcus, and whether it is in a tipped position. The view may be taken with the athlete supine and his knees flexed to 30°.[91] The cassette is placed proximal to the knees and the x-ray tube positioned between the ankles, or the film may be put in a cassette holder distal

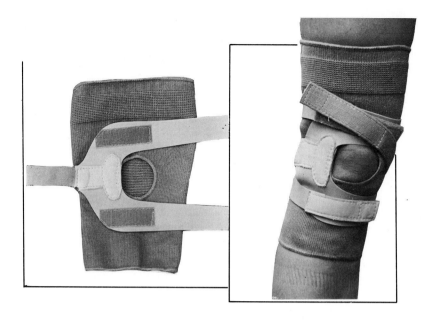

FIG. 15-10
The dynamic patellar brace is a diagnostic and therapeutic aid.

to the knees and the x-ray tube positioned proximally. If the knee is flexed more than 50° to 60°, the patella shifts away from the femur. The intercondylar sulcus may also be viewed with the athlete prone and the cassette placed under the knee with the tube positioned near the toes.[47] Although this technique is commonly used, it necessitates placing the cassette at a distorting angle, and the patella is artificially pressed into the sulcus. Instead of a set angle for the x-ray, several angles of flexion are better, including the angle of flexion where the athlete has pain.

The treatment of patellar subluxation ranges from exercises, orthotics, and braces to operative ligament releases and reconstruction of the knee. Since a youngster may outgrow the problem, the quadriceps should be strengthened and balanced with the hamstrings, and the quadriceps, hamstrings, and gastrocnemius should be stretched for flexibility. The feet of an athlete whose patella is subluxing should be checked. Excessive pronation prolongs the stance phase to allow translation of the patella. A lightweight orthosis or shoe wedge will serve to limit pronation and reduce sliding of the patella.

Recurvatum of the knee reduces the buttressing action of the lateral femoral condyle; a felt pad may be used as an external buttress. A neoprene knee sleeve that contains a buttress pad is more effective than wrapping the felt pad on with an elastic wrap, since a wrapped-on pad often slips. A dynamic patellar stabilizing brace is preferable to these padding methods.

Dynamic Patellar Stabilizing Brace

The effectiveness of the padding methods used to prevent lateral sliding of the patella is inconsistent because the pads are hard to maintain in a functional position during activity, are bulky and uncomfortable, and sometimes cause skin problems. A dynamic patellar stabilizing brace has been developed to overcome these deficiencies.[114] The brace is consistently effective throughout the full range of knee motion, is comfortable, simple to use, available in various sizes, and inexpensive. It applies an active, medially displacing force to the lateral border of the patella and improves patellofemoral seating while maintaining constant pressure during flexion, extension, and rotation.

The brace consists of an elastic sleeve with a patellar cutout and two circumferentially wrapped "live" rubber arms that apply dynamic tension to a crescent-shaped lateral patellar pad (Fig. 15-10). The arms are contoured and directed so as to avoid patellar tilting and irritation of the popliteal area. An elastic circumferential counterarm maintains the pad in proper position, preventing the brace from rotating. Each of the arms is attached by a Velcro fastener. A simple measurement for the dynamic brace is made by measuring the circumference of the athlete's knee at the kneecap, 7.5 cm (3 in) above it and 7.5 cm (3 in) below.

The dynamic brace may be used for the diagnosis, treatment, and rehabilitation of the athlete who has a subluxating patella. Its effectiveness is tested by asking the wearer to perform the activities, such as sidestep cuts, that would ordinarily cause knee pain or instability. If the brace relieves the pain or improves stability, patellofemoral dysfunction is suspected. Early use of this brace during patellofemoral development may improve patellar posture and prevent irreversible soft tissue and skeletal changes. By the time the skeletal structures mature, the subluxation may have ceased. The brace also allows skeletally immature youths who will need surgery to participate in athletics until they reach maturity and until a distal realignment is possible.

The brace can be used therapeutically to prevent contracture of the lateral retinaculum and deters stretching of the medial retinaculum, thus simulating the effect of a lateral release. It may even afford permanent relief and obviate the need for surgery. Such surgery is reserved for those athletes who do not respond to a trial of dynamic patellar bracing and vastus medialis rehabilitation. After a realignment operation, use of the brace may reduce the stresses on the realigned structures. The brace can also be used to alleviate patellar tendinitis, tibial epiphysitis, and localized chondromalacia patella. In these conditions, it acts to diminish stress on the patellar tendon and on the tendon's insertion. The brace also seems to alter the pathologic contact points of the patella, thus decreasing symptoms from localized chondromalacia patella.

Operations for Patellar Subluxation

An athlete with a recurrent painful patellar subluxation may need an operation if the quadriceps is unable to overcome the lateral capsular ligaments, especially the patellofemoral ligament that tethers the patellar laterally. The lateral tilt test may be used to check for tight lateral structures. In this test, the knee is first flexed to 45° over the examiner's knee, the examiner then uses both thumbs to push the patella medially in an attempt to seat it in its groove. If this cannot be accomplished, the lateral side is considered to be tight, and a lateral retinacular release is indicated.

When planning a lateral release, the surgeon should first assess the articular surface of the patella and analyze patellar tracking arthroscopically. If the medial facet of the patella shifts too far laterally and is soft, the surgeon makes a short skin incision lateral to the patella, dissects below the subcutaneous tissue with scissors, makes a nick in the capsule into which he inserts a straight meniscotome, and passes the meniscotome distally, lateral to the patella tendon, to release the tight lateral ligaments. He then dissects superiorly with scissors, severs the vastus lateralis tendon insertion into the patella, and continues the incision in the quadriceps 5 cm (2 in) proximal to the patella. A hemarthrosis may complicate this procedure owing to bleeding from a severed superior geniculate artery. To reduce the incidence of this complication, the surgeon may place a foam pad over the line of incision and insert a drain through a superomedial portal, removing it on the second postoperative day.

A more extensive reconstruction may occasionally be needed to correct lateral patellar subluxation, especially in athletes with ligamentous laxity or when a lateral release has proved ineffective. Reconstruction includes a lateral release, examination of the joint interior, advancement of the vastus medialis obliquus, reefing of the anteriomedial capsule, and transfer of the pes anserinus into the medial side of the patella tendon (*see* Fig. 15-11). This operation must be a meticulous one on the dynamic knee mechanism, for if the vastus medialis obliquus is advanced too distally the patella will rotate. After reconstruction, the athlete's pes is trained by conscious use during cuts to reduce the Q angle and prevent lateral patellar slide.

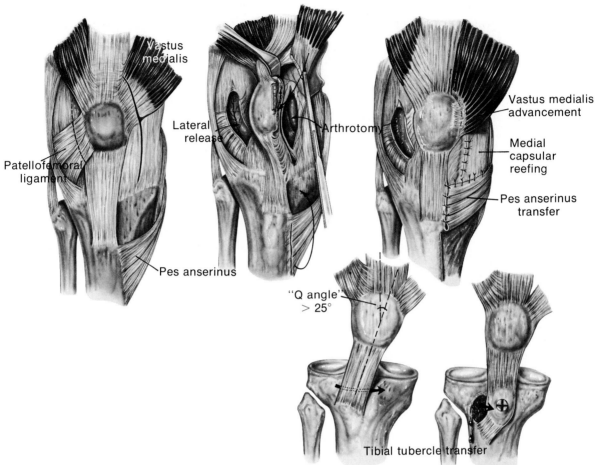

FIG. 15-11
The extensor realignment comprises a lateral release, arthrotomy,
vastus medialis advancement, medial capsular reefing, and pes
anserinus transfer. If the Q angle is greater than 25°, the tibial tubercle
is transferred medially.

Dislocated Patella

During a sidestep cut or while swinging a baseball bat, an athlete may suppose that someone
has struck his knee or that it has been hit by
the ball. What has happened is that as the quadriceps has contracted with the knee in valgus,
the kneecap has completely pulled out of its
sulcus, causing it to lodge laterally to the lateral
femoral condyle, locking the knee in flexion
(Fig. 15-12).

To reduce this dislocation, the hip is first
flexed to relax the quadriceps and the knee then
gently extended to effect reduction. To enhance
the ease of reduction, a local anesthetic may be
injected around the kneecap and into the joint.
Gentle reduction is important to allow the
kneecap to relocate without chipping off bone
or damaging articular cartilage. As the kneecap
snaps back into the intercondylar sulcus, the
lateral femoral condyle occasionally fractures,
or a medial patellar facet may be chipped off.
For this reason, the knee should be x-rayed
after reduction and checked for chips. Chips

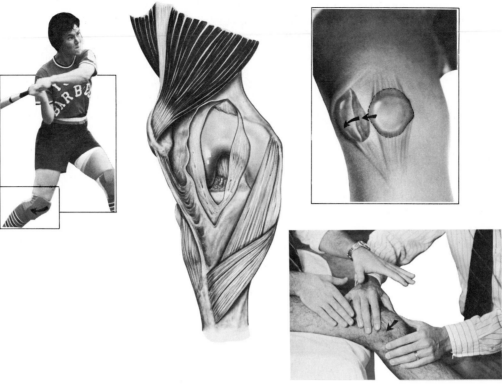

FIG. 15-12
A batter's patella may dislocate laterally during a swing, ripping the
medial capsule. To test for an unstable patella, the examiner presses it
laterally. The athlete reaches down apprehensively, feeling as if his
patella is once again dislocating.

should be replaced if they come from the buttressing area of the lateral femoral condyle or
from the medial facet of the patella.

The knee can be aspirated if it is moderately
swollen after reduction of the dislocated kneecap; this prevents further ligamentous laxity
and allows the athlete to initiate an effective
quadriceps strengthening program. He then
wears a cast for 5 weeks while starting an intensive rehabilitation program. Some surgeons
recommend acute reapproximation of the torn
capsular structures to avoid future laxity.

An athlete who has suffered recurrent dislocations of the patella may show apprehension
as the examiner presses the patella laterally to
simulate an impending dislocation. The athlete
with recurrent dislocations of the patella usually

benefits from an extensor mechanism reconstruction.

"Runner's Knee"

"Runner's knee" is a general term referring to
pain around the front of a runner's knee. Such
pain may be anteromedial, anterolateral, or behind the kneecap. Anteromedial pain may result from excessive pronation of the foot that
has a distant effect of stretching the medial knee
capsule. Anterolateral pain may result from
limited pronation with jamming of the foot and
spraining of the lateral knee capsule. Pain behind the kneecap is common in downhill running, when the runner's quadriceps tension in-

creases to keep the femur from displacing forward; however, these strong contractions also increase the patellofemoral contact forces.

Tight hamstrings, tight heel cords, and foot pronation are three factors that predispose the athlete to runner's knee.[70] The athlete's quadriceps must work hard to overcome tight hamstrings, and this increased force jams the patella against the femur. Tight heel cords mean that more knee flexion is needed to make up for the lack of shock-absorbing dorsiflexion at the ankle. Foot pronation allows the patella to translate, or shift in a horizontal plane, since the foot remains in the stance phase longer. Increased translation also accompanies congenital extensor mechanism malalignment or quadriceps muscle weakness.

Articular cartilage receives its nutrition by a diffusion of nutrients, which is enhanced by a compressive, milking action. Pressure stops absorption of nutrients into the deeper layers of the cartilage, and release of the pressure then allows an inflow of nutrients. The cartilage functions well in compression, but translation causes shearing, as in the side-to-side use of a pencil eraser. Whether caused by foot pronation, congenital malalignment, or muscle weakness, translation of the patella produces a pathologic state of articular cartilage softening or chondromalacia of the patella.[50]

Since articular cartilage is devoid of pain nerve endings, it remains unclear how the pain in chondromalacia of the patella is generated. Perhaps shearing action affects nerves in the subchondral region or cartilage waste products, lysosomes, and proteoglycans may irritate the synovium to produce the pain.

Chondromalacia of the patella may precede osteoarthritic change, but the anatomic location of the two conditions differs. The former condition is most often found near the median ridge, where the patella cartilage is thickest, and on the medial and lateral facets. In contrast, osteoarthritis first appears on the least frequently contacted area of the patella, the "odd facet" at the most medial side of the patella, which contacts the femur only during a full squat.

An athlete with chondromalacia of the patella is likely to describe pain that began or increased with downhill runs. The pain reappears during the descent and rising phases of a squat, in contrast with a meniscal tear, where the discomfort is mostly at the bottom of the squat. The examiner flexes and extends the athlete's knee, feeling for crepitus (Fig. 15-13). He then flexes the knee to 30° and places his thumbs on the lateral border of the patella. The patella is then pushed medially while being pressed into the femoral groove with the fingers. This maneuver is painless in a normal knee but hurts in one with chondromalacia. The common test of asking the athlete to contract his quadriceps while the examiner holds the patella in a distal position should be abandoned, as this test produces too many painful false-positive reactions when the sensitive synovium is trapped and pinched. Defining the area of chondromalacia by having the athlete load the knee with a slow deep bend and report when pain is felt is a better test. The examiner can also test the knee for retropatellar pain in an unloaded manner by having the athlete lie on his back, flex his hip to 90°, and then flex and extend his knee.

Runner's knee is sometimes cured by correcting abnormalities of the foot, changing training techniques, and stretching out tight structures. Flexible orthoses or wedges built into the training shoes and into everyday shoes will limit abnormal pronation, and foam rubber inserts absorb shocks and alleviate the lateral knee pain from cavus feet. The runner should avoid crowned roads and indoor banked tracks and omit downhill runs until his hamstrings and heel cords are loose.

It is very important to advise runners to stretch out their hamstrings to reduce the load on the quadriceps and the resulting patellar pressure. Heel cord flexibility will also lessen the need for shock-absorbing knee flexion and pronation of the feet.

An infrapatellar knee brace or strap, snugged over the patellar tendon, will occasionally relieve the pain behind the runner's kneecap.[76] The brace acts to displace the patella upwards and slightly anterior, altering patellofemoral

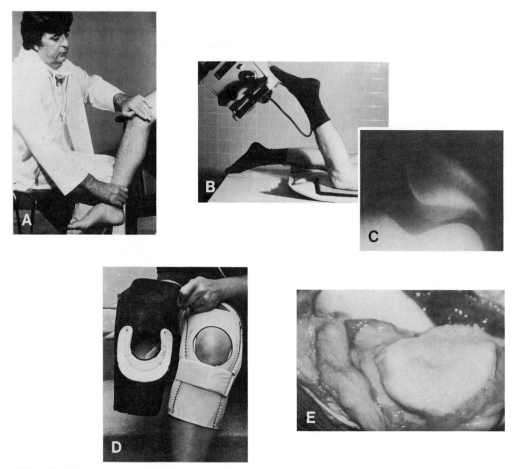

FIG. 15-13
Patella-tracking is assessed as the examiner flexes and extends the
athlete's knee (A). A "sunrise" x-ray view (B) may show "tilting" of the
patella (C) and any abnormalities of its facets or of the femoral groove.
A felt horseshoe pad (D) may prevent abnormal sideways movement of
the patella. At operation, the articular cartilage of the patella may be
soft and fibrillated (E).

relationships without impeding patellar mobility.

The rehabilitation program for an athlete with chondromalacia of the patella comprises four phases.[24] In phase I, symptomatic control is gained by activity modification and taking salicylates regularly. The athlete takes 600 mg of aspirin four times a day to arrest cartilage degradation by inhibiting proteoglycan synthesis and cathepsin.[122] Crutches may be needed until the knee pain abates. In phase II, strengthening exercises begin, starting with isometrics for the quadriceps and isotonic exercises for the hamstrings. When weight lifting is begun on a knee table, it is performed in the ranges where there is no knee pain. If the athlete has pain throughout the range of motion, resistive exercises only in full extension should be done. The first 30° usually are pain-free because the patella does not seat itself in the femoral groove until this point is reached. In phase III, the activity phase, a graduated straightahead running program begins. The program is initiated when symptoms are under control and the athlete is lifting a predetermined weight calculated from his sound side strength. Cuts, hard stops and starts, jumps, and figure-eight runs are added when the athlete has reached the weight goals. In phase IV, the athlete follows a maintenance program of resistance exercises, two or three times a week.

The soft, fibrillated articular cartilage behind a runner's kneecap may be easily shaved arthroscopically. A patellar shaving device with blade and vacuum is used for this procedure and the athlete is soon able to return to running.

A reconstructive procedure may be needed in athletes with extensor mechanism malalignment. If at surgery the cartilage surface of the patella is soft, fibrillated, or has a "crab meat" appearance (*see* Fig. 25-13E), the surgeon should remove any pieces of cartilage likely to slough and form loose bodies. Even though the surface looks smooth, the deeper layers of cartilage may have degenerated and separated to produce a "blister" effect. The shaving should not be done too deeply, as often only soft cartilage is met and the bone may soon be exposed. The realignment provided by the knee reconstruction will reduce shearing, and the improved nutrition of the cartilage will enhance its quality.

Arthritis may strike an athlete's patella, and if the odd facet is painful and badly arthritic it may be resected. When an entire major facet is arthritic and lacks cartilage cover, facet resection is preferable to patellectomy. Replacement of the patella surface with high-density polyethylene is not yet a practical procedure for the athlete.

Bipartite Patella and Patellar Fracture

Occasionally an extra ossification center of the patella may be seen in its supralateral segment on an anteroposterior x-ray film of the knee (Fig. 15-14). This segment is separated from the rest of the patella by a lucent line of fibrocartilage, producing a "bipartite patella," and the extra ossification center may sometimes be lateral or distal. Three percent of the population have separate patellar ossification centers, and 30% of this proportion have bilateral, bipartite patellae.

A bipartite patella may be painful,[139] with pain sometimes arising from direct injury to the knee, or the onset may be gradual. The quadriceps tendon usually attaches to these segments, and mobility in the synchondrosis produces pain. The segment may abut against the lateral femoral condyle or ride over it to contribute to abnormal motion of the kneecap in the intercondylar sulcus, producing chondromalacia. Kneeling hurts, and the athlete's knee-

FIG. 15-14
A bipartite patella may be painful at the fibrous union and may lead to chondromalacia because of abnormal tracking of the patella. At operation, the fibrous union may be separated (*arrows*). Note chondromalacia of the patella at the left of the arrows.

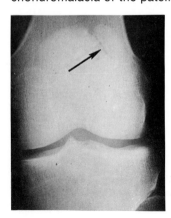 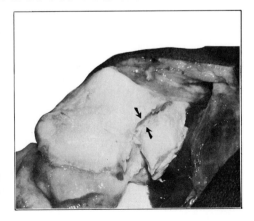

cap may catch. The area of the separate ossification center is tender, and a cylinder cast may be applied; however, if pain recurs and the area remains tender, the segment may have to be resected. A fracture line may pass through the synchondrosis of a bipartite patella, and healing with callus may occur.

The patella protects the femoral condyles. If it is struck by a baseball, for example, a stellate fracture may result. However, because cancellous bone heals quickly, early motion is allowed. Transverse fractures of the patella are not common in athletes, as they usually affect porotic bone. The tendinous extensor mechanism of the athlete will usually rupture before a transverse fracture can occur, and if there is separation or a step-off of the articular surface of a patella fracture, it should be fixed with an encircling wire or pins.

Jumper's Knee

"Jumper's knee" is a patellar or quadriceps tendinitis that results from traction stress[10] when overload produces focal degeneration of the tendon and a tearing of its fibers. There may also be some local circulatory impairment, as in the supraspinatus tendon or biceps tendon ischemia of swimmers. Some athletes also may have an aberrant immunologic response to injury that worsens the condition.

The symptoms of jumper's knee may appear after jumping or kicking, climbing or running, and although the pain may start after only one jump, it more often follows repetitive activities. The aching and tenderness reside just above the patella or inferior to the patella along the patellar tendon.

In the initial phase of jumper's knee, pain appears only after athletics, with no functional impairment.[10] In phase II, the pain occurs during the activity and persists after it, but the athlete is still able to perform at a satisfactory level. Phase III is characterized by pain that occurs during activity and is prolonged afterwards, making it difficult for the athlete to perform at his accustomed level.

To diagnose jumper's knee, the examiner feels for point tenderness near the patella and notes pain when the athlete extends his knee against manual resistance. On x-ray film, a search is made for a lucency in the inferior pole of the patella, a prolonged patellar pole, a fracture or irregularity in the inferior pole, some calcium within the tendon, or an avulsion of bone from the patella. Jumper's knee must not be seen as a benign, limited condition, for it results in some loss of continuity of fibers and then mucoid degeneration, fibrinoid necrosis, and scarred nodules may develop.[123] Soreness sometimes presages rupture of the extensor mechanism if heavy plyometric stress is applied during this period.

To treat jumper's knee in phases I and II, the athlete should warm up his knee before exercise in a warm whirlpool or with warm packs. After exercise, he should use ice massage, an ice towel, or an ice whirlpool. If he is given phenlbutazone, he should not be allowed to exercise against resistance, and he must stop plyometric exercises and running. Local steroids are effective in reducing inflammation and pain but are dangerous, as they act to degrade the collagen in the tendon. Steroids may also mask symptoms so completely that the athlete may overuse the limb, rupturing a major tendon.

A phase III jumper's knee should be rested. If pain persists while walking, curative surgery may be recommended. Granulation tissue and mucoid degeneration occasionally occupies a hole in the distal pole of the patella, a deposit similar to that residing under and in the extensor carpal radialis brevis of a tennis elbow. The material may be scraped out through a longitudinal slit in the patella tendon without otherwise disrupting the tendon. The precise area of tenderness may be located under local anesthesia, but the procedure is ordinarily done under general anesthesia.[123]

Patellar Tendon Rupture

Patellar tendon soreness sometimes precedes a catastrophic major tendon rupture, as the tendon may be pulled from its origin at the inferior pole of the patella (Fig. 15-15). Only rarely will it rupture through its midportion.

In one instance while cinematographic data were being accumulated for a biomechanical

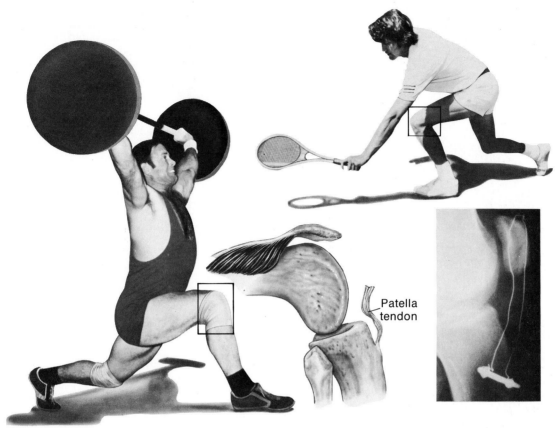

Patella
tendon

FIG. 15-15
The patella tendon may rupture during a plyometric activity with the
knee bent to about 90°. It usually rips from the patella, producing a
patella alta. Wire and bolt are used to reduce tension from the repair.

analysis of Olympic-style weight lifting, the patellar tendon rupture of an American light-heavyweight national champion was photographed.[145] The rupture occurred as he attempted to clean a weight more than twice as heavy as his body. Kinetic analysis of the lift established that when the tendon failed, patellar tendon tension was about 18 times the lifter's body weight and the angle of his knee joint was about 90°.

The best approach to major tendon rupture is a preventive one, since major tears can retire an athlete. Complete warm-up and the purest technique are encouraged, and an athlete with major tendon soreness or who is being treated with an anti-inflammatory medicine should avoid heavy training.

Major tendon tears are operated on early to allow anatomic repair before the tissue swells and weakens. The distal pole of the patella is freshened and the tendon reattached through drill holes. A pin is then placed through the tibia and a wire looped around the patella and attached to the pin to prevent any separation from occurring at the anastomosis (*see* Fig. 15-15).

Rehabilitation after a repair of the patellar tendon, as in rehabilitation after repair of a quadriceps tendon, demands a fine tuning of the flexion program. For athletes such as collegiate and free-style wrestlers, rodeo cowboys, hockey defensemen, and Olympic-style weight lifters, restoration of deep knee flexion is extremely important. Bicycle riding and contract-relax techniques are effective aids in restoring flexion.

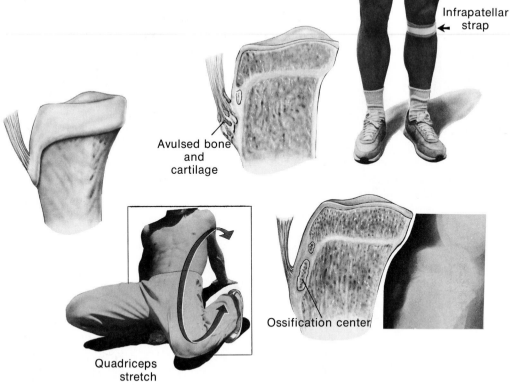

Infrapatellar strap

Avulsed bone and cartilage

Quadriceps stretch

Ossification center

FIG. 15-16
A mature tibial tubercle forms from ossification centers in the epiphysis.
Tugs by the patella tendon may avulse cartilage and bone from the
developing tibial tubercle. This irritation may be prevented by
quadriceps stretching. An infrapatellar strap may take some strain off
the tubercle.

Traumatic Tibial Epiphysitis (Osgood-Schlatter's Condition)

The powerful quadriceps complex inserts into a small area of the tibial tubercle. Sudden contraction of this complex, as in plyometric exercises, may avulse some formative tissue, and the epiphysis may separate, resulting in knee pain at the tibial tubercle and development of the "knee knob" seen in many athletically active youths.

There are four stages of change in the proximal tibial epiphysis during adolescent growth, [95] beginning with the cartilage stage followed by the apophyseal stage. In the latter stage, ossification centers form within a cartilage plate that projects down like a tongue in front of the tibia. The third phase is the epiphyseal, in which the ossification centers fuse

to the rest of the epiphysis. Stage four is closure of the growth plate.

Disruptions at the plate usually occur when girls are between the ages of 8 and 13 years and boys, between 10 and 15 years. At one time boys with tibial tubercle epiphysitis outnumbered girls with this condition, but the ratio is changing as more females participate in athletics.

To diagnose tibial epiphysitis, the examiner observes for tenderness and swelling at the tibial tubercle and for pain when the young athlete extends the knee against his manual resistance. The x-ray picture will depend on the stage of development of the epiphysis. A true lateral view of the tibial tubercle with the knee turned slightly inward should be taken.

In the early stages of tibial epiphysitis, there may be no apparent change except for swelling on x-ray. Avulsed fragments of various sizes can be observed during the apophyseal or epiphyseal stages (*see* Fig. 15-16). These findings are not the main criteria for a diagnosis or for the selection of treatment for tibial epiphysitis. X-ray films of the two knees should be compared. Although the symptomatic epiphysis looks disrupted, the opposite epiphysis will sometimes look the same. Occasionally, the worst looking x-ray changes will be on the asymptomatic side. X-ray films are still important, however, in evaluating traumatic tibial epiphysitis, since more serious conditions may cause pain, tenderness, and swelling in this region.[22] Osteomyelitis and arteriovenous malformations, for example, although uncommon may be found here, and the dreaded osteosarcoma remains a remote possibility.[22]

Ice and compression are used during the acute phase of tibial tubercle epiphysitis, and a reduction of athletic activity will usually allow healing. When the soreness leaves, quadriceps stretching is begun, and a free knee strap can then be worn over the painful region as a counterforce brace (*see* Fig. 15-16). If the young athlete will not slow down, a lightweight cylinder cast may be applied. Local steroids should not be used because these will degrade the tendon. Any avulsed piece of bone seen on x-ray film, or a palpated loose piece, should be removed. Most youngsters will have tight quadriceps from sitting all day in school. To prevent tibial tubercle epiphysitis, they should stretch their quadriceps during the warm-up before practices and games, just as they must stretch heel cords to avoid runner's bumps.

Tibial Tubercle Fractures

When a kick is interrupted by striking an opponent or by catching one's cleats in the turf, the patellar tendon may overpull and fracture the tibial tubercle. There are three types (*see* Fig. 15-17) of tibial tubercle fractures.[138] Type I is an avulsion of the tubercle, and the avulsed piece may be pulled up to the level of the knee joint. A type II fracture is a type III epiphyseal

FIG. 15-17
The tibial tubercle may be partly or completely avulsed. If fully avulsed, it should be replaced and fixed with a screw.

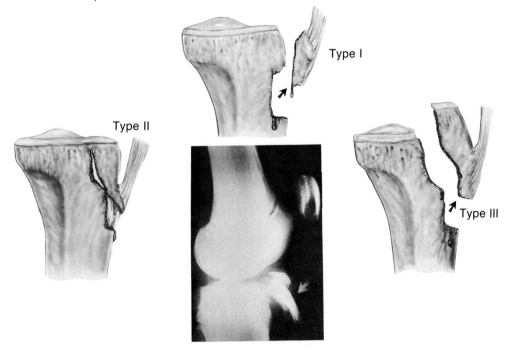

fracture that does not enter the knee joint but allows the tubercle to hinge upward. A type III tubercle fracture is a progression of a type II fracture into the knee joint. Again, the fragment may be displaced proximal to the tibia.

If a tibial fracture occurs during the cartilage stage, there may be no x-ray sign of the condition other than patella alta.[75] The radiolucent cartilage may have been pulled up to the level of the joint, and the young athlete will be unable to extend his knee. Distantly displaced avulsion fractures and displaced type III fractures require reattachment of the piece to its original site.

Lateral Side Problems

The Iliotibial Band Friction Syndrome

The iliotibial band, a thick extension of the fascia lata, is attached to the lateral intermuscular septum and the quadriceps muscle fascia, inserting at the tibial tubercle of Gerdy. With the knee extended, the iliotibial band lies anterior to the axis of knee flexion, and when the knee is flexed the band passes posterior to this axis (Fig. 15-18).

During downhill running, the iliotibial band overrides and rubs on the prominent lateral epicondyle to produce a bursitis, a condition that mostly affects distance runners and some cyclists and skiers. The runner often has bowlegs or has allowed the outer side of his shoes to wear down. The pain starts or is worsened by running on banked surfaces, where overpronation produces obligatory internal tibial rotation. The friction syndrome is less frequent in racquet sports, where running is not continuous.

Flexed-knee activities hurt, and the lateral femoral condyle is tender. The knee creaks, resembling the sound of a finger rubbing over a wet balloon.[121] For diagnosis, the knee is flexed to 90°, and the examiner presses on the lateral epicondyle or 1 cm to 2 cm proximal to it (*see* Fig. 15-18). As the knee is gradually extended, the epicondylar area will become

painful at 30°. The pain may also be produced by having the athlete support all his body weight with his knee flexed to 30°.

The athlete with iliotibial band friction should reduce his training mileage and avoid downhill runs, and the pain can be relieved by walking with the knee straight. An oral anti-inflammatory drug or a local steroid may be given. If the condition fails to respond to these measures, the posterior 2 cm of the band may have to be sectioned across the line of its fibers, leaving a gap over the epicondylar prominence at 30° of flexion.[100]

Popliteus Tenosynovitis

The popliteus muscle arises from the lateral femoral condyle as a pencil-sized, synovium ensheathed tendon. It passes deep to the fibular collateral ligament in a recess that separates the lateral meniscus from the ligament (Fig. 15-19). The tendon also attaches to the lateral meniscus and the fibula to form a conjoined tendon whose muscle belly inserts on the tibia.[73] This muscle assists the posterior cruciate in retarding forward displacement of the femur on the relatively fixed tibia during the stance phase, especially during downhill running.[5] It helps to bring about and maintain internal rotation of the tibia on the femur shortly before heel strike and continuing through three-fourths of the stance phase.[83] This action prevents the lateral femoral condyle from rotating off the lateral tibial plateau. The popliteus also retracts the posterior arch of the lateral meniscus.

Tenosynovitis of the popliteus tendon may produce pain at the lateral side of a runner's knee.[85] The subject will often relate a recent history of downhill work. Overpronation on banked surfaces produces obligatory internal tibial rotation that places more traction on the popliteus, causing backpackers, for example, to report lateral knee pain and a peculiar crunching sound while descending from mountains. Cutting athletes have pain and sometimes describe the same crunching sound during side-step cuts, when the femur is rotated internally on the tibia.

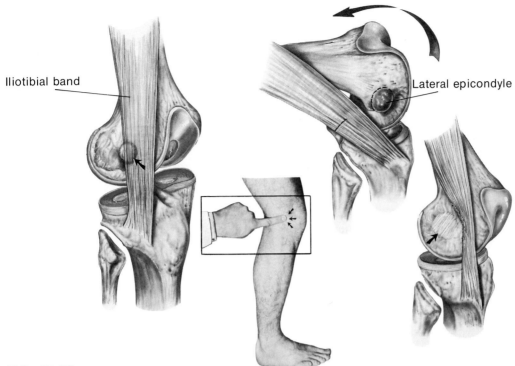

FIG. 15-18
With flexion and extension of the knee, the iliotibial band moves back and forth over the lateral epicondyle. There is tenderness over the epicondyle when the knee is flexed to 30°; the condition may be relieved by sectioning the posterior third of the band and resecting the bony prominence.

FIG. 15-19
The popliteus helps to restrict forward motion of the femur. The tendon is under increased stress and becomes irritated during downhill runs. The figure-of-four position makes the lateral collateral ligament prominent. The tender popliteus tendon lies just anterior to this ligament.

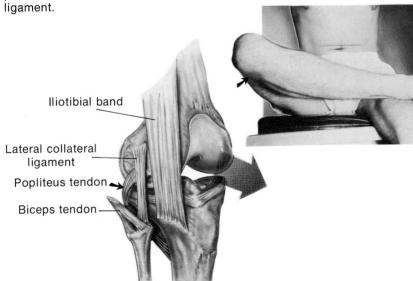

387

To diagnose popliteus tenosynovitis, the examiner should have the athlete sit in the figure-four position with the lateral side of the ankle of his affected leg resting on his opposite knee (*see* Fig. 15-19). This position makes the lateral collateral ligament prominent, and the popliteus may be palpated just anterior to the ligament and above the joint line. The symptoms of this disorder must be differentiated from those of a lateral meniscus tear. The athlete with popliteus tenosynovitis will not report the acute injury, the giving-way, or the locking that is characteristic of a torn lateral meniscus.

Oral nonsteroidal anti-inflammatory medicine may be given to an athlete with popliteus tenosynovitis, or a steroid may be instilled into the bursa about the tendon. If the athlete must run hills, he should run up the hills and ride down; changing the side of the road on which he runs may also help.

The Proximal Tibiofibular Joint

A violent twist, as in water skiing, may disrupt an athlete's proximal tibiofibular joint. The fibula may also be dislocated posteriorly when a rider's knee is caught between a gate or tree and the horse. If there is pain at the proximal fibula, it may also mean a fracture or dislocation of the upper fibula.[113]

The examiner must be especially alert for these injuries, comparing symmetrical x-ray views of both knees. If an athlete develops chronic subluxation or chronic postinjury arthritis of the proximal tibiofibular joint, the fibular head may have to be resected. Care to protect the peroneal nerves must be taken during this procedure.

Intra-Articular Disorders

The Swollen Knee

Immediate Swelling

If an athlete's knee swells with blood immediately after an injury, he probably has rup-tured his anterior cruciate ligament. Other causes of acute hemarthrosis include peripheral meniscus tears, osteochondral fractures, and grade II or grade III collateral ligament sprains. If the injury is a seemingly mild one, a bleeding diathesis must be suspected. Arthroscopic evaluation of the acutely swollen knee allows the surgeon to remove the blood, define the pathology, perform any needed repairs, and provide a prognosis for the athlete. Combinations of injuries are sometimes found, such as when a meniscus tear is associated with an anterior cruciate rupture.

Delayed Swelling

An athlete's knee may be injured and swell slowly to melon size overnight. This delayed swelling may be due to diffuse irritation of the synovium, pinching or bruising of the villi, a meniscal tear, a chondral fracture, or a grade I capsular sprain, causing the synovium to react and produce synovial fluid.

The synovium is a loose arrangement of cells: Some are synthesizing protein and glycosaminoglycans, while others are phagocytes.[125] It is highly vascular with many nerve endings, although most nerve endings at the knee are in the capsule. A knee normally contains only about 1 ml of synovial fluid. This fluid sweeps over 28 cm² (43 sq in) of synovial surface to lubricate the joint and also provides nutrition for the articular cartilage and the fibrocartilaginous menisci. Because synovial fluid does not contain fibrinogen, it normally cannot clot.

Diffuse irritation of the synovium and pinching or bruising of the villi cause the synovium to react and produce synovial fluid. Early in a traumatic effusion, the transudation of fluid into the joint is so pronounced that it outruns the hyaluronate synthesizing capacity of the lining cells; thus the viscosity of this fluid is low.

A large knee effusion inhibits quadriceps contraction and makes exercise difficult, resulting in a rapid decrease of quadriceps strength. The moderately to severely swollen knee should be sterilely aspirated to reduce capsular tension and relieve pain. This procedure also

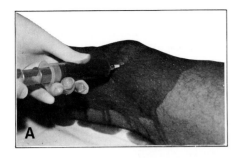

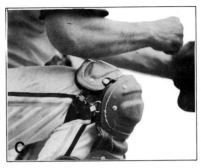

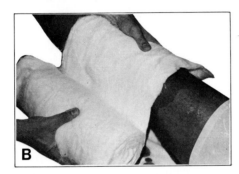

FIG. 15-20
A swollen knee joint may be aspirated with little pain through a superolateral puncture (*A*). The knee is then wrapped with a snug, but comfortable, cotton roll (*B*). Extensions from the catcher's shin guards are now available to protect the suprapatellar area of the knee (*C*).

helps to establish a diagnosis and allows early effective quadriceps exercise.

The athlete's knee is first washed with soap and prepared with iodine, as in a surgical operation. A tiny nick is then made in the skin near the supralateral pole of the patella to avoid carrying a skin plug into the joint with the needle, and an 18-guage needle is inserted through the nick and into the joint (Fig. 15-20). There is usually no need to inject local anesthetic into the skin and capsule because the aspiration causes little pain. After aspiration, the knee may be snugly wrapped in a broad, thick cotton roll for comfortable compression. The wrap is started just above the ankle and continued to the upper thigh; it is reinforced with plaster collateral strips held in place with an elastic wrap. The athlete then uses crutches and starts setting his quadriceps to pump out the remaining fluid, to prevent muscle atrophy, and to give a head start to rehabilitation. On the day after the aspiration, the compressive

cotton roll should be removed and cryotherapy begun.

In a traumatic synovitis, the aspirated fluid is initially clear and straw-colored, but during the aspiration it turns pink as blood from the needle puncture is added. If the fluid is drawn up in a plastic syringe, the walls of the syringe will give it a cloudy appearance. The fluid should be transferred to a clear test tube to allow the examiner to determine whether it is cloudy by attempting to read print through it. Because episodes of gout, pseudogout, or rheumatoid arthritis are sometimes associated with a joint injury, a wet smear should be done when fluid appears abnormal and the sample sent to the laboratory for synovianalysis. A bloody effusion indicates a damaged joint lining and possible torn ligaments. If a fracture enters the joint, fat droplets will be found in the bloody fluid. A hemarthrosis after a trivial injury should alert the examiner to the possibility of the athlete's having a bleeding diathesis.

The Knee Plica

In the embryo, a septum normally separates the suprapatellar pouch from the major part of the knee joint. This usually disappears, but in one of five knees it will persist into adult life as a fibrous band, beginning at the undersurface of the quadriceps tendon just above the patella and extending transversely in this region to insert on the medial wall of the knee joint.[119] The inner edge of the band may be round, smooth, sharp, or transparent. Loose bodies may hide behind it, but it rarely causes snapping or pain.

A medial plica is found in 50% of knees and is clinically more significant. This synvial fold begins on the medial wall of the knee joint, proceeding obliquely downwards to insert into the synovium covering the infrapatellar fat pad. Most plicas, however, are soft and pliable synovial folds that are asymptomatic. A large, thick medial patella plica is like a fibrotic shelf and may produce chondromalacia of the medial femoral condyle and of the medial facet of the patella. The athlete with a symptomatic plica will give a history of medial joint pain, but usually without injury. If injury is reported, it is usually a fall on the knee. The symptoms increase with activity, but the shelf also provokes knee pain when the athlete sits in one position for a while. It may also snap and produce pseudolocking that mimics a torn meniscus. The shelf can be felt and is tender on the thumb roll test, wherein the examiner flexes the athlete's knee to about 40° and rolls his thumb at the medial side of the patella, just above the joint line.

The presence of a shelf may be implicated by an erosion of the medial femoral condyle on the sunrise x-ray view. The outline of a shelf may also be seen on a lateral film taken during an arthrogram. If a medial fibrotic shelf is discovered during arthroscopy or arthrotomy, it should be excised, because mere division of the shelf fibrotic shelf may result in its recurrence.[115]

FIG. 15-21
Osteochondritis dissecans most often occurs on the lateral side of the medial femoral condyle, sometimes resulting in a loose body seen on x-ray that may have to be removed by operation if causing a mechanical problem.

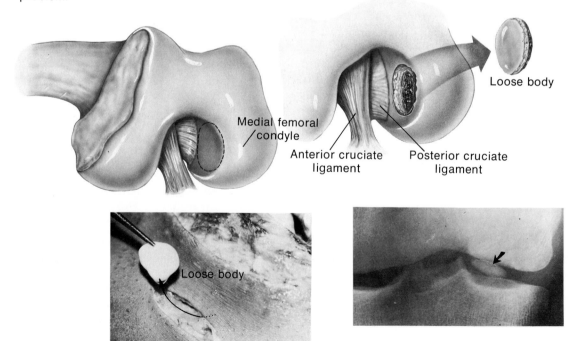

Osteochondral Fractures

When an athlete twists or cuts, falls onto a hard surface, is struck by a hard implement such as a lacrosse stick, or is kicked, a piece of bone with its overlying cartilage may be sheared off. The knee immediately swells, assuming the most comfortable, slightly flexed position. In the older athlete, only a piece of cartilage may be freed, and the subject will usually report that the twist, fall, or blow was accompanied by a "snap." Arthroscopy allows a first-hand assessment of the damage, and any associated lesions, and helps the surgeon to decide whether an operation is needed.

If the loose fragment is ignored, internal derangement and erosion of the joint surfaces is likely, whereas early operation allows easy replacement of the fragment. Pins or small screws may be used to anchor the fragment and may be removed in about 8 weeks.[79] If surgery is delayed, the configuration of the fragment's bed changes, necessitating reconstruction by trimming and using bone chips to produce an even surface. When a fragment has been sheared from the articular surface of the patella, it should be anatomically replaced to prevent fibrous tissue containing new nerve endings from filling in the defect and causing patellar pain.

Osteochondritis Dissecans

Osteochondritis dissecans is a separation of an osteocartilaginous piece of joint surface from subjacent bone (Fig. 15-21). Teenagers and adults with this condition often relate a history of knee injury,[128] such as compression fracture, when the tibial spine jams against the lateral side of the medial femoral condyle. Osteochondritic lesions are most often on the medial femoral condyle near the insertion of the posterior cruciate ligament.[112] The posterior cruciate ligament is a possible culprit, pulling up an osteochondral flap. The defect often extends to the weight-bearing surface, as if the cartilage were on a hinge. In younger children, the defects may be associated with a growth variance resulting from an obstruction to blood flow in the region.

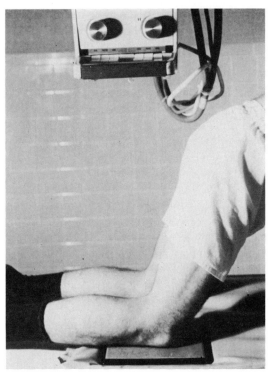

FIG. 15-22
A "tunnel view" of the knee may reveal an osteochondritis dissecans at the lateral side of the medial femoral condyle.

Athletes with osteochondritis dissecans report knee pain, catching, recurrent swelling, and occasionally a mobile loose body in the knee. The defect may often be felt and rocked on the femoral condyle with the knee acutely flexed. To aid in the diagnosis of this condition, the knee should be flexed to 90° and the tibia rotated internally as the examiner slowly extends the knee.[141] At 30° short of full extension, a pain may occur that is quickly relieved by externally rotating the tibia at the same angle of flexion. The pain presumably arises from a lesion of the medial femoral condyle that presses on the tibial spine.

On a tunnel view (notch view) of the knee, the lesion appears as a semilunar lucent line or as patchy bone (*see* Fig. 15-22). Although most of these lesions reside on the lateral side of the medial femoral condyle, others occupy the weight-bearing area of the medial femoral condyle, the lateral femoral condyle, or the patella.

If osteochondritis is diagnosed in a youth's knee, his activity should be limited. A lightweight cylinder cast or a splint may be needed that can be removed for active range-of-motion exercises. The lesion may take as long as a year to heal. In teenagers and adults, the surgeon should examine osteochondritic lesions through an arthroscope to determine the condition of the articular cartilage. If the fragment is stable, he may drill holes through it into the underlying bone under arthroscopic control to stimulate healing.[44] If the fragment is movable in its bed, it should be drilled and pinned. Long pins may be passed through the fragment and into the femoral condyle under arthroscopic control until they are felt beneath the skin. The pins should then be pulled further until they disappear just beneath the surface of the cartilage. These pins are removed readily through a nick in the skin after 8 weeks.[79]

A loose fragment that protrudes above the surrounding weight-bearing surface requires open surgery. The surgeon prepares a bed for the fragment by removing fibrous tissue and "freshening" the defect in the femoral condyle with many drill holes. If the fragment does not fit into the prepared defect, however, the bed should be packed with cancellous bone to make the fragment level with the surrounding joint surface, and the fragment should be secured with pins.

Loose Bodies

When a soft piece of articular cartilage frays off, or when a knee joint injury chips off a piece of cartilage or a chunk of cartilage and bone, the fragment may assume a life of its own, absorbing nutrients from the synovial fluid and growing in size. A loose body may also arise from an osteochondritis dissecans as a freed osteochondral disc. Such a loose body may move about in the joint, becoming a "joint mouse." Pieces of cartilage attached to the synovium receive nutrition through the synovium and sometimes have a bony center. An unattached, freely moving type of loose body, however, acquires a calcified center as it enlarges and its central part degenerates. Loose bodies may also include structures that can catch in the joint, such as synovial chondromatosis, cartilage flaps, and the ends of a torn cruciate ligament.

A loose fragment may cause the knee to catch, click, pop, lock, and give way, and its elusive symptoms may lead to a misdiagnosis of a meniscal tear. Occasionally the athlete can grasp the loose body and show it to the doctor. For diagnosis, x-ray films that include oblique views are taken to track down any loose bodies with bony or calcified centers (Fig. 15-21). The suprapatellar pouch region must be included in these x-rays films because a loose body sometimes finds its way into the pouch and then slips back into the knee.

A loose body may be located by arthroscopy or on an arthrogram. A positive-contrast arthrogram or an air arthrogram is preferable to a double-contrast arthrogram because bubbles may form during a double-contrast arthrogram and be mistaken for the loose body. The object may then be removed by arthroscopic surgery.

An elusive loose body may lodge in a recess, such as the lateral recess, or may hide under a meniscus or glide into the posteromedial part of the knee joint. The fluoroscope can be useful in locating a radio-opaque loose body.

Arthroscopic surgery obviates the need for an arthrotomy to remove a loose body. In this procedure, the skilled arthroscopist examines the knee systematically, and if he finds a single loose body he continues his search because there may be more. The loose bodies are seized with a back-biting "jaws" forceps to prevent them from squirting away. Small loose bodies are usually removed first because larger ones can be relocated to a convenient place, such as the lateral gutter, or stabbed with an 18-gauge needle and retrieved last. The larger loose body is tucked away in this manner because its early removal would generate a "fountain" of saline through the exit wound for the entire procedure.

Intercondylar Eminence Fractures of the Tibia

When a child falls from a bicycle, the anterior cruciate ligament may yank up a piece of intercondylar eminence, causing the knee to hurt,

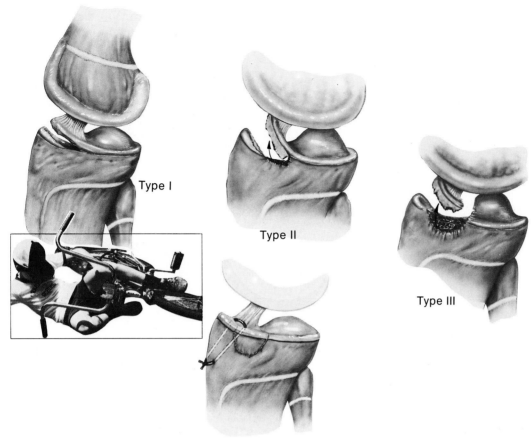

FIG. 15-23
An avulsion of the intercondylar eminence, depending on the type, may
need operative replacement.

swell, and assume a more comfortable flexed position with the hamstrings in spasm.

There are three types of intercondylar eminence fractures (*see* Fig. 15-23):[94] Type I is minimally hinged; type II has a significantly hinged beak of intercondylar eminence; and type III presents a completely displaced, rotated, free-floating anterior cruciate insertion. If a displaced avulsion fracture is overlooked on x-ray films, a serious disability may result, with instability of the knee and a mobile intercondylar piece of bone.

For nondisplaced type I fractures, the hemarthrosis is aspirated so that the knee may be extended. The aspirated blood will contain fat globules, and this type of fracture will heal in an extension cast. When the x-ray film shows a type II fracture, the knee is aspirated and immobilized in extension. These knees must be

handled carefully, as disruption of the cartilage hinge may convert a type II to the dangerous type III. If there is doubt as to whether the fracture should be graded as type II or type III, arthroscopy or an arthrotomy should be done and the piece replaced in its bed. In type III fractures, the fragment is accurately replaced into its bed and sewn in place through drill holes in the tibia.[35]

Meniscal Tears

The bowstring tear and the flap tear are the major tears of the medial meniscus. A young athlete may suffer a bowstring tear when a blow from another player buckles his knee or his foot catches in the turf as he cuts (*see* Fig. 15-24). During such cutting, the meniscus

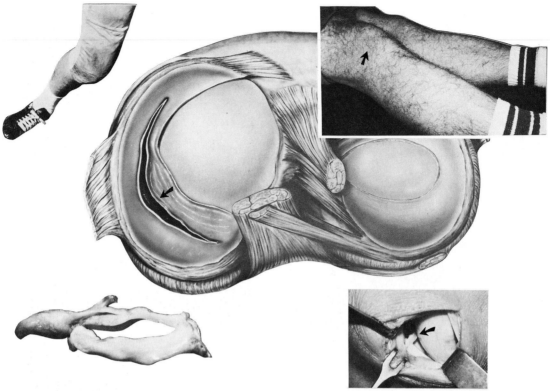

FIG. 15-24
An athlete may sustain a bowstring tear of his medial meniscus while cutting in the open field. His knee is blocked (*arrow*) from full extension by the bowstrung part of the meniscus (*arrow*). The removed meniscus may also have other rents in it besides the major tear.

twists and distorts, the anterior and posterior horns move with the tibia, but the body of the meniscus moves with the femur. The thick femoral articular cartilage drives into the meniscus, shearing it. The split meniscus may then snap back into place or block full extension of the knee joint by catching between the femur and tibia. A shorter bowstring tear may be asymptomatic until a later injury extends the tear to block extension.

In older athletes, posterior horn flap tears are common (*see* Fig. 15-25). Years of friction from the femur and tibia stress the meniscus, and those athletes who must move about in a crouched position, such as baseball catchers or collegiate and freestyle wrestlers, grind the thick posterior horn of the meniscus. The horn has trouble securing nutrients, and mucoid de-

generation occurs in its depths.[128] The underside of a degenerated meniscus may tear loose to form a flap. When this flap catches in the joint, it produces clicking, popping, giving way, slipping, and sliding. The athlete may feel as if he were walking on uneven ground or a plowed field.

Not every torn meniscus produces pain and swelling, as the meniscus itself does not contain pain fibers. If the meniscus catches in the joint, however, it tugs on the sensitive synovium and capsule to produce pain and swelling. Sometimes the torn part of the meniscus will remain in its normal position or flip back into a normal position, with no pull on the synovium and capsule. In such cases, pain and swelling may be absent, even though the athlete has a large tear of his meniscus.

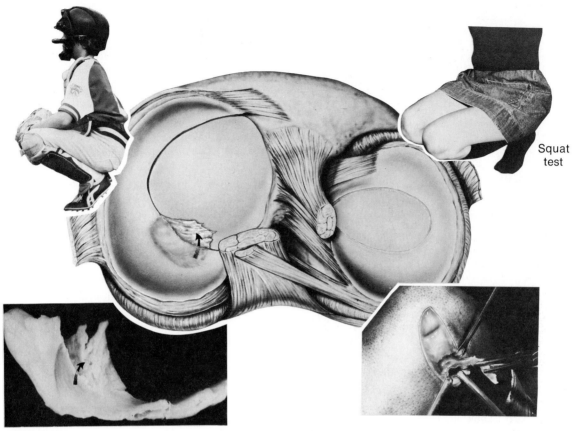

Squat
test

FIG. 15-25
Older athletes may suffer a flap tear of the medial meniscus, usually
following prolonged squatting, such as after a career of catching in
baseball. There is posteromedial knee pain at the base of a deep squat.
The separated flap can flip back and forth, causing intermittent
"clicking," "popping," and "giving way."

The most common tear of the lateral meniscus is a "parrot beak" or oblique tear (*see* Fig.
15-26). During knee rotation, the lateral meniscus does not distort like the medial meniscus, hence it tears less frequently.[73] The pain
from such a tear is usually felt laterally, but a
torn posterior horn of the lateral meniscus may
also produce medial pain.

Diagnosis

To diagnose a torn meniscus, as for any knee
injury, the examiner should ask the athlete,
"How, what, when, where?" Did the knee
twist or give way while cutting? Was there a
sharp pain or tearing sensation? Perhaps the
athlete noted a momentary locking with a quick
recovery of full extension as a bowstring
snapped back into place.

The athlete is asked whether his knee clicks,
pops, or slips. Does he feel as if he were walking on uneven ground? Such symptoms indicate catching of a meniscal flap between the
femur and tibia, particularly if the athlete squats
or changes direction. Giving way may also be
caused by weak quadriceps, a loose body, or
the proprioceptive deficiency that follows immobilization of a knee. The knee should be
x-rayed to ensure that there are no loose bodies
or fracture.

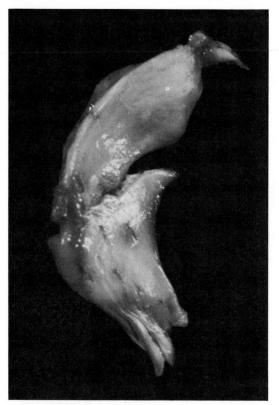

FIG. 15-26
A "parrot beak" tear of the lateral meniscus progressing to a complete transverse tear.

The examiner begins with the athlete sitting with his knee extended. If there is a rubbery block to the last 15° of extension, a freed bow-string may be interposed. The blocking, however, may also be due to hamstring strain or spasm, a loose body, or, in youths, a distal femoral growth plate fracture. The examiner then checks for tenderness over the joint line. On flexion and extension of the knee, the tender spot will move as the meniscus moves. Any tenderness will usually be posteromedial, the site of most tears.

The three main tests for a flap tear are the squat test, the click test, and the grind test. In each of these, the examiner tries to catch the torn meniscus between the femoral condyle and tibial plateau and elicit a click, pop, and pain.

The athlete does a *deep squat* (*see* Fig. 15-25). With a meniscal tear, pain occurs at the lowest part of the squat as the posterior horn is ground between the femur and tibia. Pain that occurs while going down into the squat or coming up from it suggests a patellofemoral problem.

The *click test,* or McMurray test, is performed with the athlete on his back and begins with the knee fully flexed. The examiner's fingers feel over the joint line while the foot is held by the other hand (*see* Fig. 15-27B) The leg is then rotated in an attempt to catch the flap. As the knee is extended, a click may be felt, which at times may be audible. However, any knee may be made to click or pop. A positive click test should bring pain along with the click.

The *grind test* is done with the athlete prone. The knee is flexed and traction applied to the leg, which is then rotated (Fig. 15-27C). This maneuver will usually be painless. Then, with the knee flexed, the leg is pressed down to compress the knee joint and rotated in an attempt to catch the torn meniscus between the tibia and femur (*see* Fig. 15-27D).

Total Meniscectomy

When a meniscal tear is discovered by arthrography or at arthrotomy, some surgeons remove the meniscus totally. A total meniscectomy is, however, not the solution for most meniscal lesions.

A total meniscectomy removes an important shock absorber, increasing the compressive forces on the articular cartilage. The medial meniscus normally carries 60% of the load on the medial side of the knee, and the lateral meniscus carries 75% of the lateral load.[126] If the medial meniscus is removed, the force on the condyle increases threefold. It is normally 15 kg/cm² during walking, but after a totaly meniscectomy the contact area must absorb 60 kg/cm².[97] Further, after total meniscectomy, the semimembranous insertion into the posteromedial capsular ligament and into the posterior arch of the medial meniscus is disrupted, rendering the corner lax and promoting giving-way and a feeling of instability. The integrated motion of the knee is affected, leading to later degeneration.

Whenever possible, these shock-absorbing

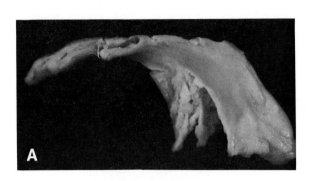

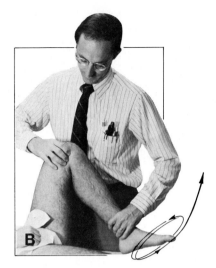

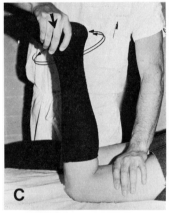

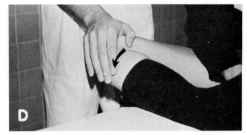

FIG. 15-27
When testing for a flap tear (A), the examiner tries to catch the flap
between the femur and the tibia. In the click test (B), the examiner first
rotates the leg and then extends it. For the grind test (C), he uses
rotation and compression. Sometimes, the pain from a torn medial
meniscus is reproduced when the knee is pressed into varus (D).

and stabilizing menisci of the knee should be
preserved. If, however, the meniscus is badly
torn or totally degenerated, contains cysts, and
has no healthy meniscal tissue, then a total
meniscectomy is indicated.

Selective Meniscectomy

The symptoms of a meniscus tear are mostly
due to the interference of the fragment with
knee mechanics. The offending flap or bowstring of the meniscus should be removed, leaving the healthy part of the meniscus remaining.

Minor splits in a meniscus unrelated to
symptoms should be left alone. In older persons, especially, a tear may be a normal degenerative sign of aging. In a postmortem study of
200 knees from persons averaging 65 years of
age, 60% of the knees had horizontal tears in
at least one meniscus.[101-104]

Only the bowstrung part of a bowstring tear
needs to be excised;[17] operative trauma is thus
reduced, postoperative bleeding is rare, con-
valescence is rapid, and the remaining part of
the meniscus serves a useful function[88]—trans-
mitting about one third of the load of a normal
meniscus across the joint.

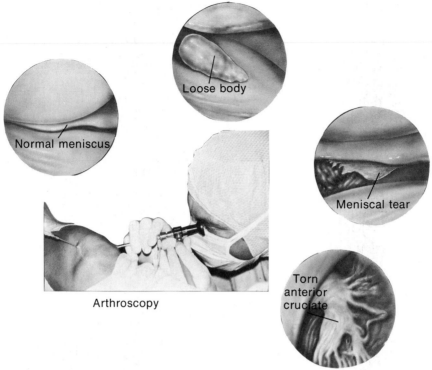

FIG. 15-28
Arthroscopy may provide an accurate diagnosis of knee injury and direct early treatment. Loose bodies, meniscal tears, and torn ligaments may be seen.

Arthroscopy

Arthroscopy enables the sports surgeon to diagnose and treat acute injuries and chronic problems accurately (Fig. 15-28). Under arthroscopic control, he may perform relatively atraumatic surgery using probes, grasper forceps, basket forceps, knives, scissors, and, occasionally, power tools. Arthroscopic surgery has a low complication rate and short rehabilitation time.[23] The arthroscopic surgeon may assess and treat extensor mechanism abnormalities, meniscal tears, and extrameniscal abnormalities, such as fibrous shelves, chondral and osteochondral fractures, osteochondritis dissecans, and loose bodies.

Meniscectomy Techniques

Arthroscopic Meniscectomy Although most procedures on menisci are still open procedures, selective arthroscopic meniscectomy should become the dominant technique as more surgeons acquire the necessary skills. The arthroscope allows the surgeon a better view of the abnormalities, and he may choose the operation to suit the lesion. Flap tears may be removed with great care to ensure that the remaining part of the meniscus is intact, healthy, and stable. After removing a bowstrung piece of meniscus, the surgeon should search for other tears, because 48% of bowstring tears are double-bowstring tears or triple tears (Fig. 15-29).[2] If a bowstring is removed and a tear remains, the knee may continue to catch and to cause pain; it may even lock. Rehabilitation is rapid after arthroscopic meniscectomy, with immediate weight-bearing and few complications. The athlete can usually return to his sport in 2 weeks.

Arthrography If the surgeon is unfamiliar with arthroscopy, he may complement his clinical examination with an arthrogram. When dye is injected into the knee joint, it may leak into a meniscal tear to provide an x-ray diagnosis.[56] Single-contrast and double-contrast arthrography with fluoroscopic and spot film techniques by experienced arthrographers have been up to 95% accurate in diagnosing meniscal tears and slightly higher for the medial meniscus.[31, 33] False-positive arthrograms are rare, but a few false-negatives do occur if a tear cannot be opened to run the dye through it.

To inject dye, the examiner should make a lateral needle puncture and aspirate the knee joint to produce a clear study. Three milliliters of a contrast medium and 30 ml of room air are then injected. If the athlete is allergic to contrast medium, an air arthrogram may be done.[31]

After injection of the dye, an elastic wrap is wound over the suprapatellar pouch to prevent the pouch from filling with contrast material. The subject then walks around with the wrap on to disseminate the dye throughout the joint before multiple views of the knee, stressed and unstressed, are taken under fluoroscopic control.

If the meniscus is intact, no air or contrast material will be seen within the meniscal substance or at its periphery (Fig. 15-30). Any dye that enters the meniscal wedge indicates a tear

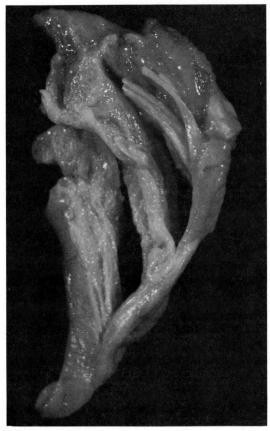

FIG. 15-29
Some bowstring tears of the medial meniscus are actually double bowstrings.

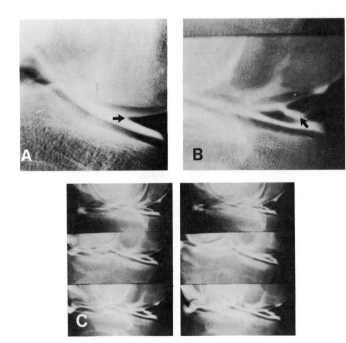

FIG. 15-30
A normal meniscus appears as an uninterrupted dark wedge (*arrow*) on an arthrogram (*A*). An arthrogram of a torn meniscus (*B*), however, shows streaks of dye (*arrow*) within the wedge. An extensive tear is revealed by streaks of dye that invade the meniscus on many views (*C*).

regardless of whether it is a large amount of dye or merely a veiled streak of contrast.

The frequently torn posterior horn of the medial meniscus is easily studied by arthrography. Although arthrography shows whether a tear exists, it is less helpful in depicting the configuration or extent of the tear. The examiner can be misled by recesses in the anterior horn of the lateral meniscus or in the posterior horn of the medial meniscus and dye collections at the popliteal sheath. The recesses are rounded, whereas tears are sharper. Collections of dye around the sheath of the popliteus tendon make posterior longitudinal tears and the common transverse tears of the middle third of the lateral meniscus more difficult to detect. [105]

The medial meniscus is usually wedge shaped, and a tear is indicated if it appears rounded. It is also wider from front to back in most persons. If its width remains the same on each film, a meniscal tear is probable. In some cases, however, menisci are not wider posteriorly, and the arthrographer can be fooled when this condition appears.

Open Medial Meniscectomy When the arthrogram shows a tear and the surgeon decides to remove it because of mechanical symptoms or pain, the knee should be examined under anesthesia and any instabilities noted. The thigh is rested on a triangular bolster so that the knee may be flexed acutely to drop the vital posterior structures out of the way during surgery.

The most common incisions used in this procedure are short anteromedial or short transverse incisions. The anteromedial incision may easily be extended if necessary, but a short transverse incision leaves less scar while affording excellent exposure. Some surgeons use an anteromedial skin incision with one vertical capsular incision anterior to the tibial collateral ligament and another behind the ligament. [11] Others prefer a horizontal skin incision and two capsular ones. [18]

After entering the knee joint, the surgeon searches for a fibrotic medial shelf, examines the articular cartilage of the patella and the femoral condyles, and analyzes the integrity of the anterior cruciate ligament. Both menisci are then examined, since the signs and symptoms of a medial meniscus tear may override those of a lateral meniscus tear. The ligamentum mucosum is pulled out of the way to enable the surgeon to look across the joint to the lateral compartment. This step demands skill and patience; sometimes, a transverse or longitudinal tear of the lateral meniscus may be seen. The medial meniscus is then inspected with a probe.

A posteromedial incision will allow an analysis of the posterior horn, where 75% of medial meniscus tears occur. This incision starts at the adductor tubercle region and extends along the

FIG. 15-31

Open total meniscectomy. The medial meniscus inserts posteriorly into a deep hole behind the intercondylar eminence (*A–C*). During an open meniscectomy, the meniscotome may not cut all of the peripheral attachments of the meniscus (*D*), and the meniscus will appear to be horizontal (*E*) when it is pulled into the notch. The surgeon sometimes is able to sever these remaining peripheral attachments by stressing the knee into valgus and inserting the meniscotome at a different angle (*F*). Once these attachments are severed, the meniscus, owing to its remaining vertical attachment, pops up (*G*). This new vertical position is called the "flip sign." The meniscus is then pulled forward (*H*), and the surgeon knows that only the vertical attachment remains because the meniscus has "flipped" (*I*). The meniscotome now fits easily around the meniscus (*J*) over its insertion into the deep hole, and the meniscectomy may then be completed. Sometimes the surgeon may complete a medial meniscectomy wherein some peripheral attachments remain intact by first cutting the vertical attachment (*K*). The meniscus may then be easily pulled forward on its peripheral attachments, whereupon these are severed. All that is left after a "total meniscectomy" is a thin rim of meniscus and a nubbin of meniscus in the deep hole (*L*).

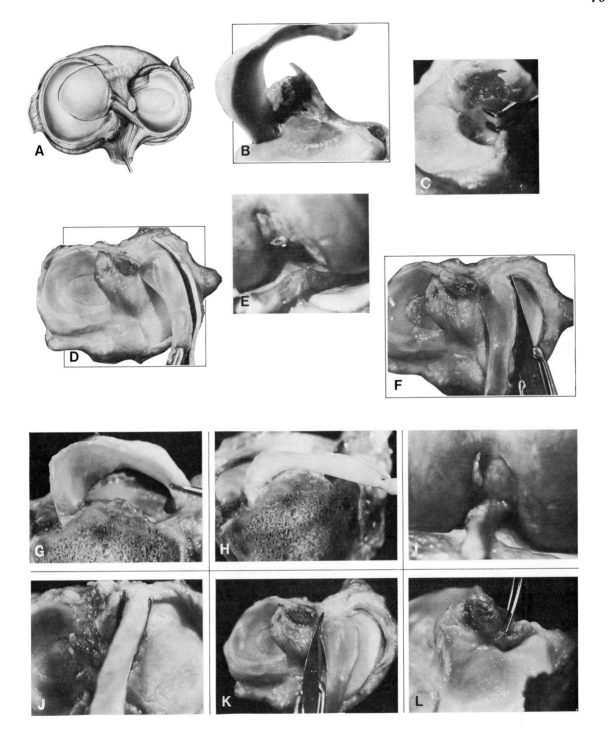

back side of the tibial collateral ligament down to the tibia. The joint is entered through a weak spot, or "back door," between the tibial collateral ligament and the posterior oblique ligament. The meniscus is then carefully separated from the deep capsular ligament, leaving a small rim or coronary ligament to help prevent anteromedial instability. Next, the meniscus is pushed out through the back door, and the meniscectomy is completed under direct vision. Free fragments that might have been left behind if an anterior approach only had been used are sometimes found.

After the meniscus has been removed, the knee is tested to see if the tear has masked any instability. If so, the surgeon must deal with the instability through an extended incision. In this procedure, before the wound is closed, the posteromedial capsular ligament is pulled forward and snugged up to provide a stable knee.[49] This step is very important to the athlete, who depends on a stable knee for cuts, jumps, and stops.

Some surgeons may use an anteromedial incision for medial meniscectomy routinely. The knee is flexed and stressed to allow more of the meniscus to be seen. After the meniscotome has been passed around the periphery of the meniscus, the meniscus is pulled into the intercondylar notch (Fig. 15-31). If it still lies horizontal when pulled into the notch, part of the posterior capsule is still attached. To facilitate removal of the meniscus, the vertical attachment is cut at the deep hole and the meniscus pulled forward on stretched synovium. It may now be removed easily under direct vision.

If the meniscus pops up into a vertical position when transferred to the notch—the "flip sign"—the surgeon knows that synovial attachments already have been severed fully. Only the strong vertical meniscal fibers now hold the meniscus and account for the vertical position. The flipped meniscus may be removed simply by placing the meniscotome horizontal to cut the vertical attachment.

In the knees of some older athletes, an exostosis extends posteriorly from the intercondylar eminence. This restrains the meniscus and keeps it from flipping, and the surgeon may think that the posterior capsular attachment remains. If he presses the meniscus posteriorly, however, it will pop free over the exostosis and may then be removed easily by severing its vertical attachment.

Open Lateral Meniscectomy A lateral meniscectomy is facilitated by acutely flexing the athlete's knee, placing his foot lateral to his opposite knee, and firmly pushing the foot toward his opposite hip, a maneuver that opens the lateral joint space.[12, 13] The meniscus is removed through an incision just anterior to the iliotibial band. Another incision may be made parallel to the popliteus tendon between the iliotibial band and the fibular collateral ligament to view the entire meniscus. Meniscal cysts and tears in the posterolateral corner may also be analyzed through this incision.

Complications of Open Total Meniscectomy The complications of open total meniscectomy may limit the future function of an athlete's knee, with complications such as instability, retained posterior horn fragments, hemarthrosis, infrapatellar numbness, and postoperative arthritis. The knee is checked for instability under anesthesia before surgery begins. After the torn meniscus has been removed, knee stability is rechecked because the meniscus may have been masking an instability.[49] To aid in preventing laxity after a total medial meniscectomy, the posteromedial corner should be advanced.

A retained posterior horn of the medial meniscus may be stable, with no attendant problems, or it may catch and tug the capsule to cause pain. The posteromedial corner should be examined through a posteromedial approach to remove these potentially catching posterior fragments.

Because hemarthrosis is common after an open meniscectomy, all bleeders should be stopped at operation and the postoperatively swollen knee aspirated early to allow effective quadriceps setting. If a painful hemarthrosis follows an open lateral meniscectomy, the surgeon should suspect that the lateral geniculate artery has been cut. This requires an operation to ligate the vessel.

The infrapatellar branch of the saphenous nerve is sometimes sectioned during an open medial meniscectomy, resulting in numbness distal to the kneecap or a painful neuroma. Athletes should be advised that such numbness may occur. Deep friction massage of the scar may prevent neuroma formation and a painful scar. If a neuroma does appear, however, it may be resected.

Half of the subjects will have normal knees after a total meniscectomy, and half will develop varying degrees of osteoarthritis (Fig. 15-32).[132] After meniscectomy at a young age, those who had undergone another arthrotomy were found to have developed cartilage damage within 2 years of the first operation.[30] This arthritic aftermath attests to both instability and increased forces on the bone and cartilage.

The athlete who develops osteoarthritis of the knee after a meniscectomy may have pain and swelling. His knee will feel insecure, and moments of instability will be painful, followed by additional aching. The narrow joint space implies a certain measure of instability, but dramatic improvement results if the athlete wears a helical glide brace.

Postmeniscectomy weight-bearing x-ray films often show compartmental narrowing, subchondral flattening of the distal end of the femur, and peripheral tibial spurring.[28] Valgus deformity often develops after a total meniscectomy in persons older than 40 years of age.[54] These persons should be followed up with weight-bearing x-ray films for early degenerative signs, since valgus proximal tibial osteotomy may add athletic life to the knee.

Discoid Meniscus

A discoid meniscus is one that lacks the normal concavity, instead covering most of the tibial plateau. This disorder is found in children but also may occur in older athletes.[9] A lateral discoid meniscus is the most common type, although a torn discoid medial meniscus may be found in some athletes. The disorder may produce a loud "clunking" at the lateral side of an adolescent female athlete's knee joint. It is more likely than is a normal meniscus to develop intrameniscal degenerative changes, tears, and cysts because it is pushed, pulled, and crimped between the tibia and femur. A meniscal cyst may be felt at the joint line as it becomes prominent with knee extension and recedes with knee flexion.[67]

Arthrography and arthroscopy are excellent diagnostic tools for discoid menisci. With arthrography, the inner border of a discoid meniscus will be seen to reside near the center of the joint.

If pain limits an athlete's activity, the discoid meniscus should be removed; however, discoid menisci are often found in autopsied knees with no history of symptoms.

Reattachment of Peripheral Tears

A peripheral tear of a meniscus may be reattached (meniscorrhaphy) if it is a vertical tear in the vascular region within 2 mm of the meniscosynovial junction, has a limited area of detachment, is accessible, and shows no dye in the rest of the meniscal body. The surgeon repairs such a tear by freshening the capsular bed and sewing the meniscus to the capsule.

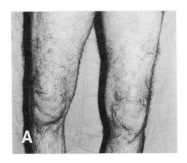
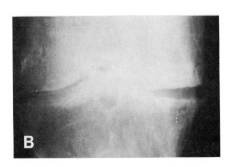

FIG. 15-32
Knee arthritis may follow meniscectomy. In this case, varus deformities (*A*) have followed medial meniscectomies. An x-ray (*B*) shows that the bone is squared-off and sclerotic and the joint space is narrowed.

The athlete wears a cast for 5 weeks and then uses crutches for 2 more weeks. Rehabilitation is similar to that after a ligamentous injury, and the athlete is allowed to run at 3 to 4 months and jump and cut at 6 months.

Postoperative Knee Rehabilitation

The Postoperative Knee Exercise Program

To achieve the goals of restoring muscular strength, power and endurance, flexibility, agility, and cardiovascular fitness after a knee operation, therapeutic exercise is the most important modality (*see* Figs. 15-33, 15-34, 15-35). The athlete should begin isometric exercises before the operation and reinstitute them in the recovery room to prevent a dissociation of quadriceps function and to ensure muscular stability of the joint.[143] Initially 50% contractions are performed for a few seconds before advancing to more forceful contractions, which are held for 6 seconds, 20 times an hour. Pillows are not permitted under the knee, which should be placed out straight while the subject reclines. Next comes active hip extension, with

FIG. 15-33
Postoperative knee exercises. The legs are squeezed against one another at varying angles to strengthen isometrically the quadriceps and hamstrings (*A–C*). The hip abductors and adductors can also be strengthened isometrically by working against hand pressure on the outside and the inside of the legs, respectively (*D, E*).

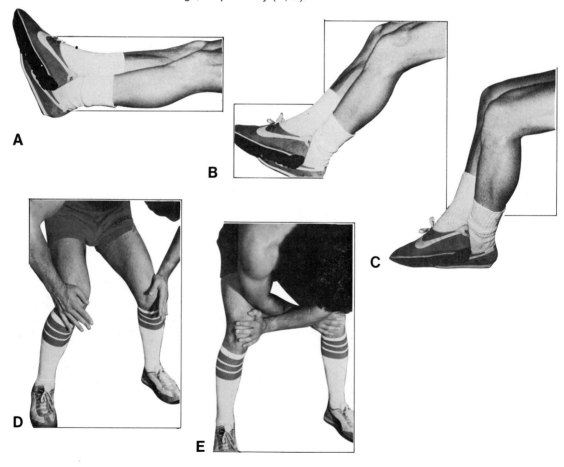

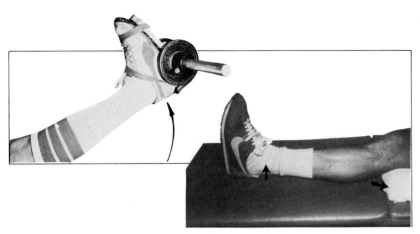

FIG. 15-34
An athlete wears a weight boot for weighted straight leg raises. A pad under the athlete's knee allows him to work on terminal extension of the knee.

the sound foot on the floor while the upper body rests, chest down, on the training table as the hip of the operated side is extended. Hip adductors may be strengthened while sitting by squeezing a basketball between the thighs, and hip adductors may be exercised by abducting the hip while lying on the unoperated side. Ankle flexion and extension and ankle circles will also provide a beneficial calf-pumping action.

Transcutaneous Electrical Nerve Stimulator

Postoperative pain before, during, and after exercise may be reduced by a transcutaneous electrical nerve stimulator (TENS).[37, 124] This is a small battery-powered device that produces a low-intensity electrical current. For hyperstimulation analgesia (*see* Chap. 8), sterile electrodes are placed on the athlete's skin near the incision site. The electrodes are then attached to the battery pack by small cables. The athlete can adjust the electrical intensity, the quality of sensation (pulse width), and the repetition rate, and the unit may be left on for short periods or all day.

The TENS allows the athlete to begin quadriceps setting and straight leg raises faster and more effectively, without excess pain, swelling, and inflammation. There is usually a dramatic

FIG. 15-35
An athlete works his knee against progressive resistance on an isotonic knee table.

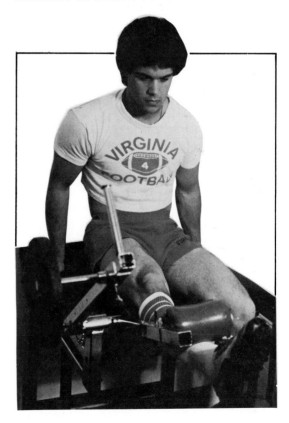

lowering in the need for pain medicines, permitting exercise with a clearer mind and without the side-effects of pain killers. The TENS may also be used for postoperative muscle stimulation, with an electrode pad placed over the vastus medialis. The athlete will be able to perform a heavier progressive resistance exercise program, and his daily activities will be more comfortable. Some athletes have even used the units during competition without apparent harm.

Straight Leg Raise

To assist himself in straight leg raising, the athlete places his sound leg under the ankle of his operated extremity. This technique will often permit an independent straight leg raise on the same day as the operation. A sling is also provided, or the leg may be held up so that the subject can lower the leg eccentrically with his hip flexors. The lowering technique is usually easier than raising the leg, since more eccentric than concentric work can be performed.

Walking

When the athlete can do a single leg lift, he is allowed to walk with two crutches, advancing to a single crutch on the sound side for 2 or 3 days after a week has passed. This aid should be used until he can walk unassisted without limping.

The athlete should never be allowed to limp, as even a slight limp will result in a longer period of rehabilitation. While using a cane or a single crutch, he should be instructed to bear as much weight as possible and to put pressure on the hand grips to prevent a limp. The knee is kept straight and locked when walking, and the athlete should concentrate on heel strike rather than walking flat-footed with his knee bent. He may usually begin jogging when he can lift 20% of his body weight and may run when he can lift 30% of his weight. If he does limp when running, his activities should be reduced.

Isotonics

Since isometric exercises build strength only at the angles used, isotonics are added as supplementary exercises. The whole limb should be exercised. An isotonic hip flexion program will serve to strengthen the quadriceps; the athlete works against a weight resting on his thigh or against a rubber tube held across his thigh. Ankle weights should be avoided because they distract the knee, which normally functions in compression.

The athlete may begin isotonic knee work on the knee table when he has no significant swelling, can flex the knee to 90°, and can straight leg raise 10% of his body weight. Active exercises and gravity, rather than manual force, are used to help him regain knee flexion.

The isotonic knee program is begun by determining the athlete's maximum lift (ML), the maximum amount of weight that he can lift once to full extension on the isotonic knee table. Repetitions start at 50% of the ML. The weight is held at full extension for 3 seconds on each repetition, with the aim of increasing to ten repetitions (Fig. 15-34). When this goal is reached, 1 or 2 more pounds are added. The hamstrings are exercised at 50% of the quadriceps working weight (25% of the quadriceps ML) and are done slowly to prevent momentum from assisting. Strength is gained from a daily workout at first, and as strength gains peak the weight training is reduced to three sets of repetitions every other day. As the athlete gains strength on this program, he may begin endurance and power work. If the knee table is being used for power work, the athlete exercises three times a week, performing three sets of the maximum number of repetitions that can be accomplished with one half of his one repetition maximum (1 RM) in 30 seconds. The exercises are done as forcibly as possible with good form, with 20 second rests between bouts.

Isokinetics

Isokinetic machines assist the athlete in power rehabilitation by allowing him to exercise his knee at fast speeds. The advantages of this type of exercise also include accommodation for fatigue or soreness, elimination of inertia, and a readout of peak torque, endurance, and total work.[11, 39]

Use of isokinetic exercises in later rehabilitation is preferable, as early exercise of weakened structures may produce edema and soreness and set back recovery if the athlete exerts too great a force. Also, the devices do not offer resistance once the joint is "locked out," which would provide a stimulus for strength gains in terminal motion. As the athlete achieves terminal knee extension, he slows down, with the result that outside stimulus is least where it is needed most. The machines also do not provide negative resistance for eccentric contraction.

Because it is a stable position, full knee extension is important. If the athlete has not achieved full extension, walking is difficult and dangerous. Terminal extension is reached by means of a limited arc technique with a bolster under the knee. If the athlete has not regained full extension, the rest of the rehabilitation program proceeds while he works on terminal extension. To avoid a flexion contracture, the leg must be supported at the ankle when the athlete sits.

The Functional Knee Program

The injured athlete may begin a functional knee rehabilitation program when he is performing advanced isotonic exercises, riding a bicycle, and starting isokinetic exercises. A graduated program will lead to the activities needed for effective competition.[8]

The functional program begins with a walk of about 2 miles. If he has no limp or pain, the athlete advances to 1 mile jogs, then walking up and down stairs, and finally jogging up stairs. He does stepups for 5 minutes a day on ordinary stairs before gradually advancing to a 45-cm (18 in) bench. Forty- and 100-yard sprints come later, and by this time, he may begin 5-minute bouts of rope skipping or isodynamic running.

In the final phase of the functional program, the athlete works in noncleated shoes on starts, stops, jumps, rounded side-step cuts, and crossover cuts before advancing to hard 90° cuts and running gradually tighter figure-eights. Defensive backs run sideways, backwards, and perform crossover steps. The athlete is now ready to demonstrate his 40-yard dash speed. Finally, he repeats the last phase in cleats. When functional test results are regarded as normal, the athlete undergoes an isokinetic strength and power analysis and returns to practice.

The Bicycle

The exercise bicycle and lightweight touring bicycle compose an important part of the knee rehabilitation program. The athlete may begin cycling when he has no significant swelling and has achieved 90° of flexion. This activity helps to restore muscular strength and muscular endurance, knee flexibility, and cardiovascular endurance and also strengthens both the quadriceps and the hamstrings. The rider's shoes should be clipped onto the pedals so that he can pull as well as push. Inactivity diminishes the oxidative enzymes in muscle fibers, and cycling stimulates and restores these mitochondrial enzyme systems.[21]

Although a low saddle promotes greater knee flexibility,[20] an athlete unaccustomed to cycling may have knee pain when he is seated too low; the seat will have to be raised for these subjects.

Early in rehabilitation the athlete clips in his sound leg and cycles one-legged.[82] Later, he clips both feet in. An isokinetic exercise bike is preferable to an isotonic one. Although inertia makes an isotonic bicycle easier to pedal, in the event of knee pain, inertia will keep the crank spinning and an injury may result. On an isokinetic bike, resistance accommodates to the force that the athlete applies, preventing inertia injuries.

Bicycle touring offers the injured athlete a pleasant means of restoring his strength, flexibility, and muscular and cardiovascular endurance. Bike rides may be split into three 20-minute periods or may be continuous for 1 hour each day.

Acute Tears of Knee Ligaments

All of the knee ligaments are involved in knee stability, and if a ligament is completely torn other supporting structures are usually damaged too. The examiner should try to gauge the extent of the damage, since early knee ligament repair is superior to later reconstruction. Occasionally, the most severe knee ligament injury does not cause much swelling, as when a tear through the capsular ligament decompresses the knee. If the knee is tense and painful, the capsule probably is intact, and if the knee swells acutely with a hemarthrosis, the athlete probably has torn his anterior cruciate ligament.

An injured knee should be examined before it swells and muscle spasm sets in. If the knee is already swollen and the muscles are in spasm, the knee can be aspirated and some local anesthetic instilled to allow a complete examination. If there is any question about the adequacy of the examination, it should be done under general anesthesia.

Diagnostic aids such as arthroscopy and arthrography are useful in many acute knee ligament injuries.[25, 111, 135] With major ligament damage, however, the instillation of an irrigant fluid into the knee joint must be done carefully because it may lead to further swelling and produce nerve and vascular damage that endangers the limb. An arthrogram is useful for collateral ligament tears during the first 48 to 72 hours, but after this time the joint seals, and dye cannot extravasate beyond the ligament. Arthrograms are not very helpful in cruciate ligament tears because the cruciates are covered by synovium, and a cruciate tear with intact synovium produce a false-negative arthrogram.

Acute Medial Ligament Tear

An acute medial knee ligament tear may be produced by forced abduction of the flexed knee with external rotation of the tibia—the "clipping" injury (see Fig. 15-36). As the knee is twisted, its capsular sleeve shortens to increase the pressure between the tibia and femur and to stop the external rotation. If external rotation stretches beyond this point, however, the medial capsular ligament tears, and the tibial collateral ligament will also tear, especially if a valgus stress is added. After the medial structures have torn, external rotation may continue along with anterior subluxation of the tibia. The anterior cruciate ligament then angles over the lateral femoral condyle and may tear, resulting in a triple lesion including tears of the deep capsular ligament, tibial collateral ligament, and anterior cruciate ligament.

The site of a medial rupture will be tender and swollen locally. The examiner tests for the integrity of the medial ligamentous structures with the athlete supine on the examining table, first examining the sound knee for baseline laxity. The knee is flexed to about 30° and valgus force applied to check the medial side (Fig. 15-37).

A slight opening of the medial side to valgus stress means a medial ligament rupture; a gross test indicates a medial ligament and either an anterior cruciate or posterior cruciate rupture. If the knee opens to abduction stress in extension, the medial ligaments and both cruciates are ruptured. The knee should be examined under anesthesia if the degree of sprain is hard to determine. A young athlete's swollen and deformed knee may be caused by a fracture of the distal femoral epiphysis; thus an x-ray film should be taken before stress tests are performed (Fig. 15-38).

Mild Medial Collateral Ligament Sprain

A mild (grade I) medial collateral ligament sprain indicates microscopic tearing of the ligament fibers without gross laxity. This is the most common knee injury in downhill skiing.[84] The inside edge of a ski catches, leaving the trailing limb with the leg rotated externally and the knee in valgus. As the skier's body continues forward, the medial side of his knee is stressed.

"Breaststroker's knee" is a grade I medial collateral ligament sprain that results from the "whip kick."[60] As the swimmer's knee moves

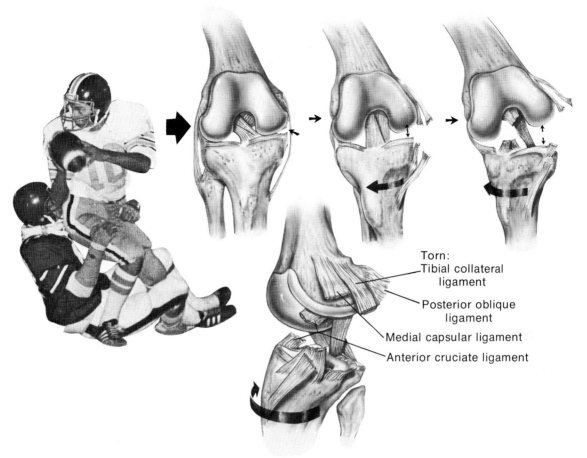

FIG. 15-36
Medial ligament tears. A ''clipping''-type injury applies a valgus force to the knee. First, the medial capsular ligament tears, then the tibial collateral, and, with further force, the anterior cruciate. The medial meniscus and the posteromedial capsular ligament also usually tear during this serious injury.

Torn:
Tibial collateral ligament
Posterior oblique ligament
Medial capsular ligament
Anterior cruciate ligament

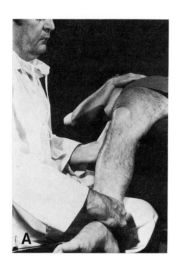

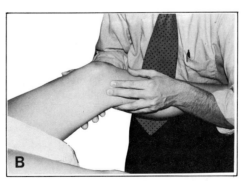

FIG. 15-37
Valgus stress is applied to the knee (*A*) as the athlete allows his leg to hang comfortably over the table. This test may also be done while one hand feels for an opening of the joint (*B*) (*arrow*).

409

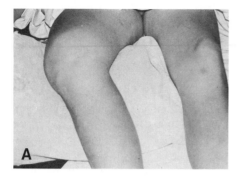 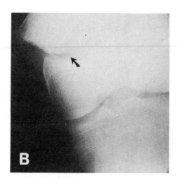

FIG. 15-38
A young athlete's swollen and deformed knee (*A*) may be caused by a fracture of the distal femoral epiphysis (*B*).

from flexion to extension during the "whip kick," his tibial collateral ligament tension increases markedly. Valgus knee stress and external rotation of the tibia accentuate the tension. The femoral origin of his tibial collateral ligament will be tender, but the knee is stable. Ice and compression are used and ultrasound will remove accumulated waste products. The athlete may then resume his flexibility and weight-lifting program while being advised to change his kick to a flutter kick for a time. The swimmer's breaststroke kick should be assessed, making sure that he is not abducting his hips during the recovery phase and then rapidly extending his knees with his legs apart during the thrust phase of the kick. Instead, his heels should be together during recovery and his knees apart only slightly during the thrust.

Moderate Medial Collateral Ligament Sprain

A moderate (grade II) medial collateral ligament sprain denotes a gross disruption of fibers and loss in integrity of the substance of the ligament. The injured ligament lengthens just enough to allow moderate instability with 5° to 15° more laxity than on the sound side; however, a definite resistance end-point is felt to valgus stress. Arthroscopy will reveal whether there are any associated injuries, such as meniscal tears.

If a knee with a grade II medial collateral ligament sprain is put in a cast, muscle function deteriorates, and the athlete suffers a major setback. Experimentally, the strength of intact or repaired dog medial collateral ligaments is influenced by exercise,[134] and immobilization means lack of strength. When the knees are exercised, the medial collateral ligaments show larger diameter collagen fiber bundles and significantly higher collagen content. Moreover, immobilization leads to significant weakening of monkey ligaments, and ligament strength will not return to normal even after 20 weeks of resumed activity.[109, 110] For these reasons, many grade II medial collateral ligament sprains are treated with a brace ·and graded exercise rather than immobilization of the knee in a cast. A functional program will give the athlete a head start toward a return to action, since the ligament is strengthened during the recovery period.

Moderate sprains fall into two groups, depending on their severity,[8] and both types are initially placed in soft casts. Within a day, the least severe sprains are put in a knee immobilizer and the more severe ones in a lightweight cast with a helical glide hinge. The latter consists of a standard hinge on the lateral side and a slotted hinge on the medial side, allowing normal external rotation of the tibia with knee extension and internal rotation with flexion. Athletes use two crutches and begin isometrics, while a maintenance strength program is begun on the sound side, along with hip flexion, extension, and abduction on the injured side. The knee immobilizer is removed three or four times a day to begin gentle knee range of motion.[26] The athlete whose knee is in a gliding-hinge cast also works on active range of motion in his cast, advancing from isometrics to isometrics against resistance about the fourth day.

He then uses one crutch on the side opposite the injury. Around the sixth day, he will no longer need the crutch, and he should then concentrate on walking without a limp while landing heel first. After 1 week, an athlete with either of these injuries is placed in a lightweight helical glide brace, and if his knee is pain-free he may begin isotonic work (*see* Fig. 15-39C).

The helical glide knee brace is designed to ensure knee stability by insisting on the helical pattern of movement rather than by shoring up the medial and lateral sides of the knee. The brace keeps the tibia on its track on the femur during running and dodging, giving the knee the feeling of being secure and free. The brace goes into action only if a deviation from the normal pattern of movement is imminent, as when the tibia threatens to run off the track. This will occur if the runner stumbles or catches his shoe, preventing the tibia from rotating inwards on the femur when the knee is bending or outwards on the femur when the knee is extending. The brace is also strong enough to counter the usual abduction and adduction strain but is not designed to withstand a heavy lateral blow to the knee.

When the athlete begins isotonic work, he may also start a bicycle program. This is prescribed because immobilization significantly depletes type I endurance muscle fibers of oxidative enzymes,[21] which drop even in well-controlled, progressive resistance exercise programs. Bicycle riding, or a high-speed isokinetic program, helps to maintain the enzyme levels. When the athlete is able to perform well on his isometric and isotonic programs, he may begin isokinetic speed work, and when the latter program is underway he may advance to graduated functional activities.

For protection against further valgus stress, a hinged, single-side knee brace has been developed that allows full flexion and extension

FIG. 15-39
A one-sided knee brace (*A*) is lightweight and resists valgus forces to the knee. A "derotation" brace (*B*) may control some instabilities but is cumbersome. The simple, lightweight helical glide brace (*C*) is effective for athletes who must cut because it restores knee synchrony and helical glide.

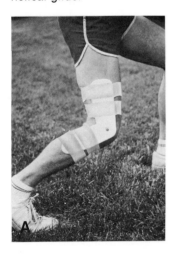

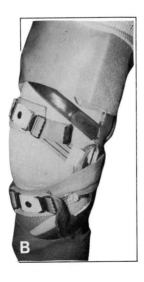

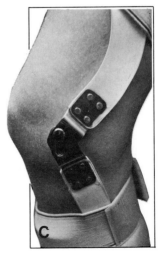

of the knee while preventing stress (*see* Fig. 15-39A).[1] This brace is designed to avoid the restrictions of mobility, speed, and performance commonly associated with cumbersome braces. It is useful when the athlete re-enters collision sports during the period of more than 1 year when the ligament remains weaker than normal.[110] If the knee is taped, the patella must be allowed to move freely, and the popliteal region is left open. Elastic tape without underwrap is usually the most secure taping method around the knee.

Pellegrini-Steida's Disease

After a partial avulsion of the medial collateral ligament from its femoral origin, heterotopic ossification may appear in the upper fibers of the medial collateral ligament.[136] Such ossification is known as Pellegrini-Steida's Disease. The new bone may appear as a hard, tender swelling at the femoral origin of the medial collateral ligament, and there is pain when the knee joint is sprung with valgus stress. A local steroid injection may relieve the symptoms, but if it fails to do so, the heterotopic bone may have to be resected.

Major Medial Collateral Ligament Sprain

A major (grade III) medial collateral ligament sprain may occur from being "clipped" in tackle football (Fig. 15-36).[117] The severe sprain produces an alarming instability with a mushy end-point, and the rupture will require surgical repair. The medial meniscus is first checked, and if it is torn peripherally it can be sutured to the capsule. All torn ligaments are replaced or reapproximated, and if the posteromedial capsular ligament is torn it is reinforced with the semimembranous or the medial head of the gastrocnemius.[48] A pes anserinus transfer is added to increase dynamic internal rotatory stability.

Pes Anserinus

The pes anserinus is the combined insertion of the sartorius, gracilis, and semitendinosus tendons that insert in a row down the proximal anteromedial face of the tibia. The tendons may be transferred to help control some rotatory instabilities of the knee and as an adjunct to extensor mechanism reconstruction (*see* Fig. 15-40A)[127] To transfer the pes, its insertion is dissected free, and the inferior portion is shifted superiorly. It is sutured to the patella tendon and under the metaphyseal flare. Such a transfer significantly increases its internal rotatory effectiveness.[108] Before transfer, the sartorius and gracilis, acting through greater moment arms over the wider proximal metaphysis than the short moment arm of the semitendinosus, provide three fourths of the rotatory force. The semitendinosus is normally the more efficient flexor of the three. After transfer, the semitendinosus becomes a better internal rotator, and the combined muscle moment arms are lengthened, almost doubling rotation forces at 30° and 60° of knee flexion.

After a pes transfer, the pes is strengthened isometrically, isotonically with a weight on a rope, and against the spring resistance of a pes plate (*see* Fig. 15-40B). Thereafter, when the athlete cuts, he consciously "thinks internal rotation" to contract his pes.

Acute Anterior Cruciate Ligament Tear

An anterior cruciate ligament may tear when an athlete cuts, decelerates, or twists (Fig. 15-41) and is the most common cause of a knee hemarthrosis. During a crossover cut, the tibia rotates internally, stressing the anterior cruciate ligament, and, if the athlete is struck from the front with his knee extended, the intercondylar shelf of his femur is driven backwards to rupture the middle third of his anterior cruciate ligament.[106] The tear may produce a loud "pop." Blood then swells the joint suddenly, and the injured athlete holds his knee in 20° to 30° of flexion, a position of comfort where it can accept the most fluid.

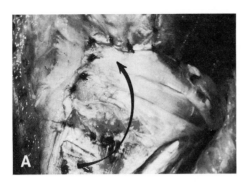

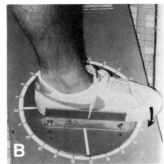

FIG. 15-40
A pes anserinus transfer includes a semitendinosis transfer to just below the metaphyseal flare of the tibia (*A*). The muscles may be restrengthened against spring resistance (*B*).

FIG. 15-41
An athlete's anterior cruciate ligament may tear with a "pop" during deceleration. In such cases, a drawer test with the knee flexed about 15° will result in the tibia's shifting forward. Some surgeons repair the tear with sutures.

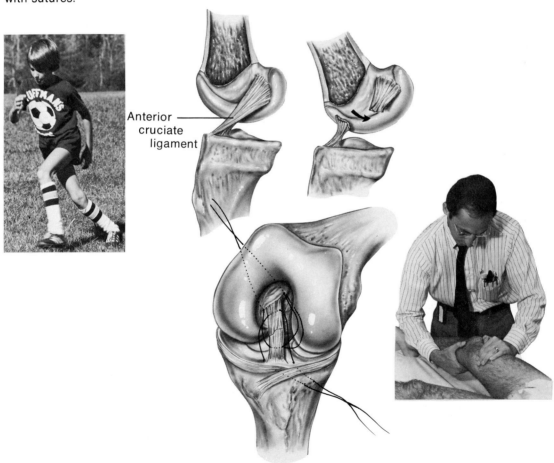

Anterior cruciate ligament

To diagnose an anterior cruciate ligament tear, the examiner should ask the athlete, "How?" "What?" "When?" "Where?" After determining the mechanism of injury, the examiner should perform an anterior drawer test with the knee in 20° flexion (Fig. 15-42). There may also be some recurvatum of the knee owing to the anterior cruciate's no longer being able to support the intercondylar shelf.[106] The customary drawer test at 90° of flexion is not as accurate because secondary restraints lend some stability.

Immediate arthroscopy provides a precise diagnosis of the type of cruciate tear and reveals unsuspected abnormalities, such as meniscal tears, accompanying almost half of the cruciate tears.[25, 111] An anterior cruciate tear gives a predictable instability that the athlete can compensate for and be functionally stable, whereas an accompanying meniscal tear produces an unpredictable instability. Intact synovium near the anterior cruciate may mislead the surgeon to assume that the ligament is intact, but an incision through the synovium may reveal the ligament to be torn completely. The cruciate ligament may even look entirely normal when the synovium is entered but may be totally incompetent owing to interstitial tearing.[109, 111]

If the surgeon finds an acutely torn anterior cruciate, what should he do?[4] When the ligament has been avulsed from its bony origin or insertion, it may be sewn back through drill holes. Ninety percent of all anterior cruciate tears, however, occur through the midportion of the ligament, and, in these cases, stitches may be passed through it and brought out through drill holes in the femur and tibia. The surgeon must preserve the infrapatellar fat pad and the ligament's synovial sheath because the blood supply to the cruciate emanates chiefly from these structures. The repair may be augmented with a strip of the medial one third of the patellar tendon or a strip of iliotibial band sutured to the anterior cruciate, forming a scaffold for vascular ingrowth.

Athletes with midsubstance repairs and augmentations may do well soon after surgery, with little functional instability. Anteromedial and anterolateral instabilities, however, often evolve later when the repair stretches out from the forces of athletic activity. One or both menisci then tear, and arthritis ensues.[4, 144] Because the natural history of repaired midsubstance tears of the anterior cruciate, augmented repairs, and unrepaired tears are about the same, some surgeons defer acute repair, re-examine the knee at 6-month intervals, and perform an extra-articular tenodesis (constructing a "lateral cruciate") if a pivot shift and functional disability develop.

Sports surgeons are sometimes noted for the rapidity with which athletes under their care are able to return safely to competition after injuries or surgery. After an anterior cruciate ligament tear, however, the damaged secondary restraints must be given about 3 months to heal. After an intra-articular cruciate ligament reconstruction, a delayed return after gradual full rehabilitation is the rule. Quadriceps work is initially deferred because it tends to pull the repair apart, and isokinetics should also be avoided because the thrust needed to kick out may rupture or stretch the repair.

Whether a torn anterior cruciate is sutured, repaired and augmented, or not repaired, the athlete must be taught new ways to land from jumps and to change direction. He must land from a jump with his knees bent. If he should land with a knee extended, it will slide out and, when flexed, will reduce and buckle. The athlete must anticipate cuts and plant only the ball of his foot to "round off the cut." If the foot is planted flat on the ground, the knee is in the unwanted position of valgus and extension.

Acute Posterior Cruciate Ligament Tear

An athlete's posterior cruciate ligament may tear when his knee is hyperextended severely (see Fig. 15-42). The anterior cruciate ligament tears first, followed by a tear in the posterior cruciate. A blow to the front of a flexed knee, a fall on the flexed knee with the ankle in plantar flexion, or a hook slide in baseball may also rupture the posterior cruciate. The ligament is usually torn from the tibia, and a bone chip visible on x-ray film may be avulsed.

The knee joint usually will not swell after a rupture of the posterior cruciate because the capsule is often damaged, allowing blood and synovial fluid to escape. The popliteal fossa will be tender and the posterior drawer test positive if both the posterior cruciate and the posterior capsule are torn. Posterior motion of the tibia on the femur is prevented mainly by the posterior cruciate, with little help from the posterior capsule. If the capsule is intact, however, there may be no posterior drawer sign.

Recurvatum of the knee is evidence of a posterior cruciate rupture, and a posterior sag with the knee flexed also indicates posterior cruciate insufficiency. The examiner should be aware that a posterior sag may masquerade as a positive anterior drawer because the tibia is being drawn forward from an already posteriorly subluxed position.

If the posterior drawer test is only up to 5 mm, an operation is not needed, as a reconstruction cannot improve on this amount of drawer. Surgery is indicated when the posterior drawer is 5 mm to 15 mm. In this procedure, the cruciate ligament is approached through a posteromedial incision and the bone fragment secured with a screw or the ligament repaired with sutures passed through drill holes in the tibia (Fig. 15-42). The repair may be augmented with the tendinous medial head of the gastrocnemius. Postoperatively, the athlete wears a knee brace with an extension stop and promptly works his quadriceps. He should refrain from early hamstring work, as the hamstrings pull the tibia backward, antagonizing the effect of the posterior cruciate that holds the tibia forward. If both anterior cruciate and posterior cruciate ligaments have been torn, a medial incision will allow repair of both structures.

FIG. 15-42
If the tibial attachment of the posterior cruciate ligament is avulsed (*A*),
it may be reattached with a screw (*B*).

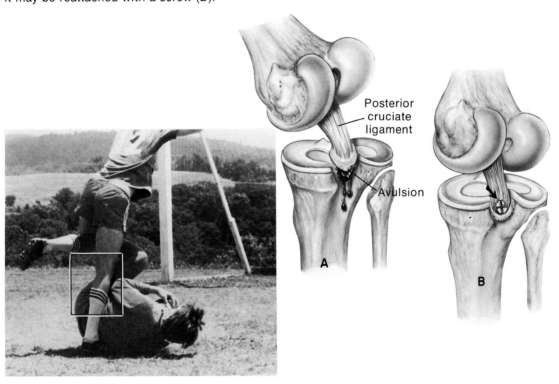

Knee Instabilities

Late Instabilities and Knee Reconstruction

An athlete's knee may become unstable months or years after a knee ligament injury, give way, and start hurting. Such instabilities are defined during an examination by the direction of the tibial displacement—the opposite of what happens in athletics, where the femur is usually moving on the fixed tibia of the planted leg. The instabilities are classified as either straight, rotatory, or combined.

If his muscles are strong enough to provide dynamic stability, an unstable knee may not bother an athlete. Surgery is reserved for functional instability, and before it is suggested the athlete should undergo a 3-month rehabilitation program of his entire lower limb while wearing a helical glide brace. This type of brace allows proper muscle action, whereas hinge braces and derotation braces decrease the athlete's mobility and do not help to guide the knee helically. Knee taping provides support but must be applied skillfully; when elastic tape must be applied frequently, it becomes very expensive. Reconstruction of the knee is indicated only if the exercise and bracing programs are unsuccessful, with the knee still painful and giving-way.

If an operation is decided on, the deficient ligament may be substituted for directly, or reinforcement may be established at a distance from the deficient ligament. In either case, adjunctive active tendon transfers are used to "back up" the repair.

Straight Instabilities

Straight instability means an instability in one plane and consists of six different kinds (*see* list). Straight anterior instability results from a tearing of the medial collateral ligament and the anterior cruciate. Straight medial instability in flexion is produced by a torn medial capsular ligament combined with a torn anterior cruciate or posterior cruciate. Straight medial instability in extension is produced by a torn medial collateral ligament and both cruciates. Straight lateral instability in flexion results from a lateral ligament tear along with an anterior cruciate or posterior cruciate rupture. Straight lateral instability in full extension means a lateral ligament tear and tears of both cruciates. This type of instability is a special hindrance to full athletic participation because the athlete must adduct his limb while running, and the lateral instability causes his supporting leg to give out.

Posterior cruciate insufficiency produces a straight posterior instability. The knee may be generally stable at examination but eventually breaks down with osteoarthritis. Even if the athlete has a posterior drawer sign, an operation

Causes of Straight Knee Instabilities

Instability	Torn or Incompetent
Anterior instability	Medial ligament and anterior cruciate
Posterior instability	Posterior cruciate
Medial instability	
Opening with valgus stress in slight flexion	Medial ligament
Opening with valgus stress in more flexion	Medial ligament and either the anterior or posterior cruciate
Opening with valgus stress in extension	Medial ligament and both cruciates
Lateral instability	
Opening with varus stress in slight flexion	Lateral ligament
Opening with varus stress in more flexion	Lateral ligament and either the anterior or posterior cruciate
Opening with varus stress in extension	Lateral ligament and both cruciates

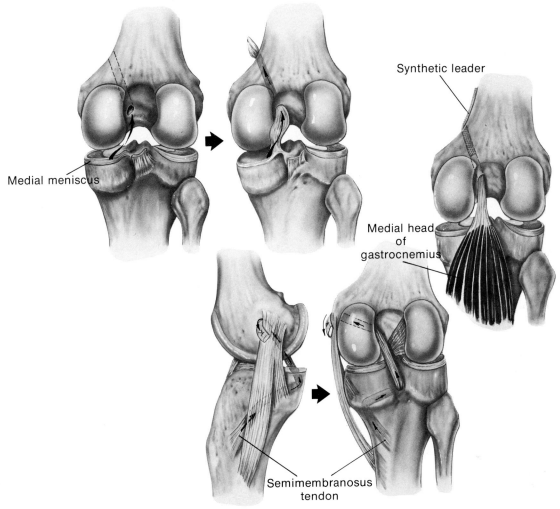

Synthetic leader

Medial meniscus

Medial head of gastrocnemius

Semimembranosus tendon

FIG. 15-43
The posterior cruciate ligament may be replaced by the medial meniscus, the tendon of the medial head of the gastrocnemius or the semimembranous tendon.

is not indicated unless he has functional instability and the drawer is more than 5 mm, since repair will not yield a result better than this.

At operation, the medial meniscus may be substituted for the posterior cruciate (*see* Fig. 15-43). Alternatively, the semitendinosus tendon may be rerouted as a cruciate substitute. Also, the medial third of the patellar tendon may serve as a replacement, since it approaches the strength of the posterior cruciate. Any one of these transfers may die, and for this reason the best replacement for the posterior cruciate

probably is the tendinous part of the medial head of the gastrocnemius, extended by an artificial leader through a hole in the femur.[142]

Because a plaster of paris cast alone will not prevent postoperative posterior sag, a Steinman pin should be placed up the center of the knee joint. In postoperative rehabilitation, the quadriceps is a dynamic stabilizer that aids the posterior cruciate in preventing the tibia from dropping backward. Thus, after replacement, the athlete should work his quadriceps but refrain from strengthening his hamstrings, as they pull the tibia backwards, antagonizing the posterior cruciate replacement.

Rotatory Instability

The rotatory instabilities of the knee include anteromedial rotatory instability, anterolateral rotatory instability, and posterolateral rotatory instability (*see* list). Whether there is such an entity as posteromedial rotatory instability is debatable.

Anteromedial Rotatory Instability

When a knee with anteromedial rotatory instability is tested, the medial tibial plateau moves anteriorly and laterally with respect to the femur. The anterior drawer test and valgus stress test in flexion are positive. Medial capsular ligament damage permits this instability, and since the anterior cruciate supports the capsular structure the instability worsens when the anterior cruciate is ruptured, too. The athlete usually walks well but is unable to sprint or cut, and in time his medial meniscus will tear. The posterior horn of the medial meniscus may block the instability, and if a total medial meniscectomy is performed the removal of this block will unveil a full-blown anteromedial rotatory instability. The examiner must be alert for this condition, as its presence makes reconstruction mandatory. The examiner should also check for an accompanying anterolateral rotatory instability in knees that show anteromedial rotatory instability.[107] To counter the instability, the posteromedial capsular ligament should be tightened and a "dynamic sling" established

by a pes anserinus transfer or an advancement of the semimembranosus.[48]

Anterolateral Rotatory Instability

Anterolateral rotatory instability refers to anterior and medial displacement of the lateral tibial plateau on the femur during testing of the knee. With an incompetent anterior cruciate ligament, the lateral femoral condyle glides posteriorly on the lateral tibial plateau. This displacement is reduced by a tightening of the iliotibial band when the knee is flexed. The athlete may report that his knee "comes apart." The midlateral capsule eventually stretches out, and the athlete's lateral meniscus may tear.

Testing for this type of instability will depend on the posterior subluxation of the lateral femoral condyle in extension and reduction of the subluxation with flexion of the knee. These tests include the pivot-shift and the jerk test, the crossover test, a side-lying test, and the flexion–rotation drawer test. All of these tests should be tried to determine which ones work best for the examiner.

To elicit a *pivot-shift,* the examiner cradles the athlete's heel with one hand and rotates the tibia internally. He also applies a valgus force to the extended knee with his other hand before passively flexing the knee while applying an axial load. At 0° to 5° of flexion, the lateral aspect of the tibia will be subluxed anteriorly, and the iliotibial band shifted forward. As the knee is flexed to 30° or 40°, the subluxation suddenly reduces with a thud or a clunk as the iliotibial band pops back into position, a movement that reproduces what the athlete feels during competition when his knee buckles.

Causes of Rotatory Knee Instabilities

Instability	Torn or Incompetent
Anteromedial rotatory instability	Medial ligament or medial ligament and anterior cruciate
Anterolateral rotatory instability	Anterior cruciate (the instability is increased by posterolateral capsular incompetence)
Posteromedial rotatory instability	Posterior cruciate and medial ligament
Posterolateral rotatory instability	Posterior cruciate and lateral ligament

The *jerk test* is a variant of the pivot-shift. "Jerk" is an engineering term for a sudden rate of change of acceleration. The examiner begins the test with the athlete's knee flexed and presses forward under the fibular head (*see* Fig. 15-44). A jerk will be felt at about 30° of knee flexion as the lateral tibial plateau subluxes anteriorly, jumping out of place when the iliotibial band shifts forward.

The *crossover test* may be used in athletes to duplicate statically a crossover cut and bring out anterolateral rotatory instability.[4] For this test, the examiner stands on the foot of the involved limb and has the subject crossover with his other leg, turning his torso as far as possible while contracting the quadriceps of the fixed limb. This test may reproduce the athlete's feeling of instability on the playing field when his quadriceps contracts, his iliotibial band slides forward, and his lateral tibial plateau subluxates.

In the *side-lying test,* the athlete first lies on his unaffected side, then rolls back about 30° and flexes the hip and knee of his uninjured leg. His weight now rests on the medial border of his heel. The examiner places one thumb behind the fibular head and the other behind the athlete's lateral femoral condyle, with his fingers over the anterior aspect. The knee is then pushed from full extension into flexion and some valgus force applied. As the knee is flexed, the tibia jumps back into a reduced position, and as the knee is extended the tibia subluxes.

To perform the *flexion–rotation drawer test,* the examiner holds the athlete's leg in a neutral position behind the calf, cradles the ankle, and lets the hip fall into external rotation. He then pulls the leg forward slightly and flexes and extends the knee with axial loading and valgus stress, movements that will accentuate the instability.

Operations designed to stabilize knees with anterolateral rotatory instability include intra-articular and extra-articular surgery. In the former procedure, the deficient cruciate may be replaced by other tissues or a ligament prosthesis. A ligament augmentation device, consisting of a braided strut of polypropylene or of carbon fibers, may be used to augment the autogenous tissue to provide a stronger intra-articular transfer.[63, 142] A prolonged rehabilitation period is needed after an intra-articular transfer. These procedures are of doubtful value for athletes because they eventually stretch out.

Extra-articular substitutions for a deficient anterior cruciate ligament include tenodeses and dynamic transfers. For a tenodesis effect, the iliotibial band may be anchored and restrained posterior to the center of knee rotation. The band may also be woven through the posterolateral capsule to strengthen and to tighten the capsule. Unfortunately, athletic activity will stretch these tenodeses, reducing or eliminating their effectiveness.

FIG. 15-44
The jerk test may be used to diagnose anterolateral rotatory instability. With this instability, the lateral tibial plateau will sublux as the examiner extends the athlete's knee.

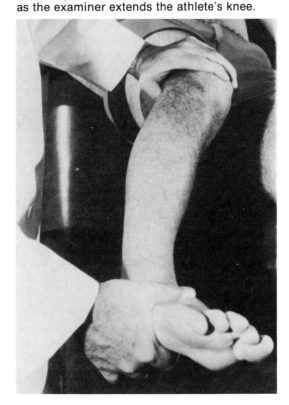

More dynamic procedures to stabilize these knees include iliotibial band reroutings and biceps femoris transfers. The iliotibial band may be passed behind and under the lateral collateral ligament and reinserted at its normal place on the tibia. As the tibia moves toward extension, the proximal lateral collateral ligament insertion then serves as an ever-tightening check rein or cam to prevent outward movement of the tibia on the femur. The defect in the iliotibial band must, of course, be repaired to prevent forward subluxation of the remaining band. A biceps tendon insertion advancement is a dynamic procedure that acts somewhat like a pes anserinus transfer does on the medial side of the knee. These dynamic transfers may help the athlete, but each replacement or shifting of knee structures will lead to other problems with the functional integration of knee motion.

Intra-articular, extra-articular, and combined transfers are being done throughout the world with varying results. Postoperatively, the athlete is often instructed to wear a hinged brace, but this is inappropriate because the knee is not a hinge joint; instead, its motion is based on Helfet's helical glide principle. A helical gliding brace will therefore allow an athlete's knee muscles to work in their normal synchronous pattern (*see* Fig. 15-39C).

Posterolateral Rotatory Instability

A tear of the arcuate complex, consisting of the arcuate and lateral collateral ligaments and the popliteus tendon, allows the athlete's lateral femoral condyle to slide backward on his convex lateral tibial plateau. The external rotation recurvatum test is used to diagnose this instability. The athlete lies relaxed on his back, and the examiner then raises the athlete's leg by his big toe. If there is posterolateral rotatory instability, the tibia will rotate externally and drop back. The knee assumes a position of recurvatum, varus, and excessive external tibial rotation, findings opposite to those in anterolateral rotatory instability.

To stabilize these knees, the popliteus tendon insertion on the lateral femoral condyle is advanced to a more proximal and anterior position. The lateral tendon of origin of the gastrocnemius is also transferred anteriorly, and because this tendon blends with the posterior capsule its advancement tightens the posterior capsule. Finally, the lateral collateral ligament and the biceps tendon are advanced. Postoperatively, the quadriceps is strengthened to hold the tibia forward. Hamstring strengthening is pursued late in rehabilitation, as early training of the hamstrings will pull the tibia backward and work against the transfer.

Combined Instabilities

The most common combined rotatory instability of the knee is anteromedial-anterolateral instability. To stabilize these knees, the tibia must be prevented from sliding both ways. A pes anserinus transfer may be performed medially. Laterally, an iliotibial band rerouting under the lateral collateral ligament acts as a check rein, preventing forward subluxation of the tibia when full extension is approached. A dynamic biceps advancement also is added on this lateral side. For combined anterolateral-posterolateral instability, a dynamic biceps femoris tendon transfer is performed, along with an advancement of the lateral collateral ligament, the popliteus tendon, and the lateral head of the gastrocnemius to tighten up the posterolateral capsule.

The Dislocated Knee

A dislocated knee is classified according to the position of the tibia in relation to the femur. Thus, an anterior dislocation of the knee means that the tibia is dislocated anterior to the femur. A dislocation may be anterior, posterior, lateral, medial, or rotatory. Anterior dislocations resulting from hyperextension of the knee are the most common type.

Many dislocated knees probably reduce spontaneously at the time of the injury, and if the knee has not already relocated it should be reduced immediately. To reduce an anterior dislocation, the examiner should apply longitudinal traction and add the appropriate push or pull. If the ligaments have been torn from the bone, there is a better chance for a stable result. Eventual stability is less likely, however, if the ligaments have ruptured in their midsubstance. Sideways dislocations will need ligament repairs, but anterior or posterior dislocations may eventually become quite stable without surgery, as the collateral ligaments remain intact and the posterior cruciate heals back to bone. In some dislocations, reduction is maintained by flexing the knee and placing a heavy pin down through the distal femur into the tibia.

A knee dislocation may result in damage to the popliteal artery, which is tethered between the adductor canal and the tendinous arch of the soleus. Although nerves may also be injured, the tibial and common peroneal nerves are more mobile than the popliteal artery and can stretch. Arterial trouble appears in about one third of knee dislocations, and about the same proportion of subjects develop nerve trouble, usually of the traction type.

After the dislocation has been reduced, the examiner should check for fullness in the popliteal area. If there is any question as to the patency of the popliteal artery, an arteriogram should be performed, and if damage is noted the vessel should be explored. An anterior dislocation of the knee is the condition most often associated with vascular problems. Even though there may be no detectable arterial damage on early examination, and the foot is warm and looks well, the intima of the vessel may be damaged. Within days an intimal flap may block the flow of blood. If an arterial procedure is needed, it is best performed under spinal anesthesia, as this provides good relaxation and the accompanying lumbar sympathetic block increases circulation to the leg.

Major ligament damage is best repaired at the time of injury. If there is vascular damage that requires attention, the experienced surgeon can take care of that simultaneously.

REFERENCES

1. ANDERSON G et al: The Anderson knee stabilizer. Phys Sportsmed 7(6):125–127, 1979
2. ANDREWS JR et al: The double bucket handle tear of the medial meniscus. Am J Sports Med 3:232–237, 1975
3. ANDREWS JR et al: The cutting mechanism. Am J Sports Med 5:111–121, 1977
4. ARNOLD JA et al: Natural history of anterior cruciate tears. Am J Sports Med 7:305–313, 1979
5. BASMAJIAN JV, LOVEJOY JF Jr: Functions of the popliteus muscle in man. J Bone Joint Surg [Am] 53:557–562, 1971
6. BEHRENS F et al: Intra-articular gluco-corticoids and cartilage damage. J Rheumatol [Suppl] 1:109, 1974
7. BENTLEY G, GOODFELLOW JW: Disorganization of the knees following intra-articular hydrocortisone injections. J Bone Joint Surg [Br] 51:498–502, 1969
8. BERGFELD J: First, second and third-degree sprains. Am J Sports Med 7:207–209, 1979
9. BERSON BL, HERMANN G: Torn discoid menisci of the knee in adults. Four case reports. J Bone Joint Surg [Am] 61:303–304, 1979
10. BLAZINA ME et al: Jumper's knee. Orthop Clin North Am 4:665–678, 1973
11. BOSWORTH DM: An operation for meniscectomy of the knee. J Bone Joint Surg [Am] 19:1113–1116, 1937
12. BROWN CW et al: Simplified operative approach for the lateral meniscus. Am J Sports Med 3:265–270, 1975
13. BRUSER DM: A direct lateral approach to the lateral compartment of the knee joint. J Bone Joint Surg [Br] 42:348, 1960
14. CAHILL BR: Stress fracture of the proximal tibial epiphysis: a case report. Am J Sports Med 5:186–187, 1977
15. CABAUD JE, SLOCUM DB: The diagnosis of chronic anterolateral rotary instability of the knee. Am J Sports Med 5:99–105, 1977
16. CABAUD HE et al: Exercise effects on the strength of the rat anterior cruciate ligament. Am J Sports Med 8:79–86, 1980
17. CARGILL AO, JACKSON JP: Bucket-handle tear of the medial meniscus: a case for conservative surgery. J Bone Joint Surg [Am] 58:248–251, 1976
18. CAVE EF: Combined anterior-posterior approach to the knee joint. J Bone Joint Surg 17:427–430, 1935
19. CHARLES CM: On the menisci of the knee joint in American whites and Negroes. Anat Rec 63:355–364, 1935
20. COOPER DL, FAIR J: Trainer's corner: stationary cycling for post-op fitness. Phys Sportsmed 4(6):129, 1976
21. COSTILL DL et al: Muscle rehabilitation after knee surgery. Phys Sportsmed 5(9):71–74, 1977

22. D'AMBROSIA RD, MacDONALD GL: Pitfalls in the diagnosis of Osgood-Schlatters disease. Clin Orthop 110:206–209, 1975

23. DeHAVEN DE, COLLINS HR: Diagnosis of internal derangements of the knee. The role of arthroscopy. J Bone Joint Surg [Am] 57:802–810, 1975

24. DeHAVEN DE et al: Chondromalacia patella in athletes. Clinical presentation and conservative management. Am J Sports Med 7:5–11, 1979

25. DeHAVEN KE: Diagnosis of acute knee injuries with hemarthrosis. Am J Sports Med 8:9–14, 1980

26. ELLSASSER JC et al: The non-operative treatment of collateral ligament injuries of the knee in professional football players. J Bone Joint Surg [Am] 56:1185–1190, 1974

27. EUCKERMAN J, STULL AG: Effects of exercise on knee ligament separation force in rats. J Appl Physiol 26:716–719, 1969

28. FAIRBANK TJ: Knee joint changes after meniscectomy. J Bone Joint Surg [Br] 30:664–670, 1948

29. FARIA IE, CAVANAGH PR: The Physiology and Biomechanics of Cycling. American College of Sports Medicine Series. New York, John Wiley & Sons, 1978

30. FOX JM et al: Multiphasic view of medial meniscectomy. Am J Sports Med 7:161–164, 1979

31. FREIBERGER RH et al: Arthrography of the knee by double contrast method. Am J Roentgenol 97:736–747, 1966

32. FUNK FJ Jr: Injuries of the extensor mechanism of the knee. Athletic Training 10:141–145, 1975

33. GAINOR BJ et al: The kick: biomechanics and collision injury. Am J Sports Med 6:185–193, 1978

34. GALWAY RD et al: Pivot shift: a clinical sign of symptomatic anterior cruciate insufficiency. J Bone Joint Surg [Br] 54:763, 1972

35. GARCIA A, NEER C II: Isolated fractures of the intercondylar eminence of the tibia. Displaced fractures reduced by extending the knee. Am J Surg 95:593, 1958

36. GASTON EA: Preventing bikers' knees. Bicycling 20(7):50–53, 1979

37. GIECK J et al: Treatment of pain in athletes by the use of transcutaneous nerve stimulation. Athletic Training 14(2):97–101, 1979

38. GINSBURG JH et al: Nutrient pathways in transferred patellar tendon used for anterior cruciate ligament reconstruction. Am J Sports Med 8:15–18, 1980

39. GLEIN GW et al: Isokinetic evaluation following leg injuries. Phys Sportsmed 6(8):75–82, 1978

40. GODSHALL RW: The predictability of athletic injuries: an 8-year study. Am J Sports Med 3:50–54, 1975

41. GOLDNER RD et al: The "blind side" of the medial meniscus. Am J Sports Med 8:337–341, 1980

42. GRANA WA, MORETZ JA: Ligamentous laxity in secondary school athletes. JAMA 240:1975–1976

43. GROOD ES, NOYES FR: Cruciate ligament prosthesis: strength, creep and fatigue properties. J Bone Joint Surg [Am] 58:1083–1088, 1976

44. GUHL JF: Operative arthroscopy. Am J Sports Med 7:328–335, 1979

45. HARDAKER WT Jr et al: Diagnosis and treatment of the plica syndrome of the knee. J Bone Joint Surg [Am] 62:221–225, 1980

46. HELLER L, LANGMAN J: The menisco-femoral ligaments in adults less than fifty-five years old. J Bone Joint Surg [Am] 59:480–482, 1977

47. HUGHSTON JC: Subluxation of the patella. J Bone Joint Surg [Am] 50:1003–1026, 1968

48. HUGHSTON JC, EILERS AF: The role of the posterior oblique ligament in repairs of acute medial collateral ligament injuries of the knee. J Bone Joint Surg [Am] 55:923–940, 1973

49. HUGHSTON JC: A simple meniscectomy. Am J Sports Med 3:179–187, 1975

50. INSALL J: "Chondromalacia patellae": patellar malalignment syndrome. Orthop Clin North Am 10:117–127, 1979

51. IRELAND J et al: Arthroscopy and arthrography of the knee: a critical review. J Bone Joint Surg [Br] 62:3–6, 1980

52. ISMAIL AM et al: Rupture of patellar ligament after steroid infiltration: report of a case. J Bone Joint Surg [Br] 51:503–505, 1969

53. JACKSON DW: Video arthroscopy: a permanent medical record. Am J Sports Med 6:213–216, 1978

54. JONES RE et al: Effects of medial meniscectomy in patients older than forty years. J Bone Joint Surg [Am] 60:783–786, 1978

55. KALENAK A, MOREHOUSE CA: Knee stability and knee ligament injuries. JAMA 234:1143–1145, 1975

56. KAYE JJ, HIMMELFARB E: Knee arthroscopy in symposium on disorders of the knee joint. Orthop Clin North Am 10:51–59, 1979

57. KEENE JS: Surgical injury to the lateral aspect of the knee—a comparison of transverse and vertical knee incisions. Am J Sports Med 8:93–97, 1980

58. KENNEDY JC: Complete dislocation of the knee joint. J Bone Joint Surg [Am] 45:889–904, 1963

59. KENNEDY JC, WILLIS RB: The effects of local steroid injections on tendons: a biomechanical and microscopic correlative study. Am J Sports Med 4:11–21, 1976

60. KENNEDY JC et al: Orthopaedic manifestations of swimming. Am J Sports Med 6:309–322, 1978

61. KENNEDY JC et al: Anterolateral rotatory instability of the knee joint. J Bone Joint Surg [Am] 60:1031–1039, 1978

62. KENNEDY JC et al: Posterior cruciate ligament injuries. Orthop Digest 7(8/9):19–31, 1979

63. KENNEDY JC et al: Presidential address: intra-articular replacement in the anterior cruciate ligament-deficient knee. Am J Sports Med 8:1–8, 1980

64. KLEIN KK: Full squats loosen the knee joint. Preventive conditioning and reduction of knee injury. Athletic J 40:7–28, 1960

65. KLEIN KK: The martial arts and the caucasian knee:

"a tiger by the tail." Am J Sports Med 3:440–447, 1975

66. KNIGHT KL: Testing anterior cruciate ligaments. Phys Sportsmed 8(5):135–138, 1980

67. KULOWSKI J, RICKETT HW: The relation of discoid meniscus to cyst formation and joint mechanics. J Bone Joint Surg 29:990–992, 1947

68. KULUND DN, BRUBAKER CE: Injuries in the bikecentennial tour. Phys Sportsmed 6(6):74–78, 1978

69. KULUND DN et al: Olympic weightlifting injuries. Phys Sportsmed 6(11):111–119, 1978

70. KULUND DN: The foot in athletics. In Helfet AJ (ed): Disorders of the Foot. Philadelphia, JB Lippincott, 1980

71. LARSON RL, OSTERNOG LR: Traumatic bursitis and artificial turf. Am J Sports Med 2:183–188, 1974

72. LARSON RL et al: The patellar compression syndrome: surgical treatment by lateral retinacular release. Clin Orthop 134:158–167, 1978

73. LAST RJ: The popliteus muscle and the lateral meniscus. J Bone Joint Surg [Br] 32:93–99, 1950

74. LEACH R et al: Obesity: its relationship to osteoarthritis of the knee. Clin Orthop 93:271–273, 1973

75. LEVI JH, COLEMAN CR: Fracture of the tibial tubercle. Am J Sports Med 4:254–263, 1976

76. LEVINE J: A new brace for chondromalacia patella and kindred conditions. Am J Sports Med 6:137–140, 1978

77. LIEB FJ, PERRY J: Quadriceps function: anatomical and mechanical study using amputated limbs. J Bone Joint Surg [Am] 50:1535–1548, 1968

78. LIEB FJ, PERRY J: Quadriceps function: an EMGic study under isometric conditions. J Bone Joint Surg [Am] 53:749–758, 1971

79. LIPSCOMB PR Jr et al: Osteochondritis dissecans of the knee with loose fragments: treatment by replacement and fixation with readily removable pins. J Bone Joint Surg [Am] 60:235–240, 1978

80. LOSEE RE et al: Anterior subluxation of the lateral tibial plateau: a diagnostic test and operative repair. J Bone Joint Surg [Am] 60:1015–1030, 1978

81. LUTTER LD: Foot-related knee problems in the long-distance runner. Foot Ankle 1:112–116, 1980

82. LYONS R: Bicycle ergometer for injured athletes. Trainer's corner. Phys Sportsmed 2(8):218, 1974

83. MANN RA, HAGY JL: The popliteus muscle. J Bone Joint Surg [Am] 59:924–927, 1977

84. MARSHALL JL, JOHNSON RJ: Mechanisms of the most common ski injuries. Phys Sportsmed 5(12):49–54, 1977

85. MAYFIELD GW: Popliteus tendon tenosynovitis. Am J Sports Med 5:31–35, 1977

86. McDANIEL WJ, DAMERON TB Jr: Untreated ruptures of the anterior cruciate ligament. J Bone Joint Surg [Am] 62:696–705, 1980

87. McDERMOTT LJ: Development of the human knee joint. Arch Surg 46:705–719, 1943

88. McGINTY JB et al: Partial or total meniscectomy. A comparative analysis. J Bone Joint Surg [Am] 59:763–766, 1977

89. McLEOD WD, BLACKBURN TA: Biomechanics of knee rehabilitation with cycling. Am J Sports Med 8:175–180, 1980

90. MEDLAR RC et al: Meniscectomies in children. Am J Sports Med 8:87–92, 1980

91. MERCHANT AC et al: Roentgenographic analysis of congruence. J Bone Joint Surg [Am] 56:1931, 1974

92. MERCHANT AC, MERCER RL: Lateral release of the patella. Clin Orthop 103:40–45, 1974

93. MEYERS E: Effect of selected exercise variables on ligament stability and flexibility of the knee. Res Q 42:4, 1971

94. MEYERS MH, McKEEVER FM: Fractures of the intercondylar eminence of the tibia. J Bone Joint Surg [Am] 41:209, 1959

95. MITAL M: Osgood-Schlatters disease: the painful puzzler. Phys Sportsmed 5(6):60–73, 1977

96. MOORE HA, LARSON RL: Posterior cruciate ligament injuries. Results of early surgical repair. Am J Sports Med 8:68–78, 1980

97. MORRISON JB: Bioengineering analysis of force rations transmitted by the knee joint. BioMed Eng 3:164, 1968

98. NICHOLAS JA, MINKOFF J: Iliotibial band transfer through the intercondylar notch for combined anterior instability. Am J Sports Med 6:341–353, 1978

99. NITTER L: Arthrosis in the knee after meniscectomy. Acta Chir Scand 93:483–494, 1946

100. NOBLE CA: Iliotibial band friction syndrome in runners. Am J Sports Med 8:232–234, 1980

101. NOBLE J: Clinical features of the degenerate meniscus with the results of meniscectomy. Br J Surg 62:977–981, 1975

102. NOBLE J, HAMBLEN DL: The pathology of the degenerative meniscus lesion. J Bone Joint Surg [Br] 57:180–186, 1975

103. NOBLE J: Lesions of the menisci: autopsy incidents in adults less than fifty-five years old. J Bone Joint Surg [Am] 59:480–482, 1977

104. NOBLE J, ERAT K: In defense of the meniscus. A prospective study of 200 meniscectomy patients. J Bone Joint Surg [Br] 62:7–11, 1980

105. NORWOOD LA Jr et al: Arthroscopy of the lateral meniscus in knees with normal arthrograms. Am J Sports Med 5:271–274, 1977

106. NORWOOD LA Jr, CROSS MJ: Anterior cruciate ligament; functional anatomy of its bundles in rotary instabilities. Am J Sports Med 7:23–26, 1979

107. NORWOOD LA Jr, HUGHSTON JC: Combined anterolateral-anteromedial rotatory instability of the knee. Clin Orthop 147:62–67, 1980

108. NOYES FR, SONSTEGARD DG: Biomechanical function of the pes anserinus at the knee and the effect of its transplantation. J Bone Joint Surg [Am] 55:1225–1241, 1973

109. NOYES FR, GROOD ES: The strength of the anterior cruciate ligament in humans and rhesus monkeys. J Bone Joint Surg [Am] 58:1074–1082, 1976

110. NOYES FR: Functional properties of knee ligaments and alterations induced by immobilization: a correlative biomechanical and histological study in primates. Clin Orthop 123:210–239, 1977

111. NOYES FR et al: Arthroscopy in acute traumatic hemarthrosis of the knee—incidence of anterior cruciate tears and other injuries. J Bone Joint Surg [Am] 62:687–695, 1980

112. O'DONOGHUE DH: Treatment of chondral damage to the patella. Am J Sports Med 9:1–10, 1981

113. OGDEN JA: Subluxation and dislocation of the proximal tibiofibular joint. J Bone Joint Surg [Am] 56:145–154, 1974

114. PALUMBO PM Jr: Dynamic patellar brace: a new orthosis in the management of patellofemoral disorders—a preliminary report. Am J Sports Med 9:45–49, 1981

115. PATEL D: Arthroscopy of the plicae: synovial folds and their significance. Am J Sports Med 6:217–225, 1978

116. PEASE RL, FLENTJE W: Rehabilitation through underwater exercise. Trainer's corner. Phys Sportsmed 4(10):143, 1976

117. PETERSON TR: Knee injuries due to blocking: a continuing problem. Phys Sportsmed 3(1):440–447, 1975

118. PEVEY JK: Out-patient arthroscopy of the knee under local anesthesia. Am J Sports Med 6:122–127, 1978

119. PIPKIN G: Knee injuries: the role of the suprapatellar plica and suprapatellar bursa in simulating internal derangements. Clin Orthop 74:161–176, 1971

120. PUDDU G: Method for reconstruction of the anterior cruciate ligament using the semitendinosus tendon. Am J Sports Med 8:402–404, 1980

121. RENNE JW: The iliotibial band friction syndrome. J Bone Joint Surg [Am] 57:1110–1111, 1975

122. ROACH JE et al: Comparison of the effects of steroid aspirin and sodium salicylate on articular cartilage. Clin Orthop 106:350–356, 1975

123. ROELS J et al: Patellar tendinitis (jumper's knee). Am J Sports Med 6:362–368, 1978

124. ROESER WM et al: The use of transcutaneous nerve stimulation for pain control in athletic medicine. A preliminary report. Am J Sports Med 4:210–213, 1976

125. SCHUMACHER HR: Traumatic joint effusion and the synovium. Am J Sports Med 3:108–114, 1975

126. SEEDHOM BB: Loadbearing function of the menisci. Rotterdam, International Congress on the Knee Joint, September 1973

127. SLOCUM DB, LARSON RL: Pes anserinus transplantation: a surgical procedure for control of rotatory instability of the knee. J Bone Joint Surg [Am] 50:226–242, 1968

128. SMILLIE IS: Injuries of the Knee Joint, 4th ed. New York, Churchill Livingstone, 1975

129. STARR W: The Strongest Shall Survive: Strength Training for Football. Annapolis, Fitness Products, 1976

130. STEADMAN JR: Rehabilitation after knee ligament surgery. Am J Sports Med 8:294–296, 1980

131. STULBERG S: Breaststroker's knee: pathology, etiology and treatment. Am J Sports Med 8:164–171, 1980

132. TAPPER EM, HOOVER NW: Late results after meniscectomy: 10–30 year follow-up after uncomplicated meniscectomy. J Bone Joint Surg [Am] 51:517–526, 1969

133. TEGTMEYER CJ et al: Arthrography of the knee: a comparative study of the accuracy of single and double contrast techniques. Radiology 132:37–41, 1979

134. TIPTON CM et al: Influence of exercise on strength of medial collateral knee ligaments of dogs. Am J Physiol 218:894–902, 1970

135. TONGUE JR, LARSON RL: Limited arthrography in acute knee injuries. Am J Sports Med 8:19–30, 1980

136. TUCKER WE: Post-traumatic para-articular ossification of medial collateral ligament of the knee. Br J Sports Med 4:212, 1969

137. WANG JB et al: A mechanism of isolated anterior cruciate ligament rupture. J Bone Joint Surg [Am] 57:411–413, 1975

138. WATSON–JONES R: Fractures and Other Bone and Joint Injuries, 2nd ed. Baltimore, Williams and Wilkins, 1941

139. WEAVER JK: Bipartite patellae as a cause of disability in the athlete. Am J Sports Med 5:137–143, 1977

140. WEAVER S: Don't wait until your knees hurt—check positioning now. Bicycling 20(7):52–53, 1979

141. WILSON JN: Wilson's sign. A diagnostic sign in osteochondritis dissecans of the knee. J Bone Joint Surg [Am] 49:477, 1967

142. WOODS GW: Proplast leader for use in cruciate ligament reconstruction. Am J Sports Med 7:314–320, 1979

143. YOCUM LA et al: The deranged knee: restoration of function. A protocal for rehabilitation of the injured knee. Am J Sports Med 6:51–53, 1978

144. YOUMANS WT: The so-called "isolated" anterior cruciate ligament tear or anterior cruciate ligament syndrome. Am J Sports Med 6:26–30, 1978

145. ZERNICKE RF et al: Human patellar-tendon rupture: a kinetic analysis. J Bone Joint Surg [Am] 59:179–183, 1977

The Leg

Running

Runners may be broadly classified as joggers, runners, sports runners, long distance runners, and marathoners.[18] The jogger runs 2 to 4 miles a day, 3 to 4 days a week at a pace just over 8 minutes per mile. A runner does a minimum of 4 miles a day at least 5 days a week at a pace faster than the jogger. The sports runner trains at 20 to 40 miles per week and competes in 3- to 6-mile races. The distance runner trains 40 to 70 miles per week at a 7- to 8-minute-per-mile pace and competes in 10,000 meter (6.2 mile) races or marathons (26.2 miles). The elite marathoner trains at 70 to 200 miles per week at a 5- to 7-minute-per-mile pace.

Athletes in other sports may also cover long distances, but their running is not at such a steady pace. A soccer midfielder, for example, may run over 7 miles in a game, and a tennis player may average almost 7 miles of walking and running in a three-set match (30 games).

Phases of Running

The phases of running include an airborne and support phase. The airborne phase consists of follow-through, forward swing, and foot descent. The foot is supinated throughout this phase. The support phase consists of heelstrike, stance, and pushoff, and as the athlete runs faster, the duration of this phase becomes shorter.

The runner's hip is adducted and his foot slightly supinated as he nears heel strike, a movement that locks the foot to stabilize it for heel strike. The landing is made on the lateral side of the heel as the leg is externally rotated. At heel strike, the anterior calf muscles contract to dorsiflex the ankle. The forces on the supporting foot at this point are three times body weight or more, depending on the terrain (four times body weight on downhill runs). There are 800 to 1000 foot strikes by each foot during each mile run. A 68-kg (150-lb) runner must therefore withstand about 120 tons of force on each foot during a mile run, and in a marathon, this force increases to 3000 tons.[18]

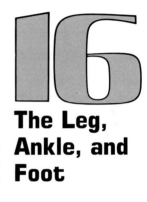

16

The Leg, Ankle, and Foot

After heel strike, the runner's foot pronates rapidly, unlocking the foot for shock absorption and surface adaptation. Pronation occurs for 55% to 70% of the support phase, and the tibia rotates internally on the talus in proportion to the amount of pronation. Shock is also absorbed at the hips and knees, with the knee flexing 30° to 40° in midstance. As the runner increases speed, the center of gravity of his body becomes lower. During stance, the anterior leg muscles continue contracting to accelerate the tibia over the foot,[81] doing so through 80% of the stance phase in running and until midswing in sprinting.

At pushoff, the foot moves from shock-absorbing pronation to supination, locking the foot for stability as a rigid lever for propulsion. The fibula shifts as the many muscles attached to it contract, and the leg rotates externally.

Proper Form

Proper running form should be taught to all school-age youths. When in good form, the runner is erect, and his jaw, neck, and shoulders are relaxed. The elbows should not be flexed more than 90°, and his hands should be kept loose, as raised shoulders, sharply flexed elbows, and clenched fists can cause pain around the shoulders. The arms should pump directly forward and backward and swing parallel to the line of progression. If the arms swing across the runner's body, pelvic rotation is accentuated to produce pain where the muscles attach to the iliac crest. The runner lands heel first in slow running and on the balls of the feet in fast running.

Running Surfaces

The ideal surface for running is flat, smooth, resilient, and reasonably soft, making the best surfaces dirt paths, grass, or wood chips. Then come composite tracks, with the least desirable surfaces being hard asphalt roads, sidewalks, and wooden tracks.

Roads are often crowned, and when the runner runs against traffic on such a road, his higher foot overpronates and his lower foot jams, stressing the foot's lateral aspect.

When running turns on the flat, the inside hip is adducted and the inside foot pronates. The outside leg has to catch up, its stride lengthens, and there is a more forceful heel strike. There is also more stress on the lateral side of the outside foot, and this stress tends to increase on banked, wooden indoor tracks, especially as a runner passes slower runners on the banked turns. The spring in the boards of wooden tracks also leads to shin splints.

Uphill runs stress the quadriceps and patella tendon. The calf muscles are stressed at pushoff, and there is increased dorsiflexion at the metacarpophalangeal joint of the great toe. The runner must lift his foot to clear the ground. Downhill runs demand a longer stride, and there is greater impact at heel strike.

An uneven surface stresses the limbs, but this also strengthens ligaments. In sidewalk running, going up and down curbs increases shock. Running in deep beach sand is unwise as well because the feet pronate markedly through the sand. Firmer sand near the water is canted like a crowned road.

The fastest tracks have a compliant surface that acts like a spring and, in some cases, can be tuned to the mechanical properties of runners to improve their times. A "tuned" indoor track with a surface of optimum compliance has been constructed, with a polyurethane surface and a wooden substructure that gives a stiffness two to three times that of the average runner.[85] This type of track reduces the usual jolt of vertical force at heel strike, the runner's stride length increases, and his contact time shortens. A runner's time improves on the tuned track, and he suffers far fewer injuries than on other kinds of tracks.

Skiing Fractures of the Tibia

When a skier falls or has a collision on the slopes, the usual mechanism of leg injury is external rotation.[130, 131] The ski becomes fixed, and the skier falls to the side and forward. Such falls often resulted in ankle fractures when skiers wore low boots, but, with today's higher, rigid, molded boots, fractures occur mostly at the junction of the middle third and lower third of the tibia—the "boot top" fracture.[41, 42, 62, 64] The "skier's fracture" is a comminuted, spiral fracture of the tibia usually accompanied by a fracture of the fibula.[133] Whereas female skiers suffer knee ligament injuries more often than do male skiers, especially grade II sprains of the medial collateral ligament, the rates of tibia and fibular fractures are about the same for men and women. The spiral fracture occurs more often in a young skier who moves slowly, with shorter skis and lower, softer boots. Although the skier's tibial fracture is usually considered to be a spiral one, oblique and double-oblique types with a butterfly are also common. Fortunately, such injuries are relatively low-energy fractures and rarely open, and internal fixation is usually not needed.

Most tibial fractures result from binding failures. This problem is aggravated when the common toe and heel release systems are poorly adjusted. When properly set, bindings can reduce ski injuries, but most skiers tend to set their bindings too tight. Since the two-mode release bindings are insensitive to several loading configurations, multimode release bindings that allow release by roll, shear, and twist methods at the heel, as well as conventional release modes (twist at the toe and forward lean at the heel), are needed. These would help protect both the knee and the leg.[63] As a practical test of bindings, the skier should be able to twist out of the bindings painlessly.

If a skier injures his leg, his boot should not be removed on the slope. Ice should be applied to the region and the leg placed into a splint. The fracture may then be reduced at the orthopedic area and a long-leg cast applied that can usually be changed to a short-leg cast relatively soon. The short cast has lateral extensions about the knee, allowing the skier to walk and permitting knee flexion and extension while keeping the knee from rotating.

The question as to when the skier may resume skiing after a fracture of the tibia and fibula must take account of the fact that the stresses of skiing make refracture a problem. Tomography may reveal gaps or defects in the cortex, and if such gaps or defects are found,

skiing may have to be proscribed for an additional 6 to 12 months.[16]

Skiers can prepare for the ski season by doing plyometric jumps in all directions over boxes, "isodynamic skiing" against the resistance of surgical tubing or a lightweight bicycle inner tube, or hiking over rough terrain. The skills of water skiing and surfing also transfer to skiing. Each of these activities demands muscular endurance, requiring the athlete to react to momentary losses of balance and shifts of his center of gravity.

Stress Fractures of the Leg

As a runner trains, osteoclasts and osteoblasts remodel his weight-bearing bones to accommodate stress. The osteoclastic action may be so rapid that a defect forms in the bone, producing a loss of continuity or a "fracture before a fracture."[43] Muscle spasm then splints the painful area. Stress fractures occur not only in beginning runners, but also in champions often after an abrupt increase in training mileage, a change in running surfaces, an injury such as an ankle sprain or a blister that changes the running gait, or a recent lay-off.

During the pushoff phase of running the leg rotates externally, and the foot supinates to become a rigid lever. The plantar flexors of the toes and the great toe flexor arise from the fibula, drawing it toward the tibia.[30, 31, 39] The fibula also moves rhythmically to and fro, especially when the runner runs on the balls of his feet on a hard surface. The point of greatest stress is near the inferior tibiofibular joint, where the cortex may break about 6 cm above the tip of the malleolus. A runner may also suffer a stress fracture through the posteromedial cortex of his upper or lower tibia.[30, 31, 40] Stress fractures are often found in the upper third of the tibia in military recruits, whereas ballet dancers usually develop stress fractures in the middle third of the tibia.[14, 39, 41, 42] Tibial stress fractures are most common in athletes with cavus feet, whereas fibular stress fractures are more common in athletes with pronated feet.

To diagnose a stress fracture of the tibia or fibula, the examiner may strike the runner's heel sharply. If there is a stress fracture, this maneuver will elicit pain at the fracture site. The bone may be tender to direct pressure as well. To check further for a fracture, the examiner may use his own knee as a fulcrum to spring the tibia. In any instance of leg pain, a stress fracture should be suspected and an x-ray film obtained. Usually no crack shows, but a callus cloud may be seen. This may not be visible immediately, but may appear about 2 weeks later under bright light as a local surface haze or even a line of condensation in the bone. If the fracture callus does not appear on the film, it may be seen on a film taken at a different angle. Soft tissue x-ray films or xeroradiographs are sometimes taken to reveal the fracture.

A technetium diphosphonate bone scan may also be done 1 to 3 hours after radionuclide injection to diagnose a stress fracture. The isotope uptake is more than 300% greater at a stress fracture site than on the sound side.[125]

If a stress fracture is suspected, the athlete should be treated as if one has been confirmed, and strapping, brace, or light cast applied. Running must not be allowed until x-ray films show healing and the bone is no longer tender. A fibular stress fracture usually takes 6 weeks and a tibial one, 8 to 10 weeks to heal. While the fracture is healing, the athlete may stay in condition by cycling and doing circuit training; he may also wear a flotation device and run in the swimming pool.

Shin Splints

Shin splints refer to a periostitis, myositis, or tendinitis, or a combination of these in an athlete's leg. There are anterior shin splints and posteromedial shin splints.

Anterior Shin Splints

The anterior tibial muscle raises the foot during each step and keeps the foot from slapping down after heel strike. This muscle action is stressful, especially in the untrained runner, whose anterior tibials are much weaker than his calf muscles. Even trained runners, however, may develop anterior shin splints if they overexert. Shin splints are common during sprinting, running uphill, and on hard surfaces and in those runners who wear stiff training shoes. In sprinting, the runner must lift the foot after a strong pushoff, and when slowing down he begins to heel run. Because this forceful heel placement leads to strain of the anterior tibial muscle, many runners have the most pain when sprinting or while slowing down after a sprint. Also, uphill cross-country running creates a tight gastrocnemius, and the forward body lean for balance increases the stress on the leg. Moreover, shin splints are likely if a runner overstrides (e.g., on downhills) or runs on hard surfaces such as asphalt. Anterior shin splints are common when the athlete changes to a hard playing surface or goes from natural grass to synthetic turf, especially if his shoes are rigid and the heel firm and not rounded. In addition, street shoes with high heels will tighten the athlete's heel cord and further stress the anterior tibial muscle.

With anterior shin splints, the runner notes pain, tenderness, and tightness along the lateral border of the tibia and at the distal third of the tibia along the medial crest. The pain increases with active dorsiflexion and passive plantar flexion of the ankle.

Anterior shin splints are treated with ice to reduce swelling, and an elastic wrap is used for compression. The runner rests while strengthening his anterior muscles and stretching his heel cords. He may dorsiflex the ankle against a weight sleeve placed over his foot, beginning with three sets of ten repetitions of 2.5 lb and working up to three sets with 10 lb. In addition, a lightweight bicycle inner tube or surgical tubing may be used to provide resistance and develop anterior tibial and peroneal strength. A plywood box measuring 12 in by 12 in by 6 in may be used for heel cord stretches for periods of 5 minutes, three times a day. Ideally, all athletes should stretch their heel cords before practice and should perform a soleus crouch to stretch the soleus component of the heel cord.

As soreness is relieved, the athlete may resume training by walking 2 miles. He then moves to a walk-and-jog, progressing to a 7.5- to 8-minute-mile pace. A flat running surface, such as grass or wood chips, is preferable, and hills should be avoided until the soreness has left. During these initial walks and runs, the leg is taped with elastic tape and the mileage increased by 5 miles per week for the next 6 weeks, up to 40 miles a week. Athletes should wear shoes with a normal height rather than high heels. If a runner's training program must be changed, the change should be gradual. He should also take time to adjust to new surfaces.

Medial Shin Splints

Medial shin splints most often affect athletes who have pronated feet and those who run on crowned roads or on an indoor track with banked turns. On turns, the inside hip is adducted, and the foot must pronate more. In addition, these athletes often have a significantly higher adduction angle of the inside leg. The uneven terrain of a cross-country course and beaches also increases such pronation.

The pain of medial shin splints is located in the posteromedial compartment, 10 cm to 15 cm proximal to the tip of the medial malleolus, and is worsened by active plantar flexion and inversion. Medial shin splints may be treated by taping the runner's arch. The toes should be flexed before the tape is applied and elastic tape placed around the arch. An orthosis will limit pronation.

The athlete strengthens the intrinsic muscles of his arch by performing 50 towel drags or towel-gathering exercises three times a day and by picking up marbles with his feet. Twenty-five repetitions of isometric dorsiflexion exercises are done three times a day, with each contraction held for 6 seconds. The exercises are done standing, as the athlete turns his foot in and pulls his arch up and inward. Occasionally, the athlete will be unable to resume running for 4 to 6 weeks. He should resume only on flat surfaces, and to take the strain off the posteromedial area he may try to run toed-in. The runner should also be taught the proper technique for running turns.

Compartment Syndromes

Anterior compartment syndrome is a dangerous complication of leg injury. It usually follows a blow or repeated blows to the shin but also may follow a heavy early training schedule. As swelling increases within the tight fascial covering that invests the muscles in the anterior compartment, the web space between the great and second toes becomes numb, and the extensor hallucis longus weakens. The condition does not improve with rest and ice application. Serial wick catheter determinations of compartmental pressure will help the physician to determine whether the condition is progressing or resolving and aid him in deciding whether a fasciotomy is needed.

A more common compartment problem in runners is chronic compartment ischemia in which the strong fascia that invests the leg muscles is unyielding. It does not accommodate to the 20% increase in muscle mass that typically occurs with heavy exercise. As the muscle volume increases, pressure in the leg compartments rises, collapsing the veins and increasing capillary resistance. Edema is produced, adding to compartmental pressure to produce an aching, ischemic pain.

Chronic compartmental ischemia may affect any of the compartments, and the onset of pain is usually gradual over 1 year or more. The runner usually must cover a certain distance to bring on the pain, which may persist into the night. The condition is usually bilateral but worse on one side than on the other. On examination, the involved muscle mass may be tender, although the runner may be asymptomatic if he has not exercised before the examination. Chronic compartmental ischemia and a stress fracture may give the same symptoms in the same area in the same type of patient. Although the bone scan in compartmental ischemia generally shows some increased uptake of isotope compared to the healthy side, it is much less than the 300% increase seen in a stress fracture. A saline technique may be used to measure superficial compartment pressure for a baseline, and the runner then runs on a treadmill until becoming symptomatic or tiring out.

The pressure is then remeasured with 30 mm Hg to 40 mm Hg, indicating a compartment syndrome.

A chronic superficial compartment syndrome in a runner is treated with a subcutaneous fasciotomy performed under local anesthesia. Three small incisions are made, and the fascia is stripped longitudinally and divided transversely at the level of the three incisions to leave a wide-open compartment. Running may be resumed in 1 week. Fasciotomy of the deep posterior compartment produces more soreness after the operation, but the runner is usually running again in 6 weeks.

"Tennis Leg"

When a middle-aged tennis player develops soreness in his calf, he may have "tennis leg,"[49, 88, 126] a strain of the medial head of the gastrocnemius near its musculotendinous junction. The gastrocnemius works across two joints, which confuses the muscle and predisposes it to tearing. A tear may occur as the player with low-heeled tennis shoes approaches the net, dorsiflexes his ankles, and suddenly extends his knees. The pain may be sharp and acute, and the player may think that a ball from an adjacent court has struck his calf. The area becomes swollen and ecchymotic, signs that years ago would have been attributed to a plantaris rupture. However, the plantaris tendon usually stays intact even if the heel cord has completely ruptured.[1, 127] The athlete with mild strain notes a generalized aching in his calf and more calf pain when he dorsiflexes his ankle. The medial belly of his gastrocnemius is tender. The soreness should be a warning that continued vigorous activity may produce complete tearing.

For mild strains, the calf is iced for 20 minutes and a strap looped around the foot for passive stretching.[89] The player stretches to discomfort, but short of pain, for 10 seconds, then relaxes for 10 seconds. This activity is continued for 10 minutes. After 5 minutes of ultrasound, the player does isometric and intermedialis exercises in a program that is repeated three times a day. An equinous taping is applied to the calf (Fig. 16-1), and the player wears a shoe with a low heel that provides comfortable calf shortening and promotes a more correct walking style than if he were to wear a higher heel. As swelling and soreness lessen, the player advances to standing calf stretches, returning to competition in about 1 week.

After a moderate strain of the medial head of the gastrocnemius, the muscle partly retracts, leaving a small gap. Soft tissue x-ray films or xerograms will show the gap and the soft tissue swelling. If the player can raise himself on the toes of his injured leg, he should wear a long leg cast for 4 weeks with his knee flexed to 60° and his ankle in gravity plantar flexion, and then wear a short leg cast in neutral position for 3 more weeks. If the medial head of the gastrocnemius has completely ruptured at the musculotendinous junction, the athlete will not be able to stand tiptoe alone on the involved leg. In addition, the gap will not fully close with knee flexion and ankle plantar flexion. These tears are repaired, and the limb is then immobilized as if for a moderate strain.

Achilles Tendon Rupture

The Achilles tendon is the conjoined tendon of the gastrocnemius and soleus muscles, the latter being the major contributor to plantar flexion strength. Much of the blood supply for the Achilles tendon reaches it through its anterior mesentery, and blood supply is poorest in the region 2 cm to 6 cm above the os calcis.[72, 127]

The normal Achilles tendon is very strong, withstanding forces up to 2000 lb during fast running.[33] The usual tearing mechanism is a stress applied to the already contracted musculotendinous unit, usually the pushoff foot, most often the left foot (Fig. 16-2). The biarticular nature of the tendon makes allowance for the athlete to push off at the ankle while extending the knee joint with the Achilles tendon unit. Rupture may occur during sudden dorsiflexion of the ankle or a moment of motor uncoordination. A football player may be pushing against the blocking sled as another athlete falls on his calf, further dorsiflexing his ankle.

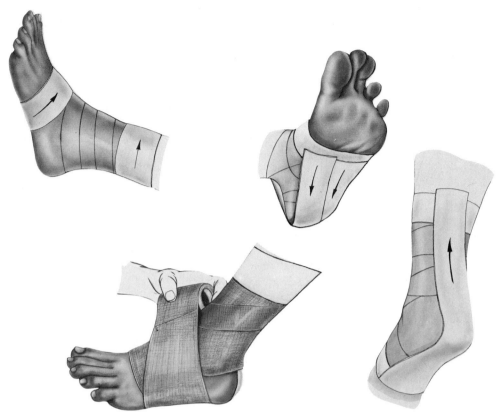

FIG. 16-1
An equinous taping takes tension off the Achilles tendon.

Ski boot pressure may cause ischemia of the Achilles tendon, and when a sudden strain is added, the tendon may rupture. A heel cord may also rupture after local injection of symptom-relieving cortisone when an athlete increases his activity as a result of feeling much better. The tendon tears in the critical zone of poor circulation 2 cm to 6 cm above the os calcis (*see* Fig. 16-2).

Athletes with Achilles tendon rupture are usually older than 30 years of age, with regressive changes in the tendon from lessened blood flow. Typically, they feel a snap during push-off, have pain, and then limp. Examination will reveal swelling, a gap, and increased passive dorsiflexion, but in about one fourth of all ruptures the diagnosis is overlooked[56] because there may have been only mild trauma and pain and the athlete may be able to stand on his toes. He can weakly plantar-flex his foot with the long toe flexors, tibialis posterior, and peroneals. The Achilles tendon appears to function normally, even if only 25% of its fibers remain in continuity. The outline of the tendon is also lost in diffuse swelling, and the gap may fill with a hematoma and be obscured. Thus a swollen lower leg should always be tested for an Achilles tendon rupture.

The "squeeze test" is the definitive test for complete rupture of the Achilles tendon (Fig. 16-3).[127] The injured athlete lies prone or kneels on a chair. The examiner squeezes the athlete's calf in the middle third, just below the place of the widest girth. The examiner's hand must be distal to the apex of the curve of the soleus because even a normal ankle will not plantar-flex if squeezed proximal to the apex of the soleus curve. If the ankle fails to plantar-flex when the calf is squeezed, the rupture is complete.

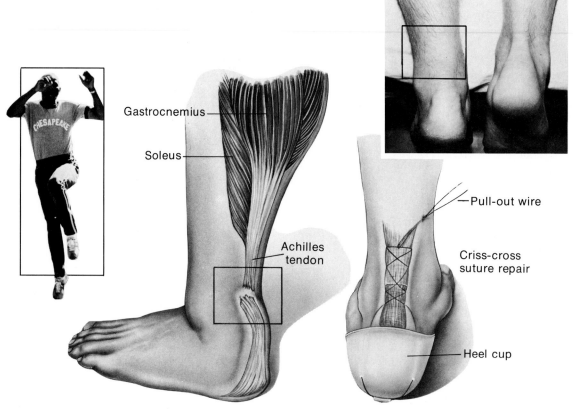

FIG. 16-2
The degenerated tendon of an older athlete may rupture during a
plyometric activity such as long jumping. It usually tears 5 cm to 10 cm
(2 in to 4 in) above its insertion into the calcaneus, and the entire
region swells, obscuring the normal tendon outline. Repair is done with
a criss-cross stitch, and the plantaris tendon is usually woven into the
repair.

Lateral x-ray films of the heel area normally
show a triangular, low-density region occupied
by fat. The triangle is bounded anteriorly by
the flexor tendons, posteriorly by the Achilles
tendon, and inferiorly by the os calcis. After a
complete rupture of the Achilles tendon, the
triangular area becomes more dense, as it does
in Achilles tendinitis and partial ruptures of the
heel cord. After a complete rupture, however,
the triangle is also distorted.[1]

Treatment of an Achilles tendon rupture is
determined on an individual basis, ranging
from nonoperative treatment to surgery.[59] The
Achilles tendon has a considerable ability to
heal itself, and if the ends are opposed it will
heal, avoiding the problems of skin slough,
tendon slough, or infection in this ideal culture
medium of edema, hematoma, and poor blood
supply.[118] If, however, the ends are not opposed, the athlete loses strength and pushoff
power and risks rerupture. It is therefore important to separate cases that will benefit from
closed treatment from those needing operation.[80]

After Achilles tendon rupture, the proximal
fragment retracts, and reduction of the tendon
requires moving *both* ends. Five milliliters of
contrast medium are injected into the gap under
fluoroscopic control, and the ankle is then exercised. The athlete rests his foot on a chair

with his ankle at 90°, a position that straightens the sheath and minimizes its tendency to collapse. The calf is next wrapped with an elastic wrap from the knee crease downwards to force the retracted upper tendon down for better contact. The athlete then lies on his side while the heel cord is fluoroscoped. If the tendon is opposed, the wrap should be removed and a long-leg gravity equinous cast applied and left on for 6 weeks, then changed to a short-leg equinous plaster for 2 weeks, followed by a short-leg walking plaster for 2 additional weeks.[74] Once out of plaster, the athlete wears a 2-cm heel lift for 3 months. Failures and poor results from closed treatment occur if the tendon ends have not been opposed, and, when opposed, if immobilization has been for too short a time.[59] If the tendon ends remain separated after the elastic wrap maneuver, the tendon should be remanipulated, or the ends are opposed operatively.

At operation, surgeons choose from medial, lateral, S-shaped, or zig-zag incisions.[100] The

FIG. 16-3
To test for a ruptured heel cord, the examiner squeezes the athlete's calf and pushes toward the knee.

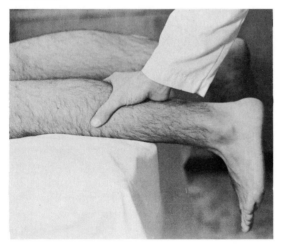

skin and subcutaneous tissue are preserved as one layer, and the laterally situated sural nerve is avoided. Vigorous retraction is also avoided, and the sheath is opened away from the line of the skin cut. On opening the sheath, the surgeon will find the tendon ends shredded into moplike frazzles. The surgeon may use a pull-out wire technique and end-to-end anastomosis along with an interwoven, distally based plantaris tendon graft to reconstruct the tendon.[32, 33, 35] Lack of tension on the muscle may cause marked calf atrophy; thus extreme plantar flexion should be avoided. The ankle is immobilized in as much dorsiflexion as the tendon suture can bear. At 3 weeks, the cast is changed and the foot dorsiflexed within the athlete's pain and motion range. This usually will place the foot at 90° to the leg, and this new cast should be worn for 4 more weeks. The pullout wire is removed at 7 weeks and a high heel worn for 2 months.

Partial Achilles Tendon Rupture

Partial rupture of the Achilles tendon may occur in young, fully grown athletes who are at their highest levels of performance.[29] It occurs especially with increased training loads, presenting as a gradual or immediate onset of sharp, stabbing pain in the lower calf. The athlete limps, and the area is tender locally.

Electrophysiologic studies may be used to diagnose partial ruptures. Potentials are reduced in the muscle of the torn tendon, and the large potentials that usually appear with moderate and strong contractions are absent.

The athlete with a partial Achilles tendon rupture is first treated with cryotherapy, strapping, and a heel lift. Steroid shots are not given because they mask symptoms and may cause a complete rupture. If the rupture is not cured by a conservative program, an operation is done to close the defect. The surgeon splits the tendon to inspect its central parts and excises pathologic granulation tissue and devitalized tissue. Multiple longitudinal incisions are also made in the tendon to encourage revascularization. Postoperatively, the athlete may exercise his ankle immediately.

Achilles Tendinitis

A runner's Achilles tendon may become inflamed if he wears high-heeled dress shoes and then trains in low-heeled shoes, or when he changes from training shoes to competition shoes without heels. It may also happen when a runner switches from cross-country running to a track with more elastic recoil. In each instance, an increased pull on the Achilles tendon occurs. Moreover, if a runner has a sore arch, his tendon may become strained as he dorsiflexes his ankle to avoid pronating his foot.

The runner with a rigid, cavus foot is predisposed to Achilles tendinitis. Uphill runs in stiff shoes will also produce the condition. On the other hand, overpronation in a shoe with a soft heel counter will twist the tendon and produce a tendinitis. The condition may also occur in cyclists who "ankle" too much, although the pain and swelling usually abate when they reduce their ankle motion while pedaling.

Repeated strains produce degeneration of the tendon and granulation tissue forms, usually about 3.75 cm (1.5 in) above the tendon's insertion into the os calcis. The degeneration may be focal or diffuse. In addition, adhesions may develop between the paratenon and the tendon, becoming constricting bands. If a steroid is injected within the paratenon, collagen synthesis is suppressed, further weakening the tendon. Moreover, pressure within the paratenon from the injected material may embarrass the tendon's blood supply and lead to ischemic necrosis. It must be kept in mind that the tendon's blood supply reaches it from its sheath and is tenuous.

A heel pad will lessen the stretching of the Achilles tendon, and a wider, or flared, cushioned heel will limit side-to-side shifting and irritation of the tendon. Arch soreness must be treated early to prevent Achilles tendon problems. If an athlete has chronic tendon pain, the surgeon may have to strip his paratenon if it is obviously diseased. Although the surface of the tendon may look perfectly normal, it should be opened longitudinally and inspected for focal degeneration and areas of degenerated granulation tissue removed.

The Ankle

The ankle works as a hinge with dorsiflexion and plantar flexion. Because the talus is wider anteriorly than posteriorly, there is some play in other planes during plantar flexion. Inversion and eversion occur at the subtalar joint.

The ligaments of the ankle include the distal tibiofibular ligaments, the deltoid ligament on the medial side, and the anterior talofibular, calcaneal-fibular, and posterior talofibular on the lateral side (*see* Fig. 16-4). The distal tibiofibular ligaments strongly bind the tibia and fibula together anteriorly and posteriorly just above the joint line. On the medial side, the deltoid ligament arises from the medial malleolus and fans out to attach on the talus and calcaneus.

The fibula provides muscular attachments and also has a weight-bearing and dynamic, stabilizing function, bearing one sixth of the weight supported by the leg. It changes position, moving to and fro and bowing to stabilize the ankle mortise in response to weight-bearing, ankle motion, and the muscular tractions of plantar flexion. The fibula is pulled distally and medially during contraction of the foot and toe flexors, a shift that deepens the ankle mortise and stabilizes the talus in stance and push-off.

The lateral ankle ligaments arise on the fibula, and the anterior talofibular ligament runs medially, reinforcing part of the weak anterior capsule. It becomes vertical during plantar flexion to serve as a collateral ligament. The distinct, cordlike calcaneal-fibular ligament lies under the sheath of the peroneal tendons. In neutral position, it is vertical and serves as a collateral ligament, but in plantar flexion it is more horizontal. This ligament stabilizes both the ankle and subtalar joints. The posterior talofibular ligament stabilizes against posterior displacement of the talus but is rarely torn unless the ankle is completely dislocated. A lateral talocalcaneal ligament lies between the anterior

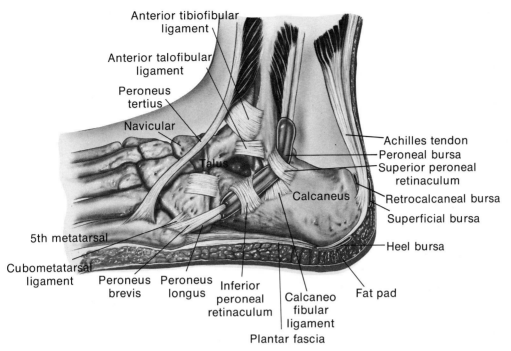

FIG. 16-4
The lateral side of the ankle and foot contains many structures that may
be injured during sports.

talofibular and the calcaneal-fibular ligament,
and its fibers blend with both of these ligaments
and the joint capsule.

Sprains

Anterior Capsular Sprain

During a hook slide in baseball or when a
player's plantar-flexed ankle suffers impact in
football, the anterior capsule may tear. This
injury produces pain on resisted dorsiflexion
and passive plantar flexion, and a long course
of rehabilitation is needed to restore full function. To prevent this type of sprain in baseball,
a lower, breakaway base with a Velcro strap
may be substituted for the standard, high, stationary base.

Medial Eversion Sprain

External rotation and abduction at the ankle
may produce a medial eversion sprain. These

sprains are less common than lateral sprains,
occurring in soccer if the player kicks an opponent and in wrestling when pushing off the
medial side of the foot. If the force is continued,
the distal tibiofibular ligament may tear, and
the interosseous ligament may be damaged. X-
ray films should be repeated 24 to 48 hours
after this injury to be certain that there is no
diastasis of the tibia and fibula. In young athletes, the deltoid ligament may snap off the
medial malleolus like a rubber band and stick
in the joint to produce a widened mortise. This
ligament must then be extracted from the joint
and replaced on the medial malleolus. For ankle
support and to keep the ankles from turning
out, wrestlers must wear high-top shoes.

Lateral Ankle Sprains

A lateral ankle sprain is the most common
sprain. As a result of the normal adduction in
running and the weaker lateral ligaments, an
athlete is more likely to turn his foot in than
out. These sprains occur commonly on an ir-

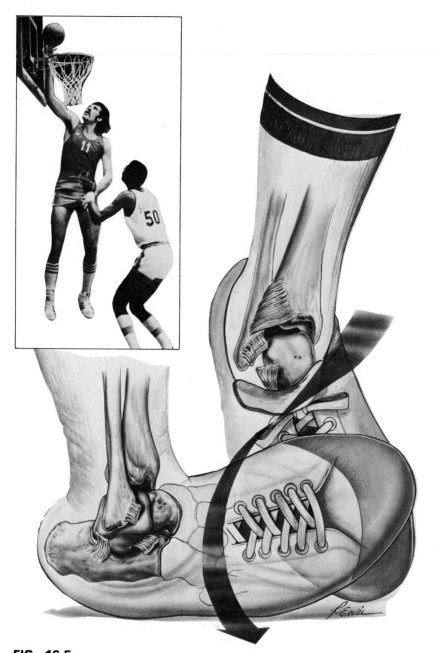

FIG. 16-5
Lateral ankle sprains. A "single-ligament sprain" occurs when the
player's plantar-flexed ankle is inverted, tearing the anterior talofibular
ligament. If the inversion continues when the whole foot has reached
the ground, the calcaneal-fibular ligament rips, producing a "double-
ligament sprain."

regular surface, such as a rutty football field or when landing on another player's foot in basketball. A tight heel cord predisposes to lateral sprains by forcing the foot into inversion and turning the lateral side of the foot under. Most lateral sprains are isolated anterior talofibular injuries.

The mild, moderate, and severe grading system for sprains is hard to apply to lateral ankle sprains because two ligaments are involved. The terms "single ligament tear" and "double ligament tear" are preferable. Lateral ankle ligaments usually tear in a predictable sequence (Fig. 16-5). With plantar flexion and inversion, the anterior talofibular ligament is vertical and tight and tears. This is a single ligament tear. With further inversion, the athlete's full body weight falls on the more dorsiflexed ankle. The calcaneal-fibular ligament is now vertical to the ground, tight, and it also tears, the combination becoming a "double ligament tear."

Signs, Symptoms, and Diagnosis In most sprains, the ankle plantar flexes and inverts. Severe sprains may be accompanied by an audible pop or tearing sensation, pain, and inability to bear weight. The skin about the lateral ligaments is loose and swells easily, and the most swollen ankle may be the least severely injured. Blood may appear around the heel or even out in the toes from leaking, damaged vessels.

Sprained ankles should be examined before swelling and muscle spasm set in to mask the signs, and the ankle should also be viewed from behind. A hemarthrosis will fill in the cavities at either side of the tendo Achilles, whereas an extra-articular hematoma will leave the tendo Achilles defined. The examiner presses on the tibia and fibula to check for fractures and also checks for tenderness at the base of the fifth metatarsal. He then palpates over the ligaments. If a palpable sulcus appears when the ankle is inverted, this is more conclusive evidence of a complete ligament tear than x-ray studies will provide. Gross instability indicates a tear of both ligaments, but the subject should always be asked whether the instability results from an old injury.

To help in giving a prognosis, the athlete should be asked to stand on his toes. If he is able to stand with ease, the prognosis is good, but if he has difficulty standing the prognosis is less promising. Proprioceptive defects are next sought with a modified Romberg test. The athlete stands on his sound foot with his eyes open and then closed, then repeats this test on the injured side. Impaired stability that is obvious to the examiner is objective evidence of a proprioceptive defect. If the athlete notes impaired stability that the examiner cannot confirm, the evidence is considered to be subjective.

X-ray films may show a flake of bone that has been avulsed from the fibula.[4] In children, a distal fibula epiphyseal fracture should be checked for, and the examiner should also look for osteochondral fractures in the talar dome. These are best seen on an internal rotation view of the ankle, mostly at the lateral side of the dome of the talus. If an athlete is not improving as well as expected after an ankle sprain, a talar dome osteochondral fracture should be suspected.

Stress tests include the anterior drawer test and talar tilt test. But because swelling and spasm may mask results from these tests, a peroneal nerve block or hematoma block may be needed.[9] The ankle anterior drawer test is similar to the anterior drawer test of the knee. The athlete sits with his knee flexed to relax his calf, and the examiner gently pulls his heel forward. In functionally normal ankles, the anterior drawer does not exceed 3 mm, and the right and left ankles are roughly equal. When the foot moves forward with crepitation at the ankle, the anterior talofibular ligament is torn, and if the test is grossly positive the calcaneal-fibular ligament is also torn.

To check for talar tilt, the examiner should let the foot fall into normal plantar flexion. The examiner then places one hand medially over the tibia while pressing the other lateral to the heel. The degree of talar tilt produced is influenced by the ankle position at the time of stress. Testing at neutral position analyzes the calcaneal-fibular ligament, whereas a plantar-flexed talar tilt test assesses the anterior talofibular ligament. There is no clear-cut amount of tilt that distinguishes between single and double ligament tears, with most results in the 10° to 20° gray zone. There is a wide normal range, with some subjects showing more than 20°. A positive test is considered to be 10° more talar tilt than is found in the normal joint,[120] although there are right and left differences with talar tilt, and the sound side may open more than the injured side.[110]

An ankle arthrogram may help in the diagnosis of double-ligament tears. The calcaneal-fibular ligament lies deep to the peroneal tendons and is closely associated with the peroneal tendon sheath. An arthrogram may show dye leaking from the joint into the peroneal sheath, indicating a calcaneal-fibular ligament tear. If the dye leaks through a large anterior talofibular tear, however, it may not pass through an associated smaller calcaneal-fibular ligament tear. To avoid this deficiency, dye may be injected directly into the peroneal sheath, along the anterior border of the peroneus brevis tendon, just behind the fibula about 4 cm proximal to the lateral malleolus.[6, 11] If the calcaneal-fibular ligament is torn, dye will pass into the ankle joint. If the arthrogram is done more than a week after the injury, however, it will be invalid because the tear will have sealed. Arthrograms are useful diagnostic adjuncts but are not as reliable as the palpation of a sulcus with the ankle inverted.

Prevention Many ankle sprains can be prevented with heel-cord stretching, proprioceptive training, and proper footwear. Sitting causes the heel cords to tighten and resist ankle dorsiflexion, whereupon the foot inverts. For this reason, all athletes should stretch their heel cords on a step or an ankle board before and after practice.

If an athlete walks and runs only on flat surfaces, a proprioceptive deficiency will develop. Proprioceptive ability can be gained by running on uneven surfaces or on a trampoline or by using a foot seesaw or wobble board each day. Although some athletes train with ankle weights, these may throw off their coordination and produce more sprains due to fatigue.

Proper footwear can also reduce the incidence of ankle sprains. Thus, training shoes should not be worn for cutting sports, as they are made for straight-ahead movement. High-top shoes are best but are not considered stylish today. Wrestlers wear them because they stay on the feet and resist abrasions to the ankle. If the athlete wears a low-cut shoe, tape may be applied firmly around it. X-ray films show that such taping lessens slipping and sliding between the foot and the shoe, making the foot and shoe a single functional unit and stimulating the stability of high-top shoes. The position of cleats on the soles also may influence ankle sprains. Cleats located a distance from the edge of the shoe offer a narrow base of support. For broader support, cleats should extend to the lateral margin of the shoe.

Routine "Preventive" Ankle Taping Adhesive tape is the biggest item in the training room, and miles of tape are used each year.[40] A hundred million dollars is spent on tape each year for high school tackle football, and its cost is soaring. Elastic tape costs even more than cloth-backed tape.

Even though taping dominates much of the trainer's time, the athlete loses support from the tape almost as soon as he walks out of the training room, and after the practice or contest the tape is discarded. Unfortunately, athletes often become psychologically dependent on taped ankles. A poor taping job can restrict the athlete's running speed and vertical jump height and may even cause injury by restricting a normal range of motion. If normal subtalar motion is blocked, its safety-valve action is compromised, and ankle sprains increase. Skillful strapping, however, may reduce such sprains.

During running, the foot comes down inverted, and the peroneus brevis contracts just before heel strike to evert the foot and to place it into a more stable position. A simple lateral loop, or a heel lock over the sock, may prevent some ankle sprains by its action on the peroneus brevis. The loop of tape may excite the peroneus brevis to contract earlier and stabilize the ankle in swing. A more complete taping job is not needed to serve this function. Routine festooning of sound, healthy ankles with adhesive tape often is unnecessary. The motto, "never sprained, never taped" makes good sense.

Playing fields should be maintained and policed so that they have no rocks, divots, or potholes. In one instance, a coach improved the condition of his field by banning local rodeos and livestock shows that had been held on the football field for decades.[134] Good maintenance of the playing field will do more to prevent ankle sprains than will taping jobs and shoe changes. With respect to indoor courts, more sprains occur on artificial floors than on wood courts, and for this reason players should wear worn gym shoes to decrease friction.

Acute Treatment of Ankle Sprains Swelling of an ankle sprain is controlled with "ICE"—*I*ce, *C*ompression, and *E*levation—and must not be accepted as a part of the injury. Wet elastic wraps kept in a bucket of ice water in an ice chest should be wrapped from the toes up over the sprain. An ice bag is then applied and kept in place with another elastic wrap over it and the leg elevated. Alternately, the ankle may be placed in a bucket of ice slush and a neoprene toecap worn to warm the toes, as the slush is shockingly cold. The ice is left on for 30 minutes, taken off for an hour, and then reapplied. A transcutaneous electrical nerve stimulator can be activated for 30 minutes during the off hour. If the ankle is very painful, a local anesthetic and aqueous steroid may be injected.[9]

A note should be sent home with the athlete describing the injury and its treatment, and the athlete and his parents should be cautioned against using a home remedy, such as hot epsom salts, which will cause the ankle to blow up. An open, basket-weave taping job is applied for support and an elastic wrap applied for compression.[79] Because the elastic wrap works best on cylinders and will not compress in the hollow about the malleous, this area should be filled with felt, or a foam horseshoe pad, to establish even compression. The elastic wrap should be removed at night because the wrap could change position and act as a tourniquet if the foot slips off the pillow. A suitcase placed under the foot of the mattress offers better elevation.

The athlete may be permitted to bear weight a bit within his pain tolerance to retain his proprioceptive sense. Also, early cryotherapy range-of-motion exercises and isometrics prevent atrophy. Contrast baths may usually begin 48 hours after the injury; they alternately dilate and constrict the vessels, producing a pumping action[22] that drains edema, lymph, and residue and relieves pain and stiffness. Moreover, blood flow is increased for 45 minutes after a treatment, helping to repair damaged tissue. Contrast treatments are given three times a day in a whirlpool or in a galvanized tub. The cold phase is in a slush made with water and ice cubes with a temperature of about 16°C (60°F). The warm phase is in water with a temperature that ranges from about 38°C to 41°C (100°F to 105°F). The athlete may follow a 10-minute program, starting with 1 minute in cold water and 3 minutes in warm water. He then does 1 minute in the cold and 2 in the warm, followed by 1 in the cold and 1 in the warm, finishing with a final minute in the cold. Cryotherapy with ice massage or in a 60-degree whirlpool will also promote recovery, and exercise may be permitted after the skin turns pink and becomes numb.

Foot and ankle exercises include foot circles and writing the alphabet with the big toe while the ankle extends over the edge of the table. For foot exercise, the athlete picks up tape rolls and other objects and pulls in a towel with his foot. As he improves, a weight may be added to the towel for resistance. Resistance exercises are begun when he has pain-free ankle motion, starting with isometrics (Fig. 16-6). He may perform these alone, and his parents or friends may also be taught to help. A lightweight bicycle inner tube may be used for isodynamic resistance. Cryotherapy permits toe raisers on a 2 inch × 4 inch board or on a step performed with the toes turned out. As swelling and soreness disappear, power work may begin on the Orthotron isokinetic unit. Isokinetic training is important because fast contractions are needed to resist inversion.

When ankle ligaments are torn, proprioceptive nerve endings are also torn. These nerves normally provide feedback that signals the need

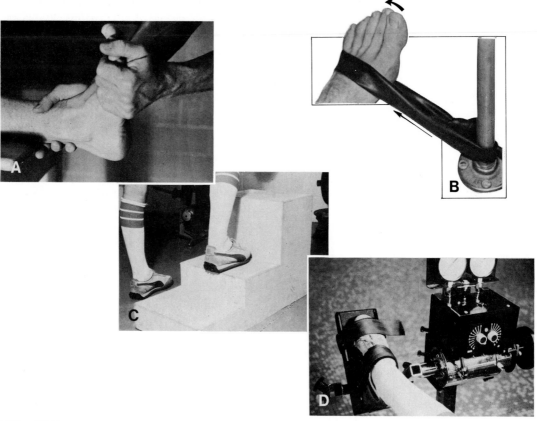

FIG. 16-6
A sprained ankle may be strengthened isometrically against the trainer's manual resistance (*A*), isodynamically (*B*), by side step-ups (*C*), and isokinetically (*D*).

for appropriate muscle action. Once torn, these nerves do not heal. The athlete may however, restore his sense of balance and coordination by a mechanism similar to that involved in learning to ride a bicycle or to walk on a tightrope. The re-education process may be performed on a seesaw block or on a tilt board curved in one plane. The board imposes passive displacements on the athlete's foot similar to uneven ground as the athlete stands at varying angles to its axis of movement. While maintaining his balance on one leg, he tries to prevent either end of the block from touching the floor. He advances next to a wobble board (*see* Fig. 16-7), a plywood disc placed on half a croquet ball or a doorknob, leaving the board free to tip in all planes. The athlete balances on the

board untaped, since the board will hit the ground before the ankle inverts too much.

The next step in rehabilitating the ankle is special training on walking style. With restricted ankle motion, the athlete will tend to abduct and rotate his leg externally with his knee extended, using his heel as a pivot point. This naturally protective gain minimizes ankle motion and allows long strides with the sound limb. To walk fast, he carries his injured limb through in abduction. The injured athlete should be taught to walk with a short step, with his feet about 10 cm (4 in) apart, and his toes pointing forward. True ankle motion is used with the heel striking first. The quadriceps and gluteus maximus waste, however, if an athlete uses this short step walk; for this reason, isomteric and resistive hip and knee extension should be added to the exercise program.

Stress can be taken off the lateral ligaments with a heel wedge. A 1.25-cm (0.5 in) lateral wedge made of felt may be placed inside the athlete's toe, or a 0.63-cm (0.25-in) neoprene lateral heel wedge may be glued in. The athlete should not wear cleats in the early rehabilitative phase, and the ankle should be taped for exercise. The athlete may begin to jog straight ahead with his ankle taped when he can walk with a normal pushoff and without a limp, taking care to walk the turns. Then, if he has no limp, he may jog the turns. When turns can be jogged without a limp, he may increase to one-half-speed runs and then full speed. When he is able to run turns without a limp, he may start running circles of progressively smaller, diameters clockwise and counterclockwise. He then runs a zigzag course and progressively tighter figure-eights. Isodynamic running is superior to running in place or jumping rope because the tubing allows body lean. Because jumping rope demands great proprioception, it is not included in the early rehabilitation of an athlete with an ankle sprain.

The advanced program includes side step-ups, progressing from 5-minute endurance bouts on a 4-inch block to the 8-inch block, the 12-inch step, and finally the 18-inch bench. Next come runs up the stadium steps sideways, half-speed cuts and finally right-angled cuts, stops, starts, and jumps. Tackle football players also use a crossover step run.

Running on the fairway of a golf course or on a cross-country course will strengthen the athlete's ankle ligaments and enhance proprioception. He should also be encouraged to ride a bicycle, and his ankle range of motion can be increased by adjusting the saddle. More plantar flexion occurs as the saddle is raised.

Protective Taping A complete rehabilitation program is the key to restoring full ankle function. Festooning the ankle with tape is not a substitute for functional strength; it gives only a false sense of security. Damaged ankles should be protectively taped for contact or heavy activity for the rest of the season, however, because the collagen in the ligaments takes about 7 months to mature. The ankle need not be taped routinely the following year, as the rehabilitation program should return it to normal. A skillful and correctly applied taping will limit abnormal extremes of motion but should not influence the normal range of motion. If normal subtalar motion is limited by taping, the ankle may be sprained again.

When a damaged ankle requires daily taping, the athlete should shave the area the night before so that the skin will not be too sensitive. If taping is needed two or three times a day, a polyurethane foam underwrap material should be applied first. Tape should be applied only to skin that is at room temperature. Taping done just after cold or heat treatment may damage the skin when the tape is removed. After the tape is removed, a skin lubricant should be used to restore moisture to the dry skin.

Standard ankle wraps do not enhance ankle stability. If they are used, benzoin should first be applied to the skin. A sock is then pulled on and sprayed with benzoin, and the ankle wrap is wrapped over the sock.

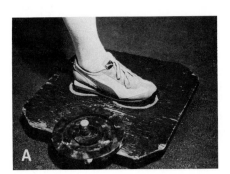 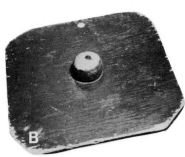

FIG. 16-7
A "wobble board" allows the athlete to regain proprioception. Weights may be added (*A*) to strengthen the ankle. The board wobbles on a doorknob or on half a croquet ball (*B*).

Surgery for an Acute Lateral Ankle Sprain
When an athlete sustains a serious double-ligament ankle sprain, he may note a tearing sensation and will have difficulty if asked to stand on his toes. The examiner can feel a gap laterally when the ankle is stressed, and the tear produces gross instability.[25, 117]

If the torn ends are not grossly separated, the sprain will heal well without operation. The ligament will fail to heal, however, if the ends are grossly separated, even if the leg is encased in plaster. Operation guarantees approximation, even when the ligament is originally grossly separated.[120]

The operation is performed through a short oblique incision and the skin gently retracted. In about one half of these cases, the surgeon will find that the torn calcaneal-fibular ligament is sufficiently approximated to have allowed healing with closed treatment. Only by exploring the region, however, can the surgeon determine whether the ligament edges are adequately opposed. Sometimes, the calcaneal-fibular ligament will be found to have pulled from its fibular attachment under the peroneal sheath to lie on top of the sheath. In such cases, closed treatment will not effect reattachment. Instead, reattachment is accomplished by means of holes drilled through the fibula. After operation, the leg is kept in a cast for 6 weeks, and the athlete then follows a rehabilitation program similar to that for the treatment of single ligament sprains.

Chronic Ankle Instability

Chronic instability in a golfer after an ankle sprain may result in his left ankle giving out or in repeated sprains in running and jumping athletes. Foot and ankle inversion before heel strike is accentuated, and the chronically unstable ankle suffers unbalanced loading. The medial aspect of the talus also develops arthritic wear.[52]

Before the surgeon decides to operate on a chronically unstable ankle, the athlete should complete a 3-month rehabilitation program while wearing proper shoes. Some athletes will have "stable instability" in which the ankle gives way during activity, although it is stable when examined. In place of surgery, neuromuscular re-education on a wobble board is needed. Surgery is also deferred if the ankle causes no functional problems but is unstable only when it is stressed. Operative repair of the ankle is indicated if it remains sore and continues to give way despite full rehabilitation.

Late direct repair, tenodesis, and reconstruction are among the procedures designed to stabilize these ankles. In late repairs, the ligaments are reefed and tightened.[5] For a tenodesis (the Evans procedure), the surgeon sections the tendon of the peroneus brevis and reroutes the distal portion of the tendon through a hole in the fibula, reattaching it to its proximal part.[43, 44] The rerouted tendon then provides a vector between the two stretched-out ligaments but does not restore the function of either directly. In most cases, the tendon will scar down as a tenodesis, but sometimes it may continue to move.

Among the reconstructive procedures performed for chronic ankle instability are the Watson–Jones operation, the modified Watson–Jones, and the Chrisman–Snook procedure. In the Watson–Jones, the surgeon transfers a one-half thickness strip of the tendon of the peroneus brevis.[48, 136] He passes the tendon strip through a hole drilled in the fibula, as in the Evans procedure. The strip is then continued through a drill hole in the talus and passed back to the fibula. In a modified Watson–Jones, instead of directing the tendon through the talar tunnel from above to below, it is brought from below to above to better resemble an anterior talofibular ligament.[52, 120, 141] If the tendon of the peroneus brevis is too small, the peroneus longus is used.

The Chrisman–Snook reconstructive procedure is a modification of the Elmslie procedure[17, 38] in which the tendon of the peroneus brevis is used rather than the fascia lata strips used in the Elmslie. The surgeon first sections the tendon of the peroneus brevis proximally and frees it to the base of the fifth metatarsal. It is next passed under the talocalcaneal ligament and sutured to remnants of the anterior talofibular ligament or passed through a slit in the anterior talofibular ligament. After feeding the tendon through a hole in the distal fibula, the surgeon brings it downward to replace the calcaneal-fibular ligament and sets it into a tunnel in the calcaneus. This reconstruction thus replaces both the anterior talofibular and the calcaneal-fibular ligaments.

After an ankle reconstruction, the athlete's leg is placed in a walking cast for 7 weeks, and the rehabilitation program should be the same as that for an athlete with a single ligament sprain.

Peroneal Tendon Dislocation

The tendons of the peroneus longus and brevis run in a groove behind the lateral malleolus. If an athlete's ankle is dorsiflexed forcefully and his peroneal tendons contract, the peroneal retinaculum may rupture about 2 mm from its insertion into the fibula, freeing the tendons. This occurs when a skier falls forward, loading the inner edge of the lower ski. This type of dislocation was more frequent when low ski boots were worn, but it still occurs when higher boots are buckled improperly.

Early diagnosis of peroneal tendon dislocation is important so that the retinaculum can be repaired.[121] It may mimic an ankle sprain, but, with the tendon dislocation, tenderness is felt behind the lateral malleolus rather than over the lateral ligaments. The examiner may even be able to reproduce the dislocation of the tendons by dorsiflexing the athlete's ankle.

An athlete with recurrent peroneal tendon dislocation reports ankle pain, snapping, and instability. In late cases, the retinaculum may be so atrophied as to be irreparable.[9] Several operations have been designed to solve this problem. A periosteal flap may be swung back over the tendons to hold them in place, or the tendons may be rerouted deep to the strong calcaneofibular ligament.[107] In the Ellis–Jones procedure, a tendon strap is constructed to hold the peroneal tendons medially.[65, 68] A strip of the Achilles tendon 5 mm wide is freed proximally and left attached to the os calcis. It is then passed over the peroneal tendons and through a hole drilled deep in the peroneal groove. The tendon strap is next sutured back

on itself and pulled snug with the ankle in dorsiflexion. Sometimes the surgeon selects the plantaris tendon as the tendon strap. If he finds that the groove for the peroneal tendons is very shallow, he may elect to deepen it.

Osteochondral Fracture of the Talus

A cross-country runner may step in a hole, twist his ankle, hear a pop, and develop ankle pain. The injury is usually treated as an ankle sprain, but later the athlete may develop a "weak ankle" with deep ankle pain, recurrent swelling, and a grating sensation. Such slow improvement or worsening after an ankle sprain may be due to an osteochondral fracture of the talus.

An osteochondral fracture in the dome of the talus may follow a compression injury to the subchondral bone.[82, 95, 140] A fragment may partly detach (stage III) and later become completely detached (stage IV). Even though it becomes completely detached, however, it may remain in place, never moving from its normal position.

Lateral lesions, produced by shearing forces, are shallow and are more likely than medial lesions to displace and to cause symptoms. They are also "wafer" shaped located in the midportion of the talus (Fig. 16-8) and are best

FIG. 16-8
Osteochondral fracture is most often seen as a "wafer" on the lateral dome of the talus.

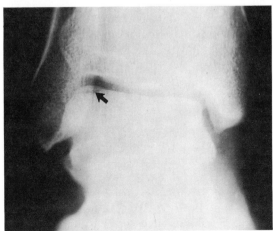

seen on an anteroposterior x-ray view with the ankle in neutral position and rotated internally about 10°. Some medial lesions probably have a traumatic origin, but others may have been present since childhood. Their depth is often greater than their width, and they are less likely to displace and are less symptomatic than lateral lesions.[3, 15] Medial lesions are cup shaped, located on the posterior surface of the talar dome and may be best seen on an anteroposterior plantar-flexed view. Tomograms are sometimes needed to discern lateral and medial osteochondral lesions.

The athlete with a stage I or stage II lateral or medial lesion should wear a cast for 12 to 18 weeks, until healing is noted between the fragment and the underlying bone. A stage III medial lesion is treated initially with a cast, but if symptoms persist the fragment is excised and the crater curetted. Early operation is indicated for stage III lateral lesions and all stage IV lateral and medial lesions. The lateral lesions are best approached through an anterolateral incision because the fibula is posterior and the lesion is in the middle third. An osteotomy of the medial malleolus may be needed to provide adequate exposure of a medial lesion.

"Footballer's Ankle"

A soccer player's ankle may be extremely plantar flexed when kicking a heavy ball on a wet pitch. He may note that his ankle becomes painful with kicking and with sudden stops and starts, and he may have swelling and tenderness at the anterior aspect of his ankle joint. An x-ray film may show that new bone has formed on the upper surface of the neck of the talus as a result of traction at the insertion of the capsule.[87, 94] Painful capsular bone spurs may be removed, as pain will be persistent and the spurs may even chip off into the joint.

To help prevent capsular sprains and the development of footballer's ankle, young players should use a number-3 ball, advance to number-4, and, finally, when their feet are large and strong, use a full-sized soccer ball.

The Feet

Evaluating the Runner

The injured runner should be required to fill out a form describing his problem and when it began. His training program should be detailed, including where he runs and any recent change in training, because more than half of all running injuries result from training errors. Such errors may include an abrupt increase in distance, duration, frequency, or intensity of training or an abrupt change in terrain or footwear. An injury may also be attributed to running when, in fact the injury has come from another activity unrelated to running.

An injury history may reveal that the runner had back or hip trouble in childhood. Just as a foot problem may cause trouble elsewhere in the body, problems at the back, hip, or knee can influence the feet. While the foot is moving and swiveling in three dimensions at the same time, the knee and hip are also moving in three planes. These joints integrate to form a pathway of motion amounting to 45 vectors that allow an almost infinite number of compensations.[21] Subclinical problems such as a pelvic tilt or a weak leg can disturb this linkage system, and the trouble is often manifested at a point far removed from the site of the problem. A leg-length difference of 0.25 in may cause sacroiliac pain, lower back pain, or greater trochanteric bursitis. If one leg is as much as 10% weaker than the other, it may disturb balance, rhythm, and gait.

The athlete to be examined stands barefoot, clad in shorts, facing the examiner, who checks for surgical scars, quadriceps alignment, bowlegs, knock-knees, and abnormal leg rotation. Does the athlete have pre-existing foot problems? Is his arch too high or too low? Is the forefoot adducted or splayed? Does he have a Morton's foot with a short hypermobile first ray? In this last case, the great toe will be shorter than the second toe. A check is made for hallux valgus, hammer toes, claw toes, or a bunionette—a prominence of the lateral side of the head of the fifth metatarsal.

With the athlete standing sideways, he is

checked for lordosis and knee recurvatum. The runner is next asked to face away from the examiner and to stand straight. The examiner's hands are placed on the runner's iliac crests to check for pelvic tilt. The runner is asked to bend over and touch the floor with his knees straight as a measure of general flexibility and to check for scoliosis. His calf muscle development is observed from behind, and the examiner checks the angle made by the long axis of the Achilles tendon with a line bisecting his os calcis.

While the runner lies supine on the examining table, the examiner checks the range of motion of his hips, hamstring flexibility, and limb lengths. The athlete then sits on the examining table as the examiner checks the area of his symptoms. If the knee is involved, each of its structures is systematically checked. The shin is exaimined for tender areas and heel-cord flexibility ascertained first with the knee bent and then with the knee extended.

The runner next kneels on the examining table with his feet extending over the side. The foot is relaxed in this position and is checked for subtalar motion and forefoot varus or valgus. The sole is examined for calluses, blisters, warts, or "athlete's foot." The impact area of the heel and the origin and course of the plantar fascia are palpated. The examiner should also feel under each metatarsal head and observes for pinch calluses medial to the metatarsal and on the medial side of the great toe that reflect hypermobility of the first ray.

The runner's training shoes, competition shoes, and everyday walking shoes are checked to determine their suitability. With the training shoes on the runner's feet, they are again checked for rearfoot and midfoot support and the toebox and the position of the underlying toes noted.

The runner should demonstrate his personal flexibility routine. Some athletes claim to be performing a full flexibility routine, but deficiencies are found when the program is demonstrated. The neck, shoulders, midsection, anterior hip capsules, adductors, quadriceps, hamstrings, iliotibial bands, and heel cords should be stretched.

The examination of a runner is not complete until his running form is evaluated for technical faults. All runners run differently, however, and even a champion runner may have an unusual running form that is perfectly normal for him. The athlete's gait may be videotaped as he runs on a treadmill, and slow-motion playback and stop action allow a complete analysis, permitting an accurate assessment of biomechanics and clues to a cure. A runner sometimes is asked to run until he is tired, and he is then put on the treadmill to note whether fatigue brings on gait abnormalities that would otherwise be unobserved; for example, a runner may be fine when he runs toed in but starts rotating out and developing knee pain when he tires.

X-ray films may be needed, including heel films, weight-bearing views in the shoes, tarsal coalition views, a skin pin x-ray, or sesamoid x-ray. After a complete examination, the runner is advised of the findings, and any necessary training changes, treatments, orthotic devices, or shoe modifications are discussed, along with the reasons for each decision.

Returning to Running After an Injury

Before an athlete returns to running after an injury, he must be *free of pain during normal daily activities* and should obtain any prescribed orthosis or shoe modification. During the layoff, he can wear a water-skiing vest and run in the deep water in the diving well of a swimming pool. His running resumes on flat terrain with low mileage every other day and builds to his normal distance and pace.

Training Shoes

Runners may be light or heavy, fast or slow and have narrow or wide, rigid or flexible feet. These differences require that training shoes have features best suited for the individual runner (*see* Fig. 16-9). The shoe should have a soft ankle collar with a well-molded Achilles pad.

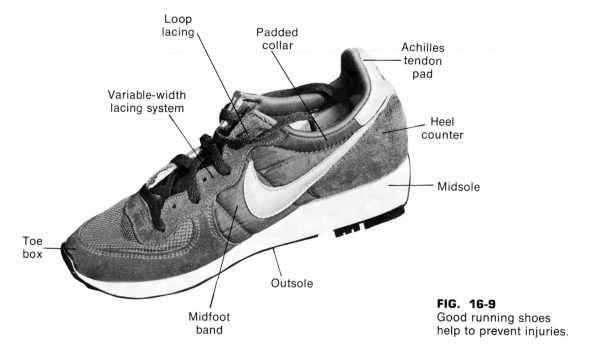

Loop lacing

Padded collar

Achilles tendon pad

Variable-width lacing system

Heel counter

Midsole

Toe box

Outsole

Midfoot band

FIG. 16-9
Good running shoes help to prevent injuries.

FIG. 16-10
The rounded heel (*A*) smooths impacts. Wedge-shaped cutouts in the heel (*B*) help to absorb shock. The widely flared heel (*C*) may help Achilles tendon problems but may lead to knee trouble and shoe breakdown between the counter and heel. The slightly flared heel (*D*) is ideal.

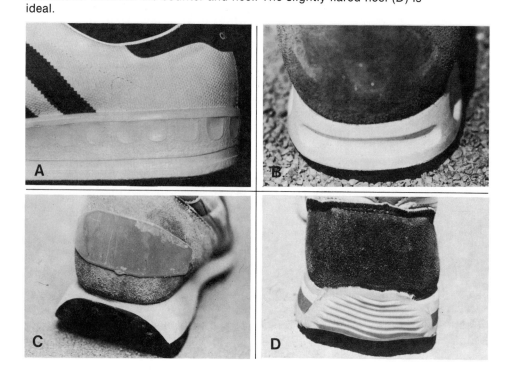

A notched counter helps to eliminate pressure on the lower Achilles. A firm heel counter stabilizes the heel from shifting and prevents shoe breakdown. In some shoes, the counter can be further snugged up through the lacing system.

A flared heel can control heel strike, decrease wobble, and dissipate forces over a broad area (*see* Fig. 16-10). Too wide a heel (more than 7.5 cm, or 3 in), however, can cause too rapid pronation, with resulting knee pain. Also, if the angle between the heel counter and the heel is too great, the shoe may break down, especially in runners who overpronate. Such runners should select a shoe with a shallow angle between the heel counter and the heel itself. The outer edge of the heel should not be allowed to wear down, and it can be reinforced with a heel plate or shoe patching material.

Shoe Lasts

Even though there is no adduction in a normal foot, most shoes are made with an inward flare. Straight last shoes (vector last) are symmetrical about the long axis of the sole (Fig. 16-11). They give extra medial support under a runner's navicular like a "Thomas heel" and are best for slower runners who land on their heels and for runners who overpronate. Curve-lasted shoes are shaped to maximize support to the outer part of the foot during faster running.

Outsole

The outsole should be tough, flexible rubber. The thickest soles are not necessarily the best shock-absorbers as shock absorption depends more on the firmness of the rubber used. The outsole may be rippled or studded, and each ripple will act to dissipate some shock while also giving good traction.

Midsole

Most training shoes have a full-length midsole and wedge, and these should be made of highly resilient material that will provide excellent shock absorption. Such shock protection is especially important for runners with rigid feet who need a well-cushioned shoe.

Innovative training and racing shoes have channels of pressurized gas encapsulated within

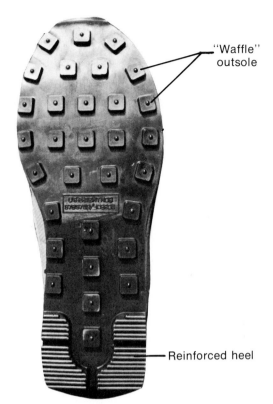

"Waffle" outsole

Reinforced heel

FIG. 16-11
This vector last (straight last) outsole has a reinforced heel and shock-absorbing "waffles."

a cushioned midsole (Fig. 16-12) to reduce heel and forefoot impact. The cushion of "air" absorbs and redistributes the energy generated with every foot strike. These lightweight shoes are especially suited for the racer with rigid feet and for hard, even training surfaces and hilly road courses. They are not recommended for very heavy runners or for those who are overpronators unless an orthotic device is worn, nor are they suited to grass or rocky or uneven terrain.

Runners with flexible feet gain extra stability with an extended medial counter, and a stability saddle will serve as a foundation to the heel cup for even greater support and stability. The overpronating runner should, however, wear stabilizing shoes several times before running in them to allow the feet to adapt to the new position.

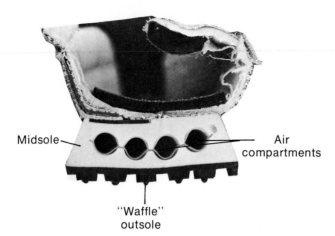

FIG. 16-12
This cutaway view of a midsole shows the air compartments.

Midsole

Air compartments

"Waffle" outsole

Boarded Last and Slip Last

A boarded last is a conventional last in which a fiber board insole makes for a stiffer shoe and the board lends stabilizing firmness and firmer heel support. This type of shoe is best for the average weight runner or the runner with a heavy heel strike. Such shoes are also good for the beginner running slowly and landing on his heel.

A slip last is sewn together like a moccasin, giving light weight and flexibility. The slip last aids fitting, as the shoe can be brought in snug. This type of shoe is recommended for runners with rigid feet and for young runners. Some shoes are partially slip lasted; they are flexible yet provide extra rearfoot stability.

Insole

An insole gives shock absorption, support, and comfort, and a foam insole can mold to the pressure pattern of the foot to give an individual fit. Removable insoles may be modified with wedges or the insole may be removed, allowing the shoe to accommodate an orthotic device. Soft rubber liners add to shock absorption and comfort. Many shoes have rubber arch cookies that give minimal support but may be in the wrong place and cause blisters.

The Midfoot and Forefoot

A midfoot band allows stability, and variable width lacing with staggered eyelets allows a snug fit, and stretchy laces prevent constriction. Vertical stabilizer straps work in conjunction with the lacing system for additional midfoot support. Nylon mesh in the forefoot region permits air circulation, and a rounded toe box prevents crowding of the toes.

Other Shoes

If shoes have grip aids, such as cleats or spikes, these should be positioned properly. If the cleats are set in too far from the sides of the shoe, the athlete's ankle may turn and sprain. The old-style tackle football shoe with seven 0.75-inch cleats was responsible for many knee injuries.[128] Today, the preferred shoe has a synthetic, molded sole with 14 short soccer-type cleats. Football and basketball shoes often have deficient insoles; thus an individually fitted foam insole may have to be added for shock absorption and comfort.[71] The shoe should be about 0.5 inches longer than the athlete's longest toe when he is bearing weight, and if the toebox rubs against his toes he should change to another style of toebox. Toe bumpers in tennis shoes are reinforced to prevent the toe of the shoe from wearing away too quickly during the service.

Selection and Care

Shoes should be tried on at the time of day that the athlete will normally be using them. Both shoes must be tried because the feet may differ in size. The runner should select a shoe based on a proper fit, comfort, and qualities that will benefit his foot, rather than choosing one because it is ranked high in a survey. Shoe ratings may give a low ranking to a durable shoe well suited for training. The athlete should not wear training shoes for other sports because they are not designed for cutting and playing tennis or basketball.

Ideally, an athlete should have two pair of shoes broken in; while one pair is in use, the other pair can be drying or airing out. When not in use, shoes may be left unlaced with absorbent foot powder sprinkled in them. If the shoes are wet after practice, they should be left in front of a fan to dry, not on a radiator, as heat will harm them. Shoes should be checked periodically and worn areas reinforced or rebuilt to prevent imbalances owing to asymmetric wear, as a breakdown of an athlete's shoes may lead to breakdown of his feet.

Problems Around the Heel

Problems affecting the athlete's heel include Achilles tendinitis, subcutaneous bursitis, "runner's bump," retrocalcaneal bursitis and bony prominence, stress fracture of the calcaneum, pinch of the os trigonum, "black dot heel," and heel bruises.[109]

Subcutaneous Bursitis

An unpadded, thin shoe counter, such as may be found in some cycling and running shoes, will irritate the subcutaneous bursa behind the lower part of the Achilles tendon, causing redness, swelling, and pain. To avoid this problem, or at the first sign of irritation in this region, the athlete should apply a Band-Aid, tape, or "second skin" and change to a shoe with a soft counter.

"Runner's Bump"

A prominence at the back of an athlete's heel may be a "runner's bump" (*see* Fig. 16-13). The bump is due to avulsions of bone flakes by his heel cord from his os calcis. A lateral x-ray film will show a stalagmite of bone extending from about 1.5 cm below the posterior-superior tip of the os calcis upward into the Achilles tendon. Once a bump has formed, it is usually

FIG. 16-13
A "runner's bump" may be caused by a bony buildup at the insertion of the Achilles tendon into the os calcis (*arrow*). A prominent posterior-superior part of the os calcis may be responsible for retrocalcaneal bursitis and irritation of the Achilles tendon. In such cases, the prominence may be resected (*dotted line*).

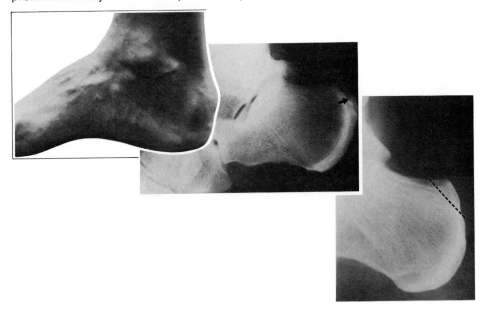

not excised for fear of weakening the heel cord. To prevent these bumps from occurring or enlarging, the athlete can work on heel cord stretching, use a heel lift, and wear shoes with a wider heel that will limit rocking..

Retrocalcaneal Bony Prominence

The heel cord begins its insertion to the os calcis about 1.5 cm distal to the uppermost posterior part of the bone. The bony area above the insertion is smooth and occupied by a retrocalcaneal bursa. This area is sometimes prominent and may rub against the bursa and the heel cord to cause pain and swelling (*see* Fig. 16-13).

To lessen this irritation, the runner can wear training shoes with a flared heel to reduce rocking at heel strike. If symptoms persist, an oblique osteotomy of the prominent bone may be performed. At operation, the surgeon retracts the heel cord and removes the bump obliquely down to the level of the heel cord insertion. Early postoperative motion is allowed, and the athlete can usually expect a good result.

Os Calcis Stress Fracture

A ballet dancer, especially one who has a long, thin os calcis, may note a gradual onset of pain and swelling at the back of her heel.[55, 135, 138] This may be caused by a stress fracture of the os calcis that can be mistaken for Achilles tendinitis. With a stress fracture, however, the bone will be tender. X-ray films of the bone may not show a fracture line initially, but one may appear later at the upper posterior margin of the os calcis, just anterior to the apophyseal plate at a right angle to the trabeculi. These fractures are immobilized in a walking plaster cast for 5 weeks.

Os Trigonum Pinch

The os trigonum is an accessory bone located just behind the talus and is found in only 10% of the population. With extreme plantar flexion, such as in ballet, jumping, or bowling at cricket, the os trigonum may be nipped like a nut in a nutcracker, producing local pain when the subject springs off his toes.[132, 135] The athlete with this disorder should rest the foot until the soreness abates. A talar spur may break off in this region, and the broken piece may have to be removed to relieve pain.

"Black Dot Heel"

Young distance runners may develop "black dot heel," a condition in which painless, irregular, black or bluish-black plaques appear on the posterior or posterolateral aspect of one or both heels (Fig. 16-14).[2, 137] The lesion is usually horizontal but may be oval or circular, lying just above the edge of the runner's thick plantar skin, which is often hyperkeratotic in this region. The plaque lies flush with the skin surface and is not palpable.

Black dot heel most likely arises from a

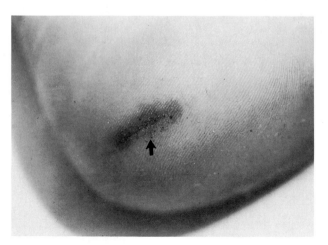

FIG. 16-14 Calcaneal petechiae (*arrow*) are noted where the plantar callus joins more normal skin.

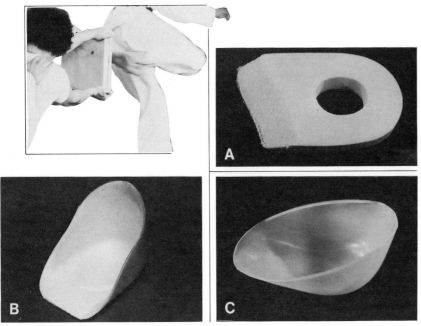

FIG. 16-15
A heel bruise may be treated with a foam donut pad (*A*), a cup of
precompressed airplane insulation (*B*), or a plastic heel cup (*C*).

shearing stress or a pinching of the heel between the counter and the sole of the shoe at
heel strike during running, producing bleeding
into the epidermis. When the lesion is pared
down with a scalpel, reddish-brown punctate
specks of dried blood are uncovered. Under a
microscope, clumps of pigment are noted in
the stratum corneum. The dark lesions may
resemble a melanoma, but individual punctate
lesions are usually discernible at the periphery
of the main mass. The lesions may also resemble a resolving verruca, but their position and
linear configuration make this diagnosis unlikely.

Black dot heel resolves spontaneously, and
recurrence may be prevented by fastening a
piece of felt inside the shoe.

Heel Bruise

The fat pad of an athlete's heel cushions his
heel at impact, but the quality of the fat pad
changes with age. In the young athlete, the fat
lobules are firm and are held between strong
septae. As he ages, the fat softens, the septae
weaken, and the pad is no longer able to cushion. Jolts may then bruise the heel and cause
subperiosteal bleeding. A tender scar sometimes forms in the damaged area. A heel bruise
may occur as runners with a short leg overstride and shock the heel, or the upper leg on
a banked track overstrides to catch up, jolting
the heel. In addition, heel bruises are not uncommon in runners who do many downhills
in shoes with sharply angled heels or heels that
are worn down.

A firm, well-fitting counter will keep the fat
pad compact to buffer the force of impact. The
athlete can further protect his heel and reduce
jolts by wearing shoes with a rounded, cushioning heel and using a donut pad or a heel cup
(*see* Fig. 16-15). The former is a foam pad that
has a hole in its center. The molded plastic heel
cup can hold the heel pad snugly. It wears well,
cushions impact, and warms the heel. The heel
cup should be worn not only in training shoes,
but also in everyday walking shoes. Everyday

shoes may have such firm heels that they may cause a heel bruise or prolong the recovery from one.

Midfoot Pain

Midfoot pain is common in those athletes who must wear lightweight shoes. Gymnasts, for example, wear only slippers but must run on a hard runway, must impact at the takeoff board, and then land forcefully. Runners and jumpers wear light and flexible competition shoes. Such light slippers or shoes may cause the feet to pronate excessively, and a midtarsal joint synovitis may develop. To help avoid and to treat this problem, the athlete can add lightweight airplane insulation inserts to the slippers or competition shoes. The runner may also wear his more supportive training shoes in competition, and the intrinsic muscles of the feet may be strengthened with "foot fists" and "towel pulls" (Fig. 16-16).

A cross-country runner may develop midfoot pain when training in cold weather on hard ground. When he runs on uneven surfaces in soft shoes, he may also sprain his calcaneonavicular ligament. This "spring ligament sprain" produces a deep medial midfoot aching. An orthosis should be provided to relieve it and the athlete advised to wear firmer, straight last shoes and to resume training on a flat surface.

Cavus Foot

High-arched, "cavus" feet are inflexible and give poor shock absorption (see Fig. 16-17). Jarring can cause arch pain, lateral knee pain, and pains extending up the lateral side of the lower extremity. Repeated tugs on the plantar fascia may produce a plantar fasciitis; however, airplane insulation inserts will cushion the feet and reduce jarring, Flexible heel cords will increase the athlete's shock-absorbing ability, and he should also stretch out his flexor hallicus longus. An athlete with cavus feet has the highest risk of rupturing his plantar fascia, as when rebounding in basketball. Such a tear can be crippling because this important supporting structure heals with scar tissue that hurts during running and jumping. Airplane insulation foam inserts should be placed in the shoes of most athletes to reduce the risk of these injuries. The inserts are especially needed in basketball sneakers, football cleats, and baseball spikes, all of which have notoriously poor arch supports. Custom-made inserts not only help to prevent plantar fascia problems, but also prevent calluses and reduce foot fatigue.[71, 75]

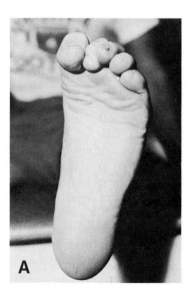 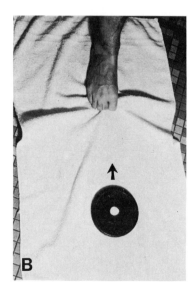

FIG. 16-16
The athlete strengthens his foot with "foot fists" (*A*) and towel-drags with weights added (*B*).

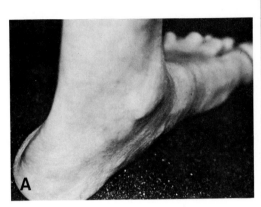
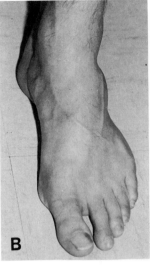

FIG. 16-17
The pronated foot is a
flat foot (*A*). Pronation
refers to dorsiflexion,
abduction, and
eversion at the subtalar
joint. A cavus foot is
high arched and rigid
(*B*).

FIG. 16-18
When the subtalar joint is opened (*A*), its complex articulations are
revealed (*B*).

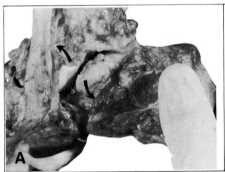
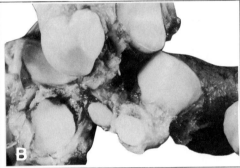

Pronated Foot

After heel strike, the runner's leg rotates internally, and his foot pronates to achieve a plantigrade position (Fig. 16-17). Pronation combines dorsiflexion, eversion, and abduction at the subtalar joint, motions that provide shock absorption (Fig. 16-18). Some pronation is normal, but limited or excessive pronation may lead to injury. Hyperpronation compensates for bowlegs, a tight Achilles tendon, rearfoot varus, and forefoot varus. The runner with a short leg will overstride on the short leg side and overpronate.

Morton's Foot

A Morton's foot may pronate excessively. The first metatarsal is short and hypermobile, with the great toe usually not projecting as far as the second toe. The hypermobile first ray takes longer to reach the ground than a normal first ray, and the foot pronates further until the first ray reaches the ground. The second metatarsal head must then bear more weight, remaining on the ground until the first metatarsal head lands, and the extra weight-bearing may cause painful callus to form under the second metatarsal head.

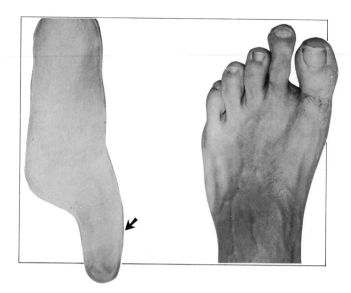

FIG. 16-19
The hyperpronation from a short and hypermobile first ray can be restricted with a Morton's extension (*arrow*) that extends under the first ray.

FIG. 16-20
A "teardrop" arch taping supports the athlete's arch and lessens tension on the plantar fascia.

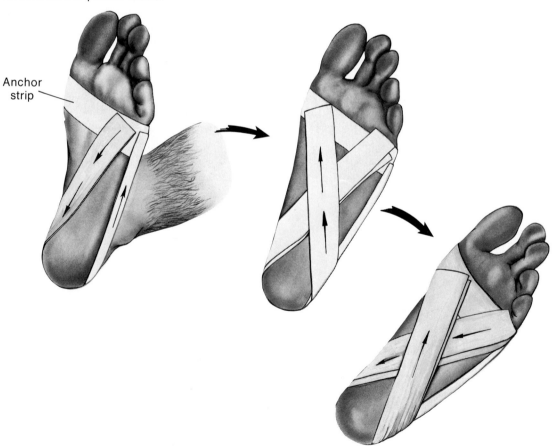

Anchor
strip

Treatment of this condition is accomplished with a Morton's extension, a pad placed under the first ray so that it need not travel as far before ground contact (Fig. 16-19). The foot may also be taped with the first ray plantar flexed (Fig. 16-20).

Plantar Fasciitis

The plantar fascia originates from the medial tuberosity of the calcaneus. Pronation causes a chronic tugging on the plantar fascia and irritates it. The periosteum is lifted and reactive bone is deposited to form a heel spur. A heel spur indicates tugging of the plantar fascia, but the spur itself is not the cause of pain.

The pronation must be limited to reduce tension on the plantar fascia. A local steroid injection is not recommended, as it treats only the inflammatory effects of the pronation and may cause tissue to degenerate at the origin of the plantar fascia, leading to a more intractable problem, or even promote plantar fascia rupture. Deep friction massage will break up adhesions, and a "toe-straight" device will bring the lesser toes into play to assume some of the stress of pushoff (Fig. 16-21). The athlete should be advised to run more toed-in and to wear a straight-last shoe, should be taped with his first ray plantar flexed, or should have his pronation reduced with an orthosis. An athlete

may have a medical problem such as gout or rheumatoid arthritis that may present as a "plantar fasciitis." A sedimentation rate, uric acid, and rheumatoid factor should be ascertained if mechanical correction does not relieve the pain.

Pronation Neuritis

Pronation neuritis may affect the posterior tibial nerve or its branches.[104] This nerve courses behind the medial malleolus, and pronation may cause irritation under its retinaculum, generating pain and tingling in the sole of the foot. When the examiner taps over the nerve, lightninglike pains advance into the foot. The numbness may be in the sensory distribution of the medial plantar, the lateral plantar, or the calcaneal branches of the posterior tibial nerve. This problem usually can be controlled by reducing pronation with an orthosis. Sometimes the surgeon elects to unroof the nerve, but, once unroofed, orthotic correction should be applied to prevent recurrence.

More commonly, calcaneal nerves are impinged upon during pronation to produce "plantar fasciitis." The fleshy abductor hallucis longus has a strong, sharp, deep fascia that rubs on the calcaneal nerves to produce a burning heel pain during pronation (Fig. 16-22). As a diagnostic procedure, the calcaneal nerves can

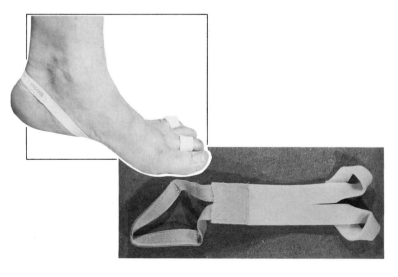

FIG. 16-21
The toe-straight device reduces plantar fascial stress and dynamically corrects claw toes.

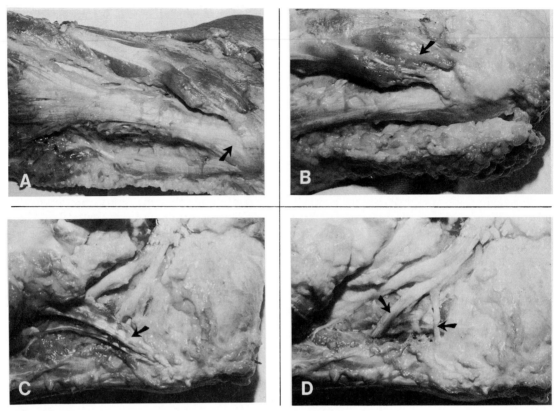

FIG. 16-22
The plantar fascia arises from the calcaneus (*A*); dorsal and medial to it
is the abductor hallucis (*B*). When the muscle belly of the abductor
hallucis is stripped away (*C*), a firm deep fascia is uncovered that
overlies the plantar nerves. When this fascia is sectioned and folded
back, the plantar and calcaneal nerves are fully seen (*D*).

be blocked with a local anesthetic that transiently relieves the pain. A steroid is then injected into the "doorway to the foot" under the
deep band, from above, to reduce the inflammation. The athlete should be advised to run
more toed-in and to wear a straight-last shoe,
and his pronation should decrease with an orthosis. If the pain persists, the deep band of the
abductor hallucis longus should be released.

Orthoses

Orthotic devices are now often used indiscrim-
inately to compensate for anatomic variations
in runners who otherwise have no injury problem. In these cases, the runner's body may have
already compensated for the abnormal patterns.
If the balance of the feet is changed, other
X-Y-Z vectors are affected, and the orthotic
may lead to injury.[21] A borderline knee problem that is not troublesome, for example, may
become painful because the foot compensation
is altered by an orthosis.

Simple measures usually cure minor injuries.
The athlete may have to alter his training program, change the surfaces he runs on, make a
shoe change, and use massage and stretching.
An inexpensive soft orthosis is sometimes used
as a trial. Such temporary orthotics may be

needed during the acute phase of an injury, and if the runner improves, a permanent device may be considered.

To make a temporary orthosis, piano felt or neoprene wedges may be glued under soft rubber inserts to make a combination that is lightweight and flexible. Unglued, loose felt pad inserts slip too easily. A typical set of inserts is a pair of soft rubber insoles with 0.25-inch neoprene medial wedges glued on. The runner's arch does not need support unless he has a problem such as a cavus foot, which demands more shock absorption and diffusion of the load. Recently available aids in dealing with an athlete's foot problems are training shoes with removable insoles that may be replaced easily by any other suitable supports, shims, lifts, or wedges.

A permanent orthosis may be flexible, semi-rigid, or rigid. Flexible supports may be made of foam rubber, cork, or leather, and a semi-rigid orthosis may be rubber or plastic. An athlete with very flexible feet may need a rigid orthosis, but these are expensive, and sending away for repairs may be inconvenient. This type of orthosis may be used in the athlete's walking shoes, but a less rigid device is desirable for his training and competition shoes.

A permanent orthosis is constructed from a mold taken with the athlete's foot in a neutral position where the talonavicular joint is congruent (Fig. 16-23).[60, 106] The neutral position is established by allowing the foot to dangle off the examining table. The head of the talus is grasped between the examiner's thumb and index finger, and the forefoot is held in the other hand. As the forefoot is rocked medially and laterally, the congruency of the talus and the navicular changes. If the talus protrudes medially, the navicular must be moved medially to gain congruency. If the talus is prominent laterally, the navicular must be shifted laterally to establish congruency. When the neutral position is found, the examiner pushes up under the fourth and fifth metatarsals, and when resistance is felt the foot is "locked" and ready for casting.

Casting begins with construction of a plaster slipper. After the plaster sets, the slipper is peeled from the foot and allowed to dry. Talcum powder is then sprinkled into the slipper to prevent the plaster of paris from sticking to the side walls, and the plaster of paris is poured into the slipper. The filled mold is then placed into a sand bin to prevent its tipping over, and the plaster is allowed to dry and set. After the mold has dried, the slipper is peeled from it and polypropylene pulled over the positive mold, trimmed, and smoothed. If needed, neoprene bumpers are glued to the orthosis, and protective plastic plates are glued to the neoprene. The orthosis is now ready to wear but should be broken in gradually to avoid painful pinch calluses. Trimming or revision of the orthosis is occasionally needed.

Corrections may also be made in a runner's shoes, as when the heel of the shoe is split and a foam rubber heel wedge inserted and cemented for Achilles tendon relief. A foam rubber rocker bottom may be inserted into the sole for metatarsal pain. Also, the counter may be reinforced with plastic, or the shoe upper on the medial side may be reinforced with leather to prevent overpronation.

The Dorsum of the Foot

On the dorsum of his foot, the athlete may suffer an instep bruise, rupture of the extensor hallucis longus tendon, pain at an os supranaviculare, fracture of the base of the fifth metatarsal bone, ski boot compression neuritis, and "surfer's knots."

Instep Bruise

If an athlete's foot is hit by a ball at cricket, struck in field hockey, or stepped on in soccer, his instep may be bruised. There is usually not much swelling, but the area is locally tender; an x-ray film should be taken to rule out a cracked bone. Ice is applied, and, in a few days, whirlpool treatments should be begun. A felt pad or a foam rubber donut pad should be

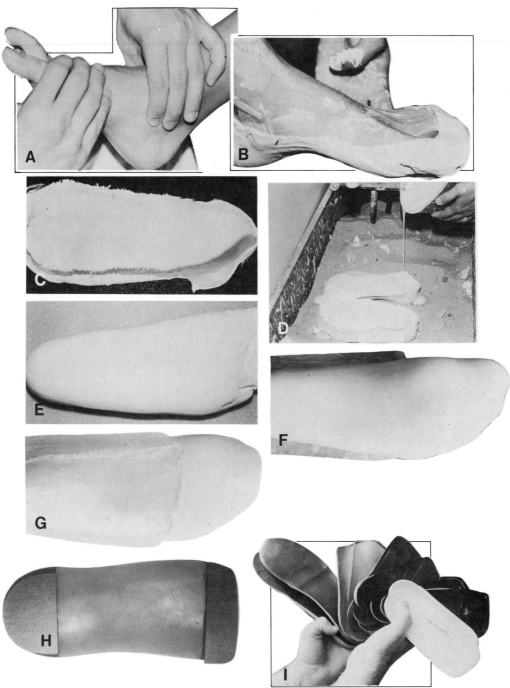

FIG. 16-23
The neutral position of the foot is ascertained (*A*). Then a plaster slipper is made (*B, C*). The slipper is filled with plaster (*D*) and allowed to stand in a sandbox. The positive (*E*) is then removed from the slipper and orthoplast pulled over it (*F*). The orthoplast is then cut out (*G*), and bumpers are affixed (*H*). This orthosis is intermediate between soft and rigid ones (*I*).

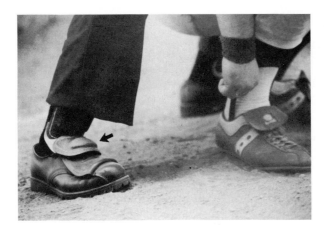

FIG. 16-24
The dorsum of the foot can be protected from bruising.

placed over the region to prevent further injury. An instep guard will prevent these bruises in baseball (Fig. 16-24).

Os Supranaviculare

Pain and swelling on the dorsum of the foot when running may be due to a mobile accessory ossification center of the navicular, the os supranaviculare. This accessary bone is located at the proximal-superior aspect of the navicular. A local xylocaine injection will relieve the pain and is also diagnostic. If the pain becomes chronic, the os supranaviculare can be resected.[142]

Fracture of the Fifth Metatarsal

The peroneus brevis, cubometatarsal ligament, lateral band of the plantar fascia, and the peroneus tertius all insert into the proximal part of the fifth metatarsal. Weight-bearing places great forces on this bone, and the injuries to it include peroneus brevis strain, hairline fracture, avulsion fracture, and the "Jones fracture."

An inversion twist of the foot may strain the tendon of the peroneus brevis. There will be local tenderness over the tendon and pain with active eversion or passive inversion. An eversion strapping is applied and then ice packs for treatment. A hairline fracture of the fifth metatarsal is caused by the same inversion twist mechanism and is also treated with an eversion strapping and ice. Casts should be avoided for these undisplaced fractures because immobilization results in a marked proprioceptive deficit

and long rehabilitation. Avulsion fractures, however, demand cast treatment. Occasionally an avulsed piece will become chronically painful and must be excised. Further, an accessory bone at the base of the fifth metatarsal, the os Vesalius, may become painful with activity and need to be resected.

The Jones fracture is a fatigue fracture in the diaphysis of the fifth metatarsal (Fig. 16-25).[66] In contrast to the injuries described above, this condition is more serious. Nonunion is frequent and may disable and retire the athlete. To compress the fracture site and avoid nonunion, the surgeon should place a malleolar lag screw across the fracture site from the styloid of the fifth metatarsal.[67] If a Jones fracture with an established nonunion is noted late, a bone graft may be needed in addition to the screw fixation.

Ski Boot Compression Neuropathy

Ski boot compression at the front of the ankle may produce a neuritis of the deep peroneal nerve and a synovitis of the extensor tendons. These structures are compressed between the tongue of the boot and the bone.[77] The condition may mimic a compartment syndrome, with decreased web space sensation and poor dorsiflexion of the toes. Boot-top pressure may also cause a numbness and tingling in the soles of the feet.[27] If a skier presents with these symptoms, his leg should be elevated and an ice pack wrapped on. Anti-inflammatory drugs or a ste-

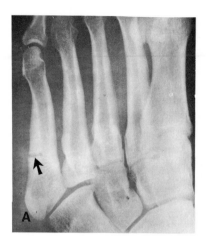

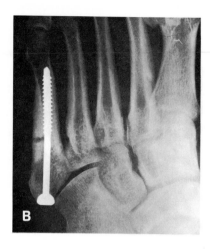

FIG. 16-25
A fracture of the diaphysis of the fifth metatarsal (*A*) may be slow healing and may need to be compressed with a lag screw (*B*).

FIG. 16-26
A metatarsal stress fracture causes the foot to swell (*A*); the fracture occurs usually through the very thin bone of the second metatarsal (*B*). It may not be visible for a few weeks on x-rays; by then callus has developed (*C*). The second metatarsal of a distance runner hypertrophies because of increased stresses on it (*D*).

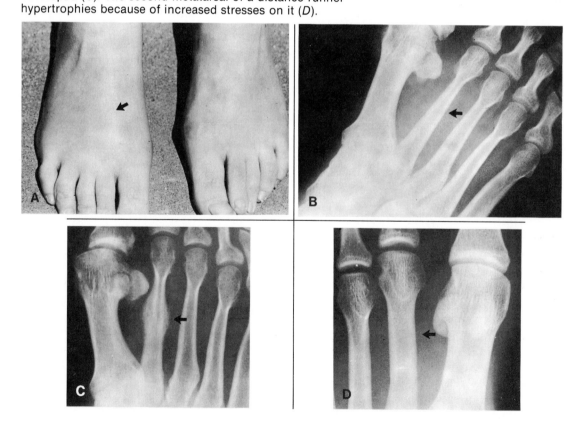

roid injection will reduce the inflammation. When the skier returns to the slopes, recurrence may be avoided by altering the pressure areas in his boots.

"Surfer's Knots"

Surfing began in Polynesia where the surfers lay prone on the surfboard when paddling out to the waves, but, in colder California waters, surfers kneel on the surfboard when paddling. Sand sticks to a waxed surfboard, and pressure and rubbing will produce hyperkeratotic skin nodules that may be found over the metatarsal-phalangeal joints of the feet and the anterior tibial surface, accompanied by swelling in the synovial sheath of the extensor digitorum longus on the dorsum of the foot. These nodules are painless and do not require treatment. Lying prone on the surfboard would prevent knots, but because they are often a status symbol it is doubtful that there will be any change in the paddling technique.

The Forefoot and Toes

Forefoot and toe problems in athletics include metatarsal stress fractures, metatarsalgia, interdigital neuromas, ganglion cysts, hallux valgus, "turf toe," sesamoiditis, sesamoid fractures, claw toes, hammer toes, "tennis toe," and ingrown toenails.

Metatarsal Stress Fracture

A runner pushes off through his second metatarsal head and second toe, and the high forces may cause a stress fracture of the thin diaphysis of his second, third, or fourth metatarsal. As a response to the repetitive forces of running, the second metatarsal of a distance runner hypertrophies to an extent where it becomes almost as broad as his first metatarsal. Despite this compensation, these runners may suffer a stress fracture if they change shoes or running surfaces, increase the intensity of their training, or run differently because of a blister. Metatarsal stress fractures are not limited to runners, however; swimmers may also develop such fractures from pushing off while practicing turns.

If an athlete sustains a stress fracture, his forefoot becomes painful and swollen (Fig. 16-26). The pain is relieved by rest but recurs with weight-bearing and pushing off. Early x-ray films may be normal, but at about 10 days a cloud of callus can usually be seen about the fracture. Treatment consists of ice, compression, and a forefoot strapping. To keep fit, the athlete wears a water-skiing vest and runs in the deep water in the diving well of a swimming pool.

Metatarsalgia

Metatarsalgia, or pain and tenderness under the metatarsal heads from bruising, is a common problem in runners. The athlete's training shoes or everyday walking shoes may have worn down, no longer providing a cushion for his metatarsal heads. Pressure builds through the day, and the area is subjected to further stress and becomes painful when the athlete trains. A 0.25-inch foam rubber rocker bottom can be inserted into the sole of the training shoes and street shoes to reduce the forces on the metatarsal heads and allow the inflammation to subside. Custom-made, shock-absorbing, airplane insulation inserts in his walking shoes, training shoes, and competition shoes can be worn to prevent this condition (Fig. 16-27).[71]

Intermetatarsal Neuritis

During pronation of the foot, the metatarsals roll, and the metatarsal heads and transverse metatarsal ligament may squeeze and pinch a nerve, especially the nerve between the third and fourth metatarsal heads. A sharp, burning pain may then strike out along the opposing surfaces of the toes. This pain is usually relieved when the athlete takes his shoe off and rests his foot. The examiner may be able to reproduce the pain by squeezing the forefoot, and a local anesthetic injected about the nerve will relieve the pain.

An orthosis to reduce pronation usually re-

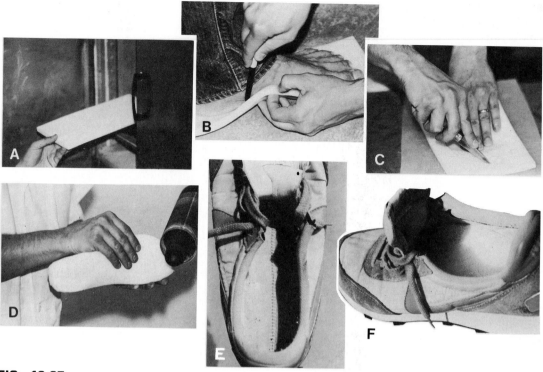

FIG. 16-27
Airplane insulation is placed into an oven (A), then allowed to cool, after which the athlete stands on it. The outline of his foot is then traced (B). The foam is cut with a knife (C) and smoothed (D). The insoles of some training shoes may be removed (E) and the custom-made airplane insulation inserted (F).

solves the problem, but sometimes a hydrocortisone shot may be needed to reduce the inflammation. The athlete should switch to shoes that are wider about the forefoot. An operation to remove the neuroma is rarely needed, and such an operation may leave a scar more painful than the neuroma. If a neurectomy is deemed necessary, the surgeon may use a dorsal approach with a small lamina spreader to spread the metatarsals for easy access to the nerve.

Ganglion Cyst

If a firm mass appears dorsally in a web space between the toes with activity and recedes after activity, the athlete may have a ganglion cyst (Fig. 16-28).[71] This arises from a flexor tendon sheath, following the path of least resistance between the toes to the dorsum of the foot. If painful, it may be removed completely after tracing it down to its origin.

Hallux Limitis, Hallux Rigidis, and Hallux Valgus

Hallux limitis refers to limited, painful motion of the metatarsophalangeal joint of the great toe (Fig. 16-29). Hallux rigidis is a rigid metatarsophalangeal joint. For best performance, an athlete needs full great-toe, metatarsophalangeal-joint motion because, during pushoff, the great toe must hyperextend about 90° on the first metatarsal. Limitation of this motion may be painful and cause a breakdown at the metatarsophalangeal joint, leading to problems in the rest of the foot.

If an athlete has limited motion in the first

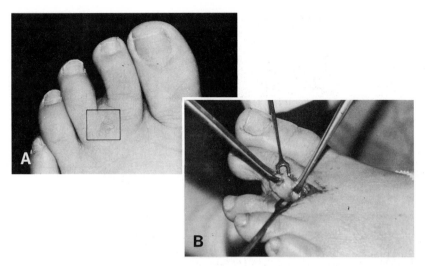

FIG. 16-28
Swelling in a webspace
(*A*) that follows activity
may be caused by a
ganglion cyst (*B*)
arising from a flexor
tendon sheath.

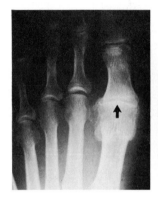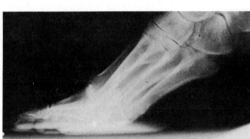

FIG. 16-29
An arthritic metatarsal-
phalangeal joint of the
great toe (*arrow*)
produces limited
dorsiflexion, "hallux
limitus."

metatarsophalangeal joint of the great toe, and motion is painful due to arthritis within the joint or a capsular sprain, he should wear a shoe with a rocker sole. Steroids should not be injected into an arthritic metatarsophalangeal joint, as they may hasten the breakdown of the articular cartilage. An arthritic metatarsophalangeal joint is sometimes resected, but this procedure can ruin the athlete's ability to push off and jump.

The athlete with hallux valgus has poor pushoff, and his shoes may irritate the bunion. He may also develop medial knee pain because of abnormal foot mechanics and a valgus stress to the knee. Daily great toe taping will usually benefit the runner with hallux valgus. An anchor strip is first placed around the great toe and another is set proximal to the bunion, these anchors are then spanned by strips of adhesive tape applied with the great toe held in a normal neutral position. An orthosis and the simple taping provides the athlete with a remarkably better gait and restores the feeling of moving straight ahead while running. A bunion splint should be worn at night to reduce progressioin of the deformity, and the athlete should wear shoes with a wider forefoot to prevent rubbing on the bunion.

To date, there is no ideal operation to correct hallux valgus in an athlete; however, releasing the adductor and applying orthotic correction to reduce the hypermobility of the first ray and pronation will halt the sesamoid shift and retard progression of the great toe deformity.

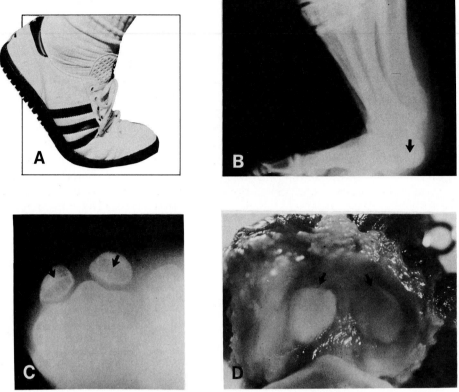

FIG. 16-30
Flexible shoes (*A*) worn on artificial turf may lead to a great toe sprain. Weight is borne on the sesamoids (*B*), small bones that can be seen on a sesamoid bone x-ray view (*C*). They reside in the tendon of the flexor brevis (*D*).

Artificial Turf Toe

In tackle football, the metatarsophalangeal joint of the great toe is often sprained, especially when players wear flexible soccer-style shoes on artificial turf (Fig. 16-30).[8, 19, 24, 45] Offensive lineman who block or push against a blocking sled and receivers and defensive backs who must cut and make quick stops may forcefully hyperextend and sprain the joint. The sprained plantar capsule of the joint will hurt, especially when the toe is extended; thus the joint should be taped to reduce its motion (Fig. 16-31). To reduce forefoot motion, players should wear a firmer shoe with a spring steel or orthoplast forefoot splint. A toe-straight device that allows the other toes to assist the great toe in pushoff may also be used (Fig. 16-21).

Sesamoiditis

The two sesamoid bones in the tendon of the flexor hallucis brevis may be irritated by pressure from a cleat under the first metatarsal head or by bowing in this area that results from faulty cleat placement (Fig. 16-30). The examiner should check the cleat position and fashion a pad that unburdens the first metatarsal head and that may relieve the pain. An orthosis to reduce pronation or a Morton's extension is sometimes curative. A 0.25-inch foam-rubber rocker bottom can be inserted into the sole of the training shoes and street shoes to reduce the forces on the sesamoids and allow the inflammation to subside. The great toe may also be strapped to limit motion, but injections are usually not helpful. In some persons with "sesamoiditis," the medial digital nerve lies just under the medial sesamoid. Their pain may be relieved by transposing this digital nerve.

Fractured Sesamoid Bone

When an athlete is down on a knee and another player lands on the back of his heel, the metatarsophalangeal joint of the great toe may be hyperextended violently, and a sesamoid bone, usually the tibial, may fracture. Treatment is identical to that for "turf toe," with ice and a strapping. Because a sesamoid is so important to weight-bearing, it should be left in place, if possible. If it is painful and suffers arthritic changes, however, it may have to be removed.

Claw Toes

Weakness or imbalance of the foot intrinsic muscles may produce a claw toe deformity. In this disorder, the metatarsophalangeal joint of the toe is extended and the proximal interphalangeal joint flexed. Athletes with this deformity are started on a muscle strengthening program that includes "foot fists," towel pulls, and picking up rolls of tape or marbles with the toes. A toe-straight device will serve as a dynamic replacement for the interosseus muscles of the foot. The device has an elastic loop that circles the heel and is connected by soft material to a loop for the second toe and one for the fourth toe. As the athlete's heel rises during walking or running, the toe-straight device prevents toe clawing by extending the proximal interphalangeal joints.

Hammer Toes

Hammer toes are flexed at the proximal interphalangeal joint and usually result from wearing ill-fitting, tight shoes and sneakers. Painful corns may form over these flexed joints. To relieve pressure on hammer toes, the athlete needs a shoe with a deep toe box. If the toes still jam, surgical excision of the diaphysis of

FIG. 16-31
"Turf toe" taping restricts the motion of the metatarsophalangeal joint of a sprained great toe.

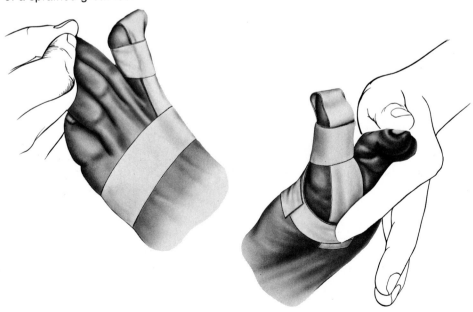

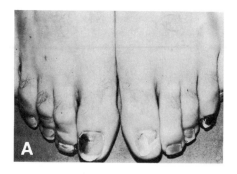
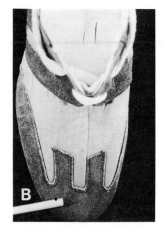
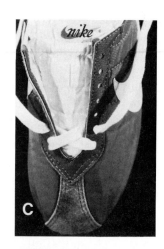
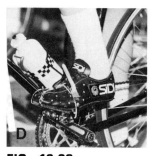
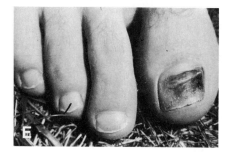
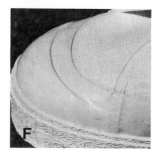

FIG. 16-32
"Marathoner's toes" (A) may be caused by rubbing from the toe box. Toe box configurations of shoes differ (B, C). Toe clips (D) may also irritate the toes. "Tennis toe" (E) may be prevented by wearing shoes with a large toe box (F).

the proximal phalanx under local anesthesia will provide complete relief.

"Tennis Toe"

Although the excellent traction of today's tennis shoes and the nonslip court surfaces stop the shoe quickly, the athlete's foot continues to move forward, and the longest toe may jam against the toe box. Such jamming may produce a subungual hematoma, and the athlete may lose his toenail (Fig. 16-32).[47]

Prevention and treatment of tennis toe requires a shoe with a larger toe box. Athletes should be advised to wear older, worn shoes when playing on nonslip surfaces so that shoes may slide a bit. If subungual blood has accumulated painfully, it may be removed by puncturing the nail with a sterilized paper clip or a small battery-powered drill point. The nail puncture should be made distally so that the nail grows out fast.

Ingrown Toenail

An ingrown toenail may develop because of pressure from poorly fitting shoes, and this disorder can bench the athlete. A player's feet grow during a high school season, and by the end of the year the shoes may be squeezing his toes. New shoes are needed before his feet outgrow the old shoes, and toenails should be left long enough to keep them from growing in along the borders. If a toenail becomes ingrown and infection appears, hot soaks are started, and the edge of the nail is lifted with a cotton bud, allowing it to grow out over the inflamed skin. The skin should be taped back to relieve pressure and to allow the nail to continue to grow. If the condition recurs, the offending portion of the nail should be removed and the nail bed revised under digital block anesthesia.

Foot Blisters

When an athlete's shoes rub and pinch his skin, the epidermis is soon sheared, and fluid accumulates to separate the epidermal layers (Fig. 16-33). Most of these blisters occur early in the season when the skin is soft or when new shoes are being broken in. The sore blister reduces the athlete's efficiency.

The key to dealing with blisters is prevention. Players may be advised to toughen their soles by going barefooted for brief periods during the off-season. Football shoes should be worn occasionally during the summer by football players and breaking-in time allowed for new shoes before formal practices begin. Wrinkles in a sock may also cause blisters, but well-fitted tube socks will help to avoid this problem. Friction may also be reduced by wearing two pairs of socks. A powder or lubricant, such as a thin coating of mineral oil or petrolatum, will aid in reducing friction between foot and shoe. Coating the feet with benzoin must be avoided because a powder and benzoin com-

FIG. 16-33
Blisters (*A*) form at friction points. "Pinch calluses" (*B*) especially affect runners with a hypermobile first ray. Warts (*C*) may masquerade as calluses, but warts show pinpoint capillaries when they are pared down. Athlete's foot (*D*) is most common in the last web space (*arrow*) but may affect the whole foot as well.

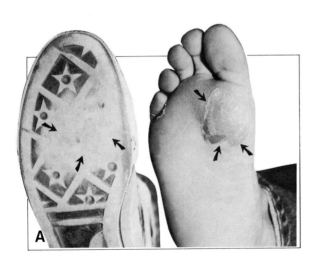

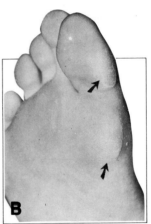

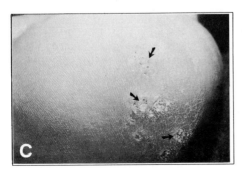

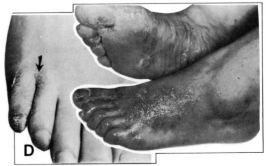

bination produces a sticky sole with lumps after the foot sweats. Calluses should be kept pared with a callus file after showering, as blisters may form under them. An ice cube may be applied to hot spots and friction areas then lubricated with a "friction fighter" to prevent progression. Hot spots behind the heel should be covered with a piece of tape or a Band-Aid, and a donut pad may be taped over a blister.

To avoid infection, blisters should not be unroofed. The blister can be aspirated of fluid with a fine-gauge needle through intact skin outside the blistered area and then covered with tape. If a decision is made to open the blister, a curved incision is made along one border of the blister and the roof left intact. Tape adherent is placed under the roof and the roof then taped down.

A broken blister may become contaminated; thus, infection must not be sealed in. A portion, of the roof is removed along with any loose skin that cannot protect the area. Dirt is then scrubbed out with soap, an antiseptic applied, and tape placed over the remaining roof for protection while allowing for some drainage.

Calluses

Calluses and corns are protective accumulations of the stratum corneum that result from pressure or pinching. Most calluses form on the ball of the foot or on the heel, and pinch-calluses frequently appear on the great toe (Fig. 16-33). Calluses lack the central thrombosed capillaries found in warts.

Calluses may be prevented by wearing cushioned shoes and by orthotically balancing the foot. In addition to his training and competition shoes, the athlete's walking shoes should be inspected, as the soles of these shoes may be too firm. If this is the case, airplane insulation inserts will distribute the pressure under the foot, thus reducing excess pressure on the callused area.

If a callus forms, it should be kept thin and massage lotion used to soften the bottom of the feet for filing. After showering, the callus may be reduced with a callus file, an emery board,

or fine sandpaper. Great-toe pinch-calluses disappear when a Morton's extension pad or a rubber forefoot wedge corrects the first ray hypermobility.

Warts

Warts are skin lesions caused by the virus *Verruca vulgaris,* which enters damaged areas such as under the metatarsal heads or at the heel. Pressure forces warts inward on the plantar surface of the foot, whereas in nonpressure areas such as the fingers the warts grow outward. To differentiate a wart from a callus or a corn, the lesion should be trimmed. The wart will show pinpoints of brown, thrombosed capillaries (Fig. 16-33), whereas a callus or a corn is clear.

Warts are treated by reducing pressure in the affected area with airplane insulation inserts that spread out the weight-bearing forces. Surface keratin is pared down with a scalpel blade, and a 40% salicylic acid plaster is then applied to the wart. The plaster is removed each day, and the dead tissue is trimmed until the wart finally pushes out. The treatment is continued until the thrombosed capillaries are no longer seen.

There are more aggressive treatments for warts, but all have disadvantages. Cantharidin therapy sometimes leaves warts developing at the edge of the lesion, and electrofulguration and dissection may result in painful scars. Liquid nitrogen or surgical incision may leave the subject with a painful scar that may be worse than the wart itself.

Athlete's Foot

Athlete's foot is an itchy, scaly infestation of the foot caused by a fungus, *Tricophyton rubrum* or *Tricophyton mentagrophytes,* or a yeast, *Candida albicans.*[91] Some persons are especially susceptible to the fungi, which are infectious and can spread from person to person with or without direct body contact. The fungi thrive in dark, warm, moist places, such as shower rooms, humid locker rooms, floors, the inside of lockers, bench surfaces, towels, and sweaty socks.

The lesions of athlete's foot may appear in many forms (Fig. 16-33). *Tricophyton rubrum* causes intertriginous scaly webs or squamous, scaly soles. *Tricophyton mentagrophytes* typically produces itchy vesicles and pustules that rupture, ooze, and macerate the skin. Other forms of athlete's foot may be hyperkeratotic and asymptomatic.

Athlete's foot should be diagnosed at the first symptom of itching or when scaly skin or cracks first appear between the toes. It frequently occurs between the fourth and fifth toes, the smallest interdigital space, which is subject to the least movement (Fig. 16-33). A scraping is taken from an active-looking skin edge and the roof of the vesicle snipped off. The examiner stains this material with potassium hydroxide and looks for hyphae in the case of the fungi or a combination of hyphae and mycelia in *Candida* infestation.

Some athletes are sensitive to the rubber in athletic shoes, which produces a contact dermatitis with a rash bilaterally over the distal forefoot and toes. Other athletes are allergic to socks or to the detergent in which the socks are cleaned. Contact dermatitis cannot be cured by a fungicidal cream, and conversely a fungal infection will worsen if it is mistaken for a contact dermatitis and treated with a steroid cream. A proper diagnosis must therefore be made by examining a potassium hydroxide preparation to assure appropriate treatment.

Infections should be treated promptly. Dead tissue is removed by careful rubbing with a soft towel, and clotrimazole or miconazole fungicidal cream or solution is then applied. These antifungal agents are also active against the yeast *Candida*. A cream or solution is best, as powder penetrates poorly. Treatment should be continued for 2 weeks; if treatment is stopped early because symptoms have disappeared the infection will recur.

To prevent athlete's foot, all locker room areas must be kept well ventilated to allow moisture to evaporate quickly. Open lockers are recommended, and a disinfectant cleaner should be used frequently. Athletes should be advised to wear rubber shoes, shower clogs, or thongs in the shower room for good foot hygiene. Feet should be dried carefully, especially between the small toes, and dusted with a medicated foot powder. Cotton placed between the toes will keep spaces dry, and clean cotton socks and porous leather shoes or sandals will help to prevent infections.

REFERENCES

1. ARNER O et al: Roentgen changes in subcutaneous rupture of the Achilles tendon. Acta Chir Scand 116:496–511, 1958/1959
2. AYRES S, MIHAN R: Calcaneal petechiac. Arch Dermatol 106:262, 1972
3. BERNDT AL, HARTY M: Transchondral fractures (osteochondritis dissecans) of the talus. J Bone Joint Surg [Am] 41:988–1020, 1959
4. BLACK HM: Roentgenographic considerations in ankle sprains. Am J Sports Med 5:238–240, 1977
5. BLACK HM: Operative treatment of ankle sprains—acute and chronic. Am J Sports Med 5:256–257, 1977
6. BLACK HM et al: Improved techniques for evaluation of ligamentous injury in severe ankle sprains. Am J Sports Med 6:276–282, 1978
7. BOSIEN WR et al: Residual disability following ankle sprains. J Bone Joint Surg [Am] 37:1237–1243, 1955
8. BOWERS KD JR, MARTIN RB: Turf-toe: a shoe surface related football injury. Med Sci Sports 8(2):81–83, 1976
9. BRADY TA, ARNOLD A: Aspiration injection treatment for varus sprain of the ankle. J Bone Joint Surg [Am] 54:1257–1261, 1972
10. BRAND RL ET AL: The natural history of inadequately treated ankle sprain. Am J Sports Med 5:248–249, 1977
11. BRAND RL et al: Repair of ruptured lateral ankle ligaments. Am J Sports Med 9:40–44, 1981
12. BRODY DM: Running injuries. Clin Symp 32:4, 1980
13. BRUBAKER CE, JAMES S: Injuries to runners. Am J Sports Med 2:189–198, 1974
14. BURROWS HJ: Fatigue infraction of the middle of the tibia in ballet dancers. J Bone Joint Surg [Br] 38:83–94, 1956
15. CANALE ST, BELDING RH: Osteochondral lesions of the talus. J Bone Joint Surg [Am] 62:97–102, 1980
16. CHRISMAN OB, SNOOK GA: The problems of refracture of the tibia. Clin Orthop 60:217–218, 1968
17. CHRISMAN OD, SNOOK GA: Reconstruction of lateral ligament tears of the ankle. J Bone Joint Surg [Am] 51:904–912, 1969
18. CLANCY WG JR: Symposium: runner's injuries. Am J Sports Med 8:137–138, 1980

19. COKER TP et al: Traumatic lesions of the metatarsophalangeal joint of the great toe in athletes. Am J Sports Med 6:326–334, 1978

20. COLLIS W, JAYSON M: Measurement of pedal pressures. Ann Rheum. Dis 31:215–217, 1972

21. CONNIFF JCG: James Nicholas: the orthopedic approach. Runner 3(5):62–65, 1981

22. COOPER DL: Contrast bath treatment for sprains. Trainer's corner. Phys Sportsmed 4(4):133, 1976

23. COOPER D, FAIR J: Ankle rehabilitation using the ankle disk. Phys Sportsmed 6(6):41, 1978

24. COOPER DL: Turf toe. Phys Sportsmed 6(9):139, 1978

25. COX JS, BRAND RL: Evaluation and treatment of lateral ankle sprains. Phys Sportsmed 5(6):51–55, 1977

26. COX JS: Surgical treatment of ankle sprains. Am J Sports Med 5:250–251, 1977

27. CRELINSTEN GL: Ski-boot neuropathy. N Engl J Med 288:240, 1973

28. DeHAVEN KE: Symposium: ankle sprains in athletes. Contemp Orthop 2:56–78, 1979

29. DENSTAD TF, ROAAS A: Surgical treatment of partial Achilles tendon rupture. Am J Sports Med 7:15–17, 1979

30. DEVAS MB, SWEETNAM R: Stress fractures of the fibula: a review of fifty cases in athletics. J Bone Joint Surg [Br] 30:818–829, 1956

31. DEVAS MB: Stress fractures of the tibia in athletes or "shin soreness." J Bone Joint Surg [Br] 40:227–239, 1958

32. DISTEFANO VJ, NIXON JE: Achilles tendon rupture: pathogenesis, diagnosis and treatment by a modified pullout wire technique. J Trauma 12:671–677, 1972

33. DISTEFANO VJ, NIXON JE: Ruptures of the Archilles tendon. Am J Sports Med 1:34–37, 1973

34. DISTEFANO VJ, NIXON JE: An improved method of taping. Am J Sports Med 2:209–211, 1974

35. DISTEFANO VJ: Ruptures of the Achilles tendon. The 1975 Schering symposium on musculotendinous injuries. Athletic Training 10:195–198, 1975

36. DREZ D JR: Metatarsal stress fracture. Am J Sports Med 8:123–125, 1980

37. DREZ D JR: Running footwear—examination of the training shoe, the foot and functional orthotic devices. Am J Sports Med 8:140, 1980

38. ELMSLIE RC: Recurrent subluxation of the ankle joint. Ann Surg 100:364–367, 1934

39. ELTON RC: Stress reaction of bone in army trainees. JAMA 204:314–316, 1968

40. EMERICK CE: Ankle taping: prevention of injury or waste of time? Athletic Training 14(3):186–188, 1979

41. ERSKINE L: The mechanics involved in skiing injuries. Am J Surg 97:667, 1959

42. ERSKINE L: Recent changes in the pattern of skiing injuries. J Trauma 14:92–93, 1974

43. EVANS DL: Recurrent instability of the ankle—a method of surgical treatment. Proc Soc Med 46:343–344, 1953

44. EVANS DL: Recurrent instability of the ankle—a method of surgical treatment. J Bone Joint Surg [Br] 39:795, 1957

45. GARRICK JG: Artificial turf, pros and cons. Phys Sportsmed 3:41–50, 1975

46. GARRICK JG: "When can I?": a practical approach to rehabilitation illustrated by treatment of an ankle injury. Am J Sports Med 9:67–68, 1981

47. GIBBS RC: Tennis toe. JAMA 228:24, 1974

48. GILLESPIE HS: BOUCHER P: Watson–Jones repair of lateral instability of the ankle. J Bone Joint Surg [Am] 53:920–924, 1971

49. GOLDING D: Tennis leg. Br Med J 4:234, 1969

50. GRAY G: Ankle rehabilitation using the ankle disk. Phys Sportsmed 6(6):141, 1978

51. HAGGMARK T, ERIKSSON E: Hypotrophy of the soleus muscle in man after Achilles tendon rupture. Am J Sports Med 7:121–126, 1979

52. HARRINGTON KD: Degenerative arthritis of the ankle secondary to long-standing lateral ligament instability. J Bone Joint Surg [Am] 61:354–361, 1979

53. HLAVAC HF: The Foot Book: Advice for Athletes. Mountain View, California, World Publications, 1977

54. HOVELIUS L, PALMGREN H: Laceration of tibial tendons and vessels in ice hockey players: three case histories of a skate boot-top injury. Am J Sports Med 7:297–298, 1979

55. HULLINGER CW: Insufficiency fracture of calcaneous similar to march fracture of metatarsal. J Bone Joint Surg [Am] 26:751–757, 1944

56. INGLIS AE: Ruptures of the tendo Achilles. J Bone Joint Surg [Am] 58:990–993, 1976

57. JACKSON DW et al: Ankle sprains in young athletes. Relation of severity and disability. Clin Orthop 101:201–215, 1974

58. JACKSON DW: Shin splints. Phys Sportsmed 6(10):51–62, 1978

59. JACOBS D et al: Comparison of conservative and operative treatment of Achilles tendon rupture. Am J Sports Med 6:107–111, 1978

60. JAMES SL et al: Injuries to runners. Am J Sports Med 6:40–50, 1978

61. JAMES S, BRUBAKER DE: Biomechanical and neuromuscular aspects of running In Exercise and Sports Sciences Reviews. Wilmore J (ed): New York, Academic Press, 1976

62. JOHNSON MD, POPE MH: Tibial shaft fractures in skiing. Am J Sports Med 5:49–62, 1977

63. JOHNSON RJ et al: Knee injury in skiing: a multi-faceted approach. Am J Sports Med 7:321–327, 1979

64. JOHNSON RJ: Trends in skiing injuries. Am J Sports Med 8:106–113, 1980

65. JONES E: Operative treatment of chronic dislocations of the peroneal tendons. J Bone Joint Surg [Am] 14:574–576, 1932

66. JONES R: Fracture of the base of the fifth metatarsal bone by indirect violence. Ann Surg 35:697–702, 1902

67. KAVANAUGH JH et al: The Jones fracture revisited. J Bone Joint Surg [Am] 60:776–782, 1978

68. KELLY RE: An operation for the chronic dislocation of the peroneal tendons. Br J Surg 7:502–504, 1926

69. KULUND DN, BRUBAKER CE: Injuries in the Bikecentennial Tour. Phys Sportsmed 6(6):674–678, 1978

70. KULUND DN et al: The long-term effects of playing tennis. Phys Sportsmed 7(4):87–94, 1979

71. KULUND DN et al: Airplane insulation for flying feet. Athletic Training 14(3):144–145, 1979

72. LAGERGREN C, LINDHOLM A: Vascular distribution in the Achilles tendon. Acta Chir Scand 116:491–495, 1958/1959

73. LAUGHMAN RK et al: Three-dimensional kinematics of the taped ankle before and after exercise. Am J Sports Med 8:425–431, 1980

74. LEA RB, SMITH L: Non-surgical treatment of tendo Achilles rupture. J Bone Joint Surg [Am] 54:7, 1972

75. LEACH R et al: Rupture of the plantar fascia in athletes. J Bone Joint Surg [Am] 60:537–539, 1968

76. LEACH R, CORBETT M: Anterior tibial compartment syndrome in soccer players. Am J Sports Med 7:258–259, 1979

77. LINDENBAUM BL: Ski boot compression syndrome. Clin Orthop 140:109–110, 1979

78. LUTTER LD: Pronation biomechanics in runners. Contemp Orthop 2:579–583, 1980

79. MacCARTEE CC: Taping treatment of severe inversion sprains of the ankle. Am J Sports Med 5:246–247, 1980

80. MacMAHON B, JOHNSON BA: Function and mechanics of rupture of tendo-Achilles. Its diagnosis and physiological repair. Orthop Rev 8(9):55–60, 1979

81. MANN RA, HAGY J: Biomechanics of walking, running and sprinting. Am J Sports Med 8:345–350, 1980

82. MARKS KL: Flake fracture of the talus progressing to osteochondritis dissecans. J Bone Joint Surg [Br] 34:90–92, 1952

83. McBRYDE AM JR: Stress fractures in athletes. Am J Sports Med 3:212–217, 1975

84. McLENNAN JG: Treatment of acute and chronic luxations of the peroneal tendons. Am J Sports Med 8:432–436, 1980

85. McHAHON TA, GREENE PR: Fast running tracks. Sci Am 239(6):148–163, 1978

86. McMASTER PE: Tendon and muscle rupture. J Bone Joint Surg [Am] 15:705–722, 1933

87. McMURRAY TP: Footballer's ankle. J Bone Joint Surg [Br] 32:68–69, 1950

88. MILLAR AP: Strains of the posterior calf musculature ("tennis leg"). Am J Sports Med 7:172–174, 1979

89. MILLER A: Rupture of the musculotendinous juncture of the medial head of the gastrocnemius muscle. Am J Sports Med 5:191–193, 1977

90. MILLER JW: Dislocation of peroneal tendons: a new operative approach. Am J Orthop 9:136–137, 1967

91. MILLIKAN LE: Athlete's foot—scratching beneath surface of fungal ailments. Phys Sportsmed 3(4):51–56, 1975

92. MITAL MA, MATZA RA: Osgood-Schlatter disease: the painful puzzler. Phys Sportsmed 5(6):60–73, 1977

93. MOORE M: Synthetic skin covers blisters, abrasions. Phys Sportsmed 8(12):15, 1980

94. MORRIS LH: "Athlete's ankle." J Bone Joint Surg [Am] 25:220, 1943

95. MUKERJEE SK, YOUNG AB: Dome fracture of the talus. J Bone Joint Surg [Br] 55:319–326, 1973

96. NAPIER J: The antiquity of human walking. Sci Am 216(4):56–66, 1967

97. NELSON R, GREGOT R: Biomechanics of distance running: a longitudinal study. Res Q 47:417–428, 1976

98. NOBLE HB, SELESNICK FH: The Thompson test for ruptured achilles tendon. Phys Sportsmed 8(8):63–64, 1980

99. PEPPARD A, RIEGLER H: Ankle reconditioning with TENS. Phys Sportsmed 8(6):105–106, 1980

100. PERCY EC, CONOCHIE LB: The surgical treatment of ruptured tendo Achillis. Am J Sports Med 6:132–136, 1978

101. PLATT H: Observations on some tendon ruptures. Br Med J 1:611–615, 1931

102. QUIGLEY TB, SCHELLER AD: Surgical repair of the ruptured Achilles tendon. Am J Sports Med 8:244–250, 1980

103. RADIN EL, PAUL IL: Importance of bone in sparing articular cartilage from impact. Clin Orthop 78:342–344, 1971

104. RASK MR: Medial plantar neuropraxia (jogger's foot): report of three cases. Clin Orthop 134:193–195, 1978

105. RASMUSSEN W: Skin splints: definition and treatment. Am J Sports Med 2:111–117, 1974

106. ROOT ML et al: Neutral position casting techniques. Los Angeles, Clinical Biomechanics, 1971

107. SARMIENTO A, WOLF M: Subluxation of peroneal tendons: case treated by rerouting tendons under calcaneofibular ligament. J Bone Joint Surg [Am] 57:115–116, 1975

108. SAVASTANO AA, LOWE EB: Surgical treatment for recurrent ankle sprains. Am J Sports Med 8:208–211, 1980

109. SEDER JI: Heel injuries incurred in running and jumping. Phys Sportsmed 4(10):70–73, 1976

110. SELIGSON D: Ankle instability: evaluation of the lateral ligaments. Am J Sports Med 8:39–42, 1980

111. SIM FH, DEWEERD JH JR: Rupture of the externsor hallucis longus tendon while skiing. Minn Med 60:789–790, 1977

112. SKEOCH DU: Spontaneous partial subcutaneous ruptures of the tendo achillis. Am J Sports Med 9:20–22, 1981

113. SLOCUM DB: Overuse syndromes of the lower leg and foot in athletes. American Academy of Orthopaedic Surgeons Instructional Course Lectures 17:359–367, 1960

114. SLOCUM DB, BOWERMAN W: Biomechanics of running. Clin Orthop 23:39–45, 1962

115. SLOCUM D, JAMES S: Biomechanics of running. JAMA 205:721–728, 1968

116. SMITH WB: Environmental factors in running. Am J Sports Med 8:138–140, 1980

117. STAPLES OS: Ruptures of the fibular collateral ligaments of the ankle: result study of immediate surgical treatment. J Bone Joint Surg [Am] 57:101–107, 1975

118. STEIN SR, LUEKENS CA: Closed treatment of Achilles tendon ruptures. Orthop Clin North Am 7:241–246, 1976

119. STEINGARD PM: Foot failures in basketball. Phys Sportsmed 2(3):64–69, 1974

120. STEWART MJ, HUTCHINS WC: Repair of the lateral ligaments of the ankle. Am J Sports Med 6:272–275, 1978

121. STOVER CN, BRYAN DR: Traumatic dislocation of the peroneal tendons. Am J Surg 103:180–186, 1962

122. SUBOTNICK SI: Orthotic foot control and the overuse syndrome. Phys Sportsmed 3(1):75–79, 1975

123. SUBOTNICK SI: Podiatric Sports Medicine. Mount Kisco, New York, Futura, 1975

124. SUBOTNICK SI: The Running Foot Doctor. Mountain View, California, World Publications, 1977

125. TELFER N: Radionuclide bone imaging in stress fractures. West J Med 129:414, 1978

126. Tennis leg (editorial). Br Med J 3:543–544, 1969

127. THOMPSON TC, DOHERTY JH: Spontaneous rupture of tendon of Achilles: a new clinical diagnostic test. J Trauma 2:126–129, 1962

128. TORG JS, QUENDENFELD T: Effect of the shoe type and cleat length on incidence and severity of knee injuries among high school football players. Res Q Am Assoc Health Phys Ed 43:203–211, 1971

129. VAINIONPAA S et al: Lateral instability of the ankle and results when treated by the Evans procedure. Am J Sports Med 8:437–439, 1980

130. VAN DER LINDEN W: The skier's boot top fracture. Acta Orthop Scand 40:797, 1970

131. VAN DER LINDEN W et al: Fractures of the tibial shaft after skiing and other accidents. J Bone Joint Surg [Am] 57:321–327, 1975

132. VERNE-HODGE N: Injuries in cricket. In Armstrong JR, Tucker WE (eds): Injury in Sport, pp 168–171. Indianapolis, Charles C Thomas, 1964

133. VINE LE: The skier's fracture: a method of treating this and similar leg injuries in country district hospitals. Med J Aust 1:1127, 1968

134. WALSH WM, BLACKBURN T: Prevention of ankle sprains. Am J Sports Med 5:243–245, 1977

135. WASHINGTON ZL: Musculoskeletal injuries in theatrical dancers: site, frequency and severity. Am J Sports Med 6:75–98, 1978

136. WATSON-JONES R: Fractures and Joint Injuries, vol 2, 4th ed. Baltimore, Williams & Wilkins, 1952

137. WILKINSON DS: Black heel: a minor hazard of sport. Cutis 20:393–396, 1977

138. WINFIELD AC, DENNIS JM: Stress fractures of the calcaneus. Radiology 72:415–418, 1959

139. WOODWARD EP: Ankle ligament surgery: experience over 18 years. Phys Sportsmed 5(8):49–55, 1977

140. YVARS F: Osteochondral fractures of the dome of the talus. Clin Orthop 114:185–191, 1976

141. ZENNIS EJ JR: Lateral ligamentous instability of the ankle: a method of surgical reconstruction by a modified Watson–Jones technique. Am J Sports Med 5:78–83, 1977

142. ZWELLING L et al: Removal of os supranaviculare from a runner's painful foot. Am J Sports Med 6:1–3, 1978

The Spectrum of Sport

Acrobatics
Alpine skiing
Angling
Archery
Auto racing
Baseball
Basketball
Baton twirling
Billiards
Bobsledding
Bowling
Bowls
Boxing
Canoeing
Cricket
Cross-country skiing
Curling
Cycling
Dancing—ballet, modern
Diving
Equestrian sports

Fencing
Field Hockey
Figure skating
Golf
Gymnastics
Handball
Horseshoe pitching
Hurling
Ice dancing
Ice hockey
Judo
Kayak
Lacrosse
Luge
Martial arts
Motorcycling
Racket sports
Road running
Rowing
Rugby
Scuba diving

Shooting
Ski jumping
Soccer
Softball
Speed skating
Surfing
Swimming
Syncronized swimming
Tackle football
Team handball
Track and field
Ultimate frisbee
Volleyball
Water polo
Water skiing
Weight lifting
Wrestling
   Freestyle
   Greco–Roman
Yachting

Appendix B

The Sports Medicine Team

The athlete
Athletic trainer
Biomechanics expert
Coach
Dentist
Equipment manager
Exercise leader
Exercise physiologist
Health educator

Kinesiologist
Masseur or masseuse
Officials
Physical educator
Physician
Podiatrist
Sports psychologist
Strength and conditioning coach

Appendix C

The Sports Medicine Curriculum

Biomechanics

Cardiac rehabilitation

Cardiopulmonary resuscitation

Drugs in athletics

Environmental stress

Evaluating fitness

Exercise physiology

Kinesiology

Injury—prevention, treatment, and rehabilitation

Medical problems

Nutrition

Officiating and rules

Preparticipation examination

Principles of training

Protective equipment

Special problems of young, female, older, and handicapped athletes

Sport Psychology

Strength training

Tactics

Transportation of the injured athlete

Warm-up

The Components of a Health-Related Physical Education Program

1. Biology of exercise
2. Benefits of regular exercise for men and women
3. How to modify coronary risk factors
4. Principles of endurance training
5. Principles of strength training
6. How to design a personal fitness program
7. Warm-up techniques
8. Nutrition
9. Injury prevention
10. First aid
11. Exposure to a wide variety of recreational and fitness activities that emphasize lifetime body sports, such as cycling, gymnastics, jogging, and swimming
12. Basic movement patterns such as throwing, changing direction (cutting and pivoting), how to land, and the stable position

Equipment for Trainers

Basic Training Room Equipment

Examination tables
Refrigerator
Sink
Whirlpool
Infrared heat lamp or hydrocollator
Scales
Weight charts
Stethoscope and blood pressure cuff
Locked cabinet for medications
Bulletin board (for emergency telephone numbers)

Trainer's Side Table (out of the way)

Gauze pads (4 in × 4 in and 2 in × 2 in)
Band-Aids
Tongue depressors
Cotton buds (Q-tips)
Buffered salt tablets
$AlCl_2$ solution (30%) (aluminum chloride)
Petrolatum
Analgesic cream (gold)
(Heavy) skin lubricant (green)
Foam pads for tapings
Tape remover
Bandage scissors
Callus file
Electric hair clipper

Trainer's Kit

Oral screw
Tongue forceps
Airways
Tourniquet
Tongue depressors
Paper bag (hyperventilation)
Contact lens case, contact lens solution, contact lens extractor
Eye cup and eye wash
Eye drops
Toothache kit
Oral thermometer
Flashlight
Scalpel
Bandage scissors
Surgical scissors
Hemostat
Forceps
Hand mirror
Safety pins
Razor with blades
Nail clippers
Callus file
Sling
Finger splints
Transcutaneous electrical nerve stimulator (TENS) unit and cream
Plastic ice bags
1-oz cups
Tape measure

Marking pen, paper, pencils
Shoe horn
Coins for pay phone
Nonadhering sterile pads
Gelfoam
Band-Aids
Butterfly closures and Steri-Strips
Roll of cotton and cotton balls
3 in × 3 in sterile gauze
2 in × 2 in nonsterile gauze
3-in roller gauze
Felt horseshoe
Tape adherent
Skin lubricant
Foam heel and lace pads
Underwrap
½-in adhesive tape
1-in adhesive tape
1½-in adhesive tape
3-inch elastic tape
Elasticon tape
Conform tape
Waterproof tape
Tape cutter
Tape remover
2-in elastic wrap
3-in elastic wrap
4-in elastic wrap
Ankle wrap
Ear drops
Nose drops
Throat lozenges
Cough syrup
Cold tablets
Aspirin
Motion sickness tablets
Antacid tablets
Salt tablets
Sun lotion
Envelopes for pills
First aid spray
Ointment for minor skin irritations
Zinc oxide ointment
Betadine
Liquid soap
Tinactin
Ethyl chloride
Ammonia capsules

Flexible collodian
Petrolatum
Saline in plastic squeeze bottle
Alcohol
Alcohol prep sponges
Cotton buds
First aid manual

Travel Trunk

Dental kit
Tongue depressors
Mouthpieces
Cotton buds
Examination gloves
Towels
Plastic ice bags
Drinking cups
Calamine lotion
Talcum powder
Analgesic balm
Telfa pads
Nonsterile gauze pads
Roller gauze
Sterile gauze roll
Assorted pieces of foam rubber
Orthopedic felt
Felt horseshoes
Tape adherent
Skin lubricant
Adhesive tape (1 in and 1½ in)
Elastic tape (3 in)
Elastic wraps (2 in, 3 in, 4 in, and 6 in)
Tape remover
Moleskin
Stockinette (3 in and 6 in)
Rolls of plaster (3 in, 4 in, and 6 in)
Neck collars
Thomas collars
Assorted protective pads
Acromioclavicular pads
Sternum pad
Thigh caps
Heel cups
Ensolite (¼ in, ⅜ in, ½ in)
Orthoplast
Slings

Rib belts
Knee immobilizer
Air splints
High-intensity lamp
Equipment hardware
Spare parts
  Chinstraps
  Shoulder pad straps
  Clips
  Screws
Pliers
Screwdrivers
Collapsible cane
Shoe horn
Coat hanger
Umbrella

Sidelines

Two spine boards, with neck traction unit or
  four 5-lb sandbags
Bolt cutter (taped to spine board)
Stretcher
Crutches
Blankets
Ice chest
Ice
"Magic sponge"
Ice water bucket
Plastic bags for ice
Water containers
Water squeeze bottles
Cups and racks

American College of Sports Medicine Position Statements

The Use and Abuse of Anabolic–Androgenic Steroids in Sports★

Based on a comprehensive survey of the world literature and a careful analysis of the claims made for and against the efficacy of anabolic-androgenic steroids in improving human physical performance, it is the position of the American College of Sports Medicine that:

1) The administration of anabolic-androgenic steroids to healthy humans below age 50 in medically approved therapeutic doses often does not of itself bring about any significant improvements in strength, aerobic endurance, lean body mass, or body weight.

2) There is no conclusive scientific evidence that extremely large doses of anabolic-androgenic steroids either aid or hinder athletic performance.

3) The prolonged use of oral anabolic-androgenic steroids (C_{17}-alkylated derivatives of testosterone) has resulted in liver disorders in some persons. Some of these disorders are apparently reversible with the cessation of drug usage, but others are not.

4) The administration of anabolic-androgenic steroids to male humans may result in a decrease in testicular size and function and a decrease in sperm production. Although these effects appear to be reversible when small doses of steroids are used for short periods of time, the reversibility of the effects of large doses over extended periods of time is unclear.

★(Med Sci Sports 9(4): XI–XIII, 1977)

5) Serious and continuing effort should be made to educate male and female athletes, coaches, physical educators, physcians, trainers, and the general public regarding the inconsistent effects of anabolic-androgenic steroids on improvement of human physical performance and the potential dangers of taking certain forms of these substances, especially in large doses, for prolonged periods.

Research Background for the Position Statement

This position stand has been developed from an extensive survey and analysis of the world literature in the fields of medicine, physiology, endocrinology, and physical education. Although the reactions of humans to the use of drugs, including hormones or drugs which simulate the actions of natural hormones, are individual and not entirely predictable, some conclusions can nevertheless be drawn with regard to what desirable and what undesirable effects may be achieved. Accordingly, whereas positive effects of drugs may sometimes arise because persons have been led to expect such changes ("placebo" effect) (8), repeated experiments of a similar nature often fail to support the initial positive effects and lead to the conclusion that any positive effect that does exist may not be substantial.

1) Administration of testosterone-like synthetic drugs which have anabolic (tissue building) and androgenic (development of male sec-

ondary sex characteristics) properties in amounts up to twice those normally prescribed for medical use have been associated with increase strength, lean body mass and/or body weight in some studies (6, 19, 20, 26, 27, 33, 34, 36) but not in others (9, 10, 12, 13, 21, 35, 36). One study (13) reported an increase in the amount of weight the steroid group could lift compared to controls but found no difference in isometric strength which suggests a placebo effect in the drug group, a learning effect or possibly a different drug effect on isotonic compared to isometric strength. An initial report of enhanced aerobic endurance after administration of an anabolic-androgenic steroid (20) has not been confirmed (6, 9, 19, 21, 27). Because of the lack of adequate control groups in many studies it seems likely that some of the positive effects on strength that have been reported are due to "placebo" effects (3, 8), but a few apparently well-designed studies have also shown beneficial effects of steroid administration on muscular strength and lean body mass. Some of the discrepancies in results may also be due to differences in the type of drug administered, the method of drug administration, the nature of the exercise programs involved, the duration of the experiment, and individual differences in sensitivity to the administered drug. High protein dietary supplements do not insure the effectiveness of the steroids (13, 21, 36). Because of the many failures to show improved muscular strength, lean body mass, or body weight after therapeutic doses of anabolic-androgenic steroids it is obvious that for many individuals any benefits are likely to be small and not worth the health risks involved.

2) Testimonial evidence by individual athletes suggests that athletes often use much larger doses of steroids than those ordinarily prescribed by physicians and those evaluated in published research. Because of the health risks involved with the long-term use of high doses and requirements for informed consent it is unlikely that scientifically acceptable evidence will be forthcoming to evaluate the effectiveness of such large doses of drugs on athletic performance.

3) Alterations of normal liver function have

been found in as many as 80 percent of one series of 69 patients treated with C_{17}-alkylated testosterone derivatives (oral anabolic-androgenic steroids) (29). Cholestatis has been observed histologically in the livers of persons taking these substances (31). These changes appear to be benign and reversible (30). Five reports (4, 7, 23, 31, 39) document the occurrence of peliosis hepatitis in 17 patients without evidence of significant liver disease who were treated with C_{17}-alkylated androgenic steroids. Seven of these patients died of liver failure. The first case of hepato-cellular carcinoma associated with taking an androgenic-anabolic steroid was reported in 1965 (28). Since then at least 13 other patients taking C_{17}-alkylated androgenic steroids have developed hepato-cellular carcinoma (5, 11, 14, 15, 16, 17, 18, 25). In some cases dosages as low as 10-15 mg/day taken for only three or four months have caused liver complications (13, 25).

4) Administration of therapeutic doses of androgenic-anabolic steroids in men often (15, 22), but not always (1, 10, 19), reduces the output of testosterone and gonadotropins and reduces spermatogenesis. Some steroids are less potent than others in causing these effects (1). Although these effects on the reproductive system appear to be reversible in animals, the long-term results of taking large doses by humans in unknown.

5) Precise information concerning the abuse of anabolic steroids by female athletes is unavailable. Nevertheless, there is no reason to believe females will not be tempted to adopt the use of these medicines. These use of anabolic steroids by females, particularly those who are either prepubertal or have not attained full growth, is especially dangerous. The undesired side effects include masculinization (2, 29, 30), disruption of normal growth pattern (30), voice changes (2, 30, 32), acne (2, 29, 30, 32), hirsutism (29, 30, 32), and enlargement of the clitoris (29). The long-term effects on reproductive function are unknown, but anabolic steroids may be harmful in this area. Their ability to interfere with the menstrual cycle has been well documented (29).

For these reasons, all concerned with advising, training, coaching, and providing medical care for female athletes should exercise all persuasions available to prevent the use of anabolic steroids by female athletes.

REFERENCES

1. AAKVAAG, A, and S. B. STROMME. The effecto of mesterolone administration to normal men on the pituitary-testicular function. *Acta Endocrinol.* 77:380–386, 1974.

2. ALLEN, D. M., M. H. FINE T. F. NECHELES, and W. DAMESHEK. Oxymetholone therapy in aplastic anemia. *Blood* 32:83–89, July 1968.

3. ARIEL, G., and W. SAVILLE. Anabolic steroids: the physiological effects of placebos. *Med. Sci. Sports* 4:124–126, 1972.

4. BAGHERI, S. A. and J. L. BOYER. Peliosis hepatitis associated with androgenic-anabolic steroid therapy. *Ann. Int. Med.* 81:610–618, 1974.

5. BERNSTEIN, M. S., R. L. HUNTER and S. YACHRIN. Hepatoma and peliosis hepatitis developing in a patient with Fanconi's anemia. *N. Engl. J. Med.* 284:1135–1136, 1971.

6. BOWERS, R. and J. REARDON. Effects of methandrostenolone (Dianabol) on strength development and aerobic capacity. *Med. Sci. Sports* 4:54, 1972.

7. BURGER, R. A. and P. M. MARCUSE. Peliosis hepatitis, report of a case. *Am. J. Clin. Path.* 22:569–573, 1952.

8. BYERLY, H. Explaining and exploiting placebo effects. *Prosp. Biol. Med.* 19:423–436, 1976.

9. CASNER, S., R. EARLY, and B. R. CARLSON. Anabolic steroid effects on body composition in normal young men. *J. Sports Med. and Phys. Fit.* 11:98–103, 1971.

10. FAHEY, T. D. and C. H. BROWN. The effects of an anabolic steroid in the strength, body composition and endurance of college males when accompanied by a weight training program. *Med. Sci. Sports* 5:272–276, 1973.

11. FARRELL, G. C., D. E. JOSHUA, R. F. UREN, P. J. BAIRD, K.W. PERKINS, and H. KRAIENBERG. Androgen-induced hepatoma. *Lancet* 1:430–431, 1975.

12. FOWLER, JR., W. M., G. W. GARDNER, and G. H. EGSTROM. Effect of an anabolic steroid on physical performance of young men. *J. Appl. Physiol.* 20:1038–1040, 1965.

13. GOLDING, L. A., J. E. FREYDINGER, and S. S. FISHEL. Weight, size and strength-unchanged by steroids. *Physician Sports Med.* 2:39–45, 1974.

14. GUY, J. T. and M. O. AUXLANDER. Androgenic steroids and hepato-cellular carcinoma. *Lancet* 1:148, 1973.

15. HARKNESS, R. A., B. H. KILSHAW, and B. M. HOBSON. Effects of large doses of anabolic steroids. *Brit. J. Sport Med.* 9:70–73, 1975.

16. HENDERSON, J. T., J. RICHMOND, and M. D. SUMER-LING. Androgenic-anabolic steroid therapy and hepatocellular carcinoma. *Lancet* 1:934, 1972.

17. JOHNSON, F. L. The association of oral androgenic-anabolic steroids and life threatening disease. *Med. Sci. Sports* 7:284–286, 1975.

18. JOHNSON, F. L., J. R. FEAGLER, K. G. LERNER, P. W. MAJEMS, M. SIEGEL, J. R. HARTMAN, and E. D. THOMAS. Association of androgenic-anabolic steroid therapy with development of hepato-cellular carcinoma. *Lancet* 2:1273–1276, 1972.

19. JOHNSON, L. C., G. FISHER, L. J. SYLVESTER, and C. C. HOFHEINS. Anabolic steroid: Effects on strength, body weight, O_2 uptake and spermatogenesis in mature males. *Med. Sci. Sports* 4:43–45, 1972.

20. JOHNSON, L. C. and J. P. O'SHEA. Anabolic steroid: effects on strength development. *Science* 164:957–959, 1969.

21. JOHNSON, L. C., E. S. ROUNDY, P. ALLSEN, A. G. FISHER, and L.J. SYLVESTER. Effect of anabolic steroid treatment on endurance. *Med. Sci. Sports* 7:287–289, 1975.

22. KILSHAW, B. H., R. A. HARKNESS, B. M. HOBSON, and A. W. M. SMITH. The effects of large doses of the anabolic steroid, methandrostenolone, on the athlete. *Clin. Endocr.* 4:537–541, 1975.

23. KINTZEN, W. and J. SILNY. Peliosis hepatitis after administration of fluoxymesterone. *Canad. Med. Assoc. J.* 83:860–862, 1960.

24. MCCREDIE, K. B. Oxymetholone in refractory anaemia. *Brit. J. of Haemtology.* 17:265–273, 1969.

25. MEADOWS, A. T., J. L. NAIMAN, and M. V. VALDES-DAPENA. Hepatoma associated with androgen therapy for aplastic anemia. *J. Pediatr.* 84:109–110, 1974.

26. O'SHEA, J. P. The effects of an anabolic steroid on dynamic strength levels of weight lifters. *Nutr. Report Internat.* 4:363–370, 1971.

27. O'SHEA, J. P. and W. WINKLER. Biochemical and physical effects of an anabolic steroid in competitive swimmers and weight lifters. *Nutr. Report Internat.* 2:351–362, 1970.

28. RECANT, L. and P. LACY. (eds.). Fanconi's anemia and hepatic cirrhosis. Clinicopathologic Conference. *Am. J. Med.* 39:464–475, 1965.

29. SANCHEZ-MEDAL, L., A. GOMEZ-LEAL, L. DUARTE, and M. GUADALUPE-RICO. Anabolic-androgenic steroids in the treatment of acquired aplastic anemia. *Blood* 34:283–300, 1969.

30. SHAHIDI, N. T. Androgens and erythropoiesis. *N. Engl. J. Med.* 289:72–79, 1973.

31. SHERLOCK, S. *Disease of the Liver and Biliary System,* 4th Edition, Philadelphia: F.A. Davis, p. 371, 1968.

32. SILINK, J. and B. G. FIRKIN. An analysis of hypoplastic anaemia with special reference to the use of oxymetholone ("Adroyd") in its therapy. *Australian Ann. of Med.* 17:224–235, 1968.

33. STANFORD, B. A. and R. MOFFAT. Anabolic steroid: effectiveness as an ergogenic aid to experienced weight trainers. *J. Sports Med. and Phys. Fit.* 14:191–197, 1974.

34. STEINBACH, M. Uber den Einfluss anabolen Wirkstoffe und Korpergewicht Muskelkraft und Muskeltraining. *Sportarzt und Sport-medizin.* 11:485–492, 1968.

35. SAMUELS, L. T., A. F. HENSCHEL, and A. KAYS. Influence of methyltestosterone on muscular work and creatine metabolism in normal young men. *J. Clin. Endocrinol. Metab.* 2:649–654, 1942.

36. STROMME, S. B., H. D. MEEN, and A. AAKVAAG. Effects of an androgenic-anabolic steroid on strength development and plasma testosterone levels in normal males. *Med. Sci. Sports.* 6:203–208, 1974.

37. WARD, P. The effect of an anabolic steroid on strength and lean body mass. *Med. Sci. Sports* 5:277–282, 1973.

38. ZAK F. G. Peliosis hepatitis. *Am. J. Pathol.* 26:1–15, 1950.

39. ZIEGENFUSS, J. and R. CARABASI. Androgens and hepatocellular carcinoma. *Lancet* 1:262, 1973.

The Recommended Quantity and Quality of Exercise for Developing and Maintaining Fitness in Healthy Adults★

Increasing numbers of persons are becoming involved in endurance training activities and thus, the need for guidelines for exercise prescription is apparent.

Based on the existing evidence concerning exercise prescription for healthy adults and the need for guidelines, the American College of Sports Medicine makes the following recommendations for the quantity and quality of training for developing and maintaining cardiorespiratory fitness and body composition in the healthy adult:

1. Frequency of training: 3 to 5 days per week.

2. Intensity of training: 60% to 90% of maximum heart rate reserve or, 50% to 85% of maximum oxygen uptake (Vo_2 max).

3. Duration of training: 15 to 60 minutes of continuous aerobic activity. Duration is dependent on the intensity of the activity, thus lower intensity activity should be conducted over a longer period of time. Because of the importance of the "total fitness" effect and the fact that it is more readily attained in longer duration programs, and because of the potential hazards and compliance problems associated with high intensity activity, lower to moderate intensity activity of longer duration is recommended for the non-athletic adult.

4. Mode of activity: Any activity that uses large muscle groups, that can be maintained continuously, and is rhythmical and aerobic in nature, e.g. running-jogging, walking-hiking, swimming, skating, bicycling, rowing, cross-country skiing, rope skipping, and various endurance game activities.

Rationale and Research Background

The questions, "How much exercise is enough and what type of exercise is best for developing and maintaining fitness?", are frequently asked. It is recognized that the term 'physical fitness' is composed of a wide variety of variables included in the broad categories of cardiovascular-respiratory fitness, physique and structure, motor function, and many histochemical and biochemical factors. It is also recognized that the adaptive response to training is complex and includes peripheral, central, structural, and functional factors. Although many such variables and their adaptive response to training have been documented, the lack of sufficient in-depth and comparative data relative to frequency, intensity, and duration of training make them inadequate to use as comparative models. Thus, in respect to the above questions, fitness will be limited to changes in Vo_2 max, total body mass, fat weight (FW), and lean body weight (LBW) factors.

Exercise prescription is based upon the frequency, intensity, and duration of training, the mode of activity (aerobic in nature, e.g. listed under No. 4 above), and the initial level of fitness. In evaluating these factors, the following observations have been derived from studies conducted with endurance training programs.

1. Improvement in Vo_2 max is directly related to frequency (2,23,32,58,59,65,77,79), intensity (2,10,13,26,33,37,42,56,77), and duration (3,14,29,49,56,77,86) of training. Depending upon the quantity and quality of training,

improvement in Vo_2 max ranges from 5% to 25% (4,13,27,31,35,36,43,45,52,53,62,71,77, 78,82,86). Although changes in Vo_2 max greater than 25% have been shown, they are usually associated with large total body mass and FW loss, or a low initial level of fitness. Also, as a result of leg fatigue or a lack of motivation, persons with low initial fitness may have spuriously low initial Vo_2 max values.

2. The amount of improvement in Vo_2 max tends to plateau when frequency of training is increased above 3 days per week (23,62,65). For the non-athlete, there is not enough information available at this time to speculate on the value of added improvement found in programs that are conducted more than 5 days per week. Participation of less than two days per week does not show an adequate change in Vo_2 max (24,56,62).

3. Total body mass and FW are generally reduced with endurance training programs (67), while LBW remains constant (62,67,87) or increases slightly (54). Programs that are conducted at least 3 days per week (58,59,61, 62,87), of at least 20 minutes duration (48, 62,87) and of sufficient intensity and duration to expend approximately 300 kilocalories (Kcal) per exercise session are suggested as a threshold level for total body mass and FW loss (12,29, 62,67). An expenditure of 200 Kcal per session has also been shown to be useful in weight reduction if the exercise frequency is at least 4 days per week (80). Programs with less participation generally show little or no change in body composition (19,25,42,62,67,84,85,87). Significant increases in Vo_2 max have been shown with 10 to 15 minutes of high intensity training (34,49,56,62,77,78), thus, if total body mass and FW reduction is not a consideration, then short duration, high intensity programs may be recommended for healthy, low risk (cardiovascular disease) persons.

4. The minimal threshold level for improvement in Vo_2 max is approximately 60% of the maximum heart rate reserve (50% of Vo_2 max) (33,37). Maximum heart rate reserve represents the percent difference between resting and maximum heart rate, adding to the resting heart rate. The technique as described by Kar-

vonen, Kentala, and Mustala (37), was validated by Davis and Convertino (14), and represents a heart rate of approximately 130 to 135 beats/minute for young persons. As a result of the aging curve for maximum heart rate, the absolute heart rate value (threshold level) is inversely related to age, and can be as low as 110 to 120 beats/minute for older persons. Initial level of fitness is another important consideration in prescribing exercise (10,40,46,75,77). The person with a low fitness level can get a significant training effect with a sustained training heart rate as low as 110 to 120 beats/minute, while persons of higher fitness levels need a higher threshold of stimulation (26).

5. Intensity and duration of training are interrelated with the total amount of work accomplished being an important factor in improvement in fitness (2,7,12,40,61,62,76,78). Although more comprehensive inquiry is necessary, present evidence suggests that when exercise is performed above the minimal threshold of intensity, the total amount of work accomplished is the important factor in fitness development (2,7,12,61,62,76,79) and maintenance (68). That is, improvement will be similar for activities performed at a lower intensity-longer duration compared to higher intensity-shorter duration if the total energy cost of the activities are equal.

If frequency, intensity, and duration of training are similar (total Kcal expenditure), the training result appears to be independent of the mode of aerobic activity (56,60,62,64). Therefore, a variety of endurance activities, e.g. listed above, may be used to derive the same training effect.

6. In order to maintain the training effect, exercise must be continued on a regular basis (2,6,11,21,44,73,74). A significant reduction in working capacity occurs after two weeks of detraining (73) with participants returning to near pretraining levels of fitness after 10 weeks (21) to 8 months of detraining (44). Fifty percent reduction in improvement of cardiorespiratory fitness has been shown after 4 to 12 weeks of detraining (21,41,73). More investigation is necessary to evaluate the rate of increase and decrease of fitness with varying training loads

and reduction in training in relation to level of fitness, age, and length of time in training. Also, more information is needed to better identify the minimal level of work necessary to maintain fitness.

7. Endurance activities that require running and jumping generally cause significantly more debilitating injuries to beginning exercisers than other non-weight bearing activities (42, 55,69). One study showed that beginning joggers had increased foot, leg, and knee injuries when training was performed more than 3 days per week and longer than 30 minutes duration per exercise session (69). Thus, caution should be taken when recommending the type of activity and exercise prescription for the beginning exerciser. Also, the increase of orthopedic injuries as related to overuse (marathon training) with chronic jogger-runners is apparent. Thus, there is a need for more inquiry into the effect that different types of activities and the quantity and quality of training has on short-term and long-term participation.

8. Most of the information concerning training described in this position statement has been conducted on men. The lack of information on women is apparent, but the available evidence indicates that women tend to adapt to endurance training in the same manner as men (8,22,89).

9. Age in itself does not appear to be a deterrent to endurance training. Although some earlier studies showed a lower training effect with middle-aged or elderly participants (4, 17,34,83,86), more recent study shows the relative change in $\dot{V}o_2$ max to be similar to younger age groups (3,52,66,75,86). Although more investigation is necessary concerning the rate of improvement in $\dot{V}o_2$ max with age, at present it appears that elderly participants need longer periods of time to adapt to training (17,66). Earlier studies showing moderate to no improvement in $\dot{V}o_2$ max were conducted over a short time-span (4) or exercise was conducted at a moderate to low Kcal expenditure (17), thus making the interpretation of the results difficult.

Although $\dot{V}o_2$ max decreases with age, and total body mass and FW increase with age, evidence suggests that this trend can be altered with endurance training (9,12,38,39,62). Also, 5 to 10 year follow-up studies where participants continued their training at a similar level showed maintenance of fitness (39,70). A study of older competitive runners showed decreases in $\dot{V}o_2$ max from the fourth to seventh decade of life, but also showed reductions in their training load (63). More inquiry into the relationship of long-term training (quantity and quality) for both competitors and non-competitors and physiological function with increasing age, is necessary before more definitive statements can be made.

10. An activity such as weight training should not be considered as a means of training for developing $\dot{V}o_2$ max, but has significant value for increasing muscular strength and endurance, and LBW (16,24,47,49,88). Recent studies evaluating circuit weight training (weight training conducted almost continuously with moderate weights, using 10 to 15 repetitions per exercise session with 15 to 30 seconds rest between bouts of activity) showed little to no improvements in working capacity and $\dot{V}o_2$ max (1,24,90).

Despite an abundance of information available concerning the training of the human organism, the lack of standardization of testing protocols and procedures, methodology in relation to training procedures and experimental design, a preciseness in the documentation and reporting of the quantity and quality of training prescribed, make interpretation difficult (62,67). Interpretation and comparison of results are also dependent on the initial level of fitness (18,74–76,81), length of time of the training experiment (20,57,58,61,62) and specificity of the testing and training (64). For example, data from training studies using subjects with varied levels of $\dot{V}o_2$ max, total body mass and FW have found changes to occur in relation to their initial values (5,15,48,50,51), i.e., the lower the initial $\dot{V}o_2$ max the larger the percent of improvement found, and the higher the FW the greater the reduction. Also, data evaluating trainability with age, comparison of the different magnitudes and quantities of effort, and comparison of the trainability of men and women may have been influenced by the initial fitness levels.

In view of the fact that improvement in the fitness variables discussed in this position statement continue over many months of training (12,38,39,62), it is reasonable to believe that short-term studies conducted over a few weeks have certain limitations. Middle-aged sedentary and older participants may take several weeks to adapt to the initial rigors of training, and thus need a longer adaptation period to get the full benefit from a program. How long a training experiment should be conducted is difficult to determine, but 15 to 20 weeks may be a good minimum standard. For example, two investigations conducted with middle-aged men who jogged either 2 or 4 days per week found both groups to improve in Vo_2 max. Mid-test results of the 16 and 20 week programs showed no difference between groups, while subsequent final testing found the 4 day per week group to improve significantly more (58,59). In a similar study with young college men, no differences in Vo_2 max were found among groups after 7 and 13 weeks of interval training (20). These latter findings and those of other investigators point to the limitations in interpreting results from investigations conducted over a short time-span (62,67).

In summary, frequency, intensity and duration of training have been found to be effective stimuli for producing a training effect. In general, the lower the stimuli, the lower the training effect (2,12,13,27,35,46,77,78,90), and the greater the stimuli, the greater the effect (2, 12,13,27,58,77,78). It has also been shown that endurance training less than two days per week, less than 50% of maximum oxygen uptake, and less than 10 minutes per day is inadequate for developing and maintaining fitness for healthy adults.

REFERENCES

1. ALLEN, T. E., R. J. BYRD and D. P. SMITH. Hemodynamic consequences of circuit weight training. *Res Q.* 43:299–306, 1976.
2. American College of Sports Medicine. *Guidelines for Graded Exercise Testing and Exercise Prescription.* Philadelphia: Lea and Febiger, 1976.
3. BARRY, A. J., W. DALY, E. D. R. PRUETT, J. R. STEINMETZ, H. F. PAGE, N. C. BIRKHEAD and K. RODAHL. The effects of physical conditioning on older individuals. I. Work capacity, circulatory-respiratory function, and work electrocardiogram. *J. Gerontol.* 21:182–191, 1966.
4. BENSETAD, A. M. Trainability of old men. *Acta. Med. Scandinav.* 178:321–327, 1965.
5. BOILEAU, R. A., E. R. BUSKIRK, D. H. HORSTMAN, J. MENDEZ and W. C. NICHOLAS. Body composition changes in obese and lean men during physical conditioning. *Med. Sci. Sports* 3:183–189, 1971.
6. BRYNTESON, P. and W. E. SINNING. The effects of training frequencies on the retention of cardiovascular fitness. *Med. Sci. Sports* 5:29–33, 1973.
7. BURKE, E. J. and B. D. FRANKS. Changes in Vo_2 max resulting from bicycle training at different intensities holding total mechanical work constant. *Res. Q.* 46:31–37, 1975.
8. BURKE, E. J. Physiological effects of similar training programs in males and females. *Res Q.* 48:510–517, 1977.
9. CARTER, J. E. L. and W. H. PHILLIPS. Structural changes in exercising middle-aged males during a 2-year period. *J. Appl. Physiol.* 27:787–794, 1969.
10. CREWS, T. R. and J. A. ROBERTS. Effects of interaction on frequency and intensity of training. *Res. Q.* 47:48–55, 1976.
11. CURETON, T. K. and E. E. PHILLIPS. Physical fitness changes in middle-aged men attributable to equal eight-week periods of training, non-training and re-training. *J. Sports Med. Phys. Fitness* 4:1–7, 1964.
12. CURETON, T. K. *The Physiological Effects of Exercise Programs upon Adults.* Springfield: C. Thomas Company, 1969.
13. DAVIES, C. T. M. and A. V. KNIBBS. The training stimulus, the effects of intensity, duration and frequency of effort on maximum aerobic power output. *Int Z. Angew. Physiol.* 29:299–305, 1971.
14. DAVIS, J. A. and V. A. CONVERTINO. A comparison of heart rate methods for predicting endurance training intensity. *Med. Sci. Sports* 7:295–298, 1975.
15. DEMPSEY, J. A. Anthropometrical observations on obese and nonobese young men undergoing a program of vigorous physical exercise. *Res. Q.* 35:275–287, 1964.
16. DELORME, T. L. Restoration of muscle power by heavy resistance exercise. *J. Bone and Joint Surgery* 27:645–667, 1945.
17. DEVRIES, H. A. Physiological effects of an exercise training regimen upon men aged 52 to 88. *J. Gerontol.* 24:325–336, 1970.
18. EKBLOM, B., P. O. ÅSTRAND, B. SALTIN, J. STERNBERG and B. WALLSTROM. Effect of training on circulatory response to exercise. *J. Appl. Physiol.* 24:518–528, 1968.

19. FLINT, M. M., B. L. DRINKWATER and S. M. HOR-VATH. Effects of training on women's response to sub-maximal exercise. *Med. Sci. Sports* 6:89–94, 1974.

20. FOX, E. L., R. L. BARTELS, C. E. BILLINGS, R. O'BRIEN, R. BASON and D. K. MATHEWS. Frequency and duration of interval training programs and changes in aerobic power. *J. Appl. Physiol.* 38:481–484, 1975.

21. FRINGER, M. N. and A. G. STULL. Changes in cardio-respiratory parameters during periods of training and detraining in young female adults. *Med. Sci. Sports* 6:20–25, 1974.

22. GETCHELL, L. H. and J. C. MOORE. Physical training: comparative response of middle-aged adults. *Arch. Phys. Med. Rehab.* 56:250–254, 1975.

23. GETTMAN, L. R., M. L. POLLOCK, J. L. DURSTINE, A. WARD, J. AYRES and A. C. LINNERUD. Physiological responses of men to 1, 3, and 5 day per week training programs. *Res. Q.* 47:638–646, 1976.

24. GETTMAN, L. R., J. AYRES, M. L. POLLOCK, J. L. DUR-STINE and W. GRANTHAM. Physiological effects of cir-cuit strength training and jogging on adult men. *Arch. Phys. Med. Rehab.,* 60:115–120, 1979.

25. GIRANDOLA, R. N. Body composition changes in women: Effects of high and low exercise intensity. *Arch. Phys. Med. Rehab.* 57:297–300, 1976.

26. GLEDHILL, N. and R. B. EYNON. The intensity of train-ing. In: A. W. Taylor and M. L. Howell (editors). *Training Scientific Basis and Application.* Springfield: Charles C. Thomas, pp. 97–102, 1972.

27. GOLDING. L. Effects of physical training upon total serum cholesterol levels. *Res. Q.* 32:499–505, 1961.

28. GOODE, R. C., A. VIRGIN, T. T. ROMET, P. CRAW-FORD, J. DUFFIN, T. PALLANDI and Z. WOCH. Effects of a short period of physical activity in adolescent boys and girls. *Canad. J. Appl. Sports Sci.* 1:241–250, 1976.

29. GWINUP, G. Effect of exercise alone on the weight of obese women. *Arch. Int. Med.* 135:676–680, 1975.

30. HANSON, J. S., B. S. TABAKIN, A. M. LEVY and W. NEDDE. Long-term physical training and cardiovascu-lar dynamics in middle-aged men. *Circ.* 38:783–799, 1968.

31. HARTLEY, L. H., G. GRIMBY, A. KILBOM, N. J. NILS-SON, I. ÅSTRAND, J. BJURE, B. EKBLOM and B. SALTIN. Physical training in sedentary middle-aged and older men. *Scand. J. Clin. Lab. Invest.* 24:335–344, 1969.

32. HILL, J. S. The effects of frequency of exercise on cardiorespiratory fitness of adult men. M. S. Thesis, Univ. of Western Ontario, London, 1969.

33. HOLLMANN, W. and H. VENRATH. Experimentelle Un-tersuchungen zur bedeutung aines trainings unterhalb and oberhalb der dauerbeltz stungsgranze. In: Korbs (editor). *Carl Diem Fetschrift.* W. u. a. Frankfurt/Wein, 1962.

34. HOLLMAN, W. Changes in the capacity for maximal and continuous effort in relation to age. *Int. Res. Sport Phys. Ed.,* (E. Jokl and E. Simon, editors). Springfield: C. C. Thomas Co., 1964.

35. HUIBREGTSE, W. H., H. H. HARTLEY, L. R. JONES, W. D. DOOLITTLE and T. L. CRIBLEZ. Improvement of aerobic work capacity following non-strenuous exer-cise. *Arch. Env. Health,* 27:12–15, 1973.

36. ISMAIL, A. H. D. CORRIGAN and D. F. MCLEOD. Effect of an eight-month exercise program on selected phys-iological, biochemical, and audiological variables in adult men. *Brit. J. Sports Med.* 7:230–240, 1973.

37. KARVONEN, M., K. KENTALA and O. MUSTALA. The effects of training heart rate: a longitudinal study. *Ann. Med. Exptl. Biol. Fenn.* 35:307–315, 1957.

38. KASCH, F. W., W. H. PHILLIPS, J. E. L. CARTER and J. L. BOYER. Cardiovascular changes in middle-aged men during two years of training. *J. Appl. Physiol.* 314:53–57, 1972.

39. KASCH, F. W. and J. P. WALLACE. Physiological vari-ables during 10 years of endurance exercise. *Med. Sci. Sports* 8:5–8, 1976.

40. KEARNEY, J. T., A. G. STULL, J. J. EWING and J. W. STREIN. Cardiorespiratory responses of sedentary col-lege women as a function of training intensity. *J. Appl. Physiol.* 41:822–825, 1976.

41. KENDRICK, Z. B., M. L. POLLOCK, T. N. HICKMAN and H. S. MILLER. Effects of training and detraining on cardiovascular efficiency. *Amer. Corr. Ther. J.* 25:79–83, 1971.

42. KILBOM, A., L. HARTLEY, B. SALTIN, J. BJURE, G. GRIMBY and I. ÅSTRAND. Physical training in sedentary middle-aged and older men. *Scand. J. Clin. Lab. Invest.* 24:315–322, 1969.

43. KNEHR, C. A., D. B. DILL and W. NEUFELD. Training and its effect on man at rest and at work. *Amer. J. Physiol.* 136:148–156, 1942.

44. KNUTTGEN, H. G., L. O. NORDESJO, B. OLLANDER and B. SALTIN. Physical conditioning through interval training with young male adults. *Med. Sci. Sports* 5:220–226, 1973.

45. MANN, G. V., L. H. GARRETT, A. FARHI, H. MURRAY, T. F. BILLINGS, F. SHUTE and S. E. SCHWARTEN. Ex-ercise to prevent coronary heart disease. *Amer. J. Med.* 46:12–27, 1969.

46. MARIGOLD, E. A. The effect of training at predeter-mined heart rate levels for sedentary college women. *Med. Sci. Sports* 6:14–19, 1974.

47. MAYHEW, J. L. and P. M. GROSS. Body composition changes in young women with high resistance weight training. *Res. Q.* 45:433–439, 1974.

48. MILESIS, C. A., M. L. POLLOCK, M. D. BAH, J. J. AYRES, A. WARD and A. C. LINNERUD. Effects of dif-ferent durations of training on cardiorespiratory func-tion, body composition and serum lipids. *Res. Q.* 47:716–725, 1976.

49. MISNER, J. E., R. A. BOILEAU, B. H. MASSEY and J. H. MAYHEW. Alterations in body composition of adult men during selected physical training programs. *J. Amer. Geriatr. Soc.* 22:33–38, 1974.

50. MOODY, D. L., J. KOLLIAS and E. R. BUSKIRK. The effect of a moderate exercise program on body weight

and skinfold thickness in overweight college women. *Med. Sci. Sports* 1:75–80, 1969.

51. MOODY, D. L., J. H. WILMORE, R. N. GIRANDOLA and J. P. ROYCE. The effects of a jogging program on the body composition of normal and obese high school girls. *Med. Sci. Sports* 4:210–213, 1972.

52. MYRHE, L., S. ROBINSON, A. BROWN and F. PYKE. Paper presented to the American College of Sports Medicine, Albuquerque, New Mexico, 1970.

53. NAUGHTON, J. and F. NAGLE. Peak oxygen intake during physical fitness program for middle-aged men. *JAMA* 191:899–901, 1965.

54. O'HARA, W., C. ALLEN and R. J. SHEPHARD. Loss of body weight and fat during exercise in a cold chamber. *Europ. J. Appl. Physiol.* 37:205–218, 1977.

55. OJA, P., P. TERASLINNA, T. PARTANER and R. KARAVA. Feasibility of an 18 months' physical training program for middle-aged men and its effect on physical fitness. *Am J. Public Health* 64:459–465, 1975.

56. OLREE, H. D., B. CORBIN, J. PENROD and C. SMITH. Methods of achieving and maintaining physical fitness for prolonged space flight. Final Progress Rep. to NASA, Grant No. NGR-04-002-004, 1969.

57. OSCAI, L. B., T. WILLIAMS and B. HERTIG. Effects of exercise on blood volume. *J. Appl. Physiol.* 24:622–624, 1968.

58. POLLOCK, M. L., T. K. CURETON and L. GRENINGER. Effects of frequency of training on working capacity, cardiovascular function, and body composition of adult men. *Med. Sci. Sports* 1:70–74, 1969.

59. POLLOCK, M. L., J. TIFFANY, L. GETTMAN, R. JANEWAY and H. LOFLAND. Effects of frequency of training on serum lipids, cardiovascular function, and body composition. In: *Exercise and fitness* (B. D. Franks, ed.), Chicago: Athletic Institute, 1969, pp. 161–178.

60. POLLOCK, M. L., H. MILLER, R. JANEWAY, A. C. LINNERUD, B. ROBERTSON and R. VALENTINO. Effects of walking on body composition and cardiovascular function of middle-aged men. *J. Appl. Physiol.* 30:126–130, 1971.

61. POLLOCK, M. L., J. BROIDA, Z. KENDRICK, H. S. MILLER, R. JANEWAY and A. C. LINNERUD. Effects of training two days per week at different intensities on middle-aged men. *Med. Sci. Sports* 4:192–197, 1972.

62. POLLOCK, M. L. The qualification of endurance training programs. *Exercise and Sport Sciences Reviews.* (J. Wilmore, editor), New York: Academic Press, pp. 155–188, 1973.

63. POLLOCK, M. L., H. S. MILLER, JR. and J. WILMORE. Physiological characteristics of champion American track athletes 40 to 70 years of age. *J. Gerontol.* 29:645–649, 1974.

64. POLLOCK, M. L., J. DIMMICK, H. S. MILLER, Z. KENDRICK and A. C. LINNERUD. Effects of mode of training on cardiovascular function and body composition of middle-aged men. *Med. Sci. Sports* 7:139–145, 1975.

65. POLLOCK, M. L., H. S. MILLER, A. C. LINNERUD and K. H. COOPER. Frequency of training as a determinant

for improvement in cardiovascular function and body composition of middle-aged men. *Arch. Phys. Med. Rehab.* 56:141–145, 1975.

66. POLLOCK, M. L., G. A. DAWSON, H. S. MILLER, JR., A WARD, D. COOPER, W. HEADLY, A. C. LINNERUD and M. M. NOMEIR. Physiologic response of men 49 to 65 years of age to endurance training. *J. Amer. Geriatr. Soc.* 24:97–104, 1976.

67. POLLOCK, M. L. and A. JACKSON. Body Composition: Measurement and changes resulting from physical training. Proceedings National College Physical Education Association for Men and Women, pp. 125–137, January, 1977.

68. POLLOCK, M. L., J. AYRES and A. WARD. Cardiorespiratory fitness: Response to differing intensities and durations of training. *Arch. Phys. Med. Rehab.* 58:467–473, 1977.

69. POLLOCK, M. L., L. R. GETTMAN, C. A. MILESIS, M. D. BAH, J. L. DURSTINE and R. B. JOHNSON. Effects of frequency and duration of training on attrition and incidence of injury. *Med. Sci. Sports* 9:31–36, 1977.

70. POLLOCK, M. L., H. S. MILLER and P. M. RIBISL. Body composition and cardiorespiratory fitness in former athletes. *Phys. Sports Med.,* 6:45–48, 1978.

71. RIBISL, P. M. Effects of training upon the maximal oxygen uptake of middle-aged men. *Int. Z. Angew. Physiol.* 26:272–278, 1969.

72. ROBINSON, S. and P. M. HARMON. Lactic acid mechanism and certain properties of blood in relation to training. *Amer. J. Physiol.* 132:757–769, 1941.

73. ROSKAMM, H. Optimum patterns of exercise for healthy adults. *Canad. Med. Ass. J.* 96:895–899, 1967.

74. SALTIN, B., G. BLOMQVIST, J. MITCHELL, R. L. JOHNSON, K. WILDENTHAL and C. B. CHAPMAN. Response to exercise after bed rest and after training. *Circ.* 37 and 38, Supp. 7, 1–78, 1968.

75. SALTIN, B., L. HARTLEY, A. KILBOM and I. ÅSTRAND. Physical training in sedentary middle-aged and older men. *Scand. J. Clin. Lab. Invest.* 24:323–334, 1969.

76. SHARKEY, B. J. Intensity and duration of training and the development of cardiorespiratory endurance. *Med. Sci. Sports* 2:197–202, 1970.

77. SHEPHARD, R. J. Intensity, duration, and frequency of exercise as determinants of the response to a training regime. *Int. Z. Angew. Physiol.* 26:272–278, 1969.

78. SHEPHARD, R. J. Future research on the quantifying of endurance training. *J. Human Ergology* 3:163–181, 1975.

79. SIDNEY, K. H., R. B. EYNON and D. A. CUNNINGHAM. Effect of frequency of training of exercise upon physical working performance and selected variables representative of cardiorespiratory fitness. In: Training Scientific Basis and Application (A. W. Taylor, ed.) Springfield: C. C. Thomas, Co., pp. 144–188, 1972.

80. SIDNEY, K. H., R. J. SHEPHARD and J. HARRISON. Endurance training and body composition of the elderly. *Amer. J. CLin. Nutr.* 30:326–333, 1977.

81. SIEGEL, W., G. BLOMQVIST and J. H. MITCHELL. Effects

of a quantitated physical training program on middle-aged sedentary males. *Circ.* 41:19, 1970.

82. SKINNER, J., J. HOLLOSZY and T. CURETON. Effects of a program of endurance exercise on physical work capacity and anthropometric measurements of fifteen middle-aged men. *Amer. J. Cardiol.* 14:747–752, 1964.

83. SKINNER, J. The cardiovascular system with aging and exercise. In: Brunner, D. and E. Jokl (editors). *Physical Activity and Aging.* Baltimore: University Park Press, 1970, pp. 100–108.

84. SMITH, D. P. and F. W. STRANSKY. The effect of training and detraining on the body composition and cardiovascular response of young women to exercise. *J. Sports Med.* 16:112–120, 1976.

85. TERJUNG, R. L., K. M. BALDWIN, J. COOKSEY, B. SAMSON and R. A. SUTTER. Cardiovascular adaptation to twelve minutes of mild daily exercise in middle-aged sedentary men. *J. Amer. Geriatr. Soc.* 21:164–168, 1973.

86. WILMORE, J. H., J. ROYCE, R. N. GIRANDOLA, F. I. KATCH and V. L. KATCH. Physiological alterations resulting from a 10-week jogging program. *Med. Sci. Sports* 2(1):7–14, 1970.

87. WILMORE, J. H., J. ROYCE, R. N. GIRANDOLA, F. I. KATCH and V. L. KATCH. Body composition changes with a 10-week jogging program. *Med. Sci. Sports* 2:113–117, 1970.

88. WILMORE, J. H. Alterations in strength, body composition, and anthropometric measurements consequent to a 10-week weight training program. *Med. Sci. Sports* 6:133–138, 1974.

89. WILMORE, J. Inferiority of female athletes: myth or reality. *J. Sports Med.* 3:1–6, 1974.

90. WILMORE, J., R. B. PARR, P. A. VODAK, T. J. BARSTOW, T. V. PIPES, A. WARD and P. LESLIE. Strength, endurance, BMR, and body composition changes with circuit weight training (Abstract) *Med. Sci. Sports* 8:58–60, 1976.

The Participation of the Female Athlete in Long-Distance Running*

In the Olympic Games and other international contests, female athletes run distances ranging from 100 meters to 3,000 meters, whereas male athletes run distances ranging from 100 meters through 10,000 meters as well as the marathon (42.2 km). The limitation on distance for women's running events has been defended at times on the grounds that long-distance running may be harmful to the health of girls and women.

*(Med Sci Sports 11(4): IX–XI, 1979)

Opinion Statement

It is the opinion of the American College of Sports Medicine that females should not be denied the opportunity to compete in long-distance running. There exists no conclusive scientific or medical evidence that long-distance running is contraindicated for the healthy, trained female athlete. The American College of Sports Medicine recommends that females be allowed to compete at the national and international level in the same distances in which their male counterparts compete.

Supportive Information

Studies (10,20,32,41,54) have shown that females respond in much the same manner as males to systematic exercise training. Cardiorespiratory function is improved as indicated by significant increases in maximal oxygen uptake (4,6,13,16,30). At maximal exercise, stroke volume and cardiac output are increased after training (30). At standardized submaximal exercise intensities after training, cardiac ouput remains unchanged, heart rate decreases, and stroke volume increases (6,30,31). Also, resting heart rate decreases after training (30). As is the case for males, relative body fat content is reduced consequent to systematic endurance training (33,35,51).

Long-distance running imposes a significant thermal stress on the participant. Some differences do exist between males and females with regard to thermoregulation during prolonged exercise. However, the differences in thermal stress response are more quantitative than qualitative in nature (36,38,47). For example, women experience lower evaporative heat losses than do men exposed to the same thermal stress (29,40,53) and usually have higher skin temperatures and deep body temperatures upon onset of sweating (3,18,45). This may actually be an advantage in reducing body water loss so long as thermal equilibrium can be maintained. In view of current findings (10,11,15,40,48, 49,50), it appears that the earlier studies which indicated that women were less tolerant to exercise in the heat than men (36,53) were misleading because they failed to consider the women's relatively low level of cardiorespiratory fitness and heat acclimatization. Apparently, cardiorespiratory fitness as measured by maximum oxygen uptake is a most important functional capacity as regards a person's ability to respond adequately to thermal stress (9,11, 15,47). In fact, there has been considerable interest in the seeming cross-adaptation of a life style characterized by physical activity involving regular and prolonged periods of exercise hyperthermia and response to high environmental temperatures (1,37,39). Women trained in long-distance running have been reported to be more tolerant of heat stress than non-athletic women matched for age and body surface area (15). Thus, it appears that trained female long-distance runners have the capacity to deal with the thermal stress of prolonged exercise as well as the moderate-to-high environmental temperatures and relative humidities that often accompany these events.

The participation of males and females in road races of various distances has increased tremendously during the last decade. This type of competition attracts the entire spectrum of runners with respect to ability—from the elite to the novice. A common feature of virtually all of these races is that a small number of participants develop medical problems (primarily heat injuries) which frequently require hospitalization. One of the first documentations of the medical problems associated with mass participation in this form of athletic competition was by Sutton and co-workers (46). Twenty-nine of 2,005 entrants in the 1971 Sydney City-to-Surf race collapsed; seven required hospitalization. All of the entrants who collapsed were males, although 4% of the race entrants were females. By 1978 the number of entrants increased approximately 10 fold with females accounting for approximately 30% of the entrants. In the 1978 race only nine entrants were treated for heat injury and again all were males (43). In a 1978 Canadian road race, in which 1,250 people participated, 15 entrants developed heat injuries—three females and 12 males,

representing 1.3% and 1.2% of the total number of female and male entrants, respectively (27). Thus, females seem to tolerate the physiological stress of road race competition at least as well as males.

Because long-distance running competition sometimes occurs at moderate altitudes, the female's response to an environment where the partial pressure of oxygen is reduced (hypoxia) should be considered. Buskirk (5) noted that, although there is little information about the physiological responses of women to altitude, the proportional reduction in performance at Mexico City during the Pan American and Olympic Games was the same for males and females. Drinkwater et al. (13) found that women mountaineers exposed to hypoxia demonstrated a similar decrement in maximal oxygen uptake as that predicted for men. Hannon et al. (23,24) have found that females tolerate the effects of altitude better than males because there appears to be both a lower frequency and shorter duration of mountain sickness in women. Furthermore, at altitude women experience less alteration in such variables as resting heart rate, body weight, blood volume, electrocardiograms, and blood chemistries than men (23,24). Although one study has reported that women and men experience approximately the same respiratory changes with altitude exposure (44), another (22) reports that women hyperventilate more than men, thereby increasing the partial pressure of arterial oxygen and decreasing the partial pressure of arterial carbon dioxide. Thus, females tolerate the stress of altitude at least as well as men.

Long-distance running is occasionally associated with various overuse syndromes such as stress fracture, chondromalacia, shinsplints, and tendonitis. Pollock et al. (42) have shown that the incidence of these injuries for males engaged in a program of jogging was as high as 54% and was related to the frequency, duration, and intensity of the exercise training. Franklin et al. (19) recently reported the injury incidence of 42 sedentary females exposed to a 12-week jogging program. The injury rate for the females appeared to be comparable to that found for males in other studies although, as the investigators indicated, a decisive interpretation of presently available information may be premature because of the limited orthopedic injury data available for women. It has been suggested that the anatomical differences between men's and women's pelvic width and joint laxity may lead to a higher incidence of injuries for women who run (26). There are no data available, however, to support this suggestion. Whether or not the higher intensity training programs of competitive male and female long-distance runners result in a difference in injury rate between the sexes is not known at this time. It is believed, however, that the incidence of injury due to running is related more to distances run in training, the running surfaces encountered, biomechanics of the back, leg and foot, and to foot apparel (28).

Of particular concern to female competitors and to the American College of Sports Medicine is evidence which indicates that approximately one-third of the competitive female long-distance runners between the ages of 12 and 45 experience amenorrhea or oligomenorrhea for at least brief periods (7,8). This phenomenon appears more frequently in those women with late onset of menarche, who have not experienced pregnancy, or who have taken contraceptive hormones. This same phenomenon also occurs in some competing gymnasts, swimmers, and professional ballerinas as well as sedentary individuals who have experienced some instances of undue stress or severe psychological trauma (25). Apparently, amenorrhea and oligomenorrhea may be caused by many factors characterized by loss of body weight (7,21,25). Running long distances may lead to decreased serum levels of pituitary gonadotrophic hormones in some women and may directly or indirectly lead to amenorrhea or oligomenorrhea. The role of running and the pathogenesis of these menstrual irregularities remains unknown (7,8).

The long-term effects of these types of menstrual irregularities for young girls that have undergone strenuous exercise training are unknown at this time. Eriksson and co-workers (17) have reported, however, that a group of 28 young girl swimmers, who underwent strenuous swim training for 2.5 years, were normal in all respects (e.g., childbearing) 10 years after discontinuing training.

In summary, a review of the literature demonstrates that males and females adapt to exercise training in a similar manner. Female distance runners are characterized by having large maximal oxygen uptakes and low relative body fat content (52). The challenges of the heat stress of long-distance running or the lower partial pressure of oxygen at altitude seem to be well tolerated by females. The limited data available suggest that females, compared to males, have about the same incidence of orthopedic injuries consequent to endurance training. Disruption of the menstrual cycle is a common problem for female athletes. While it is important to recognize this problem and discover its etiology, no evidence exists to indicate that this is harmful to the female reproductive system.

REFERENCES

1. ALLAN, J. R. The effects of physical training in a temperate and hot climate on the physiological response to heat stress. *Ergonomics* 8:445–453, 1965.
2. ÅSTRAND, P.O., L. ENGSTRÖM, B. ERIKSSON, P. KARLBERG, I. NYLANDER, and C. THORÉN. Girl swimmers. *Acta Paediat. Scand.* Suppl. 147, 1963.
3. BITTEL, J. and R. HENANE. Comparison of thermal exchanges in men and women under neutral and hot conditions. *J. Physiol. (Lond.)* 250:475–489, 1975.
4. BROWN, C. H., J. R. HARROWER, and M. F. DEETER. The effects of cross-country running on pre-adolescent girls. *Med. Sci. Sports* 4:1–5, 1972.
5. BUSKIRK, E. R. Work and fatigue in high altitude. In: *Physiology of work capacity and fatigue.* E. Simonson (Ed.), Springfield, Illinois: Charles C. Thomas, pp. 312–324, 1971.
6. CUNNINGHAM, D. A. and J. S. HILL. Effect of training on cardiovascular response to exercise in women. *J. Appl. Physiol.* 39:891–895, 1975.
7. DALE, E., D. H. GERLACH, D. E. MARTIN, and C. R. ALEXANDER. Physical fitness profiles and reproductive physiology of the female distance runner. *Phy. and Sportsmed.* 7:83–95, 1979 (Jan).
8. DALE, E., D. H. GERLACH, and A. L. WITHITE. Menstrual dysfunction in distance runners. *Obst. Gyne.* 54:47–53, 1979.
9. DILL, B. D., L. F. SOHOLT, D. C. MCLEAN, T. F. DROST, JR., and M. T. LOUGHRAN. Capacity of young males and females for running in desert heat. *Med. Sci. Sports* 9:137–142, 1977.

10. DRINKWATER, B. L. Physiological responses of women to exercise. In: *Exercise and sports sciences reviews*. J. H. Wilmore (Ed.), New York, NY: Academic Press, Vol. 1, pp. 125–153, 1973.

11. DRINKWATER, B. L., J. E. DENTON, I. C. KUPPRAT, T. S. TALAG, and S. M. HORVATH. Aerobic power as a factor in women's response to work in hot environments. *J. Appl. Physiol.* 41:815–821, 1976.

12. DRINKWATER, B. L., J. E. DENTON, P. B. RAVEN and S. M. HORVATH. Thermoregulatory response of women to intermittent work in the heat. *J. Appl. Physiol.* 41:57–61, 1976.

13. DRINKWATER, B. L., L. J. FOLINSBEE, J. F. BEDI, S. A. PLOWMAN, A. B. LOUCKS, and S. M. HORVATH. Response of women mountaineers to maximal exercise during hypoxia. *Avia. Space Environ, Med.* 50:657–662, 1979.

14. DRINKWATER, B. L., I. C. KUPPRAT, J. E. DENTON, J. L. CRIST, and S. M. HORVATH. Response of prepubertal girls and college women to work in the heat. *J. Appl. Physiol.: Respirat. Environ. Exercise Physiol.* 43:1046–1053, 1977.

15. DRINKWATER, B. L., I. C. KUPPRAT, J. E. DENTON, and S. M. HORVATH. Heat tolerance of female distance runners. *Annals NY Acad. Sci.* 301:777–792, 1977.

16. EDDY, D. O., K. L. SPARKS, and D. A. ADELIZI. The effect of continuous and interval training in women and men. *Europ. J. Appl. Physiol.* 37:83–92, 1977.

17. ERIKSSON, B. O., I. ENGSTRÖM, P. KARLBERG, A. LUNDIN, B. SALTIN, and C. THORÉN. Long-term effect of previous swimtraining in girls. A 10-year follow-up on the "Girl Swimmers." *Acta Paediat. Scand.* 67:285–292, 1978.

18. FOX, R. H., B. E. LOFSTEDT, P. M. WOODWARD, E. ERIKSSON, and B. WERKSTROM. Comparison of thermoregulatory function in men and women. *J. Appl. Physiol.* 26:444–453, 1969.

19. FRANKLIN, B. A., L. LUSSIER, and E. R. BUSKIRK. Injury rates in women joggers. *Phy. and Sportsmed.* 7:105–112, 1979 (Mar).

20. FRINGER, M. N. and G. A. STULL. Changes in cardiorespiratory parameters during periods of training and detraining in young adult females. *Med. Sci. Sports* 6:20–25, 1974.

21. FRISCH, R. E. Fatness and the onset and maintenance of menstrual cycles. *Res. In Reprod.* 6:1, 1977.

22. HANNON, J. P. Comparative altitude adaptability of young men and women. In: *Environmental stress: individual human adaptations.* L. J. Folinsbee et al. (Eds.), San Francisco: Academic Press, pp. 335–350, 1978.

23. HANNON, J. P., J. L. SHIELDS, and C. W. HARRIS. A comparative review of certain responses of men and women to high altitude. In: *Proceedings symposia on arctic biology and medicine. VI. The physiology of work in cold and altitude.* C. Helfferich, (Ed.), Fort Wainwright, Alaska: Arctic Aeromedical Laboratory, pp. 113–245, 1966.

24. HANNON, J. P., J. L. SHIELDS, and C. W. HARRIS. Effects of altitude acclimatization on blood composition of women. *J. Appl. Physiol.* 26:540–547, 1969.

25. HARRIS, D. V. (quoted in) Secondary amenorrhea linked to stress. *Phy. and Sportsmed.* 6:24, 1978 (Oct).

26. HAYCOCK, C. E., and J. V. GILLETTE. Susceptibility of women athletes to injury: Myths vs. Reality. *JAMA* 236:163–165, 1976.

27. HUGHSON, R. L. and J. R. SUTTON. Heat stroke in "run for fun." *Br. Med. J.* 2(No. 6145): 1158, 1978, (Oct).

28. JAMES, S. L., B. J. BATES, and L. R. OSTERNIG. Injuries to runners. *Am. J. Sports Med.* 6:40–50, 1978 (Mar-Apr).

29. KAWAHATA, A. Sex differences in sweating. In: *Essential problems in climatic physiology,* M. Yoshimura, K. Ogata and S. Ito (Eds.), Kyoto: Nankodo, pp. 169–184, 1960.

30. KILBOM, Å. Physical training in women. *Scand. J. Clin. Lab. Invest.* 28:1–34, Suppl. 119, 1971.

31. KOLLIS, J., H. L. BARLETT, P. OJA, and C. L. SHEARBURN. Cardiac output of sedentary and physically conditioned women during submaximal exercise. *Aust. J. Sports Med.* 9:63–68, 1977.

32. LAMB, D. R. *Physiology of exercise: responses and adaptations.* New York: Macmillan Publishing Co., Inc., p. 252, 1978.

33. MAYHEW, J. L. and P. M. GROSS. Body composition changes in young women with high resistance weight training. *Res. Q. Am. Assoc. Health Phys. Ed.* 56:433–440, 1974.

34. MOODY, D. L., J. KOLLIAS, and E. R. BUSKIRK. The effect of a moderate exercise program on body weight and skinfold thickness in overweight college women. *Med. Sci. Sports* 1:75–80, 1969.

35. MOODY, D. L., J. H. WILMORE, R. N. GIRANDOLA, and J. P. ROYCE. The effects of a jogging program on the body composition of normal and obese high school girls. *Med. Sci. Sports* 4:210–213, 1972.

36. MORIMOTO, T., Z. SLABOCHOVA, R. K. NAMAN, and F. SARGENT, II. Sex differences in physiological reactions to thermal stress. *J. Appl. Physiol.* 22:526–532, 1967.

37. NADEL, E. R., K. B. PANDOLF, M. F. ROBERTS, and J. A. J. STOLWIJK. Mechanisms of thermal acclimation to exercise and heat. *J. Appl. Physiol.* 37:515–520, 1974.

38. NUNNELEY, S. A. Physiological responses of women to thermal stress: A Review. *Med. Sci. Sports* 10:250–255, 1978.

39. PANDOLF, K. B. Effects of physical training and cardiorespiratory physical fitness on exercise-heat tolerance: recent observations. *Med. Sci. Sports* 11:60–65, 1979.

40. PAOLONE, A. M., C. L. WELLS, and G. T. KELLY. Sexual variations in thermoregulation during heat stress. *Aviat. Space Environ. Med.* 49:715–719, 1978.

41. POLLOCK, M. L. The qualification of endurance training programs. In: *Exercise and sport sciences reviews.* J. H. Wilmore (Ed.), New York, NY: Academic Press, Vol. 1, pp. 155–188, 1973.

42. POLLOCK, M. L., L. R. GETTMAN, C. A. MILESIS, M. D. BAH, L. DURSTINE, and R. B. JOHNSON. Effects of frequency and duration of training on attrition and incidence of injury. *Med. Sci. Sports* 9:31–36, 1977.

43. RICHARDS, R., D. RICHARDS, P. SCHOFIELD, V. ROSS, and J. SUTTON. Reducing the hazards in Sydney's *The Sun* City-to-Surf Runs, 1971–1979. *Med. J. Aust.* 2:453–457, 1979.

44. SHIELDS, J. L., J. P. HANNON, C. W. HARRIS and W. S. PLATNER. Effects of altitude acclimatization on pulmonary function in women. *J. Appl. Physiol.* 25:606–609, 1968.

45. STOLWIJK, J. A. J. Responses to the thermal environment. *Fed. Proc.* 36:1655–1658, 1977.

46. SUTTON, J., M. J. COLEMAN, A. P. MILLAR, L. LARARUS, and P. RUSSO. The medical problems of mass participation in athletic competition. *Med. J. Aust.* 2:127–133, 1972.

47. WELLS, C. L. Responses of physically active and acclimatized men and women to work in a desert environment. *Med. Sci. Sports* (accepted for publication, 1980).

48. WELLS, C. L. Sexual differences in heat stress response. *Phys. and Sportsmed.* 5:79–90, 1977 (Sept).

49. WELLS, C. L., and S. M. HORVATH. Metabolic and thermoregulatory responses of women to exercise in two thermal environments. *Med. Sci. Sports* 6:8–13, 1974.

50. WELLS, C. L., and A. M. PAOLONE. Metabolic responses to exercise in three thermal environments. *Aviat. Space Environ. Med.* 48:989–993, 1977.

51. WILMORE, J. H. Alterations in strength, body composition and anthropometric measurements consequent to a 10-week weight training program. *Med. Sci. Sports* 6:133–138, 1974.

52. WILMORE, J. H., and C. H. BROWN. Physiological profiles of women distance runners. *Med. Sci. Sports* 6:178–181, 1974.

53. WYNDHAM, C. H., J. F. MORRISON, and C. G. WILLIAMS. Heat reactions of male and female Caucasians. *J. Appl. Physiol.* 20:357–364, 1965.

54. YAEGER, S. A., and P. BRYNTESON. Effects of varying training periods on the development of cardiovascular efficiency of college women. *Res. Q. Am. Assoc. Health Phys. Educ.* 41:589–592, 1970.

Weight Loss in Wrestlers*

Despite repeated admonitions by medical, educational and athletic groups (2,8,17,22,23), most wrestlers have been inculcated by instruc-

*(Med Sci Sports 8(2): XI–XII, 1976)

tion or accepted tradition to lose weight in order to be certified for a class that is lower than their preseason weight (34). Studies (34,40) of weight losses in high school and college wrestlers indicate that from 3-20% of the preseason body weight is lost before certification or competition occurs. Of this weight loss, most of the decrease occurs in the final days or day before the official weigh-in (34,40) with the youngest and/or lightest members of the team losing the highest percentage of their body weight (34). Under existing rules and practices, it is not uncommon for an individual to repeat this weight losing process many times during the season because successful wrestlers compete in 15-30 matches/year (13).

Contrary to existing beliefs, most wrestlers are not "fat" before the season starts (35). In fact, the fat content of high school and college wrestlers weighing less than 190 pounds has been shown to range from 1.6 to 15.1 percent of their body weight with the majority possessing less than 8% (14,28,31). It is well known and documented that wrestlers lose body weight by a combination of food restriction, fluid deprivation and sweating induced by thermal or exercise procedures (20,22,34,40). Of these methods, dehydration through sweating appears to be the method most frequently chosen.

Careful studies on the nature of the weight being lost show that water, fats and proteins are lost when food restriction and fluid deprivation procedures are followed (10). Moreover, the proportionality between these constituents will change with continued restriction and deprivation. For example, if food restriction is held constant when the volume of fluid being consumed is decreased, more water will be lost from the tissues of the body than before the fluid restriction occurred. The problem becomes more acute when thermal or exercise dehydration occurs because electrolyte losses will accompany the water losses (16). Even when 1-5 hours are allowed for purposes of rehydration after the weigh-in, this time interval is insufficient for fluid and electrolyte homeostasis to be completely reestablished (11, 37,39,40).

Since the "making of weight" occurs by combinations of food restriction, fluid deprivation and dehydration, responsible officials should realize that the single or combined effects of these practices are generally associated with 1) a reduction in muscular strength (4, 15,30); 2) a decrease in work performance times (24,26,27,30); 3) lower plasma and blood volumes (6,7,24,27); 4) a reduction in cardiac functioning during sub-maximal work conditions which are associated with higher heart rates (1,19,23,24,27), smaller stroke volumes (27), and reduced cardiac outputs (27); 5) a lower oxygen consumption, especially with food restriction (15,30); 6) an impairment of thermoregulatory processes (3,9,24); 7) a decrease in renal blood flow (21,25) and in the volume of fluid being filtered by the kidney (21); 8) a depletion of liver glycogen stores (12); and 9) an increase in the amount of electrolytes being lost from the body (6,7,16).

Since it is possible for these changes to impede normal growth and development, there is little physiological or medical justification for the use of the weight reduction methods currently followed by many wrestlers. These sentiments have been expressed in part within Rule 1, Section 3, Article 1 of the **Official Wrestling Rule Book** (18) published by the National Federation of State High School Associations which states, "The Rules Committee recommends that individual state high school associations develop and ultilize an effective weight control program which will discourage severe weight reduction and/or wide variations in weight, because this may be harmful to the competitor . . .". However, until the National Federation of State High School Associations defines the meaning of the terms "severe" and "wide variations," this rule will be ineffective in reducing the abuses associated with the "making of weight."

Therefore, it is the position of the American College of Sports Medicine★ that the potential health hazards created by the procedures used

★The services of the American College of Sports Medicine are available to assist local and national organizations in implementing these recommendations.

to "make weight" by wrestlers can be eliminated if state and national organizations will:

1. Assess the body composition of each wrestler several weeks in advance of the competitive season (5,14,28,31,38). Individuals with a fat content less than five percent of their certified body weight should receive medical clearance before being allowed to compete.

2. Emphasize the fact that the daily caloric requirements of wrestlers should be obtained from a balanced diet and determined on the basis of age, body surface area, growth and physical activity levels (29). The minimal caloric needs of wrestlers in high schools and colleges will range from 1200 to 2400 KCal/day (32); therefore, it is the responsibility of coaches, school officials, physicians and parents to discourage wrestlers from securing less than their minimal needs without prior medical approval.

3. Discourage the practice of fluid deprivation and dehydration. This can be accomplished by:

    a. Educating the coaches and wrestlers on the physiological consequences and medical complications that can occur as a result of these practices.

    b. Prohibiting the single or combined use of rubber suits, steam rooms, hot boxes, saunas, laxatives, and diuretics to "make weight."

    c. Scheduling weigh-ins just prior to competition.

    d. Scheduling more official weigh-ins between team matches.

4. Permit more participant/team to compete in those weight classes (119-145 pounds) which have the highest percentages of wrestlers certified for competition (36).

5. Standardize regulations concerning the eligibility rules at championship tournaments so that individuals can only participate in those weight classes in which they had the highest frequencies of matches throughtout the season.

6. Encourage local and county organizations to systematically collect data on the hydration state (39,40) of wrestlers and its relationship to growth and development.

REFERENCES

1. AHLMAN, K. and M. J. KARVONEN. Weight reduction by sweating in wrestlers and its effect on physical fitness. *J. Sports Med. Phys. Fit.* 1:58–62, 1961.

2. AMA Committee on the Medical Aspects of Sports, Wrestling and Weight Control. *JAMA* 201:541–543, 1967.

3. BOCK, W. E., E. L. FOX and R. BOWERS. The effect of acute dehydration upon cardiorespiratory endurance. *J. Sports Med. Phys. Fit.* 7:62–72, 1967.

4. BOSCO, J. S., R. L. TERJUNG and J. E. GREENLEAF. Effects of progressive hypohydration on maximal isometric muscular strength. *J. Sports Med. Phys. Fit.* 8:81–86, 1968.

5. CLARKE, K. S. Predicting certified weight of young wrestlers: a field study of the Tcheng-Tipton method. *Med. Sci. Sports* 6:52–57, 1974.

6. COSTILL, D. L. and K. E. SPARKS. Rapid fluid replacement following thermal dehydration. *J. Appl. Physiol.* 34:299–303, 1973.

7. COSTILL, D. L., R. COTE, E. MILLER, T. MILLER and S. WYNDER. Water and electrolyte replacement during repeated days of work in the heat. *Aviat. Space Environ. Med.* 46:795–800, 1975.

8. ERIKSEN, F. G. Interscholastic wrestling and weight control: Current plans and their loopholes. *Proceedings of the Eighth National Conference on The Medical Aspects of Sports.* Chicago: AMA, 1967, pp. 34–39.

9. GRANDE, F., J. E. MONAGLE, E. R. BUSKIRK and H. L. TAYLOR. Body temperature responses to exercise in man on restricted food and water intake. *J. Appl. Physiol.* 14:194–198, 1959.

10. GRANDE, F. Nutrition and energy balance in body composition studies. *Techniques for Measuring Body Composition,* edited by J. Brôzek and A. Henschel. Washington, D.C., National Acad. Sci. & Nat. Res. Council, pp. 168–188, 1961.

11. HERBERT, W. G. and P. M. RIBISL. Effects of dehydration upon physical work capacity of wrestlers under competitive conditions. *Res. Quart.* 43:416–422, 1972.

12. HULTMAN, E. and L. NILSSON. Liver glycogen as glucose-supplying source during exercise. *Limiting Factors of Physical Performance,* edited by J. Keul. Stuttgart: Georg Thieme, pp. 179–189, 1973.

13. *1975 Program for the 55th State Wrestling Tournament.* Iowa High School Athletic Association, pp. 7–9.

14. KATCH, F. I. and E. D. MICHAEL, JR. Body composition of high school wrestlers according to age and wrestling weight category. *Med. Sci. Sports* 3:190–194, 1971.

15. KEYS, A. L., J. BRÔZEK, A. HENSCHEL, O. MICKELSEN and H. L. TAYLOR. *The Biology of Human Starvation.* Minneapolis: U. of Minn. Press, Vol. 1, pp. 718–748, 1950.

16. KOZLOWSKI, S. and B. SALTIN. Effect of sweat loss on body fluids. *J. Appl. Physiol.* 19:1119–1124, 1964.

17. KROLL, W. Guidelines for rules and practices. *Proceedings of the Eighth National Conference on the Medical Aspects of Sports.* Chicago: AMA, pp. 40–44, 1967.

18. *The National Federation 1974–75 Wrestling Rule Book.* The National Federation Publications. Elgin, Illinois, p. 6.

19. PALMER, W. Selected physiological responses of normal young men following dehydration and rehydration. *Res. Quart.* 39:1054–1059, 1968.

20. PAUL, W. D. Crash diets in wrestling. *J. Iowa Med. Soc.* 56:835–840, 1966.

21. RADIGAN, L. R. and S. ROBINSON. Effect of environmental heat stress and exercise on renal blood flow and filtration rate. *J. Appl. Physiol.* 2:185–191, 1949.

22. RASCH, P. G. and W. KROLL. *What Research Tells the Coach About Wrestling.* Washington: AAHPER, pp. 41–50, 1964.

23. RIBISL, P. M. and W. G. HERBERT. Effect of rapid weight reduction and subsequent rehydration upon the physical working capacity of wrestlers. *Res. Quart.* 41:536–541, 1970.

24. ROBINSON, S. The effect of dehydration on performance. *Football Injuries.* Washington: Nat. Acad. Sci., pp. 191–197, 1970.

25. ROWELL, L. B. Human cardiovascular adjustments to exercise and thermal stress. *Physiol. Rev.* 54:75–159, 1974.

26. SALTIN, B. Aerobic and anaerobic work capacity after dehydration. *J. Appl. Physiol.* 19:1114–1118, 1964.

27. SALTIN, B. Circulatory response to submaximal and maximal exercise after thermal dehydration. *J. Appl. Physiol.* 19:1125–1132, 1964.

28. SINNING, W. E. Body composition assessment of college wrestlers. *Med. Sci. Sports* 6:139–145, 1974.

29. Suggested Daily Dietary Requirements. National Research Council Data, published in Oser, B. O. *Hawk's Physiological Chemistry.* 14th Edition, New York: McGraw-Hill, pp. 1370–1371, 1965.

30. TAYLOR, H. L., E. R. BUSKIRK, J. BRÔZEK, J. T. ANDERSON and F. GRANDE. Performance capacity and effects of caloric restriction with hard physical work on young men. *J. Appl. Physiol.* 10:421–429, 1957.

31. TCHENG, T. K. and C. M. TIPTON. Iowa wrestling study: Anthropometric measurements and the prediction of a "minimal" body weight for high school wrestlers. *Med. Sci. Sports* 5:1–10, 1973.

32. TIPTON, C. M. Unpublished calculations on Iowa High School Wrestlers using a height and weight surface area nomogram. (CONSALAZIO, C. F., R. E. JOHNSON and L. J. PECORA. *Physiological Measurements of Metabolic Functions in Man.* New York: McGraw-Hill, 1963, p. 27, that was constructed from the Dubois-Meech formula published in Arch. Int. Med. 17:863–871, 1916) plus the metabolic standards for age used by the Mayo Foundation Standards that were published by Boothby, Berkson and Dunn in *Am. J. Physiol.* 116:467–484, 1936.

33. TIPTON, C. M., T. K. TCHENG and W. D. PAUL. Evaluation of the Hall Method for determining minimum wrestling weights. *J. Iowa Med. Soc.* 59:571–574, 1969.

34. TIPTON, C. M. and T. K. TCHENG. Iowa wrestling

study: Weight loss in high school students. *JAMA* 2114:1269–1274, 1970.

35. TIPTON, C. M. Current status of the Iowa Wrestling Study. *The Predicament.* 12:30–73, p. 7.

36. TIPTON, C. M., T. K. TCHENG and E. J. ZAMBRASKI. Iowa Wrestling Study: Weight classification systems. *Med. Sci. Sports* 8:101–104, 1976.

37. VACCARO, P., C. W. ZAUNER and J. R. CADE. Changes in body weight hematocrit and plasma protein concentration due to dehydration and rehydration in wrestlers. *Med. Sci. Sports* 7:76, 1975.

38. WILMORE, J. H. and A. BEHNKE. An anthropometric estimation of body density and lean body weight in young men. *J. Appl. Physiol.* 27:25–31, 1969.

39. ZAMBRASKI, E. J., C. M. TIPTON, T. K. TCHENG, H. R. JORDAN, A. C. VAILAS and A. K. CALLAHAN. Changes in the urinary profiles of wrestlers prior to and after competition. *Med. Sci. Sports.* 7:217–220, 1975.

40. ZAMBRASKI, E. J., D. T. FOSTER, P. M. GROSS and C. M. TIPTON. Iowa wrestling study: Weight loss and urinary profiles of collegiate wrestlers. *Med. Sci. Sports* 8:105–108, 1976.

Prevention of Heat Injuries During Distance Running★

Based on research findings and current rules governing distance running competition, it is the position of the American College of Sports Medicine that:

1. Distance races (>16 km or 10 miles) should *not* be conducted when the wet bulb temperature—globe temperature† exceeds 28° C (82.4° F). (1,2)

2. During periods of the year, when the daylight dry bulb temperature often exceeds 27° C (80° F), distance races should be conducted before 9:00 A.M. or after 4:00 P.M. (2,7,8,9)

3. It is the responsibility of the race sponsors to provide fluids which contain small amounts of sugar (less than 2.5 g glucose per 100 ml of water) and electrolytes (less than 10 mEq sodium and 5 mEq potassium per liter of solution.) (5,6)

4. Runners should be encouraged to frequently ingest fluids during competition and to

★(Med Sci Sports 7(1): VII–IX, 1975)

†Adapted from Minard, D. *Prevention of heat casualities in Marine Corps Recruits. Milit. Med.* 126: 261, 1961. WB-GT = 0.7 (WBT) + 0.2 (GT) + 0.1 (DBT)

consume 400–500 ml (13-17 oz.) of fluid 10-15 minutes before competition. (5,6,9)

5. Rules prohibiting the administration of fluids during the first 10 kilometers (6.2 miles) of a marathon race should be amended to permit fluid ingestion at frequent intervals along the race course. In light of the high sweat rates and body temperatures during distance running in the heat, race sponsors should provide "water stations" at 3-4 kilometer (2-2.5 mile) intervals for all races of 16 kilometers (10 miles) or more. (4,8,9)

6. Runners should be instructed in how to recognize the early warning symptoms that precede heat injury. Recognition of symptoms, cessation of running, and proper treatment can prevent heat injury. Early warning symptoms include the following: piloerection on chest and upper arms, chilling, throbbing pressure in the head, unsteadiness, nausea, and dry skin (2,9)

7. Race sponsors should make prior arrangements with medical personnel for the care of cases of heat injury. Responsible and informed personnel should supervise each "feeding station." Organizational personnel should reserve the right to stop runners who exhibit clear signs of heat stroke or heat exhaustion.

It is the position of the American College of Sports Medicine that policies established by local, national, and international sponsors of distance running events should adhere to these guidelines. Failure to adhere to these guidelines may jeopardize the health of competitors through heat injury.

RESEARCH SUPPORT FOR ACSM POSITION STATEMENT

1. ADOLPH, E. F. *Physiology of Man in the Desert.* New York Interscience, 1947.

2. BUSKIRK, E. R. and W. C. GRASLEY. Heat Injury and Conduct of Athletes. Ch. 16 in *Science and Medicine of Exercise and Sport,* 2nd Edition. W. R. Johnson and E. R. Buskirk, Editors, New York; Harper and Row, 1974.

3. BUSKIRK, E. R., P. F. IAMPIETRO and D. E. BASS. Work performance and dehydration: effects of physical conditioning and heat acclimatization. *J. Appl. Physiol.* 12:189–194, 1958.

4. COSTILL, D. L., W. F. KAMMER and A. FISHER. Fluid ingestion during distance running. *Arch. Environ. Health* 21:520–525, 1970.

5. COSTILL, D. L. and B. SALTIN. Factors limiting gastric emptying during rest and exercise. *J. Appl. Physiol.* 37(5):679–683, 1974.

6. FORDTRAN, J. A. and B. SALTIN. Gastric emptying and intestinal absorption during prolonged severe exercise. *J. Appl. Physiol.* 23:331–335, 1967.

7. MYHRE, L. G. Shifts in blood volume during and following acute environmental and work stresses in man. (Doctoral Dissertation). Indiana University: Bloomington, Indiana, 1967.

8. PUGH, L. G. C., J. I. CORBETT and R. H. JOHNSON. Rectal temperatures, weight losses and sweating rates in marathon running. *J. Appl. Physiol.* 23:347–353, 1957.

9. WYNDHAM, C. H. and N. B. STRYDOM. The danger of an inadequate water intake during marathon running. *S. Afr. Med. J.* 43:893–896, 1969.

Heat Injuries During Distance Running

The requirements of distance running place great demands on both circulation and body temperature regulation (4,8,9). Numerous studies have reported rectal temperatures in excess of 40.6° C (105° F) after races of 6 to 26.2 miles (9.6 to 41.9 kilometers) (4,8,9). Attempting to counterbalance such overheating, runners incur large sweat losses of .8 to 1.1 liters/m²/hr (4,8,9). The resulting body water deficit may total 6–10% of the athlete's body weight. Dehydration of these proportions severely limits subsequent sweating, places dangerous demands on circulation, reduces exercise capacity and exposes the runner to the health hazards associated with hyperthermia (heat stroke, heat exhaustion and muscle cramps) (2,3,9).

Under moderate thermal conditions, e.g., 65–70° F (18.5–21.3° C), no cloud cover, relative humidity 49–55%, the risk of overheating is still a serious threat to highly motivated distance runners. Nevertheless, distance races are frequently conducted under more severe conditions than these. The air temperature at the 1967 U.S. Pan American Marathon Trial, for example, was 92–95° F (33.6–35.3° C). Many highly conditioned athletes failed to finish the race and several of the competitors demonstrated overt symptoms of heat stroke (no sweating, shivering and lack of orientation).

The above consequences are compounded by the current popularity of distance running among middle-aged and aging men and women who may possess significantly less heat tolerance than their younger counterparts. In recent years, races of 10 to 26.2 miles (16 to 41.9 kilometers) have attracted several thousand runners. Since it is likely that distance running enthusiasts will continue to sponsor races under adverse heat conditions, specific steps should be taken to minimize the health threats which accompany such endurance events.

Fluid ingestion during prolonged running (two hours) has been shown to effectively reduce rectal temperature and minimize dehydration (4). Although most competitors consume fluids during races that exceed 1–1.5 hours, current international distance running rules prohibit the administration of fluids until the runner has completed 6.8 miles (11 kilometers). Under such limitations, the competitor is certain to accumulate a large body water deficit (−3%) before any fluids would be ingested. To make the problem more complex, most runners are unable to judge the volume of fluids they consume during competition (4). At the 1968 U.S. Olympic Marathon Trial, it was observed that there were body weight losses of 6.1 kg, with an average total fluid ingestion of only 0.14 to 0.35 liters (4). It seems obvious that the rules and habits which prohibit fluid administration during distance running preclude any benefits which might be gained from this practice.

Runners who attempt to consume large volumes of sugar solution during competition complain of gastric discomfort (fullness) and an inability to consume fluids after the first few feedings (4,5,6). Generally speaking, most runners drink solutions containing 5–20 grams of sugar per 100 milliliters of water. Although saline is rapidly emptied from the stomach (25 ml/min), the addition of even small amounts of sugar can drastically impair the rate of gastric emptying (5). During exercise in the heat, carbohydrate supplementation is of secondary importance and the sugar content of the oral feedings should be minimized.

Sports Medicine Journals and Organizations and Sports Associations for Handicapped Athletes

SPORTS MEDICINE JOURNALS

The American Journal of Sports Medicine
(Official publication of the American Orthopaedic Society for Sports Medicine)
The Williams and Wilkins Company
428 East Preston Street
Baltimore, Maryland 21202

Athletic Training
(Journal of the National Athletic Trainers Association)
Eastern Associates
Post Office Box 1865
Greenville, North Carolina 27834

The Journal of Orthopaedic and Sports Physical Therapy
(Official publication of the Sports Medicine Section, American Physical Therapy Association)
428 East Preston Street
Baltimore, Maryland 21202

Medicine and Science in Sports and Exercise
(Official journal of the American College of Sports Medicine)
1440 Monroe Street
Madison, Wisconsin 53706

National Strength and Conditioning Association Journal
(Official voice of the NSCA)
National Strength and Conditioning Association
211 South Stadium
Lincoln, Nebraska 68588

The Physical Education Index
Ben Oak Publishing Company
Post Office Box 474
Cape Girardeaux, Missouri 63701

The Physician and Sportsmedicine
4530 West 77th Street
Minneapolis, Minnesota 55435

Yearbook of Sports Medicine
Year Book Medical Publishers, Inc.
Chicago, Illinois, and London, England

SPORTS MEDICINE ORGANIZATIONS

American Academy of Podiatric Sports Medicine
4301 Atlantic Avenue, Suite 6
Long Beach, California, 90807

American Alliance for Health, Physical Education, Recreation and Dance
1900 Association Drive
Reston, Virginia, 22091

American College of Sports Medicine
1440 Monroe Street
Madison, Wisconsin 53706

American Orthopedic Society for Sports Medicine
70 West Hubbard, Suite 202
Chicago, Illinois 60610

American Osteopathic Academy of Sports Medicine
1551 NW 54th
Seattle, Washington, 91807

American Physical Therapy Association
1156 15th Street, NW
Washington, D.C. 20005

International Federation of Sports Medicine
c/o Allan Ryan, M.D., Secretary General
5800 Jeff Place
Edina, Minnesota 55436

National Athletic Trainers Association
131 White Building
Pennsylvania State University
University Park, Pennsylvania 16802

National Strength and Conditioning Association
211 South Stadium
Lincoln, Nebraska 68588

President's Council on Physical Fitness and Sports
400 6th Street, SW
Room 3030
Washington, D.C. 20201

NATIONAL SPORTS ORGANIZATIONS

Amateur Athletic Union
3400 West 86th Street
Indianapolis, Indiana 46268

Association for Intercollegiate Athletics for Women
1201 16th Street, NW
Washington, D.C. 20036

National Collegiate Athletic Association
Post Office Box 1906
Shawnee Mission, Kansas 66222

National Federation of State High School Athletic Associations
11724 Plaza Circle, Post Office Box 20626
Kansas City, Missouri 64195

National High School Athletic Coaches Association
3423 East Silver Springs Boulevard
Suite 9
Ocala, Florida 32670

United States Olympic Committee
1750 East Boulder Street
Colorado Springs, Colorado 80909

SPORTS ASSOCIATIONS FOR HANDICAPPED ATHLETES

American Athletic Association of the Deaf
3916 Lantern Drive
Silver Spring, Maryland 20902

American Blind Bowlers Association
150 North Bellaire
Louisville, Kentucky 40206

American Wheelchair Bowling Association
2424 North Federal Highway, Suite 109
Boynton Beach, Florida 33435

American Wheelchair Pilots Association
7008 Willetta
Scottsdale, Arizona 85257

Blind Outdoor Leisure Development, Inc. (BOLD)
533 East Main Street
Aspen, Colorado 81611

Braille Sports Foundation
Room 301, 730 Hennepin Avenue
Minneapolis, Minnesota 55402

International Council on Therapeutic Ice Skating
Post Office Box 13
State College, Pennsylvania 16801

International Sports Organization for the Disabled and International Stoke–Mandeville Games Federation
Stoke–Mandeville Spinal Injury Center
Aylesbury, England

National Amputee Golf Association
Post Office Box 9426
Solon, Ohio 44139

National Association of Sports for Cerebral Palsied
United Cerebral Palsy Association, Inc.
66 East 34th Street
New York, New York 10016

National Beep Baseball Association
3212 Tomahawk
Lawrence, Kansas 66044

National Handicapped Sports and Recreation Association
4105 East Florida Avenue
Denver, Colorado 80222

National Therapeutic Recreation Association
1601 North Kent Street
Arlington, Virginia 22209

National Wheelchair Athletic Association
4024 62nd Street
Woodside, New York 11377

National Wheelchair Basketball Association
110 Seaton Building
University of Kentucky
Lexington, Kentucky 40506

National Wheelchair Softball Association
Post Office Box 737
Sioux Falls, South Dakota 57101

New England Spinal Cord Injury Foundation (marathon racing)
369 Elliott Street
Newton Upper Falls, Massachusetts 02164

North American Riding for the Handicapped Association
Box 100
Ashburn, Virginia 22011

Paralyzed Veterans of America, Inc.
4330 East–West Highway, Suite 300
Washington, D.C. 20014

Ski for Light, Inc.
1455 West Lake Street
Minneapolis, Minnesota 55408

Special Olympics
Suite 203
1701 K Street, NW
Washington, D.C. 20006

Sport for the Physically Disabled
333 River Road
Ottawa KlL 8B9
Canada

United States Association for Blind Athletes
55 West California Avenue
Beach Haven Park, New Jersey 08008

United States Blind Golfers Association
225 Baronne Street
New Orleans, Louisiana 70112

United States Deaf Skiers Association, Inc.
9915 Good Luck Road, Apartment 103
Seabrook, Maryland 20801

Publications

National Park Guide for the Handicapped
Superintendent of Documents
U.S. Government Printing Office
Washington, D.C. 20402
Stock #2405-0286; price, 40 cents

Sports 'n Spokes (magazine for wheelchair sports)
6043 North 9th Avenue
Phoenix, Arizona 85013

Index